Smell and Taste Disorders

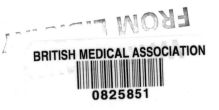

Smell and Taste Disorders

Christopher H. Hawkes, MD FRCP
Honorary Professor of Neurology and Honorary Consultant Neurologist, Neuroscience Centre, Blizard Institute,
Barts and the London School of Medicine and Dentistry, London, UK

Richard L. Doty, PhD FAAN
Professor, Department of Otorhinolaryngology: Head and Neck Surgery, and Director, Smell and Taste Center,
Perelman School of Medicine, University of Pennsylvania, Philadelphia, Pennsylvania, USA

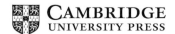

CAMBRIDGE
UNIVERSITY PRESS

CAMBRIDGE
UNIVERSITY PRESS

University Printing House, Cambridge CB2 8BS, United Kingdom

One Liberty Plaza, 20th Floor, New York, NY 10006, USA

477 Williamstown Road, Port Melbourne, VIC 3207, Australia

314–321, 3rd Floor, Plot 3, Splendor Forum, Jasola District Centre, New Delhi – 110025, India

79 Anson Road, #06–04/06, Singapore 079906

Cambridge University Press is part of the University of Cambridge.

It furthers the University's mission by disseminating knowledge in the pursuit of
education, learning, and research at the highest international levels of excellence.

www.cambridge.org
Information on this title: www.cambridge.org/9780521130622
DOI: 10.1017/9781139192446

© Cambridge University Press 2018

First published 2018

Printed in the United Kingdom by TJ International Ltd. Padstow Cornwall

A catalogue record for this publication is available from the British Library.

ISBN 978-0-521-13062-2 Paperback

....

Contents

Color plates are to be found between pp. 214 and 215.

Preface

This smell and taste disorders aims to provide neuroscientists, physicians, dentists, and psychologists with concise, practical, and authoritative information for understanding, testing, and managing disorders of taste and smell. Nearly 3 percent of Americans under the age of 65 suffer from some form of chronic olfactory or gustatory dysfunction – a percentage that rises to more than 50 percent of those over 65 years of age and is likely much higher in areas of the world where air and water pollution are prevalent. Despite such statistics, the chemical senses remain neglected by the majority of medical practitioners. Such oversight stems from a number of sources, not least of which is the lack of understanding or trivialization of these senses and the belief that their accurate assessment cannot be made in the clinic. Less-than-total dysfunction is rarely brought to the attention of the physician and, when aberrations are found, many are unsure of how to proceed.

Although practical quantitative tests of smell function are now widely available, the majority of neurologists test only cranial nerves II through XII. This continues, despite the fact that olfactory testing has been recommended by the Quality Standards Committee of the American Academy of Neurology for inclusion in the diagnostic criteria for Parkinson's disease (Suchowersky et al., 2006). Similar suggestions have been made for inclusion of smell testing as an aid in the diagnosis of Alzheimer's disease (Foster et al., 2008). There is evidence that smell tests can be useful in differential diagnosis of several disorders (e.g., depression vs. Alzheimer's disease; Parkinson's disease vs. progressive supranuclear palsy and essential tremor). Moreover, they may assist the detection of malingering. Loss of smell or taste has considerable medico-legal importance, commanding major financial compensation for those who are victims of head injury or exposure to toxic agents, particularly for the young and persons whose livelihoods depend upon chemosensation. As this book emphasizes, there are no longer excuses for neglecting the chemical senses in medical practice.

Smell and taste are regularly lumped together, particularly by lay people. While both are chemical senses and contribute to the flavor of foods and beverages, in the embryo these two systems develop independently and are completely separate at subcortical level and merge only at the anterior insula. Olfaction is seemingly more ancient, developing first phylogenetically; taste, as an oral chemosensory system, is a relatively new thalamic-dependent system. It is important to recognize, however, that both olfactory and gustatory receptor proteins are found outside of the nose and oral cavity, suggesting that these proteins are ubiquitous and have functions beyond those of transducing the conscious perception of tastes and smells. For example, olfactory receptor proteins have been found in the tongue, brain, prostate, enterochromaffin cells, pulmonary neuroendocrine cells, and spermatozoa. Taste receptors have now been reported in the epiglottis, larynx, respiratory epithelium, stomach, pancreas, and colon, where they influence such processes as digestion, chemical absorption, insulin release, and protection of the epithelium from xenobiotic agents. Olfaction is more plastic than taste, and it is damaged more readily from head trauma, viruses, and exposure to xenobiotics. Inborn mechanisms largely determine the meaning of taste experiences, whereas learning plays a much greater role for the sense of smell. Nonetheless, these primary sensory modalities intermingle both with each other and other sensory systems at the cortical level – interactions that in some cases are influenced greatly by learning. Such interplay is only just beginning to be understood.

Many chemosensory systems have evolved in mammals, including the vomeronasal system, but the senses of taste and smell are the most prominent in humans. In Chapters 1 and 2 we emphasize the anatomy and physiology of these two modalities, beginning with olfaction, which as noted above is typically more compromised than taste by injury and disease. In subsequent chapters we review methods to measure smell (Chapter 3) and taste (Chapter 4), what factors influence these modalities, and, from a clinical perspective, the nature and major causes of their dysfunction with an emphasis on neurological disorders (Chapters 5, 6, and 7). Our goal is to provide up-to-date information about these senses in health and disease, and to guide the practitioner in the assessment, treatment, and management of patients with chemosensory disturbances (Chapter 8).

We express our gratitude to the editors of Cambridge University Press who agreed to an update of our earlier work *The Neurology of Olfaction* (2009) and to include taste complaints. We hope that this compendium will serve the needs of a broad array of clinicians and scientists who recognize the unique role that the chemical senses play in medicine and everyday life.

References

Foster, J., Sohrabi, H., Verdile, G. and Martins, R., 2008. Research criteria for the diagnosis of Alzheimer's disease: Genetic risk factors, blood biomarkers and olfactory dysfunction. *International Psychogeriatrics* **20**(4), 853–855.

Hawkes, C.H., Doty, R.L., 2009. *The Neurology of Olfaction*. Cambridge, UK: Cambridge University Press.

Suchowersky, O., Reich, S., Perlmutter, J., Zesiewicz, T., Gronseth, G., Weiner, W.J., 2006. Practice parameter: Diagnosis and prognosis of new onset Parkinson disease (an evidence-based review). Report of the quality standards subcommittee of the American Academy of Neurology. *Neurology* **66**(7), 968–975.

Acknowledgments

We owe a debt of gratitude to the following who have helped with various sections of this volume:

Professor Kailash Bhatia, National Hospital for Neurology and Neurosurgery, Queen Square, London

Professor Jay Gottfried, Perelman School of Medicine, University of Pennsylvania, Philadelphia, Pennsylvania

Professor John Hardy, National Hospital for Neurology and Neurosurgery, Queen Square, London

Dr. Isabel Ubeda-Banon, Universidad de Castilla-La Mancha, Avda. de Moledores s/n, 13071, Ciudad Real, Spain.

Professor Jason Warren, National Hospital for Neurology and Neurosurgery, Queen Square, London

Chapter 1

Anatomy and Physiology of Olfaction

Introduction

The evolution of life required organisms to sense chemicals suspended or dissolved in water. Some of these chemicals provided nourishment, whereas others were destructive and had to be avoided. Single-celled organisms, such as *Escherichia coli*, developed multiple chemical receptors critical for such survival. The rotatory direction of their flagellae – whip-like appendages used to propel them through their environment – is altered by the type of chemical encountered. Thus, chemicals important for sustenance induce a counterclockwise rotation of the flagella, facilitating a smooth and somewhat linear swimming path, whereas toxic chemicals provoke a clockwise flagellar rotation, resulting in tumbling and turning away from the offending stimulus (Larsen et al., 1974).

The sense of smell is one of nature's true wonders, being ubiquitous within the animal kingdom and capable of detecting and differentiating thousands of diverse odorants at very low concentrations. Humans possess far more odorant receptor types than any other sensory system, which explains, in part, their ability to perceive such a large number of stimuli. It is now well established, as described in subsequent chapters of this book, that the olfactory system provides a unique probe into the general health of the brain. Thus, smell loss is among the first signs of neurodegenerative diseases such as Alzheimer's or Parkinson's disease and provides insight into elements of brain development. Importantly, smell loss is one of the best predictors of future mortality in older populations, being a stronger predictor than cognitive deficits, cancer, stroke, lung disease, or hypertension even after controlling for the effects of age, sex, race, education, socioeconomic status, smoking behavior, alcohol use, cardiovascular disease, diabetes, and liver damage (Wilson et al., 2011; Gopinath et al., 2012; Pinto et al., 2014; Devanand et al., 2015). In the future, screening for a range of neurological disorders by olfactory biomarkers may be commonplace and may encourage the development of protective measures that delay or prevent central nervous system (CNS) degeneration.

We now describe the detailed anatomy, physiology, and pharmacology of the olfactory pathway, followed by factors that influence olfactory input and its interpretation.

Nasal Cavity

During normal inspiration, only 5–10 percent of inhaled air reaches the olfactory epithelium. This specialized pseudostratified neuroepithelium harbors the olfactory receptors. It is found high within the nasal vault, lining sectors of the upper nasal septum, cribriform plate, superior turbinates, and, to a lesser extent, the anterior aspect of the middle turbinates

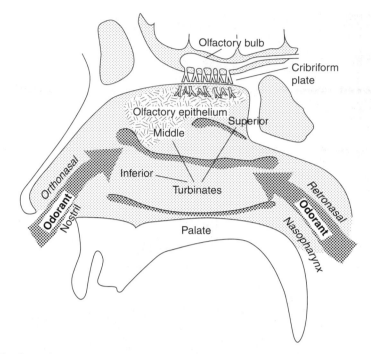

Figure 1.1 This figure shows the human nasal cavity and extent of the olfactory epithelium. Note the extension of the epithelium onto the anterior part of the middle turbinate. Odorants access the olfactory epithelium either directly through the orthonasal route (anterior arrow) or indirectly through the retronasal route as in chewing or swallowing (posterior arrow). Reproduced with permission from Rawson, N. (2000), Chapter 11, Human olfaction.

(Figure 1.1). The existence of olfactory receptor neurons (ORN) on the middle turbinate is a useful aspect of applied anatomy for those wishing to biopsy olfactory receptor cells (ORC) for culture, histology, or patch clamp studies, as it is more accessible and less risky to sample than the main olfactory area.

Sniffing. Although sniffing assists smell recognition and identification, the first awareness of a new odor can be passive; sniffing then follows in an attempt to analyze the odor further and assess its behavioral significance. Sniffing redirects up to 15 percent of the inhaled air through the olfactory meatus, a ~1 mm-wide opening leading to the uppermost sector of the nose that contains most of the olfactory epithelium. Sniffing helps to increase the number of odorous molecules that ultimately reach this region. However, molecules must absorb into the mucus that forms across the nasal mucosa to make contact with the olfactory receptor cells. In some cases – particularly in the case of hydrophobic odorants – stimuli may be carried through this mucus by specialized "odorant carrier" proteins to the receptors (Pelosi et al., 1990). It should be emphasized that without a moist mucosal surface, detection of odors is largely impossible. As mentioned in Chapter 5, diseases with excessive nasal dryness such as Sjögren's syndrome are often accompanied by smell dysfunction.

Nasal Turbinates. The nasal turbinates are highly vascularized structures that extend into the nasal cavity from its lateral wall (Figure 1.2). They can rapidly expand or contract, depending upon autonomic nervous system tone and stimulation. Exercise, hypercapnia, and increased sympathetic tone constrict their engorgement, whereas cold air, irritants, hypocapnia, and

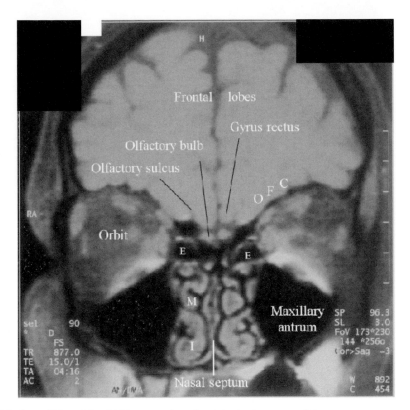

Figure 1.2 Coronal T1-weighted MRI scan to show the main structures around the nose.

increased parasympathetic tone can induce such engorgement. Turbinate engorgement can be influenced by pressure on sectors of the body, body position, or ambient temperature. Left-to-right fluctuations in relative engorgement, termed the nasal cycle, occur in many people over time, although these change with age and reciprocity is frequently the exception rather than the rule (Mirza et al., 1997). These fluctuations relate to changes in lateralized blood flow to various paired organs, including the two brain hemispheres, and belong to the basic rest-activity cycle, a continuation of the REM/non-REM sleep cycle that occurs during the daytime. Although the turbinates have never been thought relevant to the clinical neurologist, this concept may need to change given the recent suggestion that rhinorrhea, secondary to relative parasympathetic overactivity, may be a prodromal sign of Parkinson's disease (see Chapter 7 and Bower et al., 2006).

Innervation of the Nasal Cavity. In common with the nasal and oral mucosae, the olfactory epithelium also contains free nerve endings from the trigeminal nerve (CN V). Non-olfactory elements of nasal chemosensation, e.g., sharpness, coolness, warmth, and pungency, are mediated via free nerve endings of this nerve (Figure 1.3). These free nerve endings are supplied to the upper part of the nasal cavity by the anterior and posterior ethmoid nerves – branches of the nasociliary nerve which come from the ophthalmic (first division) of the trigeminal nerve. The nasopalatine nerve, a branch of the maxillary nerve (second division of the trigeminal nerve) is the source of the CN V fibers innervating the posterior nasal cavity. Most odorous compounds stimulate CN I and CN V, at least at higher

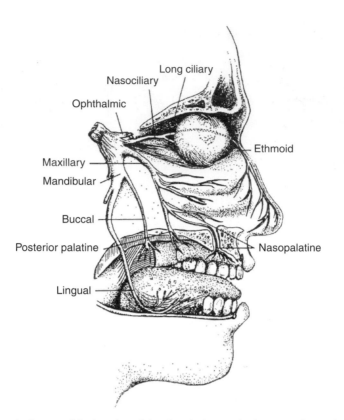

Figure 1.3 Schematic diagram of the branches of the trigeminal nerve that innervate the nasal, oral, and ocular epithelia. From Bryant & Silver (2000). Copyright © 2000, Wiley-Liss.

concentrations and/or volumes. Vanillin is one of few compounds that appear to have no perceptible CN V activity. This contrasts with ammonia, for example, which strongly stimulates the olfactory and trigeminal nerves. Thus, patients with anosmia can readily detect, via trigeminal sensation, several "impure" odors, such as menthol or camphor.

Vomeronasal Organ (VNO) and Nervus Terminalis. The VNO is a bilaterally symmetrical tubular structure located just above the palate at the base of the anterior nasal septum. This pouch-like structure is enclosed in a bony capsule and, depending upon the species, has a single opening into either the nasal or the oral cavity via the vomeronasal or nasopalatine duct, respectively. In the case of humans, the VNO is clearly vestigial and non-functional. In the developing human fetus there is a VNO which stains for gonadotropin-releasing hormone (GnRH), but its connections with the olfactory bulb disappear or become displaced and hard to locate at about 19 weeks of gestational age. In the adult human the vestigial VNO is present bilaterally on the anterior third of the nasal septum and opens through a pit about 1–2 cm behind the posterior margin of the nostril. However, VNO cells do not react to olfactory marker protein – a stain for functional olfactory neurons – and there is no neural connection to the CNS. Adult humans lack an accessory olfactory bulb, to which functional VNOs project. Moreover, most human VNO receptor genes are vestigial (pseudogenes) and the VNO-specific TRP2 cation channel critical for VNO function is lacking.

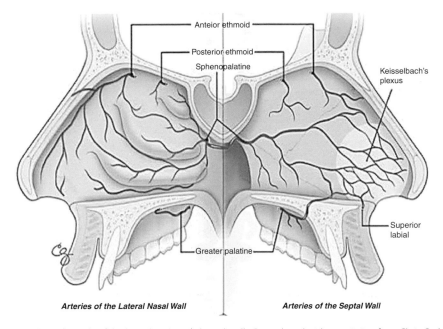

Anteior ethmoid

Posterior ethmoid

Sphenopalatine

Keisselbach's plexus

Superior labial

Greater palatine

Arteries of the Lateral Nasal Wall

Arteries of the Septal Wall

Figure 1.4 Arterial supply of the lateral and medial nasal walls. Reproduced with permission from Chris Gralapp in Medscape. (www.medscape.org/viewarticle/723327_2)

Another nerve in the noses of humans and many other vertebrates is the terminal nerve, also termed the nervus terminalis or Cranial Nerve zero. This unmyelinated and highly ganglionated nerve plexus is found within both the olfactory and non-olfactory sectors of the nasal cavity, and is the most anterior of the vertebrate cranial nerves. In some human specimens it can be seen intracranially at the base of the brain with the naked eye, lying along the inside surface of the dura mater medial to the main olfactory bulb near the cribriform plate. In the few species that have been examined, this understudied nerve releases GnRH into the region of the olfactory receptors, thereby modulating their function (Eisthen et al., 2000; Zhang & Delay, 2007). Damage to this nerve in hamsters alters copulatory behavior, presumably reflecting its close relation to the hypothalamus and its high gonadotropin-releasing hormone (GnRH) content (Schwanzel-Fukuda & Pfaff, 2003). At present, its function in humans is not known, although a sensory role, per se, is highly unlikely (Fuller & Burger, 1990).

Vascular Supply. The vascular supply of the nasal cavity comes from tributaries of the external and internal carotid arteries (Figure 1.4). The ophthalmic branch of the internal carotid artery gives rise to anterior and posterior ethmoid arteries that supply the upper part of the nasal cavity. The sphenopalatine artery, also derived from the internal carotid, feeds the posterior nasal cavity. The anterior sectors of the nasal chamber are fed by branches of the facial and internal maxillary arteries which derive from the external carotid artery. Impaired blood supply in the anterior and posterior ethmoidal arteries (branches of the ophthalmic arteries) may interfere with olfaction, as noted in Chapter 5. Thus, impairment is seen occasionally in vasculitic disorders such as systemic lupus erythematosis, giant cell arteritis, and Churg-Strauss syndrome. In

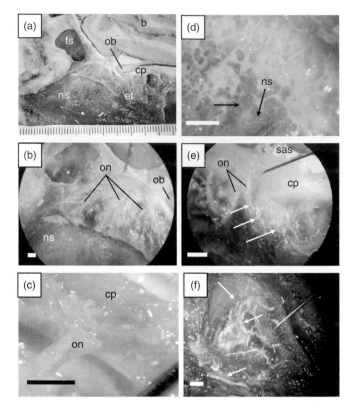

Figure 1.5 Lymphatic drainage through the nasal cavity. Silicone (Microfil) injection distribution patterns in the head of a human (a–f). All images are presented in sagittal plane with gradual magnification of the olfactory area adjacent to the cribriform plate. Reference scales are provided either as a ruler in the image (mm) or as a longitudinal bar (1 mm). Microfil introduced into the subarachnoid space was observed around the olfactory bulb (a), in the perineurial spaces of the olfactory nerves (b, c), and in the lymphatics of the nasal septum (d), ethmoid labyrinth (e), and superior turbinate (f). Some lymphatic vessels ruptured and Microfil was noted in the interstitium of the submucosa of the nasal septum (d). In (e), Microfil is observed in the subarachnoid space and the perineurial space of olfactory nerves. The perineurial Microfil is continuous with that in lymphatic vessels (arrows). Intact lymphatic vessels containing Microfil are outlined with arrows (d–f). Key to abbreviations: b – brain; fs – frontal sinus; cp – cribriform plate; et – ethmoid turbinates; ob – olfactory bulbs; on – olfactory nerves; ns – nasal septum; sas – subarachnoid space. Reproduced with permission from Johnston, Zakharov et al. (2005). (A black and white version of this figure will appear in some formats. For the color version, please refer to the plate section.)

general, there is a high rate of blood flow within the human nasal *respiratory* epithelium (~42 ml/100 g/minute), as measured by Laser-Doppler flowmetry, but the blood flow rate in the human *olfactory* epithelium is unknown.

Lymphatic Drainage. It is not widely appreciated that the nasal cavity is a major route for lymphatic drainage of cerebrospinal fluid (CSF). It is clear from observations in mice (Weller et al., 2009) and humans (Johnston et al., 2005) that CSF drains along olfactory perineural lymphatics from the subarachnoid space through the cribriform plate into the nasal cavity, terminating in cervical lymph nodes (Figure 1.5). As explained in Chapter 7, pathogens could use this drainage pathway in reverse direction to access the CSF and brain.

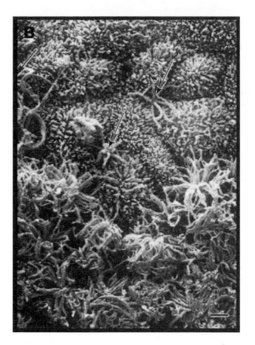

Figure 1.6 Electron photomicrograph of transition zone between the human olfactory epithelium (bottom) and the respiratory epithelium (top). Note the long olfactory receptor cell cilia compared to the cilia in the respiratory epithelium. Arrows signify two examples of olfactory receptor cell dendrites with cilia that have been cut off. Bar = 5 μm. From Menco & Morrison (2003), with permission. Copyright © 2003, Richard L. Doty.

Olfactory Receptor Cells (ORCs). In humans, the 6–10 million ORCs, collectively termed the first cranial nerve (CN I), are found at different stages of maturity in the olfactory epithelium. These bipolar cells are the first-order neurons of the system, and their central axons project directly from the nasal cavity to the olfactory bulb without an intervening synapse, making them a major conduit for CNS pathogens (Doty, 2008). When mature, each ORC projects up to 30 cilia into the mucus, which form knob-like dendritic extensions (Figure 1.6). These cells are unique in several ways. For example, they serve as sensory transducers, whereas in most other sensory systems the transducing cell is not a neuron, but it is synaptically connected to an effector sensory neuron. When damaged, ORCs, like the other cell types within the olfactory neuroepithelium, can be replenished from neuronal progenitor cells and basal stem cells located near the basement membrane (Loo et al., 1996).

Many other types of cells are located within this unique epithelium. Glial-like supporting (sustentacular) cells separate the ORCs from one another and may play some role in paracrine modulation of olfactory receptor cell activity. Another cell linked to paracrine activity is the ubiquitous microvillar cell, which is involved in modulation of ORCs via secretion of acetylcholine into the mucosa (Schiffman & Gatlin, 1993). A small number of such cells appear to project to the olfactory bulbs (Rowley et al., 1989). Most of the mucus that bathes the olfactory epithelium is derived from Bowman glands, whose ducts permeate the olfactory epithelium (Figure 1.7).

It is important to recognize that many odorants and chemicals are actively metabolized by the olfactory mucosa, being deactivated, detoxified, or, in rare cases, transformed into

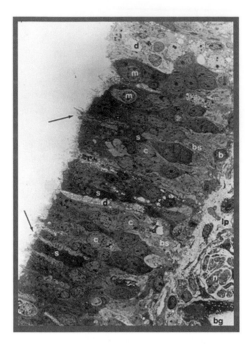

Figure 1.7 Low-power cross-section of the human olfactory neuroepithelium depicting the four major types of cells: bipolar receptor cells (arrows point to cilia at dendritic knob; c, cell body), microvillar cells (m), sustentacular cells (s), and basal cells (b). Key to abbreviations: bg – Bowman's gland; lp – lamina propria; n – collection of axons within an ensheathing cell; d – duct of Bowman's gland; bs – basal cell undergoing mitosis. Electron photomicrograph courtesy of Dr. David Moran, Longmont, Colorado.

toxic metabolites. The sustentacular cells, acinar and duct cells of Bowman glands, are enriched with xenobiotic-metabolizing enzymes. More than ten different P450 enzymes have been identified in the olfactory mucosa of mammals, including members of the CYP1A, 2A, 2B, 2C, 2E, 2G, 2J, 3A, and 4B subfamilies. Many P450s are preferentially expressed in the olfactory region, such as CYP2G1.

The ORN are among the few cells of ectodermal origin capable of regeneration. Others include cells within the subgranular zone of the hippocampal dentate gyrus, the sub-ventricular zone (SVZ) in the wall of the lateral ventricle, the organ of Corti, and the granule and periglomerular cells of the olfactory bulb (Maier et al., 2014). The latter cells arise from neuroblasts formed within the SVZ that migrate to the bulb along the rostral migratory stream. Approximately 95 percent of these neuroblasts become granule cells, whereas the remainder become GABAergic and dopaminergic periglomerular cells.

The olfactory receptor proteins are found on the cilia that, in many cases, lie along the surface of the mucus covering the epithelium. Unlike the cilia of the respiratory epithelium, these long cilia lack contractile (dynein) arms and, thus, intrinsic motility.

Olfactory Transduction

The primary second messenger for mammalian odor transduction is cAMP, whose essential function is to amplify the incoming signal from odorant receptors and ultimately facilitate release of glutamate, the primary neurotransmitter of the olfactory receptor cells. Opening

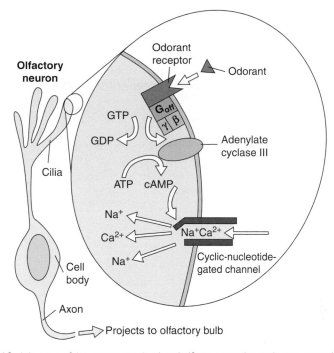

Figure 1.8 Simplified diagram of the mouse cAMP-related olfactory signal transduction cascade. Odorant binding to the olfactory receptor activates Golf. Activated Golf then dissociates from Gβγ and activates adenylate cyclase III, leading to an increase in the intracellular cAMP concentration, which in turn opens the cyclic-nucleotide-gated channels. The consequent influx of Na^+ and Ca^{2+} ions generates an action potential, which travels into the olfactory bulb. Reproduced with permission from Ebrahimi & Chess (1998).

of a cyclic nucleotide-gated channel causes movement of Na^+ and Ca^{2+} into the cell (Figure 1.8). As Ca^{2+} enters the cytoplasm of the cilium through this channel, a secondary depolarizing receptor current is activated that mediates an outward Cl^- movement in the receptor neuron. Due to the high Cl^- concentration within this neuron, an elevated reversal potential for Cl^- is induced. This increases the outward movement of Cl^- across the membrane and the induction of depolarization. Both N-methyl d-aspartate (NMDA) and non-NMDA receptors are subsequently activated by glutamate on the dendrites of the second-order neurons. Although the second messenger, inositol 1,4,5-trisphosphate (IP3), has been implicated in both invertebrate and vertebrate olfactory transduction, it appears to play a lesser role than cAMP-mediated receptor processes in mammalian olfactory signal transduction (Benbernou et al., 2011). Implementing calcium imaging, only about 5 percent of all mammalian olfactory cells utilize IP3 as a second messenger (Elsaesser et al., 2005).

Olfactory Receptor Gene Superfamily. In a 1991 landmark study that led to the 2004 Nobel Prize for Physiology or Medicine, Linda Buck and Richard Axel identified the first 18 members of the olfactory receptor gene superfamily using a degenerate polymerase chain reaction strategy (Buck & Axel, 1991). This superfamily comprises 18 gene families and 300

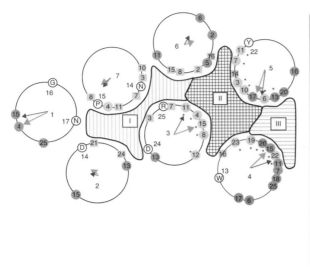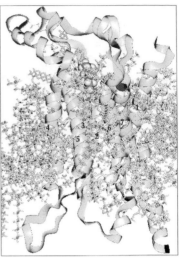

Figure 1.9 Left: Presumed odorant-binding pockets of an odor receptor protein. Overhead view of the seven transmembrane-spanning barrels of an odor receptor protein modeled against the rhodopsin G-protein coupled receptor (GPCR). Residues that are conserved among all GPCRs are shown in open circles. Colored squares and circles represent positions of conserved and variable residues, respectively, in OR proteins. Residues that align with ligand contact residues in other GPCRs are colored green and residues that do not align with such residues are colored red. The residues in each helix are numbered separately, according to the predicted transmembrane boundaries. Hypervariable residues (putative odorant-binding residues) are indicated by asterisks. Area II denotes a hypervariable pocket that corresponds to the ligand-binding pocket in other GPCRs. Reproduced from Pilpel & Lancet (1999). Right: Predicted structure for mouse olfactory receptor (OR) S25. Model depicts the putative binding pocket for the hexanol ligand (purple) to the receptor protein (side view). Each transmembrane and inter-transmembrane loop is labeled. The membrane is represented in yellow. This computed model of the S25 odorant receptor protein atoms successfully predicts the relative affinities to a panel of odorants, including hexanol, which is predicted to interact with residues in transmembranes 3, 5, and 6. Reproduced with permission from Floriano et al. (2000). (A black and white version of this figure will appear in some formats. For the colour version, please refer to the plate section.)

subfamilies (Olender et al., 2008). The receptors, like other G-protein-coupled receptors, have seven transmembrane domains with a stereotyped topology (Figure 1.9). The internal transmembrane domains, which are hypervariable in evolution, are believed to interact with odorants in a manner analogous to the α_2 adrenergic receptor-ligand interaction (Buck & Axel, 1991).

Olfactory receptors generally fall into two classes: Class I and Class II receptors (Freitag et al., 1998). The preferred odorant agonists of Class I receptors, which include receptors found mainly in fish, are generally water-soluble odorants, whereas this is not the case with Class II receptors. Amphibians and mammals express both Class I and Class II receptors.

Although humans have ~950 genes that express olfactory receptor proteins, less than 400 are functional. The remainder are pseudogenes which probably have no function – although this is not yet certain. A given olfactory receptor neuron expresses only one receptor type, resulting in ~380 different receptor elements embedded within the 6–10 million receptor cells. However, a single odorous chemical commonly binds to a subset of receptors that may overlap with additional subsets activated by other odorants. Receptor genes are found in about 100 loci spread over all chromosomes except for chromosome 20 and the Y chromosome (Olender et al., 2008) (Figure 1.10). Six chromosomes (1, 6, 9, 11, 14, 19) contain

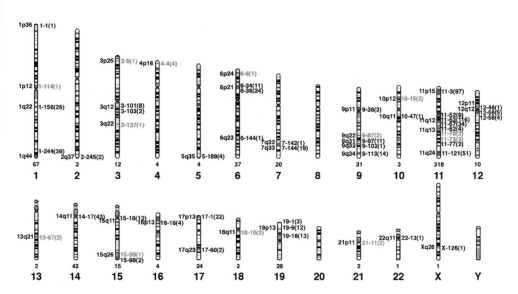

Figure 1.10 Chromosome locations of human OR genes. There were 630 OR genes that localized to 51 different chromosomal loci distributed over 21 human chromosomes. OR loci containing one or more intact OR genes are indicated in red; loci containing only pseudogenes are indicated in green. The cytogenetic position of each locus is shown on the left, and its distance in megabases from the tip of the small arm of the chromosome is shown on the right (chromosome-Mb). The number of OR genes at each locus is indicated in parentheses, and the number of OR genes on each chromosome is indicated below. Most human homologs of rodent ORs for *n*-aliphatic odorants are found at a single locus, chromosome 11p15. Reproduced with permission from Malnic et al. (2004). Since this map was published OR genes have been found on chromosome 8. (A black and white version of this figure will appear in some formats. For the color version, please refer to the plate section.)

nearly three-quarters of the receptor genes, whereas a single gene is found on chromosome 22. Chromosome 11 contains 51 percent of the receptor genes and harbors the two largest receptor gene clusters found in the mammalian genome (Olender et al., 2008). Interestingly, the olfactory subgenome spans ~30 Mb, a length that represents about 1 percent of total human genomic DNA.

The molecular phenotype of the olfactory sensory neurons is one of the most diverse in the nervous system, given the large number of different receptors, second-messenger pathways, and cell-surface antigens (Shepherd et al., 2004). At one time it was believed that all of ORN replenished themselves every 30 to 40 days, but it is now known this is incorrect (Mackay-Sim et al., 2015). Thus, long-lived receptor cells are present within the epithelium and regulatory mechanisms influence the timing and extent of receptor cell neurogenesis from the basal cell population (Hinds et al., 1984). Unfortunately, regeneration after toxic, viral, or other insults is rarely complete and, as a result, the olfactory epithelium becomes replaced and stippled by islands of respiratory-like epithelium.

Several investigators have overcome the extreme difficulty in establishing the specific ligands for olfactory receptor cells, a process termed deorphanizing the receptors (Peterlin et al., 2014). This process has been challenging, since more than one ligand can bind to a given receptor and the expressed proteins remain embedded in the plasma membrane (Lai et al., 2014). One of the more recent examples of deorphanizing olfactory receptors comes from a study by Saito et al. (2009). They deorphanized 52

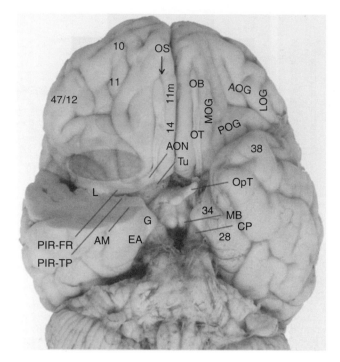

Figure 1.11 Base of human brain showing the ventral forebrain and medial temporal lobes. The blue oval area represents the monkey olfactory region, whereas the pink oval represents the probable site of the human olfactory region as identified by functional imaging studies. Modified from: Gottfried J.A., Small D.M., & Zald D.H. (2006), Chapter 6, Plate 9. Key: numbers refer to the approximate position of Brodmann areas as follows: 10 – fronto-polar area; 11/11 m – orbitofrontal/gyrus rectus region; 28 – posterior entorhinal cortex; 34 – anterior entorhinal cortex; 38 – temporal pole; 47/12 – ventrolateral frontal area. Other abbreviations: AM – amygdala; AOG/POG/LOG/MOG – anterior, posterior, lateral, medial orbital gyri; AON – anterior olfactory nucleus; CP – cerebral peduncle; EA – entorhinal area; G – gyrus ambiens; L – limen insulae; MB – mamillary body; PIR-FR – frontal piriform cortex; PIR-TR – temporal piriform cortex; OpT – optic tract; OS – olfactory sulcus; OT – olfactory tract; Tu – olfactory tubercle. (A black and white version of this figure will appear in some formats. For the color version, please refer to the plate section.)

mouse and 10 human olfactory receptors. Some were found to be tuned to a broad range of odorants ("generalists") whereas others responded to a small number of structurally related compounds ("specialists") (Saito et al., 2009). Importantly, the product of deorphanizing olfactory receptors depends upon the odorants available as ligands. Given that thousands of odorants are available, complete determination of the possible ligands for any given receptor is presently not possible. Nonetheless, understanding basic aspects of ligand-receptor interactions is an important first step for modeling stimulus-response associations and ultimately understanding odor coding.

Olfactory Bulbs

Axons of the olfactory receptor cells (ORC) ascend through the cribriform plate to make contact with the olfactory bulbs (OB). These are paired ovoid-shaped structures located immediately above the cribriform plate that lie on the undersurface of the frontal lobe (gyrus rectus; Figure 1.11). Each bulb, which develops as an outgrowth of the forebrain, has a volume of ~50 mm^3. The OBs are not simple relay stations; they are palaeocortical limbic

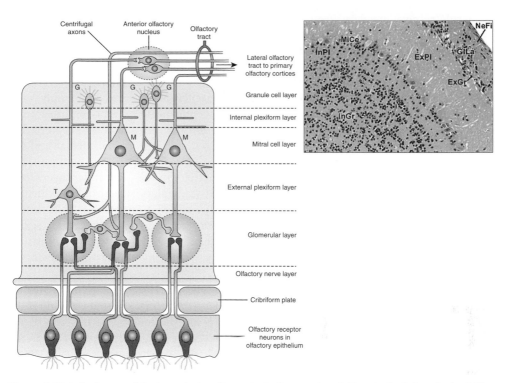

Figure 1.12 Left: diagram of the layers in the olfactory bulb. G – granule cell; M – mitral cell; T – tufted cell. The external granular layer, which is deep to the glomerular layer, is not shown for clarity. Reproduced with permission from Duda (2010). Right: Mouse olfactory bulb to show the same layers as seen with a microscope x20. Stain: hematoxylin and eosin. Key: NeFi – Nerve fiber layer; GlLa – Glomerular layer; ExGr – External granular layer; ExPl – External plexiform layer; MiCe – Mitral cell layer; InPl – Internal plexiform layer; InGr – Internal granular layer. Reproduced with permission from Texas Histopages. http://ctrgenpath.net/static/atlas/mousehistology/Windows /nervous/olf20.html.

structures that filter, integrate, and modulate information from both intrinsic and extrinsic sources. The basic olfactory bulb anatomy is shown in Figure 1.12. Unlike many cortical regions, the inter-neuronal connections within these are now well established (Shepherd, 1972).

The olfactory bulb comprises six histologically defined concentric layers that surround a seemingly vestigial evagination of the lateral ventricle. The medial-lateral symmetry observed in rodents is not seen in humans (Maresh et al., 2008).

1. **Olfactory Nerve Layer.** This is the outermost layer of the bulb – a superficial circumferential zone of unmyelinated incoming ORC fibers that interweave across the bulb's surface and ultimately defasciculate and reorganize as they penetrate radially into globe-like structures that make up the next (glomerular) layer of the bulb. There are an estimated 6 million ORC axons per side that enter into the human olfactory bulb (Moran et al., 1982).

2. **Glomerular Layer.** The globe-like glomeruli are not cells; they consist of ORC axon terminals that make contact with mitral or tufted cell dendrites, i.e., axo-dendritic synapses. In humans, each bulb has been estimated to have ~6,000 thousand glomeruli, although large individual differences have been noted (Maresh et al., 2008). Since these

glomeruli receive messages from the ~6 million olfactory axons, there is a 1000:1 convergence ratio that results in tremendous amplification of incoming signals. Many more glomeruli are present in younger than older persons, likely reflecting the decrease in trophic maintenance secondary to decline in the number of receptor cells (Smith, 1942). In addition, the elderly display more aberrant patterns of glomerular organization than the young (Maresh et al., 2008). Each glomerulus receives input only from those receptor cells that express the same type of receptor protein, implying integration of basic receptor information at this stage. In the mouse, most olfactory receptors that have been chemically identified have two target glomeruli: one in the medial and the other in the lateral wall of the bulb.

Relatively small intrinsic cells influence neural activity in the glomerular layer. Each glomerulus is surrounded by a mixed population of juxtaglomerular neurons that include periglomerular, short axon, and external tufted cells. Most periglomerular cells send a bushy dendrite into a single glomerulus and extend an axon laterally as far as five glomeruli from their origin. These cells influence the activity of neighboring glomeruli and play a significant role in odor discrimination/sharpening/contrasting the output among the glomeruli.

3. **External Plexiform Layer.** This is deep to the glomerular layer, mainly comprising (a) secondary dendrites of mitral and tufted cells, which are the primary output neurons of the bulbs, and (b) extensions from granule cells, which are the major interneurons of the olfactory bulb. It is within the external plexiform layer that reciprocal synapses between the granule and mitral/tufted cells occur. Thus, mitral cells can activate granule cells which, in turn, inhibit mitral cell activity. Importantly, centrifugal fibers from more central brain regions synapse on granule cells, thereby selectively altering mitral and tufted cell activity (Figures 1.13 and 1.14). Such influences are massive, as granule cells receive projections from olfactory cortex, basal forebrain, ventral pallidum, lateral preoptic, and rostral lateral hypothalamic areas, locus coeruleus, dorsal, and medial raphe nuclei of the midbrain (Gloor, 1997). Like ORC, many granule and periglomerular neurons can be replaced by precursors, in this case by cells that arise within the subventricular zone of the brain and migrate to the bulb via the rostral migratory stream.

4. **Mitral Cell Layer.** Mitral cells are so-called because of their resemblance to a bishop's head-dress. They make up a thin layer deep to the external plexiform layer and consist of mitral and some tufted cell bodies. Although mitral and tufted cells are histologically distinct, it is difficult to tell them apart during intracellular recordings, hence the term "mitral/tufted cell" is sometimes used.

5. **Internal Plexiform Layer.** This layer of the bulb falls between the granule and mitral cell layers. It contains a few short axon cells, peripheral dendrites of granule cells, and numerous mitral/tufted cell axons.

6. **(Internal) Granule Cell Layer.** The granule cells are small axon-less units which are the most numerous cells in the bulb. Their processes traverse several layers of the bulb, having as their primary neurotransmitter γ-aminobutyric acid (GABA).

Regeneration of Olfactory Bulb Interneurons. In the olfactory bulb of many species, the interneurons, i.e., granule and periglomerular cells, can regenerate throughout life. In contrast to embryonic interneuron progenitors that originate in the lateral ganglionic eminences, postnatal and adult progenitors originate within the subventricular zone of the lateral ventricles and must navigate migratory routes that are orders of magnitude longer than those negotiated

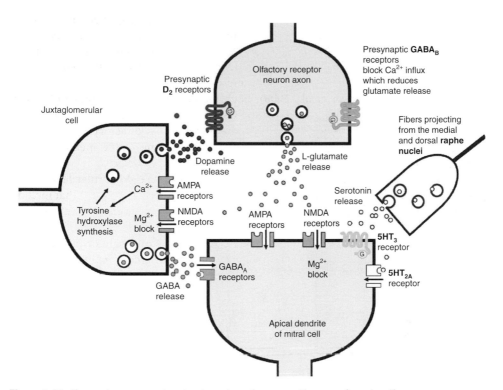

Figure 1.13 Glomerular synapses showing the variety of receptors. The axons from the olfactory receptor neurons (pink) form the olfactory nerve, which synapses on the primary apical dendrites of the mitral cells (green). L-glutamate is the primary excitatory transmitter at this synapse, which binds to AMPA and NMDA receptors on the postsynaptic membrane. Juxtaglomerular cells (blue) are inhibitory GABAergic/dopaminergic interneurons that mediate inhibition between glomeruli. Centrifugal fibers (yellow) project from the raphe nuclei to the glomeruli modulating the mitral cell activity via postsynaptic 5HT (serotonergic) receptors. Reproduced with permission from O'Connor & Jacob (2008). (A black and white version of this figure will appear in some formats. For the color version, please refer to the plate section.)

in the embryo (Lois & Alvarez-Buylla, 1994). In both cases these neuroblasts migrate toward the olfactory bulb via the rostral migratory stream. Once they reach the olfactory bulb, they spread radially to their final positions and either terminally differentiate and integrate into the circuitry or undergo apoptosis. It is not clear how much of this process occurs post-natally in large-brained mammals, given the intervening white matter tracts that may limit neuronal movement (Paredes et al., 2016). Currently the weight of the evidence is against postnatal neurogenesis in humans; possibly no more than 1 percent are replaced in adult life according to mathematical models (Bergmann et al., 2015). In addition, studies employing ^{14}C birth-dating conclude that there is little to no postnatal neurogenesis in the adult human olfactory bulb (Bergmann et al., 2015). Nonetheless, future advances in novel technology that minimizes sample variability might alter this concept (Paredes et al., 2016).

Olfactory Bulb Pharmacology

Glutamate is the main excitatory transmitter of the olfactory system and numerous mitral/tufted cell receptors are stimulated by the release of glutamate from ORC axon terminals.

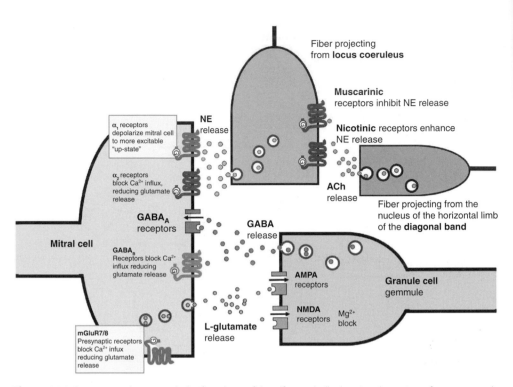

Figure 1.14 Synapses in the external plexiform layer of the olfactory bulb showing the variety of receptors and neurotransmitters. Granule cells (gray) mediate feedback and lateral inhibition between mitral cells (green) with which they form reciprocal dendro-dendritic synapses. Adrenergic and cholinergic efferent fibers project from the diagonal band (pink) and the locus coeruleus (orange), respectively. Reproduced with permission from O'Connor & Jacob (2008). (A black and white version of this figure will appear in some formats. For the colour version, please refer to the plate section.)

Mitral/tufted cells contain receptors for AMPA, kainate, GABA$_A$, 5HT, and NMDA (Figures 1.13–1.15). Excitation of mitral/tufted cells is phasic with oscillations in the theta range ~2 Hz. Part of this oscillation relates to rhythmic cycles of respiration and sniffing on ORC stimulation driven by centrifugal input. Initially, AMPA/kainate receptors depolarize mitral cells to overcome the Mg^{2+} block of the NMDA receptors. NMDA receptors then depolarize the mitral/tufted cells further, once the AMPA/kainate receptors are inactivated. The period of excitation is terminated when the mitral/tufted cells are hyperpolarized by feedback inhibition from granule cells. Each glomerulus is a functional unit receiving convergent input from ORC that express a particular receptor protein. The output from each glomerulus consists of 50–100 mitral/tufted cells whose discharge is modulated by approximately 1500–2000 juxtaglomerular cells (see Figure 1.13) which comprise (a) periglomerular cells, (b) external tufted cells, and (c) short axon cells, not all of which have been characterized pharmacologically. The population of 50–100 mitral/tufted cells that connect to a single glomerulus have synchronized response patterns facilitated by *gap junctions*, i.e., the intercellular network of protein channels that permits cell-to-cell passage of ions, hormones, and neurotransmitters. With slow oscillation, the chance of two mitral cells being synchronized by chance firing is reduced and synchronization is enhanced further because populations of mitral cells need to work in unison to overcome the Mg^{2+} NMDA block.

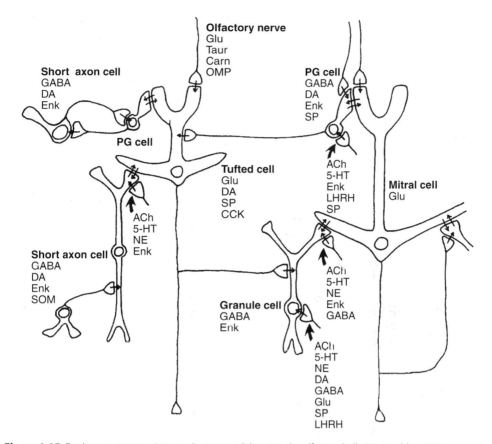

Figure 1.15 Further neurotransmitters and neuromodulators in the olfactory bulb. Key to abbreviations: ACh – acetylcholine; Carn – carnosine; CCK – cholecystokinin; DA – dopamine; Enk – enkephalin; Glu – glutamate; 5-HT – serotonin; LHRH – luteinizing hormone releasing hormone; NE – norepinephrine; OMP – olfactory marker protein; SOM – somatostatin; SP – substance P; Taur – taurine. Small arrows show the direction of synaptic transmission; solid arrows indicate centrifugal projections to the bulb. Adapted from Halasz & Shepherd (1983).

GABAergic periglomerular cells interact with olfactory nerve axon terminals and mitral/tufted cell dendrites in the glomerulus (Figure 1.13) by hyperpolarizing the mitral/tufted cell apical dendrites to abolish the stimulatory effect of L-glutamate released into the synaptic cleft by ORC. Thus, the periglomerular cell represents the first level of inhibition in the olfactory system.

Dopaminergic Neurons. The glomerular layer contains one of the largest populations of dopaminergic neurons in the brain and dopamine in the olfactory bulb is found exclusively in juxtaglomerular neurons (Figure 1.13). Dopamine released by GABAergic periglomerular cells is thought to inhibit olfactory nerve output. Both D2 and D1 receptors are expressed in the olfactory bulb but D2 receptors are most frequent and expressed in terminals of olfactory nerve axons and presynaptic components of the glomerular layer, including mitral/tufted cell dendrites and dendrites of a GABAergic/dopaminergic periglomerular cell subset. In Parkinson's disease the pathology affects mainly D1 receptors. Glutamate released from ORC axons stimulates tyrosine hydroxylase and dopamine production via NMDA receptors in the periglomerular cells.

Nitric Oxide (NO) is a transmitter present in periglomerular cells and thought to have regulatory function which is rapid because of its gaseous nature. NO may activate guanylyl cyclase and increase the production of cGMP, a process that could be involved in rapid adaptation to strong stimuli. In ORC axon terminals, the inhibitory amino acid taurine co-localizes with glutamate. Release of taurine may be initiated by NO that is present in the ORC terminals within the bulb.

Lateral dendrites of mitral/tufted cells make dendro-dendritic reciprocal synapses with granule cells (Figure 1.15). This local circuit forms the basis for reciprocal dendro-dendritic inhibition mediated by inhibitory GABA$_A$ receptors in the mitral cell. As a result of its bi-directionality, the dendro-dendritic synapse can cause mitral cells to inhibit themselves (auto-inhibition), as well as neighboring mitral cells (lateral inhibition). This interaction is responsible for generating the synchronized gamma oscillatory activity (30–70 Hz) in the olfactory bulb, thought to be important in odor detection and discrimination.

Activity in the OB can be modulated by several other neurotransmitters or hormones. *Noradrenergic* fibers from the locus coeruleus project to the granule cell layer (Figure 1.13) and reduce inhibition by granule cells on mitral cells. The net effect makes mitral cells more responsive to olfactory nerve stimuli – i.e., an alerting effect. *Cholinergic* fibers from the horizontal limb of the diagonal band project to the GCL (Figure 1.14) and may have a role in odor discrimination. In rats it has been shown that fibers containing *Orexin* A and B are distributed to the glomerular, mitral, and granule cell layers. It is suggested that this connection may allow regulation of olfactory threshold according to nutritional require-ments (Appelbaum et al., 2010). There may be a further role in maintaining alertness because in narcolepsy, where there is compulsive sleepiness, the level of Orexin A in the bulb is reduced and so is olfactory function (Baier et al., 2008). Maternal behavior in rats may be promoted by an odor-imprinting mechanism that involves *oxytocin*-mediated changes in the olfactory bulb, perhaps by influencing presynaptic release of GABA from granule cells (Yu et al., 1996).

About 80 percent of the synaptic contacts between the granule cells and the mitral or tufted cells are organized as reciprocal pairs, so that the mitral-to-tufted-to-granule synapse is excitatory and the granule-to-mitral or tufted synapse is inhibitory (Kratskin & Belluzzi, 2003). Since the latter is the only type of contact between the granule cells and the mitral or tufted cells, activation of granule cells inhibits mitral and tufted cell activity. It is noteworthy that there are between 50 and 100 granule cells for each mitral cell, and that each granule cell has at least 50 gemmules, short thorn-like extensions that are reciprocally connected to mitral or tufted cell dendrites. This arrangement provides a rich substrate for strong interactions between these cells.

The olfactory bulb receives a large number of centrifugal fibers from the primary olfactory cortex (see below) and central structures outside of this cortex (Zaborszky et al., 1986). Centrifugal inputs from the piriform cortex synapse onto granule cells to regulate dendro-dendritic inhibition of mitral cells, a process that allows lateral inhibi-tion in the olfactory bulb after sensory stimulation. While most centrifugal fibers terminate within the granule cell layer, others end in the external plexiform, internal plexiform (IPL), and glomerular layers. The IPL is largely composed of myelinated axons from the mitral and tufted cells. These axons exit from the olfactory bulb as the olfactory tract, although before leaving the bulb they distribute collaterals that terminate within the bulb's deeper regions. In the mouse, about 75 percent of the centrifugal fibers originate from olfactory cortex structures, e.g., anterior olfactory nucleus and piriform cortex. The major share of centrifugal fibers that arise from ipsilateral non-olfactory structures come from the nucleus of the horizontal limb of the diagonal band via the medial forebrain bundle (Figure 1.14), the ventral part of the nucleus of the vertical limb of the diagonal band, the substantia innominata, the ventral pallidum, the subthalamic zona incerta, and regions of the medial hypothalamus. Bilateral centrifugal projections to the bulb come from the dorsal and medial raphe nuclei and locus coeruleus (Figure 1.13). In rats, a direct dopaminergic pathway has been demonstrated from the substantia nigra (pars compacta) to the central structures of the bulb (granular cell layer, mitral cell layer, and external plexiform layer) but not peripheral structures, namely the glomerular cell layer (Höglinger et al., 2015). As discussed in Chapter 7 these routes may be used (antidromically) by various pathogens to access the brainstem – a point of possible relevance to the etiology of encephalitis and Parkinson's disease.

Central Connections

Primary Olfactory Cortex

The olfactory system is unique among sensory systems in communicating directly with the cerebral cortex without first relaying in the thalamus, although reciprocal relays do exist via the dorsomedial nucleus of the thalamus between primary and secondary olfactory cortical structures. Those areas receiving fibers directly from the olfactory bulb (OB) are known as the "primary olfactory cortex" (Figure 1.16), which consists of the following six structures: (1) anterior olfactory nucleus (AON) distributed as multiple clumps of cells within the bulb and its tract; (2) olfactory tubercle (poorly developed in humans); (3) piriform cortex – the major recipient of OB output; (4) anterior cortical nucleus of the amygdala; (5) periamygdaloid complex; and (6) the rostral entorhinal cortex. The majority of mitral and tufted cell axons enter the olfactory tract, a relatively flat structure extending back from the OB on the undersurface of the frontal lobe to a point called the olfactory trigone that lies just in front of the anterior perforated substance (Figure 1.11). As the word "trigone" implies, the tract splits into three – the medial, intermediate, and lateral olfactory striae (see Figure 1.16). According to Price (2004), in humans all fibers from the OB pass through the lateral olfactory striae and the other two striae in humans are merely vestiges. Unlike all other major sensory pathways, the main cortical projection of the bulb is ipsilateral.

Anterior Olfactory Nucleus (AON). Although the AON is outside the brain, it is a central nervous system structure that receives fibers from the bulb. It is not a true nucleus, more a transition zone of gray matter, distributed as ill-defined clumps situated in the posterior part of the OB, its tract and brain regions anterior to the piriform cortex. The AON contains pyramidal cells whose dendrites receive signals from mitral and tufted cells, the contralateral AON (via the anterior commissure), and numerous central brain structures. The pyramidal cell axons project to ipsilateral bulb neurons (mainly granule cells), the contralateral AON, the OB, and the rostral entorhinal cortex.

Piriform Cortex. The piriform cortex (PC), literally meaning "pear-shaped," is situated in the anteromedial temporal lobe (Figure 1.11) and it is the largest of the structures that

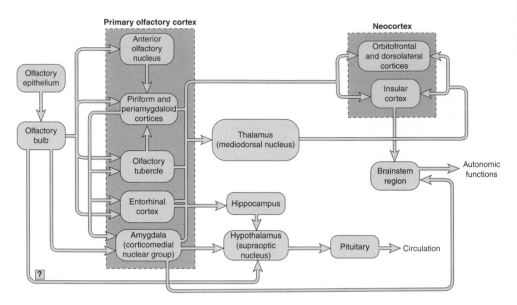

Figure 1.16 To show central olfactory projections of the olfactory system. Direct connections between the olfactory bulb and hypothalamus may not be present in humans and some other mammals. Copyright © 2010 R.L. Doty.

receive axons from the OB. Classically, it has been assumed to be *the* olfactory cortex, given that most OB projections terminate on layer I, the outermost of this three-layered paleocortex. In layer I, mitral and tufted cell axons from the olfactory bulb make contact with dendrites of pyramidal cells, whose tightly packed cell bodies are located in the main, middle zone – layer II. Layer III also contains pyramidal cells, but they are less numerous and less densely packed. Inhibitory neurons, mostly GABAergic in nature, are located within layers I and III.

The most anterior region of the piriform cortex, also named the *prepiriform, anterior piriform*, or *frontal piriform* cortex, extends from the frontotemporal junction to the caudal-most extent of the orbitofrontal cortex lateral to the olfactory tubercle and subcallosal gyrus and medial to the insular cortex (Figure 1.11). Thus, this element of the piriform cortex falls within the most caudal sector of the orbitofrontal region, and it is not a temporal lobe structure. Its more posterior region, the *temporal or posterior piriform cortex*, resides in the dorsomedial surface of the uncus, merging posteriorly with the anterior cortical nucleus of the amygdala.

Initial studies on the PC suggested that it was simply a relay station for olfactory information, but it is now known to have complex functions. The PC responds to sniffing odorless air (Sobel et al., 1998), implying that sniffing primes it for optimal reception of an odor – a concept proposed some 70 years ago by Adrian (1942). It rapidly habituates to stable but not novel odors (Poellinger et al., 2001; Sobel et al., 1999). It is responsive to odor pleasantness ("valence") (Gottfried et al., 2002), odor reward value (Gottfried & Dolan, 2003), and attention to odor (Zelano et al., 2005). It is involved in odor recognition memory and familiarity judgment (Dade et al., 2002; Plailly et al., 2005), sharpens the contrast between an odor and background odors, and probably stores olfactory traces of multisensory episodic memories (Gottfried et al., 2004). Further data suggest that the PC supports olfactory perceptual

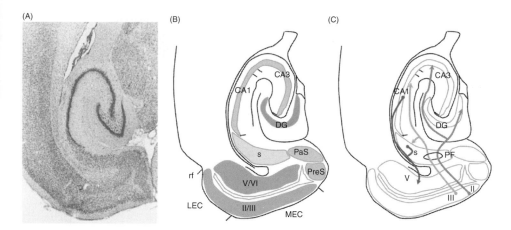

Figure 1.17 (A) Horizontal cresyl-stained section through the hippocampal formation. (B) Cytoarchitectonically defined subfields of the hippocampal formation using the same section as in (A). The rhinal fissure (rf; equivalent to the collateral sulcus in humans) delineates the entorhinal cortex from the peri-rhinal cortex. The hippocampal formation comprises the dentate gyrus (DG), the hippocampal fields CA1 and CA3, the subiculum (S), the Pre- (PreS) and Para (PaS) subiculum, and the lateral (LEC) and medial (MEC) portion of the entorhinal cortex. Within the entorhinal cortex, the deep layers V/VI are separated from the superficial ones II/III by the lamina dissecans. (C) Overall connections between the entorhinal cortex and the hippocampus use the same section as before. Cells in layer II of the EC project to both the DG and CA3 (green arrow). Cells in layer III project to the subiculum and the CA1 (orange arrows). These two groups of fibers form the perforant path. Cells in CA1 and subiculum back project to the deep layer V of the entorhinal cortex (purple arrows). Modified with permission from Coutureau & Di Scala (2009). (A black and white version of this figure will appear in some formats. For the colour version, please refer to the plate section.)

learning (Li et al., 2006). Functional magnetic resonance imaging (fMRI) experiments demonstrate that the PC becomes conditioned to the sight of food and that satiety results in reduced activity. The PC is concerned also with high-order representation of odor quality or identity. According to Gottfried et al. (2006), there is a "double dissociation" in PC whereby posterior piriform regions encode quality but not odor structure, whereas the anterior regions encode structure but not smell identity. This work suggests that we perceive most odors (which usually consist of multiple odorous molecules) as a single unified percept – a process that underlies our perception of a smell and how the brain interprets smell information. In brief, the piriform cortex does almost everything olfactory.

Entorhinal Cortex (EC). The structure and function of the EC is fairly well understood in animals but less so in humans. It occupies the most caudal zone of the primary olfactory cortex (Figure 1.17) within the rostral part of the parahippocampal gyrus (Brodmann area 28) and there are six layers in humans, although layer IV (lamina dessicans) is poorly developed. The *perforant pathway* arises in layers II and III and provides the main source of extrinsic input to sectors CAI, CA2, CA3 of the hippocampus, the subiculum, and dentate gyrus (Figures 1.17 and 1.18). Incoming fibers to EC arise from numerous cortical and subcortical areas. Input to the superficial layers (I and II) stem mainly from olfactory structures (olfactory bulb, anterior olfactory nucleus, and piriform cortex) and peri-rhinal cortex. By contrast, inputs to the deep layers (V and VI) mainly arise from the medial prefrontal cortex (prelimbic, infralimbic, and anterior cingulate cortices) and retrosplenial cortex. In rodents *olfactory input* extends to most of the entorhinal cortex surface but it is restricted to approximately 15 percent of the surface in nonhuman primates and only 4.6 percent in humans (Insausti et al., 2002). The EC receives serotonergic inputs

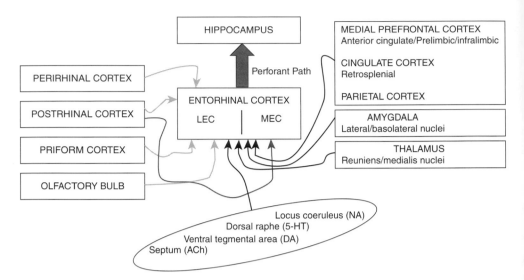

Figure 1.18 Detail of the main routes of information to the entorhinal cortex. The preferential projections to the lateral entorhinal cortex (LEC) and the medial entorhinal cortex (MEC) are shown in orange and green respectively. Fibers projecting to both the LEC and MEC are shown in black. Key to abbreviations: Ach – acetylcholine; DA – dopamine; 5-HT – 5 hydroxytriptamine; NA – noradrenaline. Modified with permission from Coutureau & Di Scala (2009).

from the dorsal raphe nucleus, dopaminergic from the ventral tegmental area, and adrenergic from the locus coeruleus. Outgoing fibers from the EC reach widespread cortical regions in particular, the peri-rhinal and prefrontal cortices. Its efferents also connect to various subcortical zones, namely the lateral septal area, amygdala, and nucleus accumbens.

Despite its widespread connections, the EC is not a simple relay station that forwards sensory information onward to the hippocampus. There is good evidence from rodent experiments that the lateral (but not medial) entorhinal cortex plays a key role in working memory (Staubli et al., 1986). Cholinergic deafferentation of the EC in rats was found to disrupt olfactory delayed non-matching to sample when the stimuli were novel, but not familiar, suggesting that sustained activity in the entorhinal cortex could provide working memory for novel stimuli (McGaughy et al., 2005).

Processing within EC probably contributes to attention, conditioning, and event and spatial cognition by compressing representations that overlap in time. These are transmitted to the hippocampus, where they are differentiated again and returned to EC (Coutureau & Di Scala G., 2009). In theory, a discrete lesion of the EC in humans would impair both semantic memory and the sense of smell, although this has yet to be shown. An adjacent area, the transentorhinal cortex, is a major source of incoming fibers to EC that is damaged very early in Alzheimer's disease and may contribute to impairment of memory and olfaction in that disorder (Braak & Braak, 1998; Chapter 7).

Amygdala. Literally meaning almond, the amygdala is a group of nuclei within the anterior temporal cortex just dorsal to the rostral hippocampus (Figure 1.19). The multiple connections are well established but its function is complex and less well defined. It is closely involved in odor perception, particularly its emotional and learning aspects (Figure 1.19). The anterior temporal lobe is divided typically into three major anatomical regions as

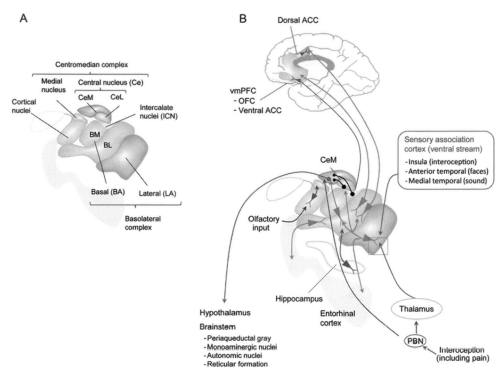

Figure 1.19 Anatomical organization and main connectivity of the amygdala. Left figure (A) shows the nuclei of the amygdala which are divided into: (1) a basolateral complex, including the lateral (LA) and basal (BA) nuclei; (2) the superficial cortex-like laminated region; and (3) the centromedial nuclear group, that includes the central (Ce) and medial nuclei plus the intercalate cell mass (IC). The BA consists of the basolateral (BL) and basomedial (BM) nuclei; the Ce comprises lateral (CeL) and medial (CeM) subdivisions. The basolateral complex and cortical nuclei resemble the cerebral cortex and contain primarily pyramidal-like projection neurons and receive inputs from unimodal cortical association areas and the thalamus; the centromedial nuclear extended amygdala resembles the striatum or globus pallidus and contains GABAergic neurons. Right figure (B). Inputs from cortical sensory areas and thalamus terminate primarily in the LA; the LA projects to the BA; the BA is interconnected with the ventromedial prefrontal cortex (vmPFC) including the orbitofrontal cortex (OFC) and ventral anterior cingulate cortex (ACC) as well as the dorsal ACC, hippocampal formation, and striatum (not shown) and projects to the CeM, which provides the main output of the amygdala to the hypothalamus and brainstem, including the parabrachial nucleus. The CeM also receives interoceptive inputs directly from the parabrachial nucleus (PBN). Reproduced and modified with permission from Benarroch (2015). (A black and white version of this figure will appear in some formats. For the colour version, please refer to the plate section.)

shown in Figure 1.19 and its legend. The *corticomedial nuclei* (shown as cortical nuclei in the figure) and periamygdaloid cortex receive most of the output from the mitral and tufted cells of the olfactory bulb. This region has strong connections to and from the olfactory bulb. Other pathways communicate with its lateral, basolateral, and central nuclei, as well as the basal ganglia, thalamus, hypothalamus, and orbitofrontal cortex.

Employing indwelling electrodes in awake humans, it was demonstrated that the amygdala is distinctly activated by odorants, producing an event-related potential similar in time course to those derived from scalp electrodes (Hudry et al., 2001). Odor-induced responses from electrodes outside the amygdala, such as those within the hippocampus and the temporal pole, were not observed. Interestingly, event-related potential latencies, but not amplitudes, decreased as a function of repeated trials, an effect that may reflect enhanced attention.

It has been suggested that the amygdala is activated chiefly in accord with the pleasantness ("valence") element of an odor (Zald & Pardo, 1997), but the situation is not clear: some experiments suggest a prime role in intensity and not valence. For example, in an fMRI study (Anderson et al., 2003), intensity and valence were dissociated by presenting one pleasant odor (citral; like lemon), and one unpleasant odor (valeric acid; like sweaty socks), each at low and high intensity. It was found that amygdala activation was related only to intensity and not valence. This concept was addressed in further experiments using neutral odors of varying intensity, in addition to pleasant and unpleasant odors (Winstonet al., 2005). Contrary to earlier work, neutral odors did not result in amygdala activation, only high-intensity pleasant or unpleasant odors did so, suggesting that the amygdala is concerned with an integrated combination of intensity and valence that reflects the overall behavioral salience (i.e., prominence) of an odor. In a further analysis, 10 subjects were asked to rate the valence of nine odors according to their pleasantness or unpleasantness and this was compared to their fMRI amygdala responses (Jin et al., 2015). It was found that the amygdala coded the complete spectrum of valence irrespective of intensity and that within-trial valence representations evolved over time, thus allowing prioritization of earlier differentiation of unpleasant stimuli.

The amygdala is involved in olfactory cross-modal recognition memory (Gottfried et al., 2004). Like the orbitofrontal cortex described in the next section, decreased functional activity in the amygdala to visual stimuli associated with food following satiety has been observed, implying that both the amygdala and the orbitofrontal cortex are a part of a structural network responsive to conditioned reward values (Gottfried et al., 2003). Behavioral studies also implicate the amygdala in memory processing specific to olfactory stimuli. For example, Buchanan et al. (2003) assessed olfactory memory in 20 patients with unilateral amygdala damage from temporal lobe resections and a single patient with selective bilateral amygdala lesions. Fifteen odors were presented without response alternatives, followed one hour later by an odor–name matching test and an odor–odor recognition test. Signal detection analysis showed that both unilateral groups were impaired in their memory for matching odors with names, but not for odor–odor recognition. The patient with bilateral amygdala damage displayed severe impairment in both odor–name and odor–odor recognition memory. None of the patients were impaired on an auditory verbal learning task, suggesting a specific impairment in olfactory memory, not merely a general memory deficit.

In common with the PC, the amygdala is probably concerned also with associative learning between olfactory and visual signals. It has been proposed that the amygdala is involved with new associations but not their long-term storage (Buchel et al., 1998; Gottfried & Dolan, 2004), a function more likely reserved for the orbitofrontal cortex as described below.

In summary, the corticomedial nucleus of the amygdala and piriform cortex have major input from the olfactory bulb and connect to multiple regions, particularly the basal ganglia, thalamus, hypothalamus, and orbitofrontal cortex. Functional imaging studies make it clear that the earlier concept of the PC as a simple relay station is incorrect. Both the amygdala and PC respond to intensity, valence, and memory components of smell to produce an olfactory percept for analysis by secondary centers, notably the orbitofrontal cortex (OFC), which in turn governs behavioral responses to a given odor.

Secondary Olfactory Cortex

Insular Cortex. This is a large chunk of cortex deep within the lateral (Sylvian) fissure and overlapped by three opercula (literal meaning: covering) from the adjacent lobes – frontal, parietal, and temporal. It contains five to six oblique gyri of variable shape, even between the two sides (Figures 1.20 and 1.21). Most parts of the insula connect reciprocally with the amygdala. Its functions are diverse with auditory, gustatory, olfactory, somatosensory, and visual components, but it may also have an important role in self-awareness (Craig, 2009).

Functional studies have confirmed much of the anatomical distribution given above. For example, Stephani et al. (2011) investigated five patients with intractable epilepsy by stimulating an array of electrodes placed over the insula (see Figure 2.8). They found somatosensory symptoms were restricted to the posterior insula with a subgroup of warmth or painful sensations in the dorsal section. Gustatory and viscerosensory symptoms (e.g., throat constriction, nausea, abdominal heaviness) occurred after stimulation of central and posterior central parts of the insula, respectively. Stimulation of the anterior insula did not show reproducible responses. Despite the strong connections between the insula cortex and amygdala, there are surprisingly few reports of olfactory sensations evoked by electrical stimulation, possibly because the olfactory fibers are located deeply within the anterior insula (Figures 1.20 and 1.21).

Orbitofrontal Cortex. The OFC is an area of prefrontal cortex commonly defined as that region in receipt of projections from the medial part of the dorsomedial thalamic nucleus. It is located above the roof of the orbit in the basal surface of the caudal frontal lobes, which includes the gyrus rectus medially and the agranular insula laterally. The putative human

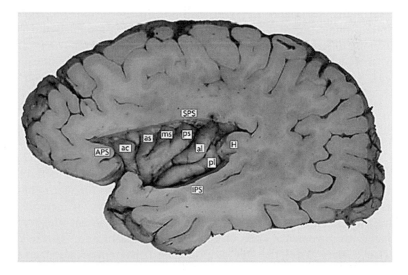

Nature Reviews | Neuroscience

Figure 1.20 Photograph of the human insular cortex viewed from its inner aspect. Key to abbreviations: APS – anterior peri-insular sulcus; ac – accessory gyrus; as – anterior short insular gyrus; ms – middle short insular gyrus; ps – posterior short insular gyrus; al – anterior long insular gyrus; pl – posterior long insular gyrus; H – Heschl's gyrus; IPS – inferior peri-insular sulcus; SPS – superior peri-insular sulcus. Reproduced with permission from Craig (2009).

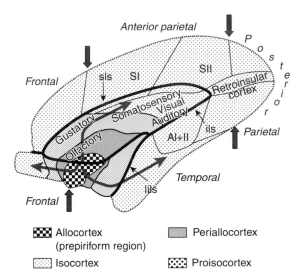

Allocortex
(prepiriform region)

Periallocortex

Isocortex

Proisocortex

Figure 1.21 Depiction of the organization of the insular cortex after opening the lateral fissure with adjoining frontal, parietal, and temporal cortices. Auditory, gustatory, olfactory, somatosensory, and visual components of the insular cortex are shown. Key to abbreviations: A1+11 – primary and secondary auditory cortex; ils – inferior limiting sulcus; lils – lateral limb of the inferior limiting sulcus; sls – superior limiting sulcus; SI – primary somatosensory cortex; SII – secondary somatosensory cortex. From: Paxinos and Mai (2004), Chapter 27: Architecture of the human cerebral cortex, page 1038.

olfactory OFC is several centimeters more rostral than the primate counterpart, as based on an imaging meta-analysis (Figure 1.11; Gottfried & Zald, 2005), implying that there may have been anterior migration of this area, or that the functions of monkey and human OFC are fundamentally different. It has two-way connections with the olfactory tubercle, piriform cortex, amygdala, and entorhinal cortex, but only input from the dorsomedial thalamic nucleus. There are other diverse connections which allow integration of sensory signals from visual, tactile, gustatory, and visceral (hypothalamic) areas, as depicted in Figure 1.22. The OFC has a lateral zone which receives taste input from the anterior insula and may constitute a tertiary taste cortex in which the reward value of taste is represented (Baylis et al., 1995). There is probably a hierarchical arrangement within OFC. The posteromedial OFC is concerned with passive smelling and odor detection. It receives signals from the amygdala and piriform cortex and transfers this information to more rostral zones of the OFC (Gottfried et al., 2006). This high-order processing zone is thought to be concerned with associative learning, working memory, and odor recognition memory. It is also proposed that there is a medial-lateral specialization, whereby pleasant odors evoke activity in the medial and ventromedial areas of OFC and unpleasant odors in the lateral zone (Gottfried et al., 2006). Thus the OFC is probably a major association area in which information about the identity and reward value of odors is represented. The diverse inputs from inferior temporal visual cortex (V5), primary somatosensory cortex, and hypothalamus allow the OFC to learn and, if needed, reject signals, e.g., visual, to which the cells would respond normally (Figure 1.22).

Initial imaging studies (Zatorre et al., 1992) suggested that the right OFC is dominant for olfaction, but this concept is probably only partially correct. Regional blood

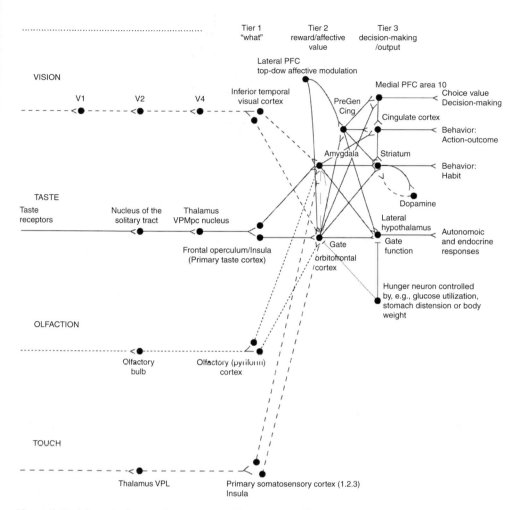

Figure 1.22 Schematic diagram showing some of the gustatory, olfactory, visual, and somatosensory pathways to the orbitofrontal cortex, and some of the outputs of the orbitofrontal cortex, in primates. The secondary taste cortex and the secondary olfactory cortex are within the orbitofrontal cortex. V1 – primary visual cortex. V4 – visual cortical area V4. PreGen Cing – pregenual cingulate cortex. "Gate" refers to the finding that inputs such as the taste, smell, and sight of food in some brain regions only produce effects when hunger is present (Rolls, 2004). Tier 1: the column of brain regions including and below the inferior temporal visual cortex represents brain regions in which whatever stimulus is present is made explicit in the neuronal representation, but not its reward or affective value, which are represented in the next tier of brain regions (Tier 2), the orbitofrontal cortex and amygdala, and in the anterior cingulate cortex. In Tier 3 areas beyond these such as medial prefrontal cortex area 10, choices or decisions about reward value are taken. Top-down control of affective response systems by cognition and by selective attention from the dorsolateral prefrontal cortex is also indicated. Medial PFC area 10 – medial prefrontal cortex area 10; VPMpc – ventralposteromedial thalamic nucleus. Reproduced with permission from Rolls (2015), Figure 1, Chapter 46.

flow studies imply that the right OFC is concerned with appraisal of the presence, intensity, hedonicity, familiarity, or potential edibility of different odorants, but it is most active when making familiarity judgements of odor, likely relying on input from the PC and least active during detection tasks (Royet et al., 2001). The left OFC is thought to be more active when making hedonic assessments, but it would appear that both OFCs have a medio-lateral specialization for hedonic variables, with pleasant odors being more represented medially within OFC. These observations, while intriguing, nonetheless should be regarded as preliminary and in need of replication. Finally, a model of parallel processing has been proposed in which the level of activity in both OFCs depends on whether the evaluation involves recognition or emotion (Royet et al., 2001). Therefore, a lesion of OFC has the potential to interfere with identification and discrimination of smell and taste signals but, contrary to earlier concepts, the damage probably has to be bilateral.

Other Central Structures Involved in Odor Processing

Dorsomedial Thalamic Nucleus (DMTN). Although the output projections of the bulb bypass the thalamus to synapse in cortical regions, the DMTN plays an important role in odor perception. The OFC has a direct input from the primary olfactory cortex (piriform cortex and amygdala), but there is a second, indirect contribution to OFC from DMTN (Figure 1.22; Rolls 2015; Tham et al., 2009), thus creating a dual access route for olfactory information. Lesions of DMTN influence odor discrimination tasks when novel or complex stimuli are employed (Eichenbaum et al., 1980). Such lesions influence the ability to unlearn previously acquired associations (Slotnick & Kaneko, 1981). Thus, in 17 patients with unilateral focal thalamic lesions, Sela et al. (2009) found an impaired ability to identify odors, but detection was intact. Only right thalamic defects reduced the pleasantness of odorants ordinarily perceived as pleasant. Additionally, those with lesions failed to modulate their sniff relative to the quality of the odorants, implying that the thalamus may play a significant role in several aspects of odor perception possibly through its cerebellar connections.

Ventrolateral Thalamic Nucleus. The ventrolateral thalamus is commonly known as the "cerebellar thalamus" because of its strong connections with the contralateral cerebellar hemisphere via the dentato-rubro-thalamic tract. Given this association and evidence of the cerebellum's role in some forms of olfactory processing as described below, Zobel et al. (2010) explored whether patients with ventrolateral thalamic lesions experience olfactory deficits. They found that detection thresholds to phenyl ethanol were significantly elevated on the side of the nose ipsilateral to the lesion, but odor detection and discrimination were not significantly affected. No patients were aware of any olfactory problem and it is not clear whether their findings were confounded by impaired sniffing.

Cerebellum. The human cerebellum contains more neurons than the rest of the brain and it is structurally connected to all major subdivisions of the central nervous system, including the basal ganglia, cerebrum, diencephalon, limbic system, brainstem, and spinal cord. The cerebellum plays a key role in modulating the act of sniffing. Apart from directing air pulses to the nasal olfactory region and modulating sniff size according to odor intensity or pleasantness, sniffing can activate independently those brain regions intimately associated with odor perception, such as the piriform and orbitofrontal cortices (Sobel et al., 1998).

The role of the cerebellum in olfaction is unclear and anatomical pathways that link olfactory areas to the cerebellum have not yet been defined (Moscovich et al., 2012). Yousem et al. (1997) showed that nasal stimulation with odors having little or no trigeminal component activated the orbitofrontal cortex markedly and the cerebellum slightly. If the odor had a trigeminal component the cerebellar activity was increased. It was suggested that the cerebellum might be involved in sensory discrimination and attention. Using fMRI, Sobel and colleagues demonstrated that the cerebellum displays olfactory-related activation mainly in the posterior lateral hemispheres (Sobel et al., 1998). The same study showed cerebellar activation (mainly in the anterior cerebellum) when odorless air was sniffed, suggesting that the cerebellum was concerned with maintenance of a feedback mechanism to regulate sniff volume. Qureshy and colleagues (Qureshy et al., 2000) mapped the human brain during olfactory processing and reported cerebellar activation during olfactory naming, implying that the cerebellum may have a role in cognitive olfactory processing. A further imaging study reported that the cerebellum is activated during odor discrimination, odor recognition memory, and passive smelling (Savic, 2002). Finally, it was demonstrated in an fMRI study of elderly volunteers that olfactory tasks activated the cerebellar lobes, especially in the superior semilunar lobule, inferior semilunar lobule, and posterior quadrangular lobule (Ferdon & Murphy, 2003). A problem with most of these studies is the confounding effect of sniffing and inadvertent trigeminal stimulation. It would be reasonable to accept that the cerebellum regulates sniffing, but whether it can directly identify odors would need more rigorously controlled experiments.

Indirect support for a role of the cerebellum in olfaction stems from reports of olfactory deficits in patients with cerebellar ataxias, as described in Chapter 7. In brief, decreased UPSIT scores have been noted in some dominant spinocerebellar ataxias (SCA) as well as the recessively inherited Friedreich's ataxia that is associated with degeneration of the afferent cerebellar pathways (Connelly et al., 2003). Thus, mild olfactory impairment is observed in the dominant spinocerebellar ataxia Type II (SCA2), but probably not in Machado-Joseph syndrome (SCA3) (Fernandez-Ruiz et al., 2003). Whether these changes relate to pathology in the cerebellum or its pathways is not established and more importantly there may be pathology in olfactory areas that has not yet been examined. Zobel et al. (2010) investigated the effects of ventrolateral thalamic lesions as described above, but they also reported contralateral deficits in odor identification and detection in patients with cerebellar lesions.

At present it may be concluded that the cerebellum regulates the intensity of sniffing. Whether it is concerned with olfactory identification as well needs further exploration.

Factors That Influence Normal Function

In light of the plasticity of the olfactory system, it is conceivable that "mere exposure" to odorants or repeated psychophysical testing may influence olfactory sensitivity. Thus, in both humans and animals, exposure or repeated testing has been reported to affect olfactory sensitivity, even where the odorant in question was initially imperceptible (Doty et al., 1981a; Doty & Ferguson-Segall, 1989; Wysocki et al., 1989; Dalton et al., 2002). The duration of these effects is debatable and in some instances the improvement may reflect training in the task rather than actual change in sensitivity (Royet et al., 2013). Spontaneous improvement in olfactory test scores occurs in those with compromised olfactory function over time, thus studies examining the exposure effects on clinical populations must include appropriate control groups (London et al., 2008). It is of interest that rodent studies show that "mere exposure" to odorants can increase neural activity within odor-specific regions of the olfactory bulb (Coopersmith et al., 1986). Despite this, long-term exposure to many odorants can either induce reversible "occupational anosmia" or long-lasting adverse influences on the ability to smell (Doty, 2015). Detailed below are non-pathological factors known to act upon human ability to smell. Pathological determinants are described in greater detail in Chapters 3 and 4.

Congenital Anosmia. This is characterized by general lack of smell function, but preservation of taste, from the time of birth. The prevalence is around 1:10,000 and in most instances the anosmia is not accompanied by other defects. An exception is the X-linked neural migration disorder, Kallman's syndrome, characterized by partial or complete loss of smell and hypogonadism. Taste sensation is normal (Hasan et al., 2007) and the olfactory receptor cells are intact (Rawson et al., 1995). In a Japanese family described by Yamamoto et al. (1966), there was tremor and either anosmia or microsmia in 14 people and it was proposed that the two traits were independent dominants. In the Faroe Islands Lygonis (1969) documented a large kindred in which 9 males and 19 females in four generations had anosmia but no other abnormality. Male-to-male transmission was witnessed several times. Singh et al. (1970) observed anosmia in six males in three generations. Mainland (1945) and Joyner (1963) recorded dominant inheritance and several instances of male-to-male transmission. One of the patients with Kallman's syndrome described by Hockaday (1966) had a father and a brother with anosmia alone. Ghadami et al. (2004) performed genome-wide linkage analysis in two large unrelated Iranian families of whom seven individuals had isolated congenital anosmia. In both families, the trait behaved as an autosomal dominant disorder with incomplete penetrance. All affected individuals shared a common haplotype in the 18p11.23-q12.2 region but no mutations were detected. Patients with congenital anosmia may have absent or reduced olfactory bulb volume, as shown in one magnetic resonance imaging (MRI) study of 25 patients (Yousem et al., 1996; Yousem et al., 2001). Anosmia from birth may be associated with congenital inability to experience pain without the expected autonomic features (Losa et al., 1989). In some families this is related to mutations in the SCN9A gene, which codes for the voltage-gated sodium channel, Nav1.7 (Goldberg et al., 2007; Nilsen et al., 2009). Feldmesser et al. (2007) performed whole-genome linkage analysis in 83 individuals from 66 families afflicted with congenital anosmia, but they were unable to find any mutation and suggested that congenital anosmia may depend on mutations in two or more genes, i.e., oligogenic inheritance. In mice, deletion of any of the three main olfactory transduction components, namely guanidine triphosphate binding protein, adenylyl cyclase, and the cyclic adenosine monophosphate-gated channel (see Figure 1.8), causes profound reduction of physiological responses to odorants. A new mutation has been found in isolated congenital anosmia (ICA). Using exome sequencing, a novel X-linked stop mutation in the cyclic nucleotide-gated channel subunit CNGA2 was discovered in two brothers with ICA (Karstensen et al., 2014). Brain MRI revealed diminished olfactory bulbs and flattened olfactory sulci.

Specific Anosmia. Usually this is defined as an inability to detect one or a few related odorants without other evidence of smell loss. It probably has a genetic basis and it is present from birth. Such anosmias should not be confused with *acquired generalized* anosmias that bring a patient to the clinic. Specific anosmias about which the subject is usually unaware are present in one form or another in a large segment of the population, and may be viewed as the olfactory equivalent of color blindness. Like color blindness there are potential risks associated with this apparently benign condition. An extreme example is specific anosmia to cyanide (almond-like), which reportedly affects about 1 percent of otherwise healthy people (Sayek, 1970). Since most so-called specific anosmias reflect markedly decreased sensitivity to an odorant, rather than complete loss, the phenomenon is best described as "specific hyposmia." In many cases, the frequency distribution of sensitivity in the population for odorants exhibiting this effect is bimodal. There are many other varieties of specific anosmias. Musk anosmia, which is probably an autosomal recessive trait, afflicts 7 percent of Caucasians but not Afro-Caribbeans (Comfort et al., 1973). No genetic locus has so far been identified. Specific anosmia to androsterone (sweaty or urinous) is also thought to be inherited, possibly X-linked, based on raised concordance in identical twins, but again no locus is presently known (Wysocki & Beauchamp, 1984). This condition affects up to 50 percent of otherwise healthy people, but some individuals with an initial specific anosmia can eventually detect the odor after repeated exposure (Wysocki et al., 1989). A similar learning process applies to furfural (almond-like) and isovaleric acid (sweaty) (Doty et al., 1981; Jacob et al., 2006; Yee & Wysocki, 2001; Jacob et al., 2006). The specific anosmia to isobutyric acid (cheesy, vomit-like smell) affects about 2.5 percent of apparently healthy individuals, whereas specific anosmia to isovaleric acid affects about 1.4 percent of Caucasians and 9.1 percent of Blacks (Amoore, 1967). There is one report of a mother and her three children, none of whom were able to perceive n-butylmercaptan (skunk odor; Patterson & Lauder, 1948). There are many other specific anosmias, although relatively little research is performed on this topic. Even though specific anosmias generally go unrecognized, they can influence the overall perception of odorants, which depend upon multiple receptors, and, in some cases, eating habits. A classic example is specific anosmia to trimethylamine, a fish-like odor. Individuals who are relatively insensitive to this chemical are more likely to ingest fish whose odors are repugnant to people with retained sensitivity.

Some of the better known specific anosmias are listed in Table 1.1.

Table 1.1. Compounds associated with specific anosmia. Adapted from Wysocki & Beauchamp, 1991.

Compound	Odor quality	Percent anosmic
Androstenone	Sweaty/urinous	47
Isobutyraldehyde	Malty	36
Cineole	Camphorous	33
Pyrroline	Spermous	12
Pentadecalactone	Musky	12
Carvone	Minty	8
Trimethylamine	Fishy	6
Isovaleric acid	Sweaty	3

Blind Smell. "Blind smell" refers to detection of a sub-threshold odor by the brain in the absence of conscious perception. It has to be distinguished from smell blindness or specific anosmia. To demonstrate this phenomenon, fMRI was used to localize brain activation induced by high and low concentrations of the putative pheromone, estratetraenol acetate (Sobel et al., 1999). Although subjects reported verbally that they were unable to detect either concentration, their forced-choice guess was better than chance for the higher concentration, and both concentrations produced significant brain activation on fMRI, mainly in the right orbitofrontal cortex. In other words, these subjects were able to detect odor at a "subconscious" level without being fully aware they could do so. These observations complement earlier work on sub-threshold visual perception and localization, termed "blind sight" (Sanders et al., 1974), where a subject correctly localizes objects that cannot be seen consciously in a blind or even a normal visual field (Weiskrantz, 1990).

Age. Reduction in smell function affects about half of the adult population between the ages of 65 and 80 years and three-quarters of those over 80 years of age (Figure 1.23; Doty et al 1984). These numbers may even be conservative depending on the criteria used for olfactory loss (Murphy et al., 2002). Not all odorants show the same degree of age-related decline. This reflects factors such as odor threshold and the nature of the function relating odorant concentration to perceived intensity. For example, it was shown that healthy control subjects over the age of 50 in general had more difficulty in identifying pleasant odors compared with less pleasant ones, an effect that may relate to the intensity of the smell in question (Hawkes et al., 2005). Such effects are complicated, given the conversion of multiple odorants into odor percepts from which individual odorant components cannot be ascertained. The age-related changes in odor identification ability, as measured by a forced-choice odor identification test, are shown in Figure 1.23. These losses are not culture specific, and are much more pronounced than the influences of gender, which are shown in the same figure.

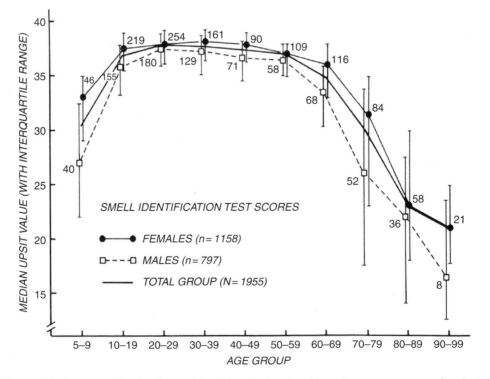

Figure 1.23 Changes in odor identification ability with age in American citizens. On average, women perform better than men at all ages on the University of Pennsylvania Smell Identification Test (UPSIT). From Doty, Shaman et al. (1984).

Age-related damage to the olfactory epithelium from environmental agents such as viruses, bacteria, toxins, and pollutants is a primary factor that influences human olfactory function. The olfactory epithelium undergoes cumulative damage throughout life, resulting in islands of respiratory-like metaplasia that begin to appear soon after birth (Nakashima et al., 1984), decreased epithelial thickness, and diminished numbers of olfactory receptors (Rosli et al., 1999). Such damage appears to be accelerated in environments containing pollutants and industrial chemicals (Hudson et al., 2006). Factors associated with age-related changes in olfactory function include: (1) an epithelium with reduced protein synthesis; (2) fewer neurotrophic factors; (3) altered vascularity; (4) decreased mitotic activity; (5) decreased intramucosal blood flow; (6) increased mucus viscosity; (7) increased secretory gland and lymphatic atrophy; (8) decreased enzymatic capacity (i.e., cytochromes) to deactivate xenobiotics; and (9) possibly neurodegenerative conditions within CNS structures, as described below and in detail in Chapter 7.

The number and cross-sectional area of the foramina of the cribriform plate decrease in some elderly people as a result of bony overgrowth, in effect pinching off the olfactory receptor axons *en route* from the nasal cavity into the brain (Krmpotic-Nemanic, 1969; Kalmey et al., 1998). The age-related decrease in ORC results in declining volume and mitral cell count, as well as reduced number of glomeruli (Hinds & McNelly, 1981). In a pioneering study, Smith (1942b) estimated age-related losses of human olfactory receptors. By counting the glomeruli in 205 olfactory bulbs of 121 cadavers over a wide age range, he concluded that loss of olfactory nerves begins soon after birth and continues throughout life at about 1 percent per year. In more recent work, Meisami & Bhatnagar (1998) measured the number of mitral cells and glomeruli in olfactory bulbs from three young adult women, three middle-aged adult women, and three aged women. The number of mitral cells and glomeruli decreased steadily with age at approximately 10 percent per decade; in the ninth and tenth decades, less than 30 percent of these structures were present. These reductions support the finding of olfactory bulb and tract volume atrophy with age (Hinds & McNelly, 1977; Yousem et al., 1998). As described in Chapter 7, older brains inevitably show pathology associated with neuro-degenerative disorders such as Alzheimer's disease and Parkinson's disease. Such pathology probably accounts for some age-related olfactory deficits seen in otherwise healthy older people. Thus, many elderly people have neurofibrillary tangles, neuropil threads, and Lewy bodies in all layers of their olfactory bulbs, with the possible exception of the olfactory nerve cell axon layer (Ohm & Braak, 1987; Kishikawa et al., 1990). In Alzheimer's disease (AD), central limbic structures that receive olfactory bulb projections have relatively high numbers of neurofibrillary tangles and neuritic plaques (Hooper & Vogel, 1976; Pearson et al., 1985; Reyes et al., 1993). Such structures include the hippocampal formation, periamygdaloid nucleus, prepiriform cortex, and entorhinal cortex. One of the earliest sites of AD change is the transentorhinal cortical region (Ferreyra-Moyano & Barragan, 1989; Jellinger et al., 1990; Braak et al., 1996), a zone containing afferent fibers *en route* from the sensory association cortex to the entorhinal cortex (Figure 1.24). It is not known to what degree such pathological entities contribute to the age-related decline in olfactory function in non-demented elderly people or whether they represent the earliest changes of disease that would be manifest clinically had the subject lived long enough.

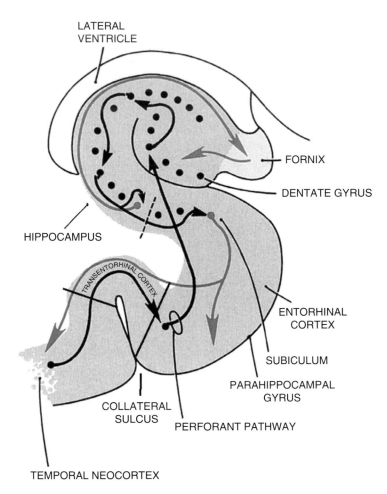

LATERAL
VENTRICLE

FORNIX

DENTATE GYRUS

HIPPOCAMPUS

TRANSENTORHINAL CORTEX

ENTORHINAL
CORTEX

SUBICULUM

PARAHIPPOCAMPAL
GYRUS

COLLATERAL
SULCUS

PERFORANT PATHWAY

TEMPORAL NEOCORTEX

Figure 1.24 Coronal section of the hippocampus to show the position of the transentorhinal cortex. This lies in the depths of the collateral sulcus between the two straight lines as shown. It is one of the first areas to be affected in Alzheimer's disease. From Braak & Braak (1998).

Hormonal Factors. On average, women outperform men on tests of odor identification, detection, discrimination, and memory. Such effects are seen across a wide range of cultures (Doty et al., 1985; Gilbert & Wysocki, 1987). It is presumed that organizational influences of reproductive hormones on the developing fetus brain is likely involved, since the sex differences appear soon after birth and no overall changes occur thereafter (Doty & Cameron, 2009). It is likely that females have more neurons and glial cells in their olfactory bulbs than males (Oliveira-Pinto et al. 2014). In their autopsy-based study, the average total number of cells in females was 16.2 million compared with 9.2 million in males, a significant difference of 43.2 percent. Presumably this dichotomy accounts for the known superiority of females in many olfactory tests.

During the menstrual cycle, women evidence three peaks in detection performance: during the latter half of menses, mid-cycle near the time of the luteinizing hormone surge, and during the mid-luteal phase see Figure 1.25 (Doty et al., 1981). The latter two

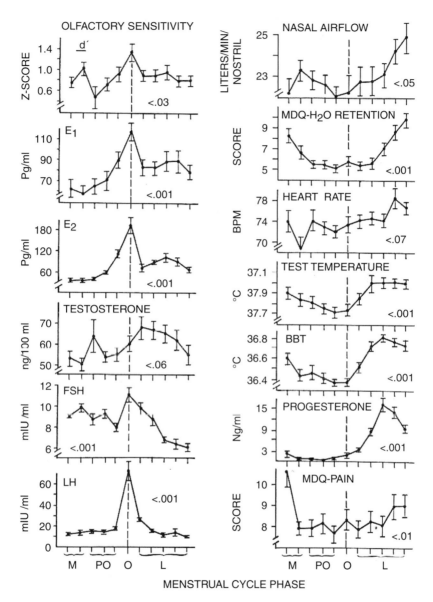

Figure 1.25 Menstrual cycle fluctuations in olfactory sensitivity, reproductive hormones, and several physiological and psychological variables. n = 17 menstrual cycles, with sensory data collected every other day. d' denotes signal detection measure reflecting distance between signal + noise and noise distributions. d' based upon 350 trials/test session. E_1 – oestrone; E_2 – estradiol; FSH – follicle stimulating hormone; LH – luteinizing hormone; MDQ – Moos' Menstrual Distress Questionnaire Items; BBT – basal body temperature. Note the strong association between circulating oestrogen levels and the olfactory sensitivity measure. From Doty et al. (1981).

changes are closely related to circulating levels of both estrone and estradiol, although they also appear in women taking oral contraceptives. Although there are anecdotal reports of heightened olfactory sensitivity during pregnancy, particularly during the first trimester (Nordin et al., 2004), empirical data on this topic are inconclusive as reviewed elsewhere (Cameron, 2014). The limited evidence suggests that during pregnancy some odors, such as clove (Gilbert & Wysocki, 1991; Laska et al., 1996), strawberry (Swallow, Lindow et al., 2005), and watermelon (Cameron, 2007) may be more readily identified, although for some odors such performance may actually be worse (Laska et al., 1996; Kolble et al., 2001; Swallow et al., 2005) or weaker (Gilbert & Wysocki, 1991).

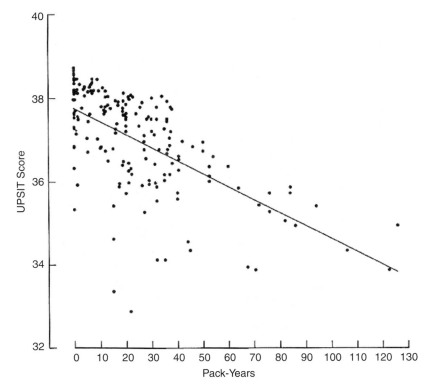

Figure 1.26 Effect of cumulative smoking dose on University of Pennsylvania Smell Identification Test (UPSIT) scores for current smokers. UPSIT scores adjusted for age and sex. The linear regression line indicates the magnitude of the smoking dose effect. Note that subjects with very high smoking doses display a 4-point difference in UPSIT scores relative to subjects with low smoking doses. From Frye et al. (1990).

Cigarette Smoking. Animal studies have found that exposure to volatiles associated with burning tobacco can cause damage to the olfactory neuroepithelium, which includes squamous metaplasia and atrophy (Vanscheeuwijck et al., 2002). Most human investigations show that tobacco smoking by itself hardly ever causes complete smell loss, although hyposmia can occur and odor identification test scores are inversely related to pack-years smoked (Figure 1.26). Previous smokers show gradual improvement of olfaction commensurate with the amount and duration of prior smoking. Thus, hyposmic current cigarette smokers can expect to improve if they give up the habit. The degree of smell identification impairment in current smokers is relatively small, around 1–2 UPSIT points, falling well behind the effect of age in those over 60 years and, to a lesser degree, the relative influence of gender (Doty et al., 1984; Frye et al., 1990). These variables may be additive; there will be a large difference (around 3–4 UPSIT points) when comparing, say, a female who has never smoked with a male current smoker of the same age. Smoking may have a protective effect against Parkinson's disease or exposure to noxious chemicals as described in Chapter 7.

Pollution. Numerous studies suggest that olfactory function can be influenced adversely by air pollution and this is described in more detail in Chapter 5 section 13.

Demography. In a massive National Geographic Magazine survey, nearly 11 million subscribers were asked about basic demography, their ability to smell, and frequency of perfume use (Gilbert & Wysocki, 1987). Identification and intensity ratings were given to the following microencapsulated odorants: androstenone (urinous), amyl-acetate (banana-like), galaxolide (musky), eugenol (cloves), mercaptans (sulphurous – often added to natural gas), and rose. With the exception of androstenone and mercaptan, all of these odors were generally rated pleasant by men and women of all nationalities. Androstenone was perceived (if at all) either as stale urine, musk-like, or sweet. People who rated androstenone as unpleasant generally gave this a high intensity rating – especially those from Europe. This observation correlates with other data suggesting that if a subject has a low threshold to androstenone it is rated unpleasant; if the threshold is high then it is rated indifferent or pleasant. Amyl acetate was given a fairly uniform hedonic rating, whereas major differences appeared for the synthetic musk, galaxolide. Galaxolide received unpleasant ratings by most Asian respondents, and pleasant ratings by Australians, 50 percent of whom indicated they would be prepared to wear it as perfume. While the majority thought that mercaptans were unpleasant, there was one exception – most people from India liked it. Many other regional differences were noted, presumably reflecting cultural and other environmental differences. Four of the six odors evoked a vivid memory, and this was true throughout the world. Galaxolide and mercaptan, to a lesser extent, were the two odorants least likely to evoke graphic memories. The ability to identify the six odors was similar worldwide. Androstenone gave most difficulty, with only 20 percent responding correctly. Likewise, Galaxolide was difficult, especially for men. This information concurs with the well-recognized specific anosmia to either androstenone or Galaxolide. Androstenone anosmia was present in 33 percent of males and 24 percent of females from America in contrast with 22 percent of males and 14 percent of females from Africa.

Summary

Apart from playing a critical role in safety, nutrition, and quality of life, olfaction provides a "health index" or probe for relatively inaccessible brain areas. Indeed, olfactory dysfunction is among the first signs of Alzheimer's disease and idiopathic Parkinson's disease. Olfaction has become a model system for neural degeneration and regeneration as it is one of few sensory systems where regeneration occurs. Olfactory ensheathing cells have axonal guidance properties that have been applied experimentally, with apparent success in one patient, to direct spinal nerve cell axons through regions of spinal cord fibrosis (Tabakow et al., 2014). The olfactory neuroepithelium, located high in the nasal cavity, contains ~6 million receptor cells on each side. Each cell expresses only one receptor type that belongs to the largest gene family in the mammalian genome. Most olfactory receptors are "generalists," responding to a range of chemical moieties. Even single-molecule odorants, which are the exception rather than the rule, are agonists for multiple receptors, indicating that the "code" for a given odorant sensation reflects a patterned combination of neural activity across different receptor types. The olfactory bulb, the first olfactory relay station in the brain, sharpens and refines the incoming signals from multiple molecules, aiding the ultimate synthesis of information from numerous peripheral inputs into single odor "percepts." Cortical regions receiving projections from the olfactory bulb include those collectively termed the "primary olfactory cortex"; namely, the anterior olfactory nucleus, piriform and peri-amygdaloid cortices, entorhinal cortex, olfactory tubercle, and corticomedial nuclear group of the amygdala. Reciprocal relationships exist among these brain regions, as well as many other brain regions. The piriform cortex is no longer viewed as a simple relay station, but, along with the amygdala, responds to odor intensity, valence, and memory. Multiple factors influence the ability to smell, including age, gender, cigarette smoking, environmental pollution, and circulating levels of reproductive hormones. Some individuals, for all practical purposes, cannot detect certain odorants, a problem termed "specific anosmia." Preferences for odors are influenced by a number of experiential factors, including cultural experiences with odors. Many disorders alter smell function, as described in detail in Chapters 5 and 7. In Chapter 3 we describe practical clinical means for quantifying smell function to help formulate a prognosis and monitor treatment efficacy.

References

Adrian, E.D., 1942. Olfactory reactions in the brain of the hedgehog. *Journal of Physiology* **100**, 459–473.

Amoore, J.E., 1967. Specific anosmia: A clue to the olfactory code. *Nature* **214**, 1095–1098.

Anderson, A.K., Christoff, K., Stappen, I., et al. 2003. Dissociated neural representations of intensity and valence in human olfaction. *Nature Neuroscience* **6**, 196–202.

Appelbaum, L., Wang, G., Yokogawa, T., et al. 2010. Circadian and homeostatic regulation of structural synaptic plasticity in hypocretin neurons. *Neuron* **68**, 87–98.

Baier, P.C., Weinhold, S.L., Huth, V., et al. 2008. Olfactory dysfunction in patients with narcolepsy with cataplexy is restored by intranasal Orexin A (Hypocretin-1). *Brain* **131**, 2734–2741.

Baylis, L.L., Rolls, E.T., Baylis, G.C., 1995. Afferent connections of the caudolateral orbitofrontal cortex taste area of the primate. *Neuroscience* **64**, 801–812.

Benarroch, E.E., 2015. The amygdala Functional organization and involvement in neurologic disorders. *Neurology* **84**, 313–324.

Benbernou, N., Robin, S., Tacher, S., et al. 2011. cAMP and IP3 signaling pathways in HEK293 cells transfected with canine olfactory receptor genes. *Journal of Heredity* **102** Suppl 1, S47–S61.

Bergmann, O., Spalding, K.L., Frisen, J., 2015. Adult neurogenesis in humans. *Cold Spring Harbor Perspectives in Biology* **7**, a018994.

Bower, J.H., Maraganore, D.M., Peterson, B.J., Ahlskog, J.E., Rocca, W.A., 2006. Immunologic diseases, anti-inflammatory drugs, and Parkinson disease: A case-control study. *Neurology* **67**, 494–496.

Braak, H., Braak, E., 1998. Evolution of neuronal changes in the course of Alzheimer's disease. *Journal of Neural Transmission* **53**, 127–140.

Braak, H., Braak, E., Yilmazer, D., et al. 1996. Pattern of brain destruction in Parkinson's and Alzheimer's diseases. *Journal of Neural Transmission* **103**, 455–490.

Bryant, B., Silver W.L. 2000. Chemesthesis: The common chemical sense. In: Finger TE, Silver WL, Restrepo, D (Eds.). *The Neurobiology of Taste and Smell.* 2nd edition. New York: Wiley-Liss, p. 73.

Buchanan, T.W., Tranel, D., Adolphs, R., 2003. A specific role for the human amygdala in olfactory memory. *Learning & Memory* **10**, 319–325.

Buchel, C., Morris, J., Dolan, R.J., Friston, K.J., 1998. Brain systems mediating aversive conditioning: An event-related fMRI study. *Neuron* **20**, 947–957.

Buck, L., Axel, R., 1991. A novel multigene family may encode odorant receptors: A molecular basis for odor recognition. *Cell* **65**, 175–187.

Cameron, E.L., 2007. Measures of human olfactory perception during pregnancy. *Chemical Senses* **32**, 775–782.

Cameron, E.L., 2014. Pregnancy and olfaction: A review. *Frontiers in Psychology* February 6(5): 67. DOI: 10.3389/fpsyg.2014.00067.

Comfort, A., Whissell-Buechy, D., Amoore, J.E., 1973. Odour-blindness to musk: Simple recessive inheritance. *Nature* **245**, 157–158.

Connelly, T., Farmer, J.M., Lynch, D.R., Doty, R. L., 2003. Olfactory dysfunction in degenerative ataxias. *Journal of Neurology, Neurosurgery, & Psychiatry* **74**, 1435–1437.

Coopersmith, R., Henderson, S.R., Leon, M. 1986. Odor specificity of the enhanced neural response following early odor experience in rats. *Brain Research* **392**, 191–197.

Coutureau, E., Di Scala G., 2009. Entorhinal cortex and cognition. *Progress in Neuro-Psychopharmacology & Biological Psychiatry* **33**, 753–761.

Craig, A.D., 2009. How do you feel now? the anterior insula and human awareness. *Nature Reviews Neuroscience* **10**, 59–70.

Dade, L.A., Zatorre, R.J., Jones-Gotman, M., 2002. Olfactory learning: Convergent findings from lesion and brain imaging studies in humans. *Brain* **125**, 86–101.

Dalton, P., Doolittle, N., Breslin, P.A. 2002. Gender-specific induction of enhanced sensitivity to odors. *Nature Neuroscience* **5**, 199–200.

Devanand, D.P., Lee, S., Manly, J., et al. 2015. Olfactory identification deficits are associated with increased mortality in a multiethnic urban community. *Annals of Neurology* **78**, 401–411.

Doty, R.L., 2008. The olfactory vector hypothesis of neurodegenerative disease: Is it viable? *Annals of Neurology* **63**, 7–15.

Doty, R.L. 2015. Neurotoxic exposure and alterations in olfaction and gustation. *Handbook of Clinical Neurology* **131**, 299–324.

Doty, R.L., Applebaum, S., Zusho, H., Settle, R. G., 1985. Sex differences in odor identification ability: A cross-cultural analysis. *Neuropsychologia* **23**, 667–672.

Doty, R.L., Cameron, E.L., 2009. Sex differences and reproductive hormone influences on human odor perception. *Physiology & Behavior* **97**, 213–228.

Doty, R.L., Ferguson-Segall, M. 1989. Influence of castration on the odor detection performance of male rats. *Behavioral Neuroscience* **103**: 691–693.

Doty, R.L., Shaman, P., Applebaum, S.L., et al. 1984. Smell identification ability: Changes with age. *Science* **226**, 1441–1443.

Doty, R.L., Snyder, P.J., Huggins, G.R., Lowry, L. D., 1981. Endocrine, cardiovascular, and psychological correlated of olfactory sensitivity changes during the human menstrual cycle. *Journal of Comparative and Physiological Physiology* **95**, 45–60.

Duda, J.E., 2010. Olfactory system pathology as a model of Lewy neurodegenerative disease. *Journal of the Neurological Sciences* **289**, 49–54.

Ebrahimi, F.A., Chess, A., 1998. Olfactory G proteins: Simple and complex signal transduction. *Current Biology* **8**, R431–R433.

Eichenbaum, H., Shedlack, K.J., Eckmann, K. W., 1980. Thalamocortical mechanisms in odor-guided behavior. I. Effects of lesions of the mediodorsal thalamic nucleus and frontal cortex on olfactory discrimination in the rat. *Brain. Behavior & Evolution* **17**, 255–275.

Eisthen, H.L., Delay, R.J., Wirsig-Wiechmann, C.R., Dionne, V.E., 2000. Neuromodulatory effects of gonadotropin releasing hormone on olfactory receptor neurons. *Journal of Neuroscience* **20**, 3947–3955.

Elsaesser, R., Montani, G., Tirindelli, R., Paysan, J., 2005. Phosphatidyl-inositide signalling proteins in a novel class of sensory cells in the mammalian olfactory epithelium. *European Journal of Neuroscience* **21**, 2692–2700.

Feldmesser, E., Bercovich, D., Avidan, N., et al. 2007. Mutations in olfactory signal transduction genes are not a major cause of human congenital general anosmia. *Chemical Senses* **32**, 21–30.

Ferdon, S., Murphy, C., 2003. The cerebellum and olfaction in the aging brain: A functional magnetic resonance imaging study. *Neuroimage* **20**, 12–21.

Fernandez-Ruiz, J., Diaz, R., Hall-Haro, C., et al. 2003. Olfactory dysfunction in hereditary ataxia and basal ganglia disorders. *Neuroreport* **14**, 1339–1341.

Ferreyra-Moyano, H., Barragan, E., 1989. The olfactory system and Alzheimer's disease. *Int. International Journal of Neuroscience* **49**, 157–197.

Floriano, W.B., Vaidehi, N., Goddard, W.A., III, Singer, M.S., Shepherd, G.M., 2000. Molecular mechanisms underlying differential odor responses of a mouse olfactory receptor. *Proceedings of the National Academy of Sciences of the United States of America* **97**, 10712–10716.

Freitag, J., Ludwig, G., Andreini, I., Rossler, P., Breer, H., 1998. Olfactory receptors in aquatic and terrestrial vertebrates. *Journal of Comparative Physiology A-:Neuroethology Sensory Neural and Behavioral Physiology* **183**, 635–650.

Fuller, G.N., Burger, P.C., 1990. Nervus terminalis (cranial nerve zero) in the adult human. *Clinical Neuropathology* **9**, 279–283.

Ghadami, M., Majidzadeh, A., Morovvati, S., et al. 2004. Isolated congenital anosmia with morphologically normal olfactory bulb in two Iranian families: A new clinical entity? *American Journal of Medical Genetics Part A* **127A**, 307–309.

Gilbert, A.N., Wysocki, C.J., 1987. The smell survey results. *National Geographic* **172**, 514–525.

Gilbert, A.N., Wysocki, C.J., 1991. Quantitative assessment of olfactory experience during pregnancy. *Psychosomatic Medicine* **53**, 693–700.

Gloor, P., 1997. *The Temporal Lobe and the Limbic System*. New York: Oxford University Press.

Goldberg, Y.P., MacFarlane, J., MacDonald, M. L., et al. 2007. Loss-of-function mutations in the Nav1.7 gene underlie congenital indifference to pain in multiple human populations. *Clinical Genetics* **71**, 311–319.

Gopinath, B., Sue, C.M., Kifley, A., Mitchell, P., 2012. The association between olfactory impairment and total mortality in older adults. *Journals of Gerontology Series A-Biological Sciences & Medical Sciences* **67**, 204–209.

Gottfried, J.A., 2010. Central mechanisms of odour object perception. *Nature Reviews Neuroscience* **11**(9), 628–641.

Gottfried, J.A., Dolan, R.J., 2003. The nose smells what the eye sees: Crossmodal visual facilitation of human olfactory perception. *Neuron* **39**, 375–386.

Gottfried, J.A., Dolan, R.J., 2004. Human orbitofrontal cortex mediates extinction learning while accessing conditioned representations of value. *Nature Neuroscience* **7**, 1144–1152.

Gottfried, J.A., O'Doherty, J., Dolan, R.J., 2002. Appetitive and aversive olfactory learning in humans studied using event-related functional magnetic resonance imaging. *Journal of Neuroscience* **22**, 10829–10837.

Gottfried, J.A., O'Doherty, J., Dolan, R.J., 2003. Encoding predictive reward value in human amygdala and orbitofrontal cortex. *Science* **301**, 1104–1107.

Gottfried, J.A., Smith, A.P., Rugg, M.D., Dolan, R.J., 2004. Remembrance of odors past: Human olfactory cortex in cross-modal recognition memory. *Neuron* **42**, 687–695.

Gottfried, J.A., Small, D.M., Zald, D.H., 2006. Chapter 6, Plate 9. In: Zald, D.H., Rauch, S.L. (Eds.) *The Orbitofrontal Cortex*. New York: Oxford University Press.

Gottfried, J.A., Winston, J.S., Dolan, R.J., 2006. Dissociable codes of odor quality and odorant structure in human piriform cortex. *Neuron* **49**, 467–479.

Gottfried, J.A., Zald, D.H., 2005. On the scent of human olfactory orbitofrontal cortex: Meta-analysis and comparison to non-human primates. *Brain Research Reviews* **50**, 287–304.

Halasz, N., Shepherd, G.M., 1983. Neurochemistry of the vertebrate olfactory bulb. *Neuroscience* **10**, 579–619.

Hasan, K., Reddy, S., Barsony, N., 2007. Taste perception in Kallmann syndrome, a model of congenital anosmia. *Endocrine Practice* **13**, 716–720.

Hawkes, C.H., Shah, M., Fogo, A., 2005. Smell identification declines from age 36 years and mainly affects pleasant odors. *Neurology* **6**(suppl. 1), 579–619.

Hinds, J.W., Hinds, P.L., McNelly, N.A., 1984. An autoradiographic study of the mouse olfactory epithelium: Evidence for long-lived receptors. *Anatomical Record* **210**, 375–383.

Hinds, J.W., McNelly, N.A., 1977. Aging of the rat olfactory bulb: Growth and atrophy of constituent layers and changes in size and number of mitral cells. *Journal of Comparative Neurology* **171**, 345–367.

Hinds, J.W., McNelly, N.A., 1981. Aging in the rat olfactory system: Correlation of changes in the olfactory epithelium and olfactory bulb. *Journal of Comparative Neurology* **203**, 441–453.

Hockaday, T.D., 1966. Hypogonadism and life-long anosmia. *Postgraduate Medical Journal* **42**, 572–574.

Hooper, M.W., Vogel, F.S., 1976. Limbic system in Alzheimers disease-neuropathologic investigation. *American Journal of Pathology* **85**, 1–13.

Höglinger, G.U., Alvarez-Fischer, D., Arias-Carrión, O., et al. 2015. A new dopaminergic nigro-olfactory projection. *Acta Neuropathologica* **130**(3), 333–348.

Hudry, J., Ryvlin, P., Royet, J.P., Mauguiere, F., 2001. Odorants elicit evoked potentials in the human amygdala. *Cerebral Cortex* **11**, 619–627.

Hudson, R., Arriola, A., Martinez-Gomez, M., Distel, H., 2006. Effect of air pollution on olfactory function in residents of Mexico City. *Chem.Senses* **31**, 79–85.

Insausti, R., Marcos, P., Arroyo-Jimenez, M.M., Blaizot, X., Martinez-Marcos, A., 2002. Comparative aspects of the olfactory portion of the entorhinal cortex and its projection to the hippocampus in rodents, nonhuman primates, and the human brain. *Brain Research Bulletin* **57**, 557–560.

Jacob, T.J., Wang, L., Jaffer, S., McPhee, S., 2006. Changes in the odor quality of androstadienone during exposure-induced sensitization. *Chemical Senses* **31**, 3–8.

Jellinger, K, Braak, H, Braak, E., Fischer, P., 1990. Alzheimer lesions in the entorhinal region and isocortex in Parkinson's and Alzheimer's diseases. *Annals of the New York Academy of Sciences* **640**, 203–209.

Jin, J., Zelano, C., Gottfried, J.A., Mohanty, A., 2015. Human Amygdala Represents the Complete Spectrum of Subjective Valence. *Journal of Neuroscience*, **35**(45), 15145–15156.

Johnston, M., Zakharov, A., Koh, L., Armstrong, D., 2005. Subarachnoid injection of Microfil reveals connections between cerebrospinal fluid and nasal lymphatics in the non-human primate. *Neuropathology and Applied Neurobiology* **31**, 632–640.

Joyner, R.E., 1963. Olfactory acuity in an industrial population. *Journal of Occupational and Environmental Medicine* **5**, 37–42.

Kalmey, J.K., Thewissen, J.G.M., Dluzen, D.E., 1998. Age-related size reduction of foramina in the cribriform plate. *The Anatomical Record* **251**, 326–329.

Karstensen, H.G., Mang, Y., Fark, T., Hummel, T., Tommerup, N., 2014. The first mutation in CNGA2 in two brothers with anosmia. *Clinical Genetics* **88**(3), 293–296.

Kishikawa, M., Iseki, M., Nishimura, M., Sekine, I., Fujii, H., 1990. A histopathological study on senile changes in the human olfactory bulb. *Pathology International* **40**, 255–260.

Kolble, N., Hummel, T., von, M.R., Huch, A., Huch, R., 2001. Gustatory and olfactory function in the first trimester of pregnancy. *European Journal of Obstetrics and Gynecology and Reproductive Biology* **99**, 179–183.

Kratskin, I.L., Belluzzi, O., 2003. Anatomy and neurochemistry of the olfactory bulb. *Neurological Disease & Therapy* **57**, 139–164.

Krmpotic-Nemanic, J., 1969. Presbycusis, presbystasis and presbyosmia as consequences of the analogous biological process. *Acta Oto-laryngologica* **67**, 217–223.

Lai, P.C., Guida, B., Shi, J., Crasto, C.J., 2014. Preferential binding of an odor within olfactory receptors: A precursor to receptor activation. *Chemical Senses* **39**, 107–123.

Larsen, S.H., Reader, R.W., Kort, E.N., Tso, W.W., Adler, J., 1974. Change in direction of flagellar rotation is the basis of the chemotactic response in Escherichia coli. *Nature* **249**, 74–77.

Laska, M., Koch, B., Heid, B., Hudson, R., 1996. Failure to demonstrate systematic changes in olfactory perception in the course of pregnancy: A longitudinal study. *Chemical Senses* **21**, 567–571.

Li, W., Luxenberg, E., Parrish, T., Gottfried, J.A., 2006. Learning to smell the roses: Experience-dependent neural plasticity in human piriform and orbitofrontal cortices. *Neuron* **52**, 1097–1108.

Lois, C., Alvarez-Buylla, A., 1994. Long-distance neuronal migration in the adult mammalian brain. *Science* **264**, 1145–1148.

London, B., Nabet, B., Fisher, A.R., et al. 2008. Predictors of prognosis in patients with olfactory disturbance. *Annals of Neurology*, **63**(2), 159–166.

Loo, A.T., Youngentob, S.L., Kent, P.F., Schwob, J.E., 1996. The aging olfactory epithelium: Neurogenesis, response to damage, and odorant-induced activity. *International Journal of Developmental Neuroscience* **14**, 881–900.

Losa, M., Scheier, H., Rohner, P., et al. 1989. [Long-term course in congenital analgesia]. *Schweizerische medizinische Wochenschrift* **119**, 1303–1308.

Lygonis, C.S., 1969. Familiar absence of olfaction. *Hereditas* **61**, 413–416.

Mackay-Sim, A., St.John, J., Schwob, J.E., 2015. Neurogenesis in the olfactory epithelium. In: R. L. Doty (Ed.), *Handbook of Olfaction and Gustation*. New York: Wiley-Liss, pp. 135–158.

Maier, E.C., Saxena, A., Alsina, B., Bronner, M. E., Whitfield, T.T., 2014. Sensational placodes: Neurogenesis in the otic and olfactory systems. *Developmental Biology* **389**, 50–67.

Mainland, R.C., 1945. Absence of olfactory sensation. *Journal of Heredity* **36**, 143–144.

Malnic, B., Godfrey, P.A., Buck, L.B., 2004. The human olfactory receptor gene family. *Proceedings of the National Academy of Sciences of the United States of America* **101**, 2584–2589.

Maresh, A., Rodriguez, G.D., Whitman, M.C., Greer, C.A., 2008. Principles of glomerular organization in the human olfactory bulb – Implications for odor processing. *PLoS One* **3**, e2640.

McGaughy, J., Koene, R.A., Eichenbaum, H., Hasselmo, M.E., 2005. Cholinergic deafferentation of the entorhinal cortex in rats impairs encoding of novel but not familiar stimuli in a delayed nonmatch-to-sample task. *Journal of Neuroscience* **25**, 10273–10281.

Meisami, E., Bhatnagar, K.P., 1998. Structure and diversity in mammalian accessory olfactory bulb. *Microscopy Research and Technique* **43**, 476–499.

Menco, B.P., Morrison, E.E., 2003. Morphology of the mammalian olfactory epithelium: Form,

fine structure, function, and pathology. *Neurological Disease and Therapy* **T7**, 17–50.

Mirza, N., Kroger, H., Doty, R.L., 1997. Influence of age on the "nasal cycle." *Laryngoscope* **107**, 62–66.

Moran, D.T., Rowley, J.C., III, Jafek, B.W., Lovell, M.A., 1982. The fine structure of the olfactory mucosa in man. *Journal of Neurocytology* **11**, 721–746.

Moscovich, M., Munhoz, R.P., Teive, H.A., et al. 2012. Olfactory impairment in familial ataxias. *Journal of Neurology, Neurosurgery, & Psychiatry* **83**, 970–974.

Murphy, C., Schubert, C.R., Cruickshanks, K.J., et al. 2002. Prevalence of olfactory impairment in older adults. *JAMA* **288**, 2307–2312.

Nakashima, T., Kimmelman, C.P., Snow, J.B., Jr., 1984. Structure of human fetal and adult olfactory neuroepithelium. *Archives of Otolaryngology* **110**, 641–646.

Nilsen, K.B., Nicholas, A.K., Woods, C.G., et al. 2009. Two novel SCN9A mutations causing insensitivity to pain. *Pain* **143**, 155–158.

Nordin, S., Broman, D.A., Olofsson, J.K., Wulff, M., 2004. A longitudinal descriptive study of self-reported abnormal smell and taste perception in pregnant women. *Chemical Senses* **29**, 391–402.

O'Connor, S., Jacob, T.J., 2008. Neuropharmacology of the olfactory bulb. *Current Molecular Pharmacology* **1**, 181–190.

Ohm, T.G., Braak, H., 1987. Olfactory bulb changes in Alzheimer's disease. *Acta Neuropathologica* **73**, 365–369.

Olender, T., Lancet, D., Nebert, D.W., 2008. Update on the olfactory receptor (OR) gene superfamily. *Human Genomics.* **3**, 87–97.

Oliveira-Pinto, A.V., Santos, R.M., Coutinho, R.A., et al. 2014. Sexual dimorphism in the human olfactory bulb: Females have more neurons and glial cells than males. *PloS One*, **9**(11), p.e111733.

Paredes, M.F., Sorrells, S.F., Garcia-Verdugo, J. M., Alvarez-Buylla, A., 2016. Brain size and limits to adult neurogenesis. *Journal of Comparative Neurology* **524**, 646–664.

Patterson, P. M., Lauder, B. A., 1948. The incidence and probable inheritance of smell blindness; To normal Butyl mercaptan. *Journal of Heredity* **39**, 295–297.

Paxinos, G., Mai, J.K., 2004. *The Human Nervous System.* 2nd edition. San Diego & London: Elsevier Academic Press.

Pearson, R.C., Esiri, M.M., Hiorns, R.W., Wilcock, G.K., Powell, T.P., 1985. Anatomical correlates of the distribution of the pathological changes in the neocortex in Alzheimer disease. *Proceedings of the National Academy of Sciences* **82**, 4531–4534.

Pelosi, P., Maremmani, C., Muratorio, A., 1990. Purification of an odorant binding protein from human nasal mucosa. *NATO ASI Series H* **39**, 125–130.

Peterlin, Z., Firestein, S., Rogers, M.E., 2014. The state of the art of odorant receptor deorphanization: A report from the orphanage. *Journal of General Physiology* **143**, 527–542.

Pilpel, Y., Lancet, D., 1999. The variable and conserved interfaces of modeled olfactory receptor proteins. *Protein Science* **8**, 969–977.

Pinto, J.M., Wroblewski, K.E., Kern, D.W., Schumm, L.P., McClintock, M.K., 2014. Olfactory dysfunction predicts 5-year mortality in older adults. *PLoS One* **9**, e107541.

Plailly, J., Bensafi, M., Pachot-Clouard, M., et al. 2005. Involvement of right piriform cortex in olfactory familiarity judgments. *Neuroimage* **24**, 1032–1041.

Poellinger, A., Thomas, R., Lio, P., et al. 2001. Activation and habituation in olfaction: An fMRI study. *Neuroimage* **13**, 547–560.

Price, J.L., 2004. The Olfactory System. In: Paxinos G., Mai J.M. (Eds.), *The Human Nervous System,* 2nd edition. Academic Press, pp. 1198–1212.

Qureshy, A., Kawashima, R., Imran, M.B., et al. 2000. Functional mapping of human brain in olfactory processing: A PET study. *Journal of Neurophysiology* **84**, 1656–1666.

Rawson, N., 2000. Human olfaction. In: Finger T.E., Silver W.L., and Restrepo, D. (Eds.) *The Neurobiology of Taste and Smell.* Canada: Wiley-Liss.

Rawson, N.E., Brand, J.G., Cowart, B.J., et al. 1995. Functionally mature olfactory neurons from two anosmic patients with Kallmann syndrome. *Brain Research* **681**, 58–64.

Reyes, P.F., Deems, D.A., Suarez, M.G., 1993. Olfactory-related changes in Alzheimer's disease: A quantitative neuropathologic study. *Brain Research Bulletin* **32**, 1–5.

Rolls, E.T., 2004. The functions of the orbitofrontal cortex. *Brain and Cognition* **55**, 11–29.

Rolls, E.T., 2015. Neural integration of taste, smell, oral texture, and visual modalities. Figure 1, Chapter 46. In: Doty, R.L. (Ed.), *Handbook of Olfaction and Gustation.* Hoboken, NY: John Wiley & Sons.

Rosli, Y., Breckenridge, L.J., Smith, R.A., 1999. An ultrastructural study of age-related changes in mouse olfactory epithelium. *Journal of Electron Microscopy (Tokyo)* **48**, 77–84.

Rowley, J.C., III, Moran, D.T., Jafek, B.W., 1989. Peroxidase backfills suggest the mammalian olfactory epithelium contains a second morphologically distinct class of bipolar sensory neuron: The olfactory microvillar cell. *Brain Research* **502**, 387–400.

Royet, J.P., Hudry, J., Zald, D.H., et al. 2001. Functional neuroanatomy of different olfactory judgments. *Neuroimage* **13**, 506–519.

Royet, J.P., Plailly, J., Saive, A.L., Veyrac, A., Delon-Marin, C. 2013. The impact of expertise on olfaction. *Frontiers in Psychology* **4**, 938, DOI: 10.3389/fpsyg.2013.00928.

Saito, H., Chi, Q., Zhuang, H., Matsunami, H., Mainland, J.D., 2009. Odor coding by a Mammalian receptor repertoire. *Science Signaling* **2**, ra9.

Sanders, M.D., Warrington, E.K., Marshall, J., Wieskrantz, L., 1974. "Blindsight": Vision in a field defect. *Lancet* **1**, 707–708.

Savic, I., 2002. Imaging of brain activation by odorants in humans. *Current Opinion in Neurobiology* **12**, 455–461.

Sayek, I., 1970. The incidence of the inability to smell solutions of potassium cyanide in the rural health center of Ortabereket. *The Turkish Journal of Pediatrics* **12**, 72–75.

Schiffman, S.S., Gatlin, C.A., 1993. Sweeteners: State of knowledge review. *Neuroscience & Biobehavioral Reviews* **17**, 313–345.

Schwanzel-Fukuda, M., Pfaff, D.W., 2003. The structure and function of the nervus terminalis.

In: R.L. Doty (Ed.), *Handbook of Olfaction and Gustation*. New York: Marcel Dekker, pp. 1001–1026.

Sela, L., Sacher, Y., Serfaty, C., et al. 2009. Spared and impaired olfactory abilities after thalamic lesions. *Journal of Neuroscience* 29, 12059–12069.

Shepherd, G.M., 1972. Synaptic organization of the mammalian olfactory bulb. *Physiological Reviews* 52, 864–917.

Shepherd, G.M., Chen, W.R., Greer, C.A., 2004. Olfactory bulb. In: G. M. Shepherd (Ed.), *The Synaptic Organization of the Brain*. New York: Oxford University Press, pp. 165–216.

Singh, N., Grewal, M.S., Austin, J.H., 1970. Familial anosmia. *Archives of Neurology* 22, 40–44.

Slotnick, B.M., Kaneko, N., 1981. Role of the mediodorsal thalamic nucleus in olfactory discrimination learning in rats. *Science* 214, 91–92.

Smith, C.G., 1942. Age incident of atrophy of olfactory nerves in man. *Journal of Comparative Neurology* 77, 589–594.

Sobel, N., Prabhakaran, V., Hartley, C.A., et al. 1998. Odorant-induced and sniff-induced activation in the cerebellum of the human. *Journal of Neuroscience* 18, 8990–9001.

Sobel, N., Prabhakaran, V., Hartley, C.A., et al. 1999. Blind smell: Brain activation induced by an undetected air-borne chemical. *Brain* 122(2): 209–217.

Staubli, U., Fraser, D., Kessler, M., Lynch, G., 1986. Studies on retrograde and anterograde amnesia of olfactory memory after denervation of the hippocampus by entorhinal cortex lesions. *Behavioral and Neural Biology* 46, 432–444.

Stephani, C., Fernandez-Baca, V.G., Maciunas, R., Koubeissi, M., Luders, H.O., 2011. Functional neuroanatomy of the insular lobe. *Brain Structure and Function* 216, 137–149.

Swallow, B.L., Lindow, S.W., Aye, M., et al. 2005. Smell perception during early pregnancy: No evidence of an adaptive mechanism. *BJOG.* 112, 57–62.

Tabakow, P., Raisman, G., Fortuna, W., et al. 2014. Functional regeneration of supraspinal connections in a patient with transected spinal cord following transplantation of bulbar olfactory ensheathing cells with peripheral nerve bridging. *Cell Transplant* 23, 1631–1655.

Tham, W.W., Stevenson, R.J., Miller, L.A., 2009. The functional role of the medio dorsal thalamic nucleus in olfaction. *Brain Research Reviews* 62, 109–126.

Vanscheeuwijck, P.M., Teredesai, A., Terpstra, P.M., et al. 2002. Evaluation of the potential effects of ingredients added to cigarettes. Part 4: Subchronic inhalation toxicity. *Food and Chemical Toxicology.* 40, 113–131.

Weiskrantz, L., 1990. The Ferrier lecture, 1989. Outlooks for blindsight: Explicit methodologies for implicit processes. *Proceedings of the Royal Society of London B: Biological Sciences* 239, 247–278.

Weller, R.O., Djuanda, E., Yow, H.Y., Carare, R. O., 2009. Lymphatic drainage of the brain and the pathophysiology of neurological disease. *Acta Neuropathologica* 117, 1–14.

Wilson, R.S., Yu, L., Bennett, D.A., 2011. Odor identification and mortality in old age. *Chemical Senses* 36, 63–67.

Winston, J.S., Gottfried, J.A., Kilner, J.M., Dolan, R.J., 2005. Integrated neural representations of odor intensity and affective valence in human amygdala. *Journal of Neuroscience* 25, 8903–8907.

Wysocki, C.J., Beauchamp, G.K., 1984. Ability to smell androstenone is genetically determined. *Proceedings of the National Academy of Sciences* 81, 4899–4902.

Wysocki, C.J., Beauchamp, G.K., 1991. Individual differences in human olfaction. *Chemical Senses* 3, 353–373.

Wysocki, C.J., Dorries, K.M., Beauchamp, G.K., 1989. Ability to perceive androstenone can be acquired by ostensibly anosmic people. *Proceedings of the National Academy of Sciences* 86, 7976–7978.

Yamamoto, K., Ito, K., Yamaguchi, M., 1966. A family showing smell disturbances and tremor. Jinrui idengaku zasshi. *The Japanese Journal of Human Genetics* 11, 36–38.

Yee, K.K., Wysocki, C.J., 2001. Odorant exposure increases olfactory sensitivity: Olfactory epithelium is implicated. *Physiology & Behavior* 72, 705–711.

Yousem, D.M., Geckle, R.J., Bilker, W., McKeown, D.A., Doty, R.L., 1996. MR evaluation of patients with congenital hyposmia or anosmia. *American Journal of Roentgenology* **166**, 439–443.

Yousem, D.M., Geckle, R.J., Bilker, W.B., Doty, R.L., 1998. Olfactory bulb and tract and temporal lobe volumes: Normative data across decades. *Annals of the New York Academy of Sciences* **855**, 546–555.

Yousem, D.M., Oguz, K.K., Li, C., 2001. Imaging of the olfactory system. *Seminars in Ultrasound, CT and MRI* **22**(6), 456–472.

Yousem, D.M., Williams, S.C., Howard, R.O., et al. 1997. Functional MR imaging during odor stimulation: Preliminary data. *Radiology* **204**, 833–838.

Yu, G.Z., Kaba, H., Okutani, F., Takahashi, S., Higuchi, T., 1996. The olfactory bulb: A critical site of action for oxytocin in the induction of maternal behaviour in the rat. *Neuroscience* **72**, 1083 1088.

Zaborszky, L., Carlsen, J., Brashear, H.R., Heimer, L., 1986. Cholinergic and GABAergic afferents to the olfactory bulb in the rat with special emphasis on the projection neurons in the nucleus of the horizontal limb of the diagonal band. *Journal of Comparative Neurology* **243**, 488–509.

Zald, D.H., Pardo, J.V., 1997. Emotion, olfaction, and the human amygdala: Amygdala activation during aversive olfactory stimulation. *Proceedings of the National Academy of Sciences of the United States of America* **94**, 4119–4124.

Zatorre, R.J., Jones-Gotman, M., Evans, A.C., Meyer, E., 1992. Functional localization and lateralization of human olfactory cortex. *Nature* **360**, 339–340.

Zelano, C., Bensafi, M., Porter, J., et al. 2005. Attentional modulation in human primary olfactory cortex. *Nature Neuroscience* **8**, 114–120.

Zhang, W., Delay, R.J., 2007. Gonadotropin-releasing hormone modulates voltage-activated sodium current and odor responses in Necturus maculosus olfactory sensory neurons. *Journal of Neuroscience Research* **85**, 1656–1667.

Zobel, S., Hummel, T., Ilgner, J., et al. 2010. Involvement of the human ventrolateral thalamus in olfaction. *Journal of Neurology* **257**, 2037–2043.

Anatomy and Physiology of Gustation

Introduction

Relatively few clinicians test the sense of taste, i.e., the perception of sweet, sour, bitter, salty, and umami tastes, and, largely for this reason, quantitative clinical data on taste function are limited. This is in spite of estimates from the National Health and Nutrition Examination Survey (NHANES) that around 20.5 million Americans over the age of 40 years likely have chronic taste problems, a figure somewhat lower than that estimated for chronic olfactory problems (26.3 million) (Liu et al., 2016). In the NHANES study, ethnicity, heavy alcohol consumption, and a history cardiovascular disease were associated with a higher prevalence of disordered taste. Other studies suggest that taste disorders are much less prevalent than olfactory disorders. For example, in one study of 750 consecutive patients presenting with chemosensory complaints to the University of Pennsylvania Smell and Taste Center, whole-mouth taste deficits were found in only 4% compared to ~70% of those with olfactory deficits (Deems et al., 1991). Such disparities relative to the NHANES survey reflect, in part, the type of taste tests that were administered.

Apart from taste, it should be emphasized that smell, texture, and temperature all play a decisive role in determining whether a potential foodstuff is ingested or rejected (Scott & Mark, 1987). The human taste system has multiple receptors specifically tuned to detect healthy nutrients such as calorie-dense sugars, starches, and unhealthy toxins like bitter tasting alkaloids or sour tasting acids. Analogous to olfaction, learning plays a major role in establishing food preferences, even prenatally (see below), and these can be long lasting (Stein et al., 1996; Mennella, 2009; Stein et al., 2012).

In addition to differentiating nutrients from toxins, the gustatory system prepares the body for the arrival and utilization of foods via so-called cephalic phase reflexes (Berthoud et al., 1981). These include changes in the output and character of gastric, salivary, and pancreatic secretions, as well as cardiovascular and thermoregulatory responses. Some digestive and homeostatic responses readily become conditioned to external stimuli, as described classically by Pavlov for salivary secretions. In the infant, sucrose and other tastants that are inherently pleasant evoke ingestive responses that begin with rhythmic mouth movements and oral response patterns that end up in swallowing. In contrast, quinine and other aversive stimuli induce rejection responses, including gagging, drooling, and spitting. Since these responses also occur in decerebrate animals and anencephalic infants, they likely originate within the brainstem. Learned responses require connections with higher brain centers.

We describe below the gross and microscopic anatomy of the peripheral taste structures and how they function. This is followed by sections on cortical taste pathways and their function, and how taste appreciation are influenced in outwardly healthy people.

Anatomy and Distribution of Taste Buds

The oral taste receptors are found within taste buds, structures named by early anatomists because of their resemblance to a flower bud (Figure 2.1). These structures, which number on average around 7,500 in humans, are comprised of distinct clusters of epithelial cells on the tongue, soft palate, epiglottis, larynx, and oral pharynx. Each taste bud has an apical opening, termed the taste pore, through which stimuli enter from the oral epithelial surface into a lumen called the taste pit (Figure 2.2). As depicted in Figure 2.1, elongated cells are present within each test bud that have been classified, on the basis of histological appearance, as Types I (dark), II (light), and III (intermediate) (Murray, 1973). The basal and marginal cells are designated Types IV and V, respectively. The narrow neck of Type I cells interweaves around Type II cells. In contrast, Type II cells have a short, thick, and straight neck, and have a plasma membrane that is thicker than that of Type I cells (Murray & Murray, 1967). Their microvillae project deeper within the taste pit than those of Type I

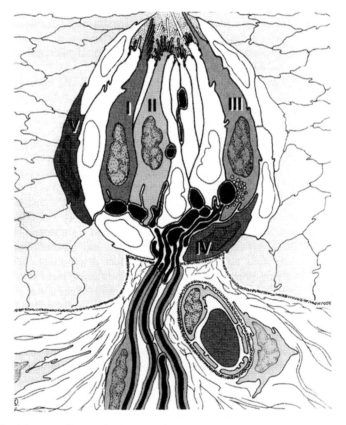

Figure 2.1 Idealized drawing of longitudinal section of mammalian taste bud. Cells of Type I, II, and III are elongated and form the sensory epithelium of the bud. These cells have different types of microvillae within the taste pit and may reach the taste pore. Type IV are basal cells and Type V are marginal cells. Synapses are most apparent at the bases of Type III cells. The connecting taste nerves have myelin sheaths. Reproduced with permission from Witt et al. (2003).

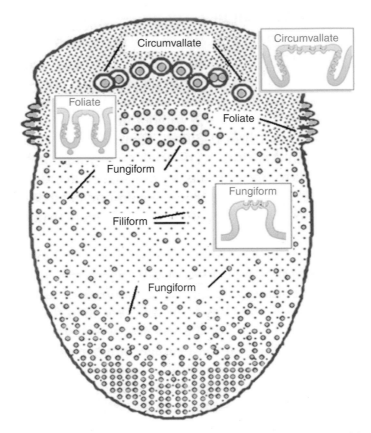

Figure 2.2 Schematic representation of the tongue demonstrating the relative distribution of the four main classes of papillae. Note that the fungiform papillae can vary considerably in size, and that they are typically most dense on the anterior and lateral regions of the tongue. Copyright © 2006 Richard L. Doty.

cells. Tight junctions seal the elements of the taste bud from the bud's pit, so only the tips of the cells are exposed to tastants.

Lingual taste buds are located mainly within protuberances termed papillae (Figure 2.2). Papillae vary considerably in size and shape, but can be classified into four major types. The largest, the *circumvallate* papillae (literally meaning a battlement surrounded by a moat) make up the "chevron" of the posterior tongue. Humans typically have, on average, nine of these papillae which, in extreme cases, can harbor more than a thousand taste buds apiece (Miller, 1988). The secretions around these large structures and in the valleys between them come largely from the intralingual salivary glands, termed von Ebner's glands. Each of the *fungiform* (mushroom-shaped) papilla, found primarily on the tip and sides of the tongue, contains an average of six to nine taste buds (Segovia et al., 2002). The leaf-like *foliate papillae* consist of ridges ("folia") and valleys along the postero-lateral margin adjacent to the third molar teeth. Although marked variation is evident, as is the case with taste buds in other oral regions, the average number of foliate buds is estimated at 1,300 per tongue. The relatively small and pointed *filiform papillae* (thread-like) contain no taste buds and serve to move and abrade food particles during swallowing. They are located mainly in the central

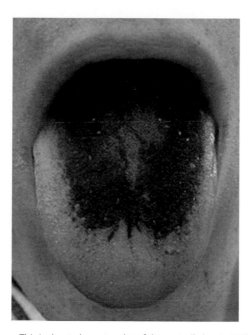

Figure 2.3 Black hairy tongue. This is due to hypertrophy of the centrally located filiform papillae which become yellow or black from contact with food or tobacco. Note the filiform papillae are not involved with taste; they help move and abrade food. From Wikipedia. (A black and white version of this figure will appear in some formats. For the color version, please refer to the plate section.)

region of the tongue (Figure 2.2). Hypertrophy of these papillae results in "hairy tongue," which becomes yellow or black from contact with food or tobacco (Figure 2.3).

Like epithelial cells in general, the elements of the taste bud, including its receptor cells and supporting structures, die and become replaced at various intervals by stem cells located near the base of the bud in the stratum germinativum (Beidler & Smallman, 1965). Although many taste bud cells, notably the receptor cells, turn over about every 10 days (Beidler & Smallman, 1965), some are long lived (Hamamichi et al., 2006), just like some olfactory receptor cells (Hinds et al., 1984). In contrast with olfactory receptor cells, taste receptor cells are not neurons as they synapse with the projection neurons that make up the taste nerves.

There are large individual differences in terms of sensitivity to sweet-, sour-, bitter-, and salty-tasting stimuli across tongue regions. Although some textbooks suggest that various tongue regions are individually responsible for each of the basic taste qualities, with sweet best at the front and bitter best at the back, this is an oversimplification and probably wrong. Recent work suggests that, in general, all tongue regions are responsive to sweet, sour, bitter, and salty sensations, although age-related changes are clearly evident – see Figure 2.4 (Doty et al., 2016). Note that in all cases, the front of the tongue is the most sensitive to the taste stimuli, as well as to low levels of electrical stimulation.

Depending upon its location, a given test bud is innervated by branches from one of four nerves (Figure 2.5). The first of these nerves, the *chorda tympani* nerve, supplies the anterior foliate papillae and the lingual fungiform papillae in the anterior two-thirds of the tongue. Centripetal taste signals in the chorda tympani join other elements of the facial nerve (CN VII) in the middle ear. Its cell bodies are in the geniculate ganglion, thus its signals traverse

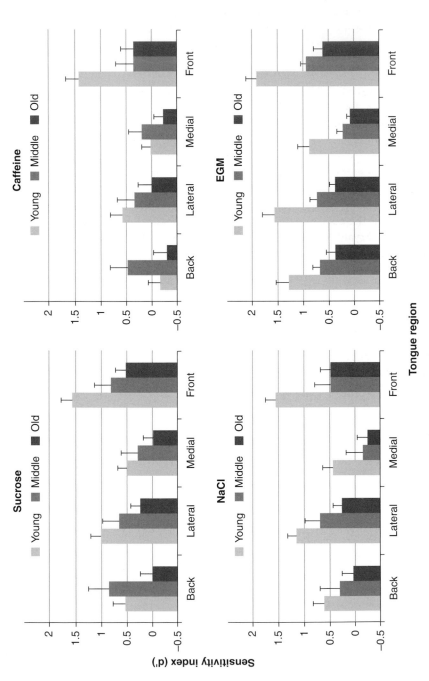

Figure 2.4 Criterion-free signal detection measures (d') of taste sensitivity to four types of taste stimuli as a function of age and tongue region. Larger numbers indicate greater sensitivity. Note the similarity of the relative pattern of sensitivity across tongue regions and the very large age-related decrements in such sensitivity on all tongue regions. From Doty et al. (2016).

the geniculate ganglion (without relay) to accompany the nervus intermedius within the internal auditory meatus and terminate in the rostral part of the solitary tract nucleus. The second nerve, the *greater (superficial) petrosal* nerve, supplies the taste buds of the soft palate. This nerve also has its cell bodies in the geniculate ganglion and transfers taste input via the nervus intermedius to the central portion of the solitary tract nucleus. The third nerve, a branch of the *glossopharyngeal nerve* (CN IX), innervates the posterior foliate and circumvallate papillae located in the posterior third of the tongue. The taste signals travel via the pharyngeal branches of CN IX to the inferior glossopharyngeal (petrosal) ganglion where its cell bodies lie. Its central limb enters the medulla and terminates in the middle sector of the solitary tract nucleus. The fourth nerve that supplies taste buds is the *vagus nerve* (CN X). This innervates the root of tongue and upper esophagus via its superior laryngeal branch. Centripetal signals ascend through the inferior (nodose) ganglion and terminate in the caudal part of the solitary tract nucleus (Figure 2.5).

The maxillary and mandibular branches of the trigeminal nerve (CN V) mediate touch, pain, and temperature throughout the nasal and oral epithelia, contributing to the sensation of flavor. For example, the coolness and fizziness of carbonated drinks largely depend on this nerve (Komai & Bryant, 1993; Bryant & Moore, 1995). Interestingly, there is now evidence that CN IX may extend fine branches into sectors of the lateral anterior tongue normally innervated by CN VII, although it is unknown whether these branches innervate taste buds (Doty et al., 2009). The multiple and spatially segregated neural innervations of the taste buds provide considerable spare capacity ("redundancy") in case of injury or damage to any one or subset of nerves. Conversely, the pathway for olfaction is more unitary and therefore more vulnerable.

Saliva. Before a tastant can be perceived, it must first be in liquid form. Saliva dissolves most taste substances and aids in their movement to and from the taste buds. It is secreted from multiple sources within the oral cavity, but most come from the parotid, submandibular, and sublingual glands (Bradley & Beidler, 2003). Dryness of the mouth, as seen in Sjögren's syndrome, is associated with impaired taste. Hypogeusia can also occur in cystic fibrosis, where saliva is more viscous. In addition to water, saliva contains electrolytes, diverse proteins, and peptides critical for lubrication and protection of the oral cavity. Amylase and lipase break down starch and fat for digestion. There is evidence that components of saliva may directly alter taste, as discussed in Chapter 5.

Growth Factors. Among the agents for repair and maintenance of the oral epithelium are Epidermal Growth Factor (EGF), Nerve Growth Factor (NGF), and Transforming Growth Factor-alpha (Bodner, 1991; Noguchi et al., 1991; Schultz et al., 1991; Humphreys-Beher et al., 1994). In rats, taste buds atrophy following removal of the submandibular and sub-lingual salivary glands – a process that can be prevented by adding EGF to their drinking water (Morris-Witman et al., 2000). Gene knockout experiments in mice show that the development of taste buds and somatic tongue innervation is heavily dependent on two other growth factors: Brain Derived Neurotrophic Factor (BDNF) and Neurotrophin 3 (NT3). If BDNF is not expressed there is a reduction in taste bud number and impaired taste perception. Absence of NT3 results in severe loss of somatosensory innervation to the mouth and tongue. Deficiency of BDNF may have relevance to familial dysautonomia (see Chapter 6) where there is loss of taste and marked reduction of taste bud number. Another growth factor, mischievously termed Sonic Hedgehog (Shh), is important for the develop-ment of taste buds. Shh is expressed exclusively in Type IV taste cells (Figure 2.1), the

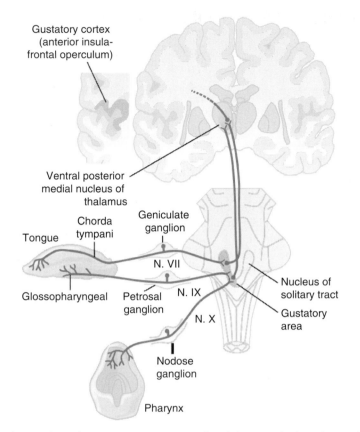

Figure 2.5 Distribution of cranial nerves to gustatory regions. Signals from taste buds on the anterior two-thirds of the tongue and soft palate travel with CN VII, through the geniculate ganglion, to the anterior portion of the solitary tract nucleus (STN). For clarity, fibers of the greater superficial petrosal nerve (CN VII) are not shown. Signals from foliate, circumvallate papillae, and pharyngeal taste buds pass through the petrosal ganglion of CN IX to the mid-section of STN. Taste buds on the epiglottis, larynx, and esophagus send their afferents through the nodose ganglion of CN X to the inferior sector of STN. Note: there is no relay in any of the three ganglia (geniculate, petrosal, and nodose). These ganglia contain the cell bodies of the respective bipolar gustatory neurones. See text for description of the central pathway. Reproduced and modified with permission from Buck & Bargmann (2013), Figure 32–13, Chapter 32.

undifferentiated basal cells and precursors of the three types of taste receptor cells. Deficiency of Shh has not been associated with any human gustatory disease so far, but such deficiency may be induced by immunotherapy. Thus, patients with advanced basal cell carcinoma who are treated with Vismodegib, a new hedgehog-pathway inhibitor, may have taste problems. This compound inhibits Shh-mediated stimulation of taste bud stem cells, resulting in reduced taste bud cell growth, dysgeusia, or ageusia in about 50 percent of cases (Basset-Seguin et al., 2015).

The vital moist environment of the mouth is controlled by the superior and inferior salivatory nuclei. These nuclei are located in the rostral part of the dorsal vagal nucleus in the medulla and their efferents travel in the chorda tympani and glossopharyngeal nerves. Thus, damage to the salivatory nuclei or their secretomotor fibers will create a dry mouth and impairment of taste.

Taste Receptors and Peripheral Neural Coding

Even though more than 2,000 genes have been associated with taste buds in primates (Hevezi et al., 2009), fewer than 50 taste receptor genes have been identified. The Type II cells harbor G-protein-coupled receptors (GPCRs) – T1R1, T1R2, and T1R3 – that mediate *sweet* and *umami* (monosodium glutamate-like) sensations, as well as a family of about 30 GPCRs that convey *bitter*. In most cases, the G proteins exert their effects through second messengers acting on specific intracellular targets such as kinases or basolateral channels. Several "bitter" receptors can be expressed on the same cell and respond to multiple bitter-tasting substances. Receptors that have been identified for taste are listed in Table 2.1. As shown, many tastants, such as quinine and caffeine, are agonists for numerous bitter receptors (bolded for these two compounds in Table 2.1). *Salty taste* is mediated mainly by Type I cells, which play a role in neurotransmitter clearance, ion redistribution, and transport (Chaudhari & Roper, 2010). Such sensations depend upon the entry of Na^+ ions into the cells via specialized membrane channels such as the amiloride-sensitive Na^+ channel. *Sour taste* is conveyed by hydrogen ions in Type III cells by passage through specialized proton channels (Chang et al., 2010). Members of the TRP and the KCNK two-pore potassium channel families are likely responsible for transduction of many CN V-mediated sensations (Gerhold & Bautista, 2009), although CO_2 sensing also occurs via carbonic anhydrase 4, a glycosylphosphatidyl-inositol-anchored enzyme found on taste cells sensitive to sour tastants (Chandrashekar et al., 2009).

In addition to the classic receptors described in Table 2.1, there is evidence that taste buds contain receptors specifically tuned to fatty substances such as long-chain fatty acids. In the past, it was assumed that fat was detected mainly via textural or olfactory cues, but a large behavioral and physiological literature has emerged suggesting this is not the case. For example, rodent taste cells have been identified that are activated by essential cis-polyunsaturated fatty acids and long-chain fatty acids (for reviews, see Khan & Besnard, 2009; Mattes, 2011; Steinert & Beglinger, 2011). Linoleic acid, a long-chain unsaturated free fatty acid, depolarizes mouse taste cells and elicits a robust intracellular calcium rise via activation of a G-protein-coupled receptor associated with the transient receptor potential channel type M5 (TRPM5) (Liu et al., 2011). Mice lacking TRPM5 channels were found to exhibit lessened sensitivity and no taste preferences for linoleic acid. These findings suggest that fatty acids activate some taste cells in a manner analogous to that of other G-protein-coupled receptors.

Coding of Taste Quality. Historically there have been two opposing theories for taste quality coding – the "across fiber" theory and "labeled line" theory. In the across fiber concept it is proposed that quality is coded by the pattern of activity across neurons. The labeled line scheme suggests that taste neuron types are specific coding channels for taste quality. Individual taste receptor cells probably do not code for just one class of tastants in humans, although they do in some invertebrates and fish. More likely they code for several stimulant classes (across fiber or broad tuning), although it is suspected they show preference for one class over another. There is probably some crude taste appreciation from bare lingual nerve endings located on the tongue surface and because of central convergence there are thalamic neurons that respond to both taste and touch signals. There is also considerable modification of afferent taste signals both peripherally and centrally.

Hitherto, most electrophysiological studies supported broad tuning of cortical taste neurons (Carleton et al., 2010) and this was the consensus view until subsequent work by

Table 2.1. Examples of receptors identified for transduction of major taste qualities. Bitter compounds known to bind three or more types of receptors are presented in bold in the right-hand column. Data from Chandrashekar et al. (2006) and Roudnitzky et al. (2011).

Taste quality	Receptor(s)	Tastant class	Examples of tastants
Sweet	$T_1R_2 + T_1R_3$	Sugars[*]	Glucose, Fructose, Maltose, Sucrose
		Artificial sweeteners	Aspartame[**], Acesulfame-K, Cyclamate[**], Saccharin
		d-Amino acids	D-Phenylalanine, D-Alanine, D-Serine (also some selective L-Amino acids)
		Sweet proteins[**]	Curculin, Monellin, Thaumatin
Bitter	T2R1		**Amarogentin, Arborescin, Cascarillin, Chloramphenicol**, Dextromethorphan, **Diphenylthiourea, Humulone isomers, Parthenolide, Picrotoxinin**, Sodium cyclamate, Sodium thiocyanate, Thiamine, **Yohimbine**
	T2R3		**Chloroquine**
	T2R4		**Amarogentin, Arborescin, Artemorin, Azathioprine, Campher, Colchicine, Dapsone, Denatonium, Diphenidol, Parthenolide**, Propylthiouracil, **Quassin, Quinine**
	T2R5[***]		Cyclohexamide
	T2R7		**Caffeine, Chloroquine**, Chlorpheniramine, **Chomolyn, Diphenidol**, Papaverine, **Quinine, Strychnine.**
	T2R8[***]		Denatonium, **Saccharin**
	T2R10		**Arborescin**, Arglabin, **Artemorin**, Brucine, **Campher, Caffeine, Cascarillin, Chloramphenicol, Chloroquine**, Chlorpheniramine, Coumarin, Cucurbitacin B, Cucurbitacin E, Cycloheximide, **Dapsone, Denatonium**, Dextromethorphan, **Diphenidol**, Erythromycin, Famotidine, Haloperidol, Papaverine, **Parthenolide, Picrotoxinin, Quassin, Quinine, Strychnine**, Thujon (-)-a-, **Yohimbine**
	T2R13		**Diphenidol**, Denatonium benzoate
	T2R14		**Arborescin**, Arglabin, Aristolochic acid, **Artemorin, Azathioprine**, Benzamide, Benzoin, **Campher, Caffeine**, Carisoprodol, **Cascarillin**, Chlorhexidine,

Gymnema tea has been used as an Indian folk-remedy for diabetes as it slows the absorption of sugar in the gut as well as reducing the sweet taste of food, thus acting as an appetite suppressant. Sodium salts and a mixture of lactoglobulin with phosphatidic acid can block the bitterness of caffeine or quinine. If table salt is sprinkled on pineapple segments or similar bitter-tasting fruit, the bitterness (from citric acid) is lessened. Blockers for *sour* and *umami* tastes are not known as yet. Umami taste is thought to be transduced by both receptors and apical ion channels (Figure 2.7). Synaptic neurotransmitters or neuromodulators released at synapses in taste buds have not yet been identified with certainty. The best evidence is for serotonin but adrenergic, cholinergic, and peptidergic transmitters are also involved. For example, subsets of taste receptor cells have been found to express such gut peptides as ghrelin, GLP-1, neuropeptide Y, and vasoactive intestinal peptide (VIP). The secretion patterns of some such peptides correlate with specific taste qualities, implying a role in taste quality coding (Geraedts & Munger, 2013).

Central Nervous System Taste Structures

Central Innervation

The central gustatory afferent path is complex with initial relays in the thalamus, unlike the olfactory pathways. The first segment of the taste with initial relays is *completely separate from the olfactory pathway* but the two modalities converge in the anterior insula. In this section we review the main aspects of the central taste pathway. The reader is referred elsewhere for more detailed accounts of this anatomy of both human and non-human species (Pritchard, 2012).

Brainstem and Thalamus

The three major taste nerves (CN VII, IX, and X) terminate in the nucleus of the solitary tract (NST), a segment of the medulla located between the spinal nucleus of CN V laterally and the dorsal nucleus of CN X medially (Figure 2.5). The NST is divided into 10 subnuclei in humans, of which at least one contains gustatory neurons – the interstitial nucleus (Pritchard, 2012). Topographically, the tongue is arranged in a rostro-caudal fashion within the NST with the tip of the tongue most superior. Thus, fibers from the chorda tympani (CN VII) terminate in the rostral section of the NST, those from CN IX go to the mid portion, and those from CN X end in the caudal part, although there is overlap. Importantly, neurons from CN VII, IX, and X also terminate within the marginal subdivision of the spinal trigeminal nucleus and in the dorsal horn as far as the third cervical segment. They are involved with common sensation in the oral cavity (Norgren, 1981) and permit integration of taste with somatosensory input from the mouth. The marginal zone of the spinal trigeminal nucleus projects to the NST, whose neurons in turn project directly and ipsilaterally via the central tegmental tract to the thalamus (Figure 2.5). This contrasts with the situation in rodents and other non-primates that have an indirect thalamic taste projection that relays within the parabrachial nucleus of the pons.

The superior and inferior salivatory nuclei are concerned with maintaining a moist environment within the oral cavity. These nuclei are situated in the rostral part of the dorsal vagal nucleus in the medulla and their secretomotor efferents travel in the chorda tympani and glossopharyngeal nerves. Damage to the salivatory nuclei or their secretomotor fibers will create a dry mouth that can impair taste in the absence of any problem with taste innervation.

Thalamus. The thalamic gustatory nucleus is the parvicellular portion of the ventroposteromedial nucleus (VPMpc), logically placed as a medial extension of that portion of VPM in receipt of the main somatosensory trigeminal input (Figure 2.5). When the human VPMpc is stimulated, the evoked taste sensations are ipsilateral (Lenz et al., 1997) but some clinical studies with MRI correlation suggest that the taste pathway crosses just before terminating in the thalamus (Onoda et al., 2012). Interestingly, damage to the left, but not the right, insula produces a *bilateral* deficit in the verbal recognition of tastes, implying that projections from both sides of the tongue may project through this site to the left hemisphere language area. In contrast, both right and left lesions influence the ipsilateral, but not contralateral, perceived intensity of taste on the tongue (Pritchard et al., 1999). To be resolved, this problem will require further clinic-pathological studies. The consensus view is that the human taste pathway is mostly ipsilateral right up to the cortical centers, but there is a degree of bilateral cortical representation.

Insular Cortex. As explained in Chapter 1, the insula has direct and reciprocal connections with the *frontal* (opercular, premotor, and medial regions), *temporal* (auditory cortex, polar, and superior temporal sulcus), *parietal* (primary and secondary sensory areas), and *caudolateral orbitofrontal cortices*. There are indirect connections with the hypothalamus, hippocampus, and striatum (see Figures 1.21 and 1.22.). Links to the amygdala, basal ganglia, and entorhinal cortex are also present, although there are very few taste-responsive cells in the amygdala (Pritchard & Scott, 2015). In humans, the insula consists of five to six oblique gyri (see Figures 1.20 and 1.21). Cortical regions that receive primary gustatory projections from the VPMpc are the granular neurons located within the anterior insula/inner operculum and the outer operculum of the frontal lobe, which lie just dorsal to the olfactory input (see Figure 1.21). This region probably constitutes the primary cortical taste center. It connects to the nearby dysgranular and agranular regions of the insula which comprise the secondary gustatory cortices. Projections extend from this zone to the lateral orbitofrontal cortex (OFC). The OFC joins the limbic system via projections to the amygdala and lateral hypothalamus (see Figure 2.9).

A detailed human *in vivo* study of taste localization within the insula was undertaken by Stephani et al. (2011) in five patients with intractable epilepsy. Multiple sites in the insula were stimulated during awake surgery. They found subjective reports of taste in the central regions of the insula (Figure 2.8), which is slightly posterior to the location suggested by Paxinos and Mai (2004), although their diagram of electrode positions indicate that only one anterior area was stimulated.

Other regions of the insula are likely involved in the perception of taste mixtures and the inter-sensory coding of "flavor," integrating taste sensations with those of touch and smell. Importantly, the insular cortex is involved in the development and maintenance of conditioned taste aversions and, in part, mediates phobias to novel tastes (Schier et al., 2014). It also plays a significant role in taste-related attentional mechanisms, increasing activity in exploratory tasks where attempts to detect a taste are performed when no tastant is present. The amygdala, in conjunction with the orbitofrontal cortex, plays a significant role in interpretation of tastes, which require memory processing and cognition, forming complex intermodal and hedonic associations necessary for the overall appreciation of flavor (Rolls, 2011).

On the basis of predominantly non-primate work, it is proposed that there is a dual pathway for taste: one for the common sensory aspect and another for the hedonic aspects (Sewards, 2004). Clearly, hedonic aspects of taste would involve the limbic system, but it is

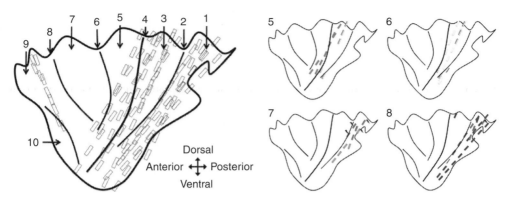

Figure 2.8 Localizations of those electrode contacts that evoked clinical responses with electrocortical stimulation. Left: Anatomical landmarks of the insula are indicated by numbers: 1 posterior long gyrus of the insula, 2 postcentral insular sulcus, 3 anterior long gyrus of the insula, 4 central insular sulcus, 5 Posterior short gyrus of the insula, 6 precentral insular sulcus, 7 middle short gyrus of the insula, 8 short insular sulcus, 9 anterior short gyrus of the insula, 10 accessory gyrus of the insula. Right: responses were grouped into gustatory (figure 5, blue): viscerosensory (figure 6, yellow), warmth or pain (figure 7, red), and general somatosensory (figure 8, green). Composite color bars indicate qualitatively inconsistent or ambiguous symptoms after stimulation. Reproduced with permission from Figures 4–8 in Stephani et al. (2011). (A black and white version of this figure will appear in some formats. For the colour version, please refer to the plate section.)

doubtful there is a direct projection from the nucleus of the solitary tract to the hypothalamus and amygdala. More likely, the pathway travels initially via the insular cortex.

Orbitofrontal Cortex and Taste

The orbitofrontal cortex (OFC) receives taste input from the primary taste cortex (insula), as well as visual information from the temporal lobe (V5, fusiform gyrus), piriform nucleus (for olfaction), and somatosensory cortex. The OFC in turn projects to the anterior cingulate cortex which is a tertiary taste cortical area (Figure 2.9) as suggested by Rolls and Grabenhorst, 2008). PET and fMRI studies suggest that neurons, primarily in the caudal and lateral orbitofrontal cortex, are activated by taste and are separate from olfactory responsive cells (Figure 2.10) (Small & Prescott, 2005). According to Rolls (2011), olfactory–taste and visual–taste association learning takes place in the human orbitofrontal cortex to build representations of flavor. In turn this allows a decision to be made about palatability of ingested food.

Taste is considered to be a "primary reinforcer," i.e., a stimulus that is innately rewarding or punishing without learning. Thus, initial exposure in the newborn to a sweet taste will be accepted, whereas the first time that a bitter taste is encountered it will be rejected (Rolls & Grabenhorst, 2008). Conversely, olfaction is not a primary reinforcer; any reward/punishment behavior has to be acquired (Rolls, 2011). It is proposed that genes coding for taste receptors are connected by labeled lines to appropriate brain areas where they are represented according to their reward value (Rolls & Grabenhorst, 2008). These authors also suggested that, in the primate taste system, the first stage at which this occurs is in the OFC.

Factors That Influence Taste in Normal People

Considerable variation in taste sensitivity is present in healthy people and this relates to multiple influences such as age, gender, past stimulus familiarity, smoking, and genetic differences in the number of receptors, ion channels, and their afferent neurons. Experience

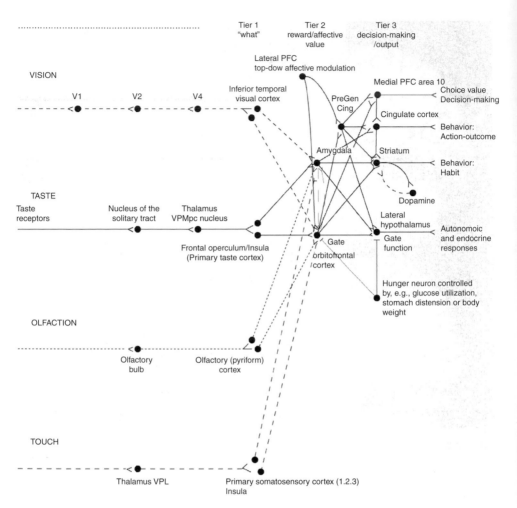

Figure 2.9 Diagram showing some of the gustatory, olfactory, visual, and somatosensory pathways to the orbitofrontal cortex, and some of the outputs of the orbitofrontal cortex, in primates. The secondary taste cortex and the secondary olfactory cortex are within the orbitofrontal cortex. V1 – primary visual cortex. V4 – visual cortical area. PreGen Cing – pregenual cingulate cortex. "Gate" refers to the finding that inputs such as the taste, smell, and sight of food in some brain regions only produce effects when hunger is present (Rolls & Grabenhorst, 2008). **Tier 1**: the column of brain regions including and below the inferior temporal visual cortex represents brain regions in which a "what" stimulus is present in the neuronal representation, but not its reward or affective value which are represented in the next tier of brain regions (**Tier 2**), the orbitofrontal cortex and amygdala, and in the anterior cingulate cortex. In **Tier 3** areas beyond these such as medial prefrontal cortex area 10, choices or decisions about reward value are taken. Top-down control of affective response systems by cognition and by selective attention from the dorsolateral prefrontal cortex is also indicated. Medial PFC area 10 – medial prefrontal cortex area 10; VPMpc – ventralposteromedial thalamic nucleus. Reproduced with permission, from Rolls (2015), Figure 1, Chapter 46.

is critical, since taste thresholds to many chemicals may improve after repeated exposure, a phenomenon seen in other sensory systems, e.g., olfactory and somatosensory. Although there is considerable variability among subjects, the threshold for stimulation of sour taste by hydrochloric acid is on average 0.0009M; for salt by sodium chloride 0.01M; for sweet by sucrose 0.01M; and for bitter by quinine 0.000008M. Thus the threshold for bitter is much

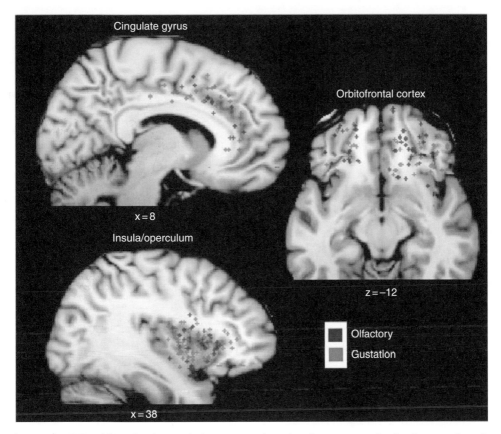

Figure 2.10 PET and fMRI plots from multiple sources to show that chemosensory stimuli activate a variety of regions within the insula, anterior cingulate, and orbitofrontal cortex, and that most respond to both gustatory and olfactory stimulation. Taste stimuli tend to activate the caudal and lateral orbitofrontal cortex; whereas olfactory stimuli do not (especially in the right hemisphere). In contrast, olfactory stimuli activate the most ventral insular region, which is continuous with the primary olfactory cortex; whereas gustatory stimuli do not. Reproduced with permission from Small & Prescott (2005). (A black and white version of this figure will appear in some formats. For the color version, please refer to the plate section.)

lower and this has probably developed for protective purposes because most poisonous substances have a bitter taste. Not all bitter or sour compounds have the same intensity and the relative degree of bitterness etc. can be measured. The threshold for a given tastant varies according to its quality (bitter, sour etc.) as well as the nature of the chemical itself (Table 2.2).

Specific Ageusia

Some call this "taste blindness." It refers to the inherited impairment of taste detection for certain chemicals in the presence of preserved taste for other compounds. This is the taste equivalent of specific anosmia and color blindness. In contrast to specific anosmias, there have been far fewer reports of specific ageusias in humans. Despite this, inherited ageusia is of major interest because of the prospect that genetic studies might lead to the identification of further specific taste receptors and their associated genes. The best documented example of largely genetically determined taste sensitivity is the relative ability to detect phenyl thiocarbamide

Table 2.2. Relative taste indices (the reciprocal of thresholds) of various substances. The intensities of the four primary sensations of taste are referred respectively to the intensities of taste of hydrochloric acid, quinine, sucrose, and sodium chloride, each of which is considered to have a taste index of 1. From Guyton & Hall (1996), Chapter 53.

Sour substances	Index	Bitter substances	Index	Sweet substances	Index	Salty substances	Index
Hydrochloric acid	1	Quinine	1	Sucrose	1	NaCl	1
Formic acid	1.1	Brucine	11	1-Propoxy-2-amino-4-nitrobenzene	5000	NaF	2
Chloracetic acid	0.9	Strychnine	3.1	Saccharin	675	CaCl$_2$	1
Acetyllactic acid	0.85	Nicotine	1.3	Chloroform	40	NaBr	0.4
Lactic acid	0.85	Phenylthiourea	0.9	Fructose	1.7	NaI	0.35
Tartaric acid	0.7	Caffeine	0.4	Alanine	1.3	LiCl	0.4
Malic acid	0.6	Veratrine	0.2	Glucose	0.8	NH$_4$Cl	2.5
Potassium H tartrate	0.58	Pilocarpine	0.16	Maltose	0.45	KCl	0.6
Acetic acid	0.55	Atropine	0.13	Galactose	0.32		
Citric acid	0.46	Cocaine	0.02	Lactose	0.3		
Carbonic acid	0.06	Morphine	0.02				

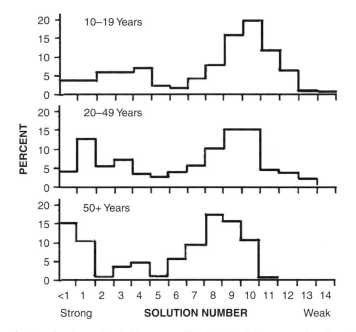

Figure 2.11 Distribution of PTC taste thresholds measured by the Harris Kalmus procedure. N = 441 men. Modified from Harris & Kalmus (1949).

(PTC), a bitter agent and one of the most widely studied inherited traits in humans (Wooding, 2006). The serendipitous discovery (Fox, 1931) that some people can taste PTC and others gave rise to a basic classification into PTC "tasters" and "non-tasters." While this simple division served an important role, it is an over-simplification. There is, in fact, a wide spectrum of sensitivities to these and related compounds, as shown in Figure 2.11, where the influences of age and the bimodal nature of PTC thresholds are apparent. Like PTC, age-related changes of 6-n-propylthiouracil (PROP) bitter sensitivity have been noted for some T2R38 haplotype combinations, particularly heterozygotes (Mennella et al., 2010). To address this issue further, some investigators have subdivided respondents into "non-tasters," "medium tasters," and "super-tasters" (Hayes et al., 2008).

Although a simple autosomal recessive model was initially proposed to explain the PTC taster/non-taster dichotomy (Snyder, 1931), subsequent work revealed more complexity (Olson et al., 1989; Reddy & Rao, 1989). In 1993, mutations in the T2R38 taste receptor gene (Table 2.1) on chromosome 7q were associated with the ability to taste PTC (Kim et al., 2003). Five worldwide haplotypes (i.e., a group of genes on one chromosome) have since been identified that account for 55–85 percent of the variance in PTC sensitivity (Kim & Drayna, 2005). However, these polymorphisms (normal variants) alone do not fully explain the range of sensitivities exhibited to PTC, PROP, and related bitter tastants. The multiplicity of receptor genes identified for bitter tasting agents likely contributes to this diversity (Table 2.1) (Reed et al., 1999; Bufe et al., 2005). Furthermore, PTC and PROP tasters, particularly those at the high end of the sensitivity distribution, so called "supertasters," have on average, more fungiform papillae than non-tasters (Bartoshuk et al., 1994). Individuals sensitive to PROP are also more sensitive to the bitterness or burning of caffeine, potassium chloride, capsaicin (chili, pepper) saccharine, and the sweet taste of saccharine and sucrose (Hayes et al., 2008). Importantly, those with most sensitivity to PROP may be more sensitive to the tactile properties of some taste stimuli, thereby influencing more than taste per se (Green & George, 2004).

There is marked ethnic variability in PTC sensitivity. Employing the taster/non-taster concept, non-tasters are reportedly more frequently represented in persons of northern European ancestry (about 30%), followed by Asians (about 10%) and Afro-Caribbeans (about 3%) (Sato et al., 1997; Kim & Drayna, 2005). PTC non-tasters are insensitive to other bitter compounds, including PROP, an agent used medically as a thyroid hormone blocker. Inadvertently, non-tasters may consume isothiocyanates and goitrins, which are bitter tasting compounds found in cabbage, broccoli, or sprouts, and develop a thyroid goiter. Conversely, those who *are* able to taste PTC and PROP have a lower incidence of thyroid deficiency. In Ecuadorian Andean communities where goiter is endemic, PTC tasters avoid maize that contains a bitter goitrogen and do not develop goiters (Greene, 1974). However, these individuals are more susceptible to malaria, unlike their non-tasting counterparts, thus conferring a survival advantage to the non-tasters.

In a classic study, Fischer et al. (1961) found a statistically significant inverse correlation between the percentage of foods disliked on a 118-item food questionnaire and taste thresholds for both quinine and PROP. Taste thresholds for sucrose, sodium chloride, and hydrochloric acid were not related to the reported dislikes.

Conditioned Taste Aversions

The decision to consume a particular food depends on the ability to discriminate various tastants. Animals and humans can be taught to avoid certain flavors by pairing the taste with gastrointestinal malaise, such as that experimentally induced by endotoxins (Grigoleit et al., 2012). Following such learning, the degree to which aversion applies to other stimuli can indicate the taste similarity of various tastants. For example, an animal taught to avoid sucrose, without conditioning, will also avoid fructose, glucose, and saccharine. Some reactions are thought to be innate, i.e., not requiring conditioning. Thus premature babies show pleasure with sweet tastes and dislike for bitter tastes in the absence of prior experience. It is presumed this response is hard-wired into the nervous system for protection in that many harmful substances are bitter. Beyond this initial predisposition, preferences can be strengthened or weakened by repeated exposure. On first sampling, chili is found unpleasant and burning in quality. Through repeated exposure some people come to like it despite the fact that it still produces burning sensations. The palatability of a compound may vary according to satiety. For example, when a sweet substance is eaten it is initially reported pleasant but on multiple repeated exposure, as long as the sweet substance is swallowed, the taste becomes unpleasant. Conditioning may play a role in the weight loss associated with anorexia nervosa, cancer, or depression. One theory proposes that in anorexia nervosa increased production of estrogen at puberty causes food aversion. Indeed, there is evidence from animals that estrogens suppress appetite. Taste preferences and aversions probably relate to plastic changes in taste responsive cells of the OFC and their connections with the amygdala and visual cortex (see Figure 2.9).

Age

The ability to taste is well developed in the fetus and becomes increasingly sophisticated as the individual matures. As shown in Figure 2.4, decrements in taste function occur across time that are noticeable even in middle age (Doty et al., 2016). Such reductions are most evident when small regions of the tongue are evaluated.

Taste in the Fetus and Premature Infants. Taste papillae can be identified in the human fetus by six to seven weeks of gestation, and as early as 8 weeks, synapses to nerve fibers by early taste bud primordia can be identified. The circumvallate papillae generally develop earlier than the fungiform papillae. By 10 to 14 weeks, taste pores are visible, although most pores develop around 14–15 weeks (Witt & Reutter, 1997). The human fetus can chew, swallow, and even regurgitate during the second half of pregnancy. At term, the fetus swallows 70 to 260 ml of amniotic fluid/kilogram of body weight each day (Pritchard, 1965). Such swallowing plays an important role in the development of the gastrointestinal tract and somatic growth. It is probably the only mechanism for fetal resorption of the principal amniotic fluid electrolytes (Ross & Nijland, 1997).

Tastants introduced into the amniotic fluid alter the frequency of swallowing in the fetus and taste-induced behavioral responses are present in premature infants six to nine months of gestational age. These include facial expressions associated with pleasure or displeasure (Steiner, 1974). Reflex salivation and, in some cases, retching occurs when a drop of lemon juice is placed in the mouth of premature infants (Eckstein, 1927). Sucking frequency is increased by sucrose and decreased by low concentrations of quinine. Salt induces variable responses. In one study, for example, 0.9 percent NaCl was presented orally to 20 premature infants. While most would not ingest the solution, four (20 percent) readily did so (Martin due Pan, 1955).

Studies of facial reactions to tastants indicate that newborn babies can clearly perceive sweet-, sour-, bitter-, salty-, and umami-tasting stimuli. Automatic lip licking and rhythmic sucking, followed by relaxation of the facial muscles and smiling responses, occur in response to sweet- and umami-tasting substances. In contrast, bitter-tasting agents produce mouth corner depression, eye closure, flat tongue protrusions, head turning and shaking, and drooling (Steiner, 1979). Like premature infants, a number of neonates either reject or show indifference to moderate concentrations of sodium chloride (0.1 M–0.2 M). By four months of age, such salt concentrations are generally preferred to water (Beauchamp et al., 1986). Negative responsiveness to salt ingestion appears to develop between 4 and 24 months of age.

Although babies become exposed to more varied taste experiences during the neonatal period than in utero, pre-natal factors, such as pregnancy-related electrolyte imbalances and dehydration of the mother, can influence post-natal responses to tastes and flavors (Leshem, 1998). In one study, 4-month-old babies of mothers who had experienced varying degrees of vomiting during pregnancy more readily accepted 0.1 and 0.2 M solutions of NaCl than did babies of mothers who had no vomiting (Crystal & Bernstein, 1995). Such effects appear to be long lasting. Thus, in another study, adolescents whose mothers had experienced marked morning sickness exhibited, relative to adolescents whose mothers had no such experiences, (a) greater self-reported use of salt, (b) greater intake of salt in the laboratory, and (c) stronger preferences for salty snack food (Leshem, 1998).

During the neonatal period babies become exposed to a wide range of flavors and reinforcements that can have long-lasting effects on their ingestion habits and preferences. Suckling responses and the amount of milk that is ingested can be influenced by the taste of the mother's milk, which in turn can be influenced by the mother's diet. Such influences are multimodal and largely dependent upon odor-related cues. For example, a garlic-like smell is present in milk from lactating mothers who eat garlic (Mennella et al., 1995). Breast-feeding infants with no prior experience of such milk spend more time suckling than infants without such exposure (Mennella & Beauchamp, 1993), conceivably reflecting the novelty of the flavor.

Taste in Children. Although children have similar numbers of taste buds as neonates, the size and distribution of the papillae and associated taste buds only reach adult levels in the late teenage years. By 8–10 years, the anterior tongue attains adult size. The posterior tongue, which contains fewer fungiform papillae, continues to grow until 15 to 16 years (Temple et al., 2002). Eight- to nine-year-old boys have higher densities of both taste papillae and taste pores than do adult males, although, on average, both groups have the same number of taste pores per papilla. The papillae of boys are rounder and smaller than those of men, whose papillae take on the characteristic mushroom-like shape (Temple et al., 2002).

Children are more sensitive than adults when small regions of the tongue are tested, presumably because receptor density is greater in the regions tested (Segovia et al., 2002). Such differences are rarely observed for whole-mouth tests. Indeed, whole-mouth sucrose thresholds may be somewhat elevated in 3- to 6-year-old children (Visser et al., 2000). One study compared the whole-mouth detection thresholds for sucrose, sodium chloride, citric acid and caffeine of 68 children aged 6–8 years to those of 61 young adults (James et al., 1997). The thresholds of the girls were the same as those of the adults of both sexes. However, the thresholds of the boys were higher for all stimuli than those of the adults, save caffeine, where thresholds were similar to those of men but worse than those of women. The boys were less sensitive than the girls to sucrose and sodium chloride. These findings led the authors to conclude that "the taste sensitivity of 8–9-year old males, although well developed, has not fully matured" (page 193).

Cultural and experiential factors influence food preferences of children and teenagers. Novel foods become acceptable upon repeated exposure, even when initially distasteful. In one study, four- to five-year-olds were repeatedly exposed over several weeks to either plain tofu or tofu made sweet or salty (Sullivan & Birch, 1990). When tested months later, the children preferred the tofu to which they were exposed. The preference did not generalize to other foods of similar color and texture (e.g., ricotta) that possessed similar sweetness or saltiness. In first- and second-generation Chinese adolescent immigrant boys to Canada (Hrboticky & Krondl, 1984), the second-generation boys gave higher hedonic flavor and prestige ratings to the Canadian deserts, snack, and fast foods, and discriminated better among nutrient rich and poor foods. Culture also influences cognitive and inter-sensory associations, such as those between taste and vision. For example, the majority of British subjects associated brown-colored drinks with "cola" flavor and none with "grape" flavor. In contrast, approximately half of the Taiwanese subjects connected brown-colored drinks with grape flavor and none with cola flavor (Shankar et al., 2010).

Taste in Adults. Apart from modification by experience and context, taste in early adulthood is similar to that of the teenage years. As in children, taste sensitivity is correlated with the number of receptors that are stimulated. On the anterior tongue, threshold and suprathreshold taste measurements correlate with the number of fungiform papillae and taste buds (Smith, 1971; Miller & Reedy, Jr., 1990; Zuniga et al., 1993; Doty et al., 2001; Miller et al., 2002; Segovia et al., 2002).

Taste function declines in later life, particularly after the age of 65 years, just like olfaction, but at a slower pace. Age-related deficits have been noted for a broad array of tastants, including caffeine, citric acid, hydrochloric acid, magnesium sulfate, propylthiourea, quinine, sodium chloride, sucrose, tartaric acid, and a large number of amino acids (Schiffman et al.,

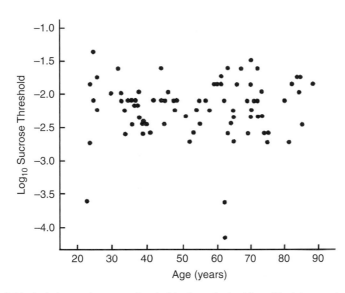

Figure 2.12 Individual whole-mouth sucrose threshold values obtained from 81 adult normal subjects using the 2-down, 1-up single staircase procedure. Modified from Weiffenbach et al. (1982).

1979; Bartoshuk et al., 1986; Matsuda & Doty, 1995; Stevens et al., 1995; Mojet et al., 2001). Sweet tastes are less ravaged by age than salt, bitter, and sour (Weiffenbach et al., 1986), conceivably reflecting the number of afferent fibers involved in their transduction.

Age-related deficits are not so obvious when measured by whole-mouth techniques compared to regional testing and they are greater for most tastants other than sweet (Baker et al., 1983). This change may be detected by electrogustometry, a process that measures the threshold to a weak DC signal applied to the tongue (Chapter 4) (Coates, 1974; Grant et al., 1987). Examples of whole mouth changes in the elderly are shown for sucrose and NaCl in Figures 2.12 and 2.13, respectively. Note the clear age-related effect for NaCl, but not for sucrose. When small regions of the tongue are tested, as shown in Figure 2.14, marked decrements with advancing years are apparent, in this case to NaCl. The R-index depicted in Figure 2.14 is a non-parametric signal detection sensitivity measure, derived from hit and false alarm rates established for each subject at a particular tongue location (Brown, 1974). These data are derived from 120 test trials, namely 60 of distilled water and 20 each of the three NaCl concentrations, with water rinses between stimulus presentations (Matsuda & Doty, 1995).

Several factors are associated with taste impairment in the elderly, including: (1) fewer taste buds, (2) decreased number of functioning receptors within taste buds, (3) variation in responsivity of taste nerves, (4) alterations in CNS pathways, and (5) changes in salivary constituents and volume (Doty, 2001). Thus, Mochizuki (1939) reported that the mean number of buds per circumvallate papilla in healthy people was 248 in those aged 0–20 years, 206 at 20–70 years, falling to just 88 in those aged 74–85 years. In a similar study, 242 buds were found in the circumvallate papillae of individuals aged 0–20 years, 196 at 21–60 years, and just 116 in people aged 61–80 years (Arey et al., 1935). Furthermore, a statistically significant age-related decrement in taste bud numbers within the epiglottis is reported (Kano et al., 2007).

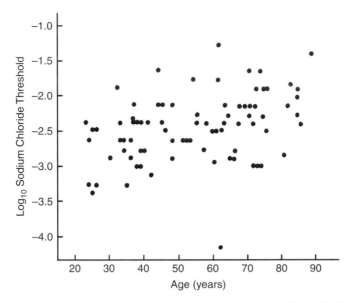

Figure 2.13 Individual whole-mouth NaCl threshold values obtained from 81 adult normal subjects using the 2-down, 1-up single staircase procedure. Modified from Weiffenbach et al. (1982).

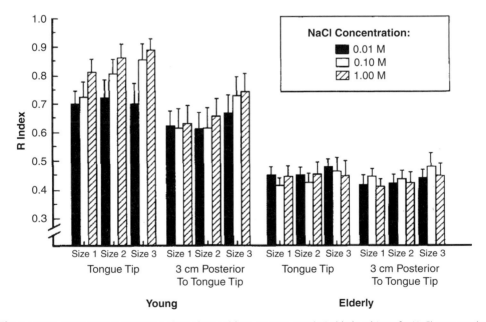

Figure 2.14 Mean (±SEM) sensitivity values obtained from 12 young and 12 elderly subjects for NaCl presented to two tongue regions for three stimulation areas (12.5, 25, and 50 mm²) and three concentrations (0.01 M, 0.10 M & 1.00 M). Sensitivity was measured by a non-parametric signal detection analysis sensitivity measure derived from hit and false alarm rates (R-index). Note that the sensitivity of the older subjects was markedly reduced in all tongue regions and for all stimulus areas assessed. Unlike the young subjects, greater sensitivity was not seen on the tongue tip than on a more posterior tongue site. Reproduced from Matsuda & Doty (1995).

Unlike circumvallate papillae, the number of taste buds within *fungiform* papillae appears not to decline with age. At autopsy, there was no age or sex difference in taste bud numbers in 182 fungiform papillae from 22 persons aged 2 to 90 years (Arvidson, 1979). Miller (1988) similarly found no statistically meaningful connection between age and taste bud densities on either the tip or the mid-region of tongues from young adults (22–36 years, $n = 5$), middle-aged adults (50–63 years, $n = 7$), and old adults (70–90 years, $n = 6$), although the sample sizes were small and there was marked variability in taste bud number between subjects. One group studied older Fischer 344 rats and found decreased electrophysiological responses to some salts, acids, and sugars from the chorda tympani nerves (McBride & Mistretta, 1986), but they saw no meaningful change in taste bud numbers within the fungiform papillae (Mistretta & Oakley, 1986), thus supporting the human findings described above.

Gender

Numerous studies confirm that men and women differ in terms of taste preferences and their ability to detect or resolve slight differences in tastant concentration, whether at threshold or suprathreshold level (for review of the early literature, see Doty, 1978). Any observed sex differences usually relate to non-sweet-tasting agents, as in the case of aging. When whole-mouth testing is performed, sex differences are often not observed, except for the sour-tasting citric acid (Figure 2.15). As shown, women have lower whole-mouth thresholds than men to this agent, although there is considerable overlap.

The degree of gender-related taste differences depends upon the tongue region evaluated (Figure 2.16), as in the case of aging. Using a set of 8 mm diameter filter papers, Sato et al., (2002) determined detection thresholds for stimuli representing sweet, sour, bitter, and salt.

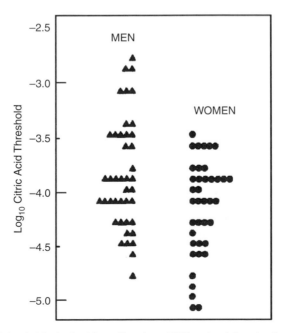

Figure 2.15 Citric acid thresholds obtained from 42 male and 39 female adults using the 2-down, 1-up single staircase procedure. Modified from Weiffenbach et al. (1982).

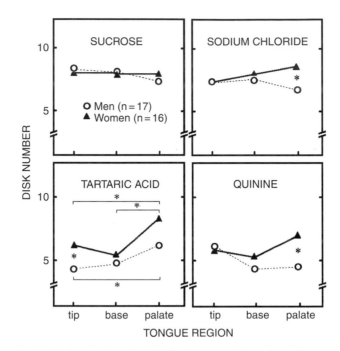

Figure 2.16 Mean threshold values for 17 male and 16 female non-smokers at four different tongue locations. The stimuli were presented on 8 mm filter paper disks placed on the extended tongue. Concentrations represent binary dilution steps, such that 10 = a 10% solution for sucrose, a 5% solution for NaCl, a 2% solution for tartaric acid, and 0.25% solution for quinine. * indicates statistically significant differences at the 0.05 α level with Bonferroni correction. Modified from Sato et al. (2002).

Women exhibited significantly lower thresholds than men on the soft palate for sodium chloride (salt) and quinine (bitter) and on the tip of the tongue for sour (tartaric acid). Both sexes were less sensitive to sour on the soft palate than on the tip, presumably because the soft palate contains fewer taste buds.

It is not well established how much sex differences in sensitivity to taste quality influence food likings, although men tend to favor more bitter tasting foods and have stronger preferences for sweet stimuli than women. Women, in turn, report larger numbers of food aversions than men.

Cigarette Smoking

There is a large and somewhat conflicting literature on the influences of smoking on taste perception. In general, smoking raises electrogustometric thresholds (Coates, 1974; Grant et al., 1987). Additionally, smoking impairs common sensation over the tongue (Said et al., 2010). Some find that whole-mouth smoking-related deficits are restricted to bitter or salty tastants (Perrin et al., 1961; Suliburska et al., 2004), whereas others do not (Pepino & Mennella, 2007). As expected, whole-mouth procedures reveal less smoking-related changes on thresholds for sweet than for non-sweet stimuli. In general, whole-mouth procedures are less sensitive to smoking effects than regional evaluation. Conversely, one investigation of smokers compared to never-smokers documented a modest elevation of whole-mouth thresholds for sucrose (Figure 2.17), which correlated with lifetime smoking dose measured in pack years (Figure 2.18).

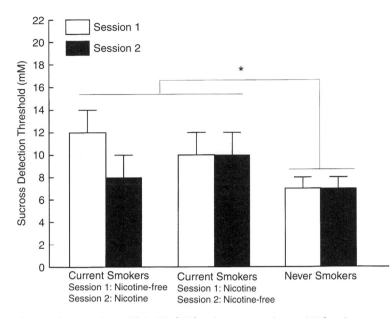

Figure 2.17 Sucrose detection thresholds (mM) of 27 female current smokers and 22 female never-smokers during first (white bar) and second (black bar) test session. Fourteen of the current smokers smoked nicotine-free cigarettes 30 minutes prior to measuring detection thresholds during Session 1 and nicotine cigarettes during Session 2. The order was reversed for the remaining 13 smokers. The group of never-smokers did not smoke and procedures were identical during Sessions 1 and 2. Data are presented as means (±SEM). * signifies current smokers significantly different from never smokers at p < 0.05 level. From Pepino & Mennella (2007).

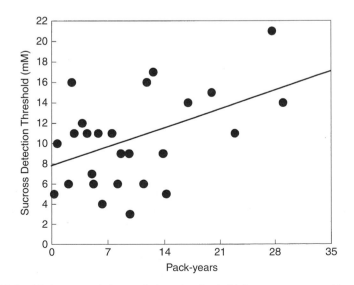

Figure 2.18 Relationship between whole-mouth detection thresholds for sucrose measured by a staircase procedure and cigarette smoking in 27 female current smokers. r = 0.46, p < 0.02. From Pepino & Mennella (2007).

Summary

In this chapter we provided an overview of the basic anatomy and physiology of the human gustatory system. Notable advances have occurred in the discovery of taste receptors that mediate the basic taste qualities of sweet, sour, bitter, salt, and umami, as well as fatty acids and other lipids that fall outside the four classic taste qualities. Several genes are now known to be involved directly in the development of taste papillae or indirectly with taste perception. Reflecting the sense of smell, the ability to taste is influenced by age, gender, and smoking behavior.

References

Arey, L.B., Tremaine, M.J., Monzingo, F.L.,1935. The numerical and topographical relations of taste buds to human circumvallate papillae throughout the life span. *Anatomical Record* **64**, 9–25.

Arvidson, K., 1979. Location and variation in number of taste buds in human fungiform papillae. *Scandinavian Journal of Dental Research* **87**, 435–442.

Baker, K.A., Didcock, E.A., Kemm, J.R., Patrick, J.M., 1983. Effect of age, sex and illness on salt taste detection thresholds. *Age Ageing* **12**, 159–165.

Bartoshuk, L.M., Duffy, V.B., Miller, I.J., 1994. PTC/PROP tasting: anatomy, psychophysics, and sex effects. *Physiology & Behavior* **56**, 1165–1171.

Bartoshuk, L.M., Rifkin, B., Marks, L.E., Bars, P., 1986. Taste and aging. *Journal of Gerontology* **41**, 51–57.

Basset-Seguin N., Hauschild A., Grob J.J., et al. 2015. Vismodegib in patients with advanced basal cell carcinoma (STEVIE): a pre-planned interim analysis of an international, open-label trial. *Lancet Oncology* **16**(6), 729–736.

Beauchamp, G.K., Cowart, B.J., Moran, M., 1986. Developmental changes in salt acceptability in human infants. *Developmental Psychobiology* **19**, 17–25.

Beidler, L.M. Smallman, R.L., 1965. Renewal of cells within taste buds. *The Journal of Cell Biology* **27**, 263–272.

Berthoud, H.R., Bereiter, D.A., Trimble, E.R., Siegel, E.G., Jeanrenaud, B., 1981. Cephalic phase, reflex insulin secretion. Neuroanatomical and physiological characterization, *Diabetologia* **20** *Suppl*, 393–401.

Bodner, L., 1991. Effect of parotid submandibular and sublingual saliva on wound healing in rats. *Comparative Biochemistry and Physiology Part A: Physiology* **100**, 887–890.

Bradley, R.M. Beidler, L.M., 2003. Saliva: its role in taste function. In Doty, R.L. (Ed.), *Handbook of Olfaction and Gustation*, 2nd edition, pp. 639–650. New York: Marcel Dekker.

Brown, J., 1974. Recognition assessed by rating and ranking. *British Journal of Psychology* **65**, 13–22.

Bryant, B.P., Moore, P.A., 1995. Factors affecting the sensitivity of the lingual trigeminal nerve to acids. *American Journal of Physiology-Regulatory, Integrative and Comparative Physiology* **268**, R58–R65.

Buck, L.B., Bargmann, C.I. 2013. Figure 32–13, Chapter 32. In Kandel, E.R., Schwartz, J.H., Jessell, T.M., Siegelbaum, S.A., Hudspeth, A.J. (Eds.), *Principles of Neural Science*. 5th edition.

Bufe, B., Breslin, P.A., Kuhn, C., et al. 2005. The molecular basis of individual differences in phenylthiocarbamide and propylthiouracil bitterness perception. *Current Biology* **15**, 322–327.

Carleton, A., Accolla, R., Simon, S.A., 2010. Coding in the mammalian gustatory system. *Trends in Neurosciences* **33**, 326–334.

Chandrashekar, J., Hoon, M.A., Ryba, N.J., Zuker, C.S., 2006. The receptors and cells for mammalian taste. *Nature* **444**, 288–294.

Chandrashekar, J., Yarmolinsky, D., von, B.L., et al. 2009. The taste of carbonation, *Science* 443–445.

Chang, R.B., Waters, H., iman, E.R., 2010. A proton current drives action potentials in genetically identified sour taste cells. *Proceedings of the National Academy of Sciences* **107**, 22320–22325.

Chaudhari, N., Roper, S.D., 2010. The cell biology of taste. *Journal of Cell Biology* **190**, 285–296.

Chen, X., Gabitto, M., Peng, Y., Ryba, N.J., Zuker, C.S., 2011. A gustotopic map of taste qualities in the mammalian brain. *Science* **333**, 1262–1266.

Coates, A.C., 1974. Effects of age, sex, and smoking on electrical taste threshold. *Annals of Otology, Rhinology & Laryngology* **83**, 365–369.

Crystal, S.R., Bernstein, I.L., 1995. Morning sickness: Impact on offspring salt preference. *Appetite* **25**, 231–240.

Deems, D.A., Doty, R.L., Settle, R.G., et al. 1991. Smell and taste disorders, a study of 750 patients from the University of Pennsylvania Smell and Taste Center. *Archives of Otolaryngology – Head and Neck Surgery* **117**, 519–528.

Doty, R.L., 1978. Gender and reproductive state correlates of taste perception in humans. In McGill, T.E., Dewsbury, D.A., Sachs, B.D. (Eds.), *Sex and Behavior: Status and Prospectus*. New York: Plenum Press, New York, pp. 337–362.

Doty, R.L., 2001. Olfaction and gustation in normal aging and Alzheimer's disease. In Hof P. R., & Mobbs, C.V. (Eds.), *Functional Neurobiology of Aging*. San Diego: Academic Press, pp. 647–658.

Doty, R.L., Bagla, R., Morgenson, M., Mirza, N., 2001. NaCl thresholds: relationship to anterior tongue locus, area of stimulation, and number of fungiform papillae. *Physiology & Behavior* **72**, 373–378.

Doty, R.L., Cummins, D.M., Shibanova, A., Sanders, I., Mu, L., 2009. Lingual distribution of the human glossopharyngeal nerve. *Acta Otolaryngologica* **129**, 52–56.

Doty, R.L., Heidt, J.M., MacGillivray, M.R., et al. 2016. Influences of age, tongue region, and chorda tympani nerve sectioning on signal detection measures of lingual taste sensitivity. *Physiology & Behavior* **155**, 202–207.

Eckstein, A., 1927. Zur Physiologie der Geschmacksempfindung und des Saugreflexes bei Sauglingen. *Z. Kinderheilk*, **45**, 1–18.

Eyman, R.K., Kim, P.J., Call, T. 1975. Judgment error in category vs magnitude scales. *Perceptual and Motor Skills* **40**, 415–423.

Fischer, R., Griffin, F., England, S., Garn, S.M., 1961. Taste thresholds and food dislikes. *Nature* **191**, 1328.

Fox, A.L., 1931. Six in ten "tasteblind" to bitter chemical. *The Science News-Letter* **9**, 249.

Frank, M.E., Bieber, S.L., Smith, D.V. 1988. The organization of taste sensibilities in hamster chorda tympani nerve fibers. *Journal of General Physiology* **91**, 861–896.

Geraedts, M.C., Munger, S.D., 2013. Gustatory stimuli representing different perceptual qualities elicit distinct patterns of neuropeptide secretion from taste buds. *Journal of Neuroscience* **33**, 7559–7564.

Gerhold, K.A., Bautista, D.M., 2009. Molecular and cellular mechanisms of trigeminal chemosensation *Annals of the New York Academy of Sciences* **1170**, 184–189.

Grant, R., Ferguson, M.M., Strang, R., Turner, J. W., Bone, I., 1987. Evoked taste thresholds in a normal population and the application of electrogustometry to trigeminal nerve disease. *Journal of Neurology, Neurosurgery, & Psychiatry* **50**, 12–21.

Green, B.G. George, P., 2004. "Thermal taste" predicts higher responsiveness to chemical taste and flavor. *Chemical Senses* **29**, 617–628.

Greene, L.S. 1974. Physical growth and development, neurological maturation, and behavioral functioning in two Ecuadorian Andean communities in which goiter is endemic. II. PTC taste sensitivity and neurological maturation. *American Journal of Physical Anthropology* **41**, 139–151.

Grigoleit, J.S., Kullmann, J.S., Winkelhaus, A., et al. 2012. Single-trial conditioning in a human taste-endotoxin paradigm induces conditioned odor aversion but not cytokine responses. *Brain, Behavior, and Immunity* **26**, 234–238.

Guyton, A.C., Hall, J.E. 1996. *Textbook of Medical Physiology*, 9th edition, Chapter 53. WB Saunders Company.

Hamamichi, R., Asano-Miyoshi, M., Emori, Y., 2006. Taste bud contains both short-lived and long-lived cell populations. *Neuroscience* **141**, 2129–2138.

Harris, H., Kalmus, H., 1949. The measurement of taste sensitivity to phenylthiourea (PTC). *Annals of Eugenics* **15**, 24–31.

Hayes, J.E., Bartoshuk, L.M., Kidd, J.R., Duffy, V.B., 2008. Supertasting and PROP bitterness depends on more than the TAS2R38 gene. *Chemical Senses*, 33, 255–265.

Hevezi, P., Moyer, B.D., Lu, M., et al. 2009. Genome-wide analysis of gene expression in primate taste buds reveals links to diverse processes. *PLoS One* 4, e6395.

Hinds, J.W., Hinds, P.L., McNelly, N.A., 1984. An autoradiographic study of the mouse olfactory epithelium: Evidence for long-lived receptors. *Anatomical Record* 210, 375–383.

Hrboticky, N., Krondl, M., 1984. Acculturation to Canadian Foods by Chinese immigrant boys: Changes in the perceived flavor, health value and prestige of foods. *Appetite* 5, 117–126.

Humphreys-Beher, M.G., Macauley, S.P., Chegini, N., et al. 1994. Characterization of the synthesis and secretion of transforming growth factor-alpha from salivary glands and saliva. *Endocrinology* 134, 963–970.

James, C.E., Laing, D.G., Oram, N., 1997. A comparison of the ability of 8–9-year-old children and adults to detect taste stimuli. *Physiology & Behavior* 62, 193–197.

Jiang, P., Josue, J., Li, X., et al. 2012. Major taste loss in carnivorous mammals. *Proceedings of the National Academy of Sciences of the United States of America* 109, 4956–4961.

Kano, M., Shimizu, Y., Okayama, K., Kikuchi, M., 2007. Quantitative study of ageing epiglottal taste buds in humans. *Gerodontology* 24, 169–172.

Khan, N.A., Besnard, P., 2009. Oro-sensory perception of dietary lipids: New insights into the fat taste transduction. *Biochimica et Biophysica Acta* 1791, 149–155.

Kim, U.K., Drayna, D., 2005. Genetics of individual differences in bitter taste perception: Lessons from the PTC gene. *Clinical Genetics* 67, 275–280.

Kim, U.K., Jorgenson, E., Coon, H., Leppert, M., Risch, N., Drayna, D., 2003. Positional cloning of the human quantitative trait locus underlying taste sensitivity to phenylthiocarbamide, Science 21 Feb 2003: Vol. 299, Issue 5610, pp. 1221–1225.

Komai, M., Bryant, B.P., 1993. Acetazolamide specifically inhibits lingual trigeminal nerve responses to carbon dioxide. *Brain Research* 612, 122–129.

Lenz, F.A., Gracely, R.H., Zirh, T.A., et al. 1997. Human thalamic nucleus mediating taste and multiple other sensations related to ingestive behavior. *Journal of Neurophysiology* 77, 3406–3409.

Leshem, M., 1998. Salt preference in adolescence is predicted by common prenatal and infantile mineralofluid loss. *Physiology & Behavior* 63, 699–704.

Li, X., Li, W., Wang, H., et al. 2005. Pseudogenization of a sweet-receptor gene accounts for cats' indifference toward sugar. *PLoS Genetics* 1, 27–35.

Liu, G., Zong, G., Doty, R.L., Sun, Q., 2016. Prevalence and risk factors of taste and smell impairment in a nationwide representative sample of the US population: a cross-sectional study. *BMJ Open*, 6, e013246.

Liu, P., Shah, B.P., Croasdell, S., Gilbertson, T.A., 2011. Transient receptor potential channel type M5 is essential for fat taste. *Journal of Neuroscience* 31, 8634–8642.

Martin due Pan, R., 1955. Le role du gout et de l'odorat dans l'alimentation due nourrisson. *Pediatrie* 10, 169–176.

Matsuda, T. Doty, R.L. 1995. Regional taste sensitivity to NaCl: Relationship to subject age, tongue locus and area of stimulation. *Chemical Senses* 20, 283–290.

Mattes, R.D., 2011. Accumulating evidence supports a taste component for free fatty acids in humans. *Physiology & Behavior* 104, 624–631.

McBride, M.R., Mistretta, C.M., 1986. Taste responses from the chorda tympani nerve in young and old Fischer rats. *Journal of Gerontology* 41, 306–314.

Mennella, J.A., 2009. Flavour programming during breast-feeding. *Advances in Experimental Medicine and Biology* 639, 113–120.

Mennella, J.A., Beauchamp, G.K., 1993. The effects of repeated exposure to garlic-flavored milk on the nursling's behavior. *Pediatric Research* 34, 805–808.

Mennella, J.A., Johnson, A., Beauchamp, G.K., 1995. Garlic ingestion by pregnant women alters the odor of amniotic fluid. *Chemical Senses* **20**, 207–209.

Mennella, J.A., Pepino, M.Y., Duke, F.F., Reed, D.R., 2010. Age modifies the genotype-phenotype relationship for the bitter receptor TAS2R38. *BMC Genetics* **11**, 60.

Miller, I.J., 1988. Human taste bud density across adult age groups. *Journals of Gerontology* **43**, 826–830.

Miller, I.J., Reedy, F.E., Jr., 1990. Variations in human taste bud density and taste intensity perception. *Physiology & Behavior* **47**, 1213–1219.

Miller, S.L., Mirza, N., Doty, R.L., 2002. Electrogustometric thresholds: Relationship to anterior tongue locus, area of stimulation, and number of fungiform papillae. *Physiology & Behavior* **75**, 753–757.

Mistretta, C.M., Oakley, I.A., 1986. Quantitative anatomical study of taste buds in fungiform papillae of young and old Fischer rats. *Journal of Gerontology* **41**, 315–318.

Mochizuki, Y., 1939. Studies on the papilla foliate of Japanese. 2. The number of taste buds. *Okajimas Folia Anatomica Japonica* **18**, 369.

Mojet, J., Christ-Hazelhof, E., Heidema, J. 2001. Taste perception with age: generic or specific losses in threshold sensitivity to the five basic tastes? *Chemical Senses* **26**, 845–860.

Morris-Witman, J., Sego, R., Brinkley, L., Dolce, C., 2000. The effects of sialoadenectomy and exogenous EGF on taste bud morphology and maintenance. *Chemical Senses* **25**, 9–19.

Murray, R.G., 1973 The ultrastructure of taste buds. In: Friedmann, I. (ed.) *The Ultrastructure of Sensory Organs*. North Holland, Amsterdam, pp. 1–81.

Murray, R.G., Murray, A., 1967. Fine structure of taste buds of rabbit foliate papillae. *Journal of Ultrastructure Research* **19**, 327–353.

Noguchi, S., Ohba, Y., Oka, T., 1991. Effect of salivary epidermal growth factor on wound healing of tongue in mice. *The American Journal of Physiology* **260** E620–E625.

Norgren, R., 1981. The central organization of the gustatory and fisceral afferent systems in the nucleus of the solitary tract. In Katsuki, Y. Norgren, R., & Sato, M. (Eds.), *Brain Mechanisms in Sensation*. New York: John Wiley and Sons, pp. 173–186.

Olson, J.M., Boehnke, M., Neiswanger, K., Roche, A.F., Siervogel, R.M., 1989. Alternative genetic models for the inheritance of the phenylthiocarbamide taste deficiency. *Genetic Epidemiology (Suppl)*, **6**, 423–434.

Onoda, K., Ikeda, M., Sekine, H., Ogawa, H., 2012. Clinical study of central taste disorders and discussion of the central gustatory pathway. *Journal of Neurology* **259**, 261–266.

Paxinos G., Mai J.K., 2004. *The Human Nervous System*. Amsterdam: Elsevier Academic Press.

Pepino, M.Y., Mennella, J.A., 2007. Effects of cigarette smoking and family history of alcoholism on sweet taste perception and food cravings in women. *Alcoholism: Clinical & Experimental Research* **31**, 1891–1899.

Perrin, M., Krut, L.H., Bronte-Stewart, B. 1961. Smoking and food preferences. *British Medical Journal.*, **1**, 387–388.

Pritchard, J.A., 1965. Deglutition by normal and anencephalic fetuses. *Obstetrics and Gynecology* **25**, 289–297.

Pritchard, T.C., 2012. Gustatory system. In Mai, J.K., & Paxinos, G. (Eds.), *The Human Nervous System*, 3rd edition. Elsevier, New York, pp. 1187–1218.

Pritchard, T.C., Macaluso, D.A., Eslinger, P.J., 1999. Taste perception in patients with insular cortex lesions. *Behavioral Neuroscience* **113**, 663–671.

Pritchard, T.C., Scott, T.R., 2015. Functional organization of the gustatory system in macaques. In Doty, R.L. (Ed.), *Handbook of Olfaction and Gustation*. John Wiley & Sons, Hoboken, pp. 983–1003.

Reddy, B.M., Rao, D.C., 1989. Phenylthiocarbamide taste sensitivity revisited: Complete sorting test supports residual family resemblance. *Genetic Epidemiology (Suppl)*, **6**, 413–421.

Reed, D.R., Nanthakumar, E., North, M., et al. 1999. Localization of a gene for bitter-taste perception to human chromosome 5p15 [letter]. *The American Journal of Human Genetics* **64**, 1478–1480.

Rolls, E.T., 2011. Chemosensory learning in the cortex. Amsterdam: North Holland Publishers,

Rolls et al Journal is: Frontiers in Systems Neuroscience, Sept. 16; 5:78

Rolls, E.T., 2015. Neural integration of taste, smell, oral texture, and visual modalities. In: Doty, R.L. (Ed.), *Handbook of Olfaction and Gustation*. Hoboken, New Jersey: John Wiley & Sons.

Rolls, E.T., Grabenhorst, F., 2008. The orbitofrontal cortex and beyond: from affect to decision-making. *Progress in Neurobiology* **86**, 216–244.

Ross, M.G., Nijland, M.J., 1997. Fetal swallowing: Relation to amniotic fluid regulation. *Clinical Obstetrics and Gynecology* **40**, 352–365.

Roudnitzky, N., Bufe, B., Thalmann, S., et al. 2011. Genomic, genetic and functional dissection of bitter taste responses to artificial sweeteners. *Human Molecular Genetics* Volume **20**, Issue 17, 1 September 2011, Pages 3437–3449.

Yekta, S.S., Luckhoff, A., Ristic, D., Lampert, F., Ellrich, J., 2010. Impaired somatosensation in tongue mucosa of smokers. *Clinical Oral Investigations* **16**(1), 39–44.

Sato, K., Endo, S., Tomita, H., 2002. Sensitivity of three loci on the tongue and soft palate to four basic tastes in smokers and non-smokers. *Acta Oto-Laryngologica* **122**, 74–82.

Sato, T., Okada, Y., Miyamoto, T., Fujiyama, R., 1997. Distribution of non-tasters for phenylthiocarbamide and high sensitivity to quinine hydrochloride of the non-tasters in Japanese. *Chemical Senses* **22**, 547–551.

Schier, L.A., Hashimoto, K., Bales, M.B., Blonde, G.D., Spector, A.C., 2014. High-resolution lesion-mapping strategy links a hot spot in rat insular cortex with impaired expression of taste aversion learning. *Proceedings of the National Academy of Sciences* **111**, 1162–1167.

Schiffman, S.S., Hornack, K., Reilly, D., 1979. Increased taste thresholds of amino acids with age. *American Journal of Clinical Nutrition* **32**, 1622–1627.

Schultz, G., Rotatori, D.S., Clark, W., 1991. EGF and TGF-alpha in wound healing and repair. *Journal of Cellular Biochemistry* **45**, 346–352.

Scott, T.R., Mark, G.P., 1987. The taste system encodes stimulus toxicity. *Brain Research* **414**, 197–203.

Segovia, C., Hutchinson, I., Laing, D.G., Jinks, A.L., 2002. A quantitative study of fungiform papillae and taste pore density in adults and children. *Developmental Brain Research* **138**, 135–146.

Sewards, T.V., 2004. Dual separate pathways for sensory and hedonic aspects of taste. *Brain Research Bulletin* **62**, 271–283.

Shankar, M.U., Levitan, C.A., Spence, C., 2010. Grape expectations: The role of cognitive influences in color-flavor interactions. *Consciousness and Cognition* **19**, 380–390.

Small, D.M., Prescott, J., 2005. Odor/taste integration and the perception of flavor. *Experimental Brain Research* **166**, 345–357.

Smith, D.V., 1971. Taste intensity as a function of area and concentration: Differentiation between compounds. *Journal of Experimental Psychology* **87**, 163–171.

Snyder, L.H., 1931. Inherited taste deficiency. *Science* **74**, 151–152.

Stein, L.J., Cowart, B.J., Beauchamp, G.K., 2012. The development of salty taste acceptance is related to dietary experience in human infants: A prospective study. *American Journal of Clinical Nutrition* **95**, 123–129.

Stein, L.J., Cowart, B.J., Epstein, A.N., et al. 1996. Increased liking for salty foods in adolescents exposed during infancy to a chloride-deficient feeding formula. *Appetite* **27**, 65–77.

Steiner, J.E., 1974. Discussion paper: Innate, discriminative human facial expressions to taste and smell stimulation. *Annals of the New York Academy of Sciences* September 27; **237**, 229–233.

Steiner, J.E., 1979. Human facial expressions in response to taste and smell stimulation. *Advances in Child Development & Behavior* **13** 257–295.

Steinert, R.E., Beglinger, C., 2011. Nutrient sensing in the gut: Interactions between chemosensory cells, visceral afferents and the secretion of satiation peptides. *Physiology & Behavior* **105**, 62–70.

Stephani, C., Fernandez-Baca, V.G., Maciunas, R., Koubeissi, M., Luders, H.O., 2011. Functional neuroanatomy of the insular lobe. *Brain Structure and Function* **216**, 137–149.

Stevens, J.C., Cruz, L.A., Hoffman, J.M., Patterson, M.Q., 1995. Taste sensitivity and aging: high incidence of decline revealed by repeated threshold measures. *Chemical Senses* 20, 451–459.

Suliburska, J., Duda, G., & Pupek-Musialik, D. 2004. [Effect of tobacco smoking on taste sensitivity in adults]. *Przegląd Lekarski* 61, 1174–1176.

Sullivan, S.A., Birch, L.L. 1990. Pass the sugar, pass the salt: Experience dictates preference. *Developmental Psychology* 26, 546–551.

Temple, E.C., Hutchinson, I., Laing, D.G., Jinks, A.L., 2002. Taste development: Differential growth rates of tongue regions in humans. *Developmental Brain Research* 135, 65–70.

Visser, J., Kroeze, J.H., Kamps, W.A., Bijleveld, C.M., 2000. Testing taste sensitivity and a version in very young children: Development of a procedure. *Appetite* 34, 169–176.

Weiffenbach, J.M., Baum, B.J., Burghauser, R., 1982. Taste thresholds: Quality specific variation with human aging. *Journal of Gerontology* 37, 372–377.

Weiffenbach, J.M., Cowart, B.J., Baum, B.J. 1986. Taste intensity perception in aging. *Journal of Gerontology* 41, 460–468.

Witt, M., Reutter, K., 1997. Scanning electron microscopical studies of developing gustatory papillae in humans. *Chemical Senses* 22, 601–612.

Witt, M., Reutter, K., Miller Jr, I.J., Doty, R.L., 2003. Morphology of the peripheral taste system. In Doty, R.L. (Ed.), Handbook of Olfaction and Gustation. Marcel Dekker, New York, 651–677.

Wooding, S. 2006. Phenylthiocarbamide: A 75-year adventure in genetics and natural selection. *Genetics* 172, 2015–2023.

Zhao, H., Zhou, Y., Pinto, C.M., et al. 2010. Evolution of the sweet taste receptor gene Tas1r2 in bats. *Molecular Biology and Evolution* 27, 2642 2650.

Zuniga, J.R., Davis, S.H., Englehardt, R.A., et al. 1993. Taste performance on the anterior human tongue varies with fungiform taste bud density. *Chemical Senses*, 18, 449–460.

Measurement of Olfaction

Chemosensory testing is critical for establishing the nature and validity of a patient's complaint. Patient self-reports are notoriously inaccurate (Stinton et al., 2010) and, in some cases, considerable return of function may have occurred without patient awareness until they are tested formally (London et al., 2008). Quantitative testing establishes a baseline for monitoring of functional changes, e.g., the effects of pharmacological, surgical, or immunological interventions. Importantly, such testing may detect malingering (Doty & Crastnopol, 2010) and provide an accurate basis for disability compensation.

Many physicians still evaluate smell and taste by simply asking the patient to identify common odorants (e.g., coffee, tobacco) or to detect sugar or salt placed in the mouth. These approaches are inadequate: they are non-quantitative, have no normative referents, and can be faked easily by malingerers. They are as crude as testing visual acuity by shining a light in the eye. As shown later in this chapter, there are practical means for accurate and inexpensive assessment of smell function in the clinic.

Most patients with chemosensory disturbances have olfactory, not gustatory, deficits. This is in spite of presenting with apparent loss of taste (Figure 3.1). Such complaints, unless reported directly as involving the basic taste qualities of sweet, sour, bitter, or salt, typically reflect confusion between taste, per se, and flavor. Flavor depends upon retronasal stimulation of the olfactory receptors during chewing and swallowing, not simply the stimulation of taste buds. As apparent from Figure 3.1, relatively few patients actually have taste dysfunction, as measured objectively by tests in which the stimulus is swilled within the whole mouth.

This chapter will address the psychophysical, electrophysiological, and psychophysiological methods of olfactory measurement followed by structural and functional imaging techniques.

Olfactory Testing

Basic Considerations

As noted in Chapter 1, the human olfactory system can detect thousands of odorants, a fact that might appear to prohibit meaningful assessment. It must be remembered that (a) olfaction is a synthetic sense, i.e., it typically blends together inputs from molecules that individually have different odors into a single overall smell perception ("percept"), save when only a few distinct components are present (Laing & Francis, 1989); (b) most odorant receptors respond to multiple chemicals (Duchamp-Viret et al., 1999); and (c) there is considerable spatial intermingling of receptor-related information within the olfactory

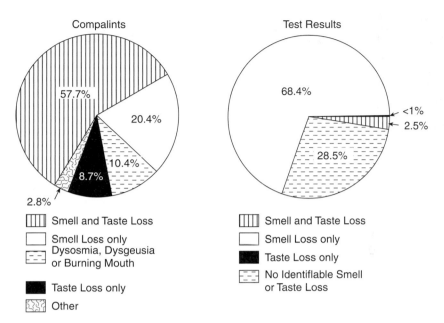

Figure 3.1 Left: Primary complaints of 750 consecutive patients presenting to the University of Pennsylvania Smell and Taste Center. Right: Test results. The complaint categories of smell loss, taste loss, and smell and taste loss include some patients with secondary complaints of chemosensory distortion and burning mouth. From Deems et al. (1991).

epithelium, bulb, and cortex (Wilson, 2001). Thus, lesions within any segment of the olfactory system generally affect more than a single stimulus or odor quality. Presumably this explains, in part, why most measures of olfactory function are correlated with one another and why, for example, individuals who have elevated thresholds for one odorant have raised thresholds for another. Hence, determining a threshold for one stimulus provides an index of a subject's general olfactory sensitivity, assuming the absence of specific anosmias or hyposmias.

Before any type of olfactory test can be performed, an odor stimulus must be presented to the nose in a reliable manner. Numerous approaches to this end have been developed (Figure 3.2). Some deliver odorants via glass or plastic bottles, alcohol pads, felt-tipped pens, glass rods, wooden sticks, "scratch and sniff" labels, or strips of blotter paper dipped into liquids. Other media include mechanical devices, termed olfactometers. These range from the simple draw tube olfactometer of Zwaardemarker (Zwaardemaker, 1889; Zwaardemaker, 1925) to relatively complex computer-controlled air-dilution olfactometers that employ flow meters or mass flow controllers to provide accurate stimulus concentrations of specified durations (Kobal & Plattig, 1978; Punter, 1983 Doty et al., 1988; Lorig et al., 1999). Most clinical tests require only that a uniform stimulus is presented from trial to trial in a reliable manner. Recent developments include olfactometers that permit threshold tests to be self-administered and automatically scored and simple odor wands that provide odorants upon the touch of a button (Figure 3.3).

Odorants can be presented bilaterally (both nostrils simultaneously) or unilaterally (one nostril at a time, usually with the contralateral nostril occluded). Unilateral smell loss will go undetected if only bilateral testing is performed, since bilateral testing largely reflects the better functioning side. Also, odorants may be injected intravenously – so-called intravenous

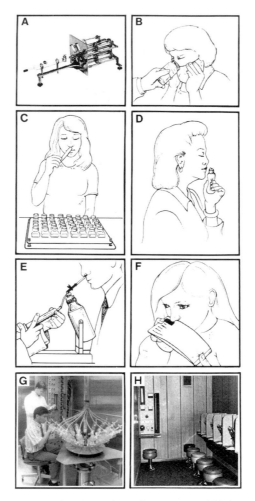

Figure 3.2 Procedures for presenting odorants to subjects for assessment. (A) Laboratory version of the draw-tube olfactometer of Zwaardemaker. In its simplest version, an outer tube, made of rubber or another odorous material, slides along a calibrated inner tube, which is connected to a sniffing tube. When the odorized tube is slid toward the patient, less of its internal surface is exposed to the inspired airstream, resulting in a weaker olfactory sensation. In the pictured version, several stimuli can be presented simultaneously at varying concentrations. (B) Sniff bottle. (C) Perfumer's strip. (D) Squeeze bottle. (E) Blast injection device. The experimenter injects a given volume of air into the odorant-containing bottle and releases the pressure by squeezing a clamp on the tube leading to the nostril, producing a stimulus pulse. (F) Microencapsulated "scratch-and-sniff" test. (G) An air-dilution olfactometer connected to sniff ports located on a rotating table. (H) An odor evaluation room where subjects sit in front of sniff ports to sample odorants. Copyright © 2006, Richard L. Doty.

olfaction. Thiamine propyldisulfide (Alinamin; Prosultiamine) is a typical stimulus. It produces a garlic-like sensation and has potential value to measure olfaction when the airway is blocked (see Takagi, 1989, for review). Although it is often assumed that the injected odorant reaches the olfactory receptors directly from blood vessels, the stimulus may also reach the receptors via diffusion through nasal capillaries, lung air, or both (Maruniak et al., 1983). These uncertainties have led to a decline in its use.

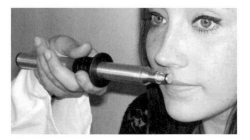

Figure 3.3 A modern pen-like device, termed the Snap & Sniff® wand, by which odorants can be presented for sampling using a simple sliding mechanism. This set of devices comes in multiple odorant configurations. Photo courtesy of Sensonics International, Haddon Heights, NJ, USA. Copyright © 2014 Sensonics International.

Although olfactory function can be tested retronasally by introducing odors into the mouth, it is extremely difficult to equate the amount of stimulus reaching the receptors by the oral route to that reaching the receptors by the front of the nose. Sniffing influences stimulus concentration from the front of the nose, whereas mouth movements, such as chewing and swallowing, influence stimulus concentration via flows from the oral cavity through the rear of the nose. Airflow is not the same for the two different directions, in part because of variation in anatomy and the involved pressures and flows. The amount of absorption on the walls of the nose and oral cavity changes according to variable anatomy and flow patterns induced by sniffing and swallowing.

Types of Olfactory Tests

Olfactory tests can be divided into three major classes: psychophysical, electrophysiological, and psychophysiological.

Psychophysical Tests provide direct information about a subject's perceptual experience when presented with olfactory stimuli. Among these nominally disparate tests are those of odor detection, identification, discrimination, and memory. Such procedures are analogous to those developed for measurement of hearing and vision. Other measures employ strategies developed by psychologists for assessment of memory and discrimination.

Electrophysiological Tests measure alterations in electrical activity from the brain or olfactory receptors using electrodes placed on the scalp or inside the nose. The commonest procedure assesses *Odor Event-Related Potentials* (OERPs). These are far-field potentials, detected from the scalp, that reflect summated cortical neural activity induced by repeated presentation of an odorant. The next most frequently used electrophysiological investigation is the electro-olfactogram (EOG), a measure obtained from electrodes placed inside the nose on the surface of the olfactory epithelium. The EOG consists of odor-induced summated receptor potentials.

Psychophysiological Tests rely on reflex or reflex-like reactions to odors from the autonomic nervous system, such as changes in body temperature, heart rate, respiration rate, palmar sweating, and blood pressure. Unfortunately, many of these responses are highly variable and influenced by co-stimulation of the intranasal trigeminal system, limiting their usefulness in terms of measuring olfaction, per se.

The integrity and function of the central olfactory system can be measured by *structural and functional imaging*. This includes computerized tomography (CT), magnetic resonance imaging (MRI), positron emission tomography (PET), single photon emission tomography (SPECT), and magneto-encephalography (MEG). *Functional measures of nasal patency and airflow*, such as acoustic rhinometry and anterior rhinomanometry, may be useful in some instances to determine whether odors are actually reaching the olfactory receptors. Details of these and other means for addressing olfactory dysfunction are described in the following sections.

Psychophysical Tests

Largely as a result of funding from the US National Institutes of Health in the early 1980s, there was an explosion in development of clinically applicable olfactory tests in the United States which led to further development elsewhere, particularly in Europe. The psychometric properties of such tests have been established, thus permitting comparisons of their utility (Table 3.1). Since nominally disparate psychophysical tests rely on several odorants at variable concentrations, and typically have different cognitive demands (Doty et al., 1995; Hedner et al., 2010) and reliabilities (Hummel et al., 1997), any change in their findings must be interpreted cautiously. For example, Hedner et al. (2010) demonstrated, for the Sniffin' Sticks test, that demographic and cognitive factors accounted for 9% of the variation in threshold values, 23% of the variance in discrimination values, and 15% in identification values. While it is a popular assumption that threshold detection procedures evaluate primarily the olfactory bulb and nasal epithelium, whereas measures of discrimination, identification, or memory assess central structures, evidence for this concept is conflicting. Moreover, operational terms used to describe such experiments, e.g., detection, discrimination or identification, are probably not representative of independent physiologic or psychologic chemosensory processes. For example, if an odor is to be identified or remembered, it must first be detected. The ability to remember odor qualities is a prerequisite for discriminating among them, assuming they are of equivalent intensity. Even threshold tests in which a choice is made between an odor and a blank requires short-term memory and the ability to discriminate subtle elements of smell.

In accord with such concepts, the scores of nominally distinct olfactory tests correlate with one another, as indexed by strong loadings on a common factor in principal component analyses (Doty et al., 1994; Tourbier & Doty, 2007; Lotsch et al., 2008). In such analyses, secondary factors have been observed that reflect response bias measures, suprathreshold pleasantness measures, and some other task-related factors that reflect some degree of independence from measures represented by the common primary factor. For example, in a pioneering study, Doty et al. (1994) performed a principal component (PC) analysis of nine tests of olfactory function, including measures of odor detection, identification, discrimination, memory, suprathreshold intensity scaling, and identification. After controlling for gender, smoking, and education, the major PC, which accounted for 30% of the total variance, was loaded most strongly by tests of identification, memory, and threshold. A second PC, which accounted for 13.5% of the variance, represented loadings from suprathreshold odor-identification test rating scales and a bias measure derived from signal detection theory. This is of interest, since suprathreshold rating measures do not control for response biases, unlike forced-choice tests of identification, discrimination, memory, and threshold. The remaining two factors largely reflected odorant pleasantness ratings (9.6% of the variance) and a non-forced choice test of threshold detection (9.0% of the

Table 3.1. Clinical olfactory tests. Commercially available tests are shaded gray.

Test	Type of test	Number of odors or items	Test-retest reliability coefficient	Estimated test duration	Availability of norms
Alberta Smell Test (Green & Iverson, 1998)	ID	8	Not Reported	10 min	NO
Alcohol Sniff Test (Davidson & Murphy, 1997; Davidson et al., 1998).	Detection Threshold	1	0.30	<5 min	NO
Amoore Threshold Test (Amoore & Ollman, 1983)	Detection Threshold	1	0.70	<10 min	NO
Barcelona Smell Test (Cardesin et al., 2006)	Detection & Recognition	24	Not Reported	~30 min	NO
Biolfa® Olfactory Test (Bonfils et al., 2004)	Detection & Recognition	3 & 8	Not Reported	~30 min	NO
Brief Smell ID Test™ (also known as Cross-Cultural Smell ID Test) (Doty et al., 1996; Liu et al., 1995)	ID	12	0.73	<5 min	YES
CCCRC Test (Cain et al., 1983)	ID & Detection	10 ID 1 Threshold	ID: 0.60 Threshold: 0.36	~30 min	Limited
Combined Olfactory Test (COT) (Robson et al., 1996)	ID & Detection	9 ID	0.87	10 min 1 Detect	NO
Dusseldorf Odour Discrimination Test (Weierstall & Pause, 2012)	Discrimination	15**	0.66	15 min	NO
European Test of Olfactory Capabilities (ETOC) (Thomas-Danguin et al., 2003)	ID & Detection	16	0.90	< 20 min	NO

Table 3.1. (cont.)

Test	Type of test	Number of odors or items	Test-retest reliability coefficient	Estimated test duration	Availability of norms
Italian Olfactory Identification Test (IOIT) (Maremmani et al., 2012)	ID	33	0.96 & 0.99***	10–15 min	Limited
Jet Stream Olfactometer (Ikeda et al., 1999)	ID	8	Not Reported	<5 min	NO
Jones' Ascending Series Threshold Tests (Jones, 1955a; Jones, 1955b)	Recognition Threshold	3	n-butanol: 0.82 safrol: 0.77 n-butyric acid: 0.80	20–25 min	NO
Kremer Olfactory Test (Kremer et al., 1998)	ID	6	Not Reported	<5 min	NO
Le Nez du Vin (McMahon & Scadding, 1996)	ID	6	Not Reported	<5 min	NO
Monell Extended Sniffin' Sticks Identification Test (MONEX-40) (Freiherr et al., 2012)	ID	40	0.68	~15 min	NO
Odor Confusion Matrix (OCM) (Wright, 1987; Kurtz et al., 2001)	ID	10	0.94	~1 hr	NO
Odor Identification Test for Children (Laing et al., 2008)	ID	16	Not Reported	~5 min	Limited
Odor Discrimination / Memory Test™ (ODMT) (Choudhury et al., 2003; Bromley & Doty, 1995)	Discrimination & Short-term Odor Memory	12	0.68	15 min	YES
Odor Stick ID Test Hashimoto et al., 2004; Saito et al., 2006)	ID	13	0.77	<15 min	Limited

Test	Measure	Number	Reliability	Time	Pediatric
Pediatric Smell Wheel (Cameron & Doty, 2013)	ID	11	0.70	< 5 min	YES
Pocket Smell Test™ (PST) – (Duff et al., 2002; Solomon et al., 1998; Rawal et al., 2015)	ID	3 & 4	0.80 &.85	< 1 min	NO
Quick Smell Test (Q-SIT) (Jackman & Doty, 2005)	ID	3	0.87	< 1 min	NO
Quick Sniff Test (Gilbert et al., 2002)	ID & Intensity	1	ID Not Reported Intensity: 0.51	< 1 min	NO
San Diego Odor ID Test (Anderson et al., 1992; Krantz et al., 2009)	ID	6	0.85	~10 min	NO
Scandinavian Odor ID Test (SOIT) (Nordin et al., 1999)	ID	16	0.79	10–15 min	Limited
Smell Diskettes (Simmen et al., 1999)	ID	8	Not Reported	< 5 min	NO
Snap & Sniff® Threshold Test (Doty, 2015)	Detection Threshold	1	~0.90	~20 min	YES
Smell Threshold Test™ (Doty, 2000)	Detection Threshold	1	0.88	~30 min	YES
Sniffin' Sticks Test – Identification (Hummel et al., 1997; Hummel et al., 2001; Haehner et al., 2009a; Hummel et al., 1997)	Identification	12 / 16 / 32	0.77 / 0.73 / 0.88	10–20 min	YES
Sniffin' Sticks Test – Identification, Discrimination & Threshold (Hummel et al., 1997; Haehner et al., 2009a)	Threshold, Detection & Identification	16 / 32 / Threshold:16	0.54 / 0.80 / 0.61 & 0.92	30 minutes to one hour for whole test	YES

Table 3.1. (cont.)

Test	Type of test	Number of odors or items	Test-retest reliability coefficient	Estimated test duration	Availability of norms
T&T Olfactometer Test (Takagi, 1989)	Recognition Threshold	5	0.22–0.45	15–30 min	Limited
University of Pennsylvania Smell Identification Test (UPSIT; also known as Smell Identification Test) (Doty et al., 1984a;Doty, 1995)	ID	40	0.94	10–15 min	YES
Utrecht Odor ID Test (Geur Identificatie Test Utrecht (GITU)) (Hendriks, 1988)	ID	18 or 36	0.68–0.77	30–45 min	NO
Viennese Odor Test (Lehrner & Deecke, 2000)	ID	20	0.75	15 min	NO

Key: ID = identification. D=discrimination T= threshold.
Note: duration of test assumes a healthy cooperative subject.

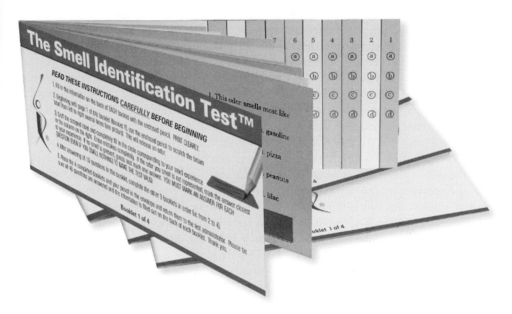

Figure 3.4 The University of Pennsylvania Smell Identification Test (known commercially as the Smell Identification Test™). This test consists of 4 test booklets, each containing 10 odors with 4 corresponding response alternatives. Norms based upon ~1,000 Americans permit accurate assessment of smell loss in both an absolute sense and in terms of age- and sex-related normative values for this country. Variations can occur in non-North American populations, necessitating adjustments based upon local norms. Photograph courtesy of Sensonics International, Haddon Heights, NJ, USA.

variance), respectively. In essence, a test of odor identification will reflect changes in threshold and discrimination. It is probably not necessary to administer multiple tests.

Odor Identification Tests. The most widely used olfactory tests are straightforward multiple-choice smell identification tests, several of which are commercially available (Table 3.1). One of the most popular is the University of Pennsylvania Smell Identification Test (UPSIT), a forced-choice 40-item identification test that employs microencapsulated "scratch and sniff" odorants (Doty et al., 1984; Doty, 1995) (Figure 3.4). The UPSIT is reliable (test-retest r = 0.94), and can be self-administered and sent through the post, thereby making it amenable to epidemiological and follow-up studies (see, e.g., Siderowf et al., 2007; London et al., 2008). This test provides an index of absolute dysfunction (e.g., anosmia, severe microsmia, moderate microsmia, mild microsmia, anosmia), with an indication of relative dysfunction based upon age- and gender-adjusted normative percentile ranks (Doty, 1995). Malingering may be suspected on the basis of improbable responses (Doty & Crastnopol, 2010). Since there are four forced-choice response alternatives, someone with true anosmia should score, on average, ~10 (25%). An individual who scores four or less is probably malingering, as discussed in detail in Chapter 8. Although the North American UPSIT version has some items that are not well known in Europe and elsewhere (e.g., "pumpkin pie," "skunk," and "gasoline"), the test is available in some 30 other languages and culturally familiar response alternatives are given, as well as a few culture-relevant odorant substitutions (see, e.g., Fornazieri et al., 2013). Outside North America, indeed in general, use of local control data for tests like the UPSIT circumvents the problem of smell unfamiliarity at the expense of slight loss in sensitivity.

As indicated in Table 3.1, shorter versions of the UPSIT have been developed, including a widely employed 12-item version, termed the Brief Smell Identification Test, and two shorter versions, the Quick Smell Identification Test (Q-SIT; three odors) and the Pocket Smell Test (PST; four odors). In keeping with many odor identification tests and most other psychophysical measures, the UPSIT and its shorter clones may assess indirectly some elements of cognitive function unrelated to olfaction. Thus, even a healthy subject may be certain they can detect an odor but may not identify it correctly simply because it is unfamiliar. Use of a small number of alternative response categories for each odor in part circumvents this potential problem, although the smarter individual may select the correct answer by a process of elimination. Cognitive impairment also may be a relevant confounder for many other sensory investigations, including odor detection threshold tests (Doty et al., 2015), highlighting the point that psychophysical testing involves multiple brain processes. Confounding from cognitive dysfunction can be controlled for by excluding those with such impairment on basic screening tests such as the Mini-Mental State Examination (MMSE). Although some investigators eliminate patients with MMSE scores below 25, this may be too conservative and we suggest a minimum score of 27/30. Alternatively, there is a 40-item visual test (Picture Identification Test), analogous to the UPSIT, to ensure that the basic concepts underlying the investigation are understood (Vollmecke & Doty, 1985).

A popular odor identification test, particularly in Europe, is the Sniffin' Sticks Test (SST). The identification element of this test battery is available in three versions: a 12-item "screening" test, a 16-item test (most widely used), and a 32-item test (Figure 3.5). The identification varieties employ felt tip pens saturated with odorants (Kobal 1996). The reliability of this procedure is comparable to that of the 12-odorant B-SIT (Hummel, 1997). Thus, when the

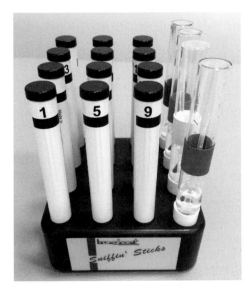

Figure 3.5 The 12-odorant Sniffin' Sticks Olfactory Screening Test. This contains 12 felt-tip pens filled with odors. The subject is asked to smell the tip of the pen and name the odor from a multiple-choice list containing four items for each pen. Note: The four tubes on the right of the holder are supra-threshold taste sprays, now replaced with taste strips. For more detailed testing an "extended" test is available which has 48 sticks. This produces a Threshold, Discrimination, and Identification score (TDI index).

16-stick SST was compared directly to the UPSIT (Wolfensberger, 2000; Silveira-Moriyama, 2008), the correlation between them was moderately strong (r= 0.75), likely reflecting the reliability of the shorter test (SST) (Kobal, 1996). The test-retest reliability for identification of the 16- and 32-odor version is reportedly higher (0.88) (Haehner et al., 2009).

The full, i.e., "extended," version of the SST test includes measures of threshold detection, discrimination, and identification. The test scores of each are added in linear fashion, resulting in the "TDI" index. Normative data are available for this index based upon several thousand healthy subjects (Hummel et al., 2007). Its claimed advantage is that olfaction is measured from several aspects and there should be coherence between the three main parameters (assuming that the three modalities are inter-dependent). Potentially, this association could help to identify a malingerer who may deliberately score badly on one component of the extended SST. The information derived from assessing three components of olfaction is clearly of interest from the research perspective given that some believe threshold defects characterize peripheral lesions and identification problems point to a cognitive (central) defect. As discussed above, the existence of such central/peripheral dichotomy is disputed and many consider that most olfactory tests are inter-related (Doty, 1994)

The TDI score has a number of shortcomings. If it is assumed, as do the investigators who developed the test, that the elements to be combined are, in fact, measuring different entities, i.e., threshold, discrimination, and identification (Lotsch et al., 2008), then one person may do well, for example, on identification but poorly on detection, and another may do well on detection but poorly on identification, with both ending up with the same combined score for quite different reasons. Moreover, simply adding test scores together results in differential arbitrary weightings of the test components for each subject, because the distribution of each test measure differs. Importantly, the tests within the composite have diverse non-olfactory test demands, employ different stimuli, have dissimilar reliabilities, and have varying levels of chance performance. The proper statistical solution, if such data are to be combined, would be to convert the scores of each test to standardized z-scores and then perform the addition or averaging of the scores. However, there is still the issue of knowing the relative contributions of the various tests for a given TDI score.

The standard 12- or 16-odor SST is rapid, inexpensive, and can be self-administered (Mueller, 2006), but the extended version, which requires threshold measurement, is more time consuming (30 minutes or more depending on subject cooperation) and has to be administered by a trained technician. A potential problem with the identification component of the SST, which is shared by other odor identification tests and mentioned briefly above, is that some subjects may actually smell a given stimulus, but they are unable to assign a name to it. This can happen if the odor is unfamiliar (e.g., due to age or cultural factors) or because of cognitive problems, such as difficulties in memory, recall, or agnosia. Forced-choice responses common to all three procedures (a) minimize this problem through the process of elimination, (b) increase test reliability, and (c) allow for the detection of malingering. It may be useful to record, in addition to the forced-choice response, whether there is "something smelled" or "nothing smelled" to ascertain whether the aberrant response is truly one of no function.

Until recently there was no commercially available test for those children who are too young to read or may have insufficient vocabulary to complete adult designed identification tests. The Pediatric Smell Wheel is a commercially available game-like test for evaluating olfaction in young children that overcomes some of these problems (Cameron and Doty, 2013). A rotating cardboard disk exposes one of 11 odors at a time

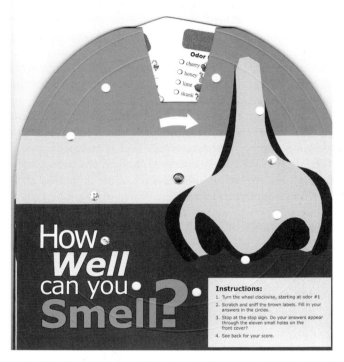

Figure 3.6 Photograph of the front of the Smell Wheel, a game-like rotating odor identification test. This forced-choice test was designed to capture the child's imagination and to provide a standardized test measure with a minimum number of trials and odors known to young children. Copyright @ 2012 Sensonics International, Haddon Heights, NJ, USA.

for sampling. Multiple-choice alternatives use both words and pictures of the stimuli, increasing the likelihood that a child understands the concept to be explored (Figure 3.6). The subjects' answers, which are made next to the words and pictures, rotate around and appear in small holes at the front of the test after all items are answered. The number of correct answers is the sum of the holes that appear filled in.

Odor Discrimination Tests. Odor discrimination procedures establish how well a subject can differentiate various odorant qualities. Such tests do not require naming or formal identification of the odors. They are widely employed in the food and beverage industry, but less so in clinical testing. For example, a manufacturer may be interested in changing an expensive ingredient for a less costly one and wishes to establish whether any difference is discerned in the food flavor.

There are numerous odor discrimination test paradigms. In a same/different test, a subject indicates on each of a series of trials whether two stimuli are the same or different. The number of same-odor and different-odor trials that are correctly differentiated serves as the dependent measure, although values based upon signal detection analysis can be employed as well (O'Mahony et al., 1979; Potter & Butters, 1980). Other variations of this general theme include picking the "odd" stimulus in a set from which only the "odd" stimulus differs, such as the triangle test and the match-to-sample discrimination test, where the subject must determine from a set of foils (i.e., confounding odors) which odor smells the same as a target odorant (Frijters, 1980).

Perhaps the most complex odor discrimination test is that of *multidimensional scaling* (MDS) (Schiffman et al., 1981). In one application of this procedure, similarity ratings are made for all possible pairs of stimuli presented to a subject. Correlations among the ratings are then subjected to an algorithm that places the stimuli into two- or three-dimensional space relative to their perceived similarities. The perceptual ability of participants is established by the amount of odorant groupings that correspond spatially to normal subjects. MDS is seldom used in the clinic because it is time consuming and there are no well-validated norms. It is interesting that stimulus spaces derived from similarity ratings of odor names are essentially identical to those derived from actually smelling the same odors, suggesting the close association of semantic representations with odors, per se (Carrasco & Ridout, 1993). A picture showing the three-dimensional MDS solution for odor similarity judgments for a subset of UPSIT odorants is shown in Figure 3.7. Olfactory stimuli that are closest in space are odorants with the most similar smells.

Odor Threshold Tests. Odor threshold tests seek to define the lowest concentration of an odor that is perceived or can be discerned from a standard. Like identification tests, some of these tests are commercially available (Table 3.1; Figure 3.8). The *absolute or detection threshold* is the lowest odorant concentration where some sensation is perceived, usually not odor quality. The *recognition threshold* is the lowest concentration where odor quality can be discerned, e.g., like a banana, at a level higher than chance. The *difference threshold* (also termed the differential threshold) is the smallest amount by which a stimulus can be perceived stronger or weaker than another concentration of the same odor, i.e., the "just noticeable difference," or JND. Within much of the stimulus continuum, the increment in odorant concentration (ΔI) needed to produce a JND increases as the comparison concentration (I) increases, with the ratio approximating a constant (Weber's law; $\Delta I / I = K$; Weber, 1834).

Detection thresholds are generally preferred in clinical assessment to both recognition and differential thresholds as they are more reliable and take less time. It should be emphasized that there is no such thing as "the threshold value" for a given odorant for all persons, despite the insistence and practical need of regulatory agencies in defining such measures. Establishing useful odor or taste threshold guidelines applicable to large groups of subjects for aesthetic or other purposes in environmental situations is challenging and contentious, given the costs involved in completely eliminating odors or tastants from urban air or water to levels that no one can detect them at all times (see, e.g., Burlingame, 2015) Threshold tests provide relative values that depend upon multiple factors, including: (a) age and gender, (b) whether detection or recognition is assessed, (c) the size of concentration steps used in testing, (d) the type of dilution medium employed (e.g., air or liquid), (e) stimulus volume, (f) time between trials, (g) number of choices at each step (e.g., target

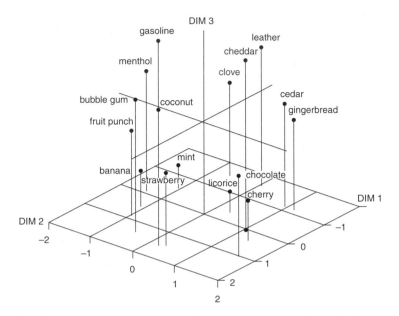

Figure 3.7 Three-dimensional space representation of selected UPSIT odors based on multidimensional scaling of similarity judgments. DIM denotes stimuli, e.g. some patients with schizophrenia dimension as follows: DM1, fruitiness/pleasantness; DM2, strength; DM3 familiarity/spiciness. Odors that are closest in 3-dimensional space smell were rated more alike than those farther apart. From Carrasco & Ridout (1993). Copyright 1993 by the American Psychological Association, Inc.

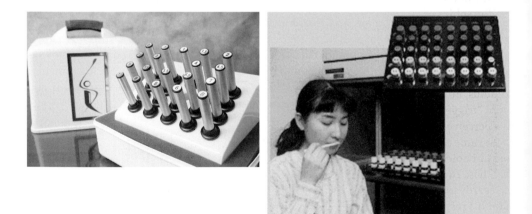

Figure 3.8 Two commercially available threshold test kits. Left: The Snap & Sniff® Threshold Test (Sensonics International, Haddon Heights, NJ, USA). The rose-like odorant, phenylethyl alcohol, is provided in 15 half-log concentration steps ranging from −9 log vol/vol to −2 log vol/vol, although custom odors are also available. The stimulus is delivered via smell "wands" and a single staircase method is used to present the stimuli. Right: The T & T Olfactometer (Daiichi Yakuhin Sangyo Co. Ltd, Tokyo, Japan). This is a non-forced-choice test of odor recognition and detection thresholds for 5 different odorants. These are presented to the subject on perfumer's blotter strips, which are dipped into the test solution for each trial and then discarded.

odorant vs. one or more blank foils), and (h) the psychophysical algorithm employed (e.g., the number of trials can greatly alter the threshold value). Although there are reports that threshold values exhibit untoward variability (Brown et al., 1968; Yoshida, 1984; Stevens et al., 1998), such variability is not the norm when the subject is given appropriate instructions and a sufficient number of forced-choice trials are used.

The two most common means of presenting different concentrations of odorants for threshold testing are the ascending method of limits procedure (AML) and the initially ascending single staircase procedure (ASP). Odorants are presented sequentially from low to high concentrations in the AML, with estimates of the transition point between detection and no detection (Cain et al., 1983). In the ASP, the stimulus series commences below the threshold range as in the AML. Once above-chance performance appears, the next lower concentration of odorant is then presented. A series of "staircase" reversals are subsequently collected, with decreases in concentration made for the next trial or trial sequence when correct detection occurs. Increases in concentration are employed when incorrect responses are reported. The ASP, which has numerous variants, achieves a reliable threshold estimate with relatively few trials. One version of this procedure – the maximum-likelihood adaptive staircase procedure –evaluates the probable threshold continuously from prior responses (Linschoten et al., 2001). On a given trial, a computer establishes the tentative threshold value. The next trial is then made that approximates this value. Although this procedure results in a quicker convergence onto the threshold value than the AST, it requires a computer to calculate the concentration to be presented on each trial and in practice it produces thresholds analogous to those using the AST procedure.

Threshold values are not static entities and some question whether the threshold concept is even valid. Adherents to signal detection theory view perception of weak signals from a different standpoint. According to their thinking, the detection situation comprises two processes: the sensitivity of the system in discerning a signal from background of noise and the liberalness or conservativeness of the subject in reporting the presence of the signal, i.e., the subject's response criterion. The latter includes the influence of subject expectancy and reward regarding the presence or absence of a signal. Although forced-choice procedures control to a large degree the response criterion, SDT provides a measure of both the subject's sensory sensitivity and the response criterion (Tanner, Jr. & Swets, 1954). For example, two individuals may experience the same subtle degree of sensation from a weak stimulus, but one may report a sensation and the other may not. The former person may be more "trigger happy" than the second who may wish to be absolutely certain the stimulus was perceived correctly. In this hypothetical example, the stimulus may have been detected to the same degree, but the two subjects had different reporting criteria. In a traditional non-forced-choice detection threshold paradigm, the investigator would incorrectly conclude that these two subjects differed in sensitivity to the stimulus, when, in fact, they only differed in regards to their response criterion (Figure 3.9). Apart from providing an estimate of the subject's response criterion, signal detection measurement can detect subtle variations in an individual's sensitivity that are difficult to detect by other means, for example, the small changes in olfactory sensitivity that occur across phases of the menstrual cycle (Doty et al., 1981). It is rarely used clinically because stable measurements typically require a large number of trials and normative data are lacking.

Odor Memory Tests. The goal of an odor memory test is to measure how much a memory of a recently experienced odor is retained over time. This is not straightforward for several

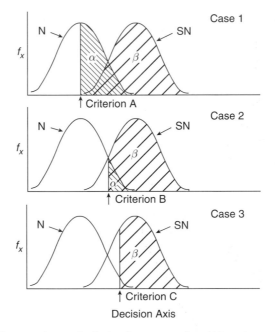

Figure 3.9 The distance between the two distributions is a measure of sensitivity and termed d′. In these examples, the sensitivities remain constant but different response criteria are denoted. Thus, the distance between the noise (N) and signal plus noise (SN) distributions are similar. In Case 1, a liberal criterion was chosen by the subject in which a relatively large number of false positive responses occurred (i.e., α, reports of the presence of an odor when a blank which represents noise (N) is presented). In Cases 2 and 3, more conservative criteria were chosen, decreasing both the number of false positives (α) and hits (β). Traditional threshold measures confound the influences of sensory or perceptual sensitivity and the setting of the response criterion. From [Doty 1976]. Copyright © 1976, Academic Press, Orlando, Florida.

reasons. First, recall in general may be the factor that is being assessed, not just odor memory. Second, subjects have a strong tendency to assign a name (label) to an odor, e.g., "chocolate," and then remember that name or label. In fact, they are just retrieving a concept or label from long-term memory and attaching it to the stimulus, reflecting the fact that they already know the smell of chocolate. When the chocolate odor is experienced again, they remember having smelled the odor of chocolate – an odor and association that was present in long-term memory during the entire process. Thus, an ideal odor memory test would employ unfamiliar odors that are not easily labeled or recalled from long-term memory. This is a daunting task given that so few of such odorants exist and even when labels are not readily applied, hedonic, or other semantic labels are assigned. Both short- and long-term odor recognition is facilitated by such verbal encoding (Jehl et al., 1997), providing one explanation why women, unlike men, exhibit better odor memory on the left side of the nose, conceivably by accessing left hemisphere verbal resources (Doty & Kerr, 2005).

Operationally, odor memory tests require a subject to smell a target stimulus (or set of target stimuli) and after variable delay, identify the target stimulus from foils (confounders). For example, one odor memory test (Figure 3.10) has 12 microencapsulated odors that are smelled individually and the subject must select, after 10-, 30-, or 60-second intervals, the target odorant from a set of four alternatives (Doty, 2003). During the delay periods, the subject is required to count aloud backwards in threes from 260 in an effort to minimize the rehearsal of any verbal labels the subject may apply to the target stimulus. The

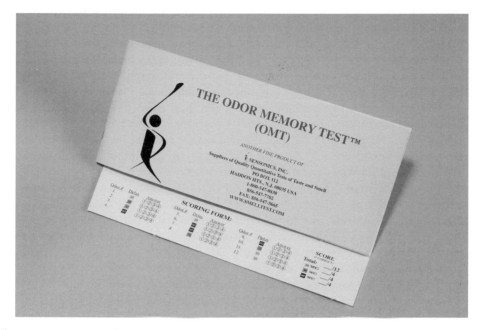

Figure 3.10 A commercially available odor memory/discrimination test. A page containing a single microencapsulated odor strip is scratched with a pencil tip and smelled by the subject, who then counts backwards in steps of three from 260. After delays of 10, 30, or 60 seconds, the volunteer is shown four written odor choices on the same page and asked which of the four corresponds to the initial stimulus. The responses are recorded on a fold out tab on the bottom of the last page of the booklet, as shown for of the test booklet above. Copyright © 2012 Sensonics International.

dependent measures are the proportion of trials where correct performance occurs at each delay interval, as well as the total number of correct trials. The overall score is influenced by sex and age, like tests of threshold and odor identification. Measures on this test may be more sensitive to the influence of drugs, such as alcohol, than scores on odor identification and detection threshold procedures (Patel et al., 2004).

As noted earlier in this chapter, poor performance on an odor memory test must be interpreted cautiously, because anyone with a deficit in odor detection or discrimination will, of necessity, show an overall deficit on odor memory tests. Thus, from a purist's perspective, a delay interval effect is needed to infer that some change in memory is present. Normal people show little decline in remembering odors over several days in some instances (Engen & Ross, 1973; Engen et al., 1973). Hence, when no delay interval effects are seen on a test such as that shown in Figure 3.10, the test score may, in fact, simply represent a test score from a match-to-sample discrimination test.

Suprathreshold Rating and Scaling Procedures. Perception of the strength of suprathreshold attributes such as odor quality, intensity, and pleasantness can be measured easily. Such characteristics are often assessed as a function of concentration, since this is one of few physical olfactory dimensions that can be varied reliably. Theoretically, ratings of odorant intensity, for example, could reflect the extent of neural damage present in the afferent pathway, given that the intensity of a stimulus is related in most sensory systems to the number of recruited neurons and the frequency at which they fire (Drake et al., 1969). Since suprathreshold ratings of intensity appear to be less sensitive to olfactory dysfunction than odor identification and threshold test measures, they have rarely been used clinically. Importantly, intensity ratings are relatively insensitive to the olfactory losses of age (Rovee et al., 1975). It is possible that such ratings are detecting elements of normal function that are missed by other procedures. Most PD patients, for example, report some type of smell on the majority of UPSIT items, but they are unable to identify them, suggesting that suprathreshold odor intensity is not the factor that is most affected in this disease.

The attributes of odors can be assessed using straightforward rating scales. Such measurements have been employed throughout history and notably by Sir Francis Galton (McReynolds & Ludwig, 1987). Today, two rating scales are in common use: category scales and visual analog or line scales. In category scaling, the subject specifies the perceived amount of attribute by indicating which of a discrete set of categories describes it best, whereas in visual analog scales the participant indicates the value by placing a mark along a line. Usually descriptors, such as "no smell" and "extremely strong smell," are placed at the ends of the line, although there are many variations on this theme. To overcome a tendency of subjects to bunch responses at the extremes of the scale and to provide more ratio-like responses, descriptors have been added along the scale to mimic better the geometric progression of suprathreshold intensity sensations noted by other methods (e.g., Neely et al., 1992; Green et al., 1996). Examples of various forms of rating scales are presented in Figure 3.11.

One scaling technique that attempts to mitigate non-linearity in rating responses is known as cross-modal matching. The most popular procedure assigns numbers in relative proportion to the perceived attribute under study, usually intensity, where the goal is to establish ratio relationships among the perceived characteristics. In the "free modulus" method, the subject assigns a number to the first stimulus presented. All values allotted to stimuli after this are made in proportion to the intensity of the other stimuli. For example, if the subject allocates the first stimulus number 20, when a subsequent concentration is presented that smells half as strong, the number 10 would be assigned. A stimulus that is 10 times as strong would be given the number 200, and so on. In some cases, the subject is provided with a standard ("fixed modulus") for which a number has been allocated (often the middle stimulus of the series) in an effort to provide more reliable responses. In general, absolute values of the numbers are not important, only the ratios between them, although on average, stronger stimuli are initially assigned larger numbers than weaker stimuli.

Results from magnitude estimation procedures are usually plotted on log-log coordinates (log magnitude estimates on the vertical axis and log odorant concentrations on the horizontal axis), where they typically are reasonably linear. The best fit line is determined using linear regression. The resulting function, $\log P = n \log \Phi + \log k$, where P = perceived intensity, k = the Y intercept, Φ = stimulus concentration, and n = the slope, can be represented in its exponential form as a power function, $P = k\Phi^n$. The slope serves as the index of sensory function. The larger the value of n, i.e., the steeper the slope, the greater the increase in perceived intensity as concentration is increased. This value varies from odor to odor, but for olfaction rarely exceeds 1. An example of magnitude estimates of coffee odor in a pioneering study by Reese and Stevens is presented in Figure 3.12.

Unlike intensity, magnitude estimates of odor pleasantness or unpleasantness ("valence") are often not monotonic as a function of concentration. In some cases, odors are pleasant at lower concentrations but are unpleasant at higher concentrations. To obtain magnitude estimates in such cases, one can assign negative numbers to the unpleasant concentrations and positive numbers to pleasant concentrations and employ ratio estimates separately for each end of the

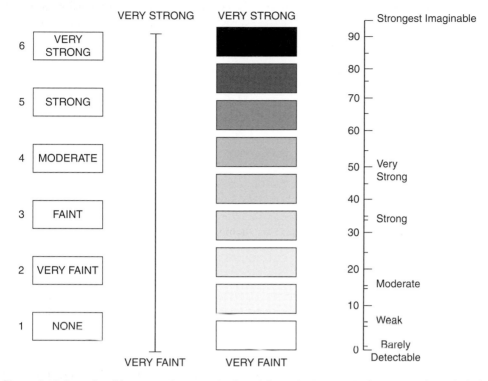

Figure 3.11 Examples of four types of rating scales. From left to right: (a) A standard category scale in which the subject provides answers in discrete categories; (b) a visual analog or graphic scale with anchors (descriptors) at each end; (c) a category scale with logarithmic visual density referents to denote non-linear increasing magnitudes of sensation, with verbal anchors at each end; (d) a labeled magnitude scale with labels or anchors positioned in logarithmic fashion. In these examples the scales are oriented in a vertical position; in many cases, such scales are presented in a horizontal (left: right) configuration. Copyright © 2002, Richard L. Doty.

valence continuum. Examples of changes that occur for a number of odorants in both intensity and hedonics as a function of odorant concentration are shown as log-linear plots in Figure 3.13.

Magnitude estimation is rarely employed in the clinic, despite its theoretical appeal. Not all subjects consistently provide ratio estimates of stimuli or understand the concept of producing sensory ratios. Accurate responses require a good memory for the prior stimulus. If too much time elapses between stimulus presentations, memory of the prior stimulus fades. If too little time passes, adaptation can distort the relationship. Line scales are superior to magnitude estimation and category scales when such factors as variability, reliability, and ease of use are taken into consideration (Lawless, 1986a 1986b). Line scales that employ descriptors placed at logarithmic intervals along its path are now widely used and, on several grounds, are preferable to classic scaling paradigms (Figure 3.12).

Regardless of the scaling procedure employed, suprathreshold judgments of trait magnitudes are relative and influenced by such factors as context, e.g., a moderately intense odor is reported more intense when presented with weak comparison stimuli than with strong comparison stimuli (Helson, 1964; Eyman, 1975). Theoretically, the influences of context are of little concern in clinical tests so long as standardized stimulus presentation procedures

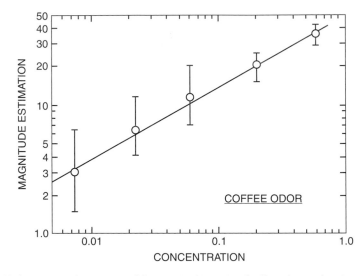

Figure 3.12 Median magnitude estimates of the perceived intensity of coffee odor as a function of concentration plotted on a log/log scale. Interquartile ranges indicated by vertical lines. From Reese and Stevens (1960).

are followed and normative data are available based on such procedures. Unfortunately, normative data are lacking for suprathreshold scaling measures.

The choice of test largely depends on whether smell function is to be measured for basic clinical screening, medicolegal purposes, or detailed research. We suggest that tests of identification are the most suitable for screening in a non-research setting. The time available to a clinician is a highly relevant factor and *the* major reason why objective measurement is rarely undertaken. In a busy hospital clinic where time is very limited, brief tests employing three or four scratch and sniff odorants are useful as they take a minute or less to complete, are inexpensive, and are sufficiently reliable for rapid screening and some survey work. For screening purposes, all odors should be identified correctly to be certain a patient's smell function is normal. Any mistake warrants further investigation with longer tests. Such brief tests have been used not only for screening, but in surveys and experimental studies. For example, the four-item Pocket Smell Test (PST) was incorporated into the US National Health and Nutrition Examination Survey (NHANES), in which large numbers of the US population are periodically evaluated for their general health (Rawal et al., 2015).

If more time is available, or if more certainty is needed regarding the degree of dysfunction, longer tests should be administered (see Table 3.1). Some, such as the 40-item UPSIT or its 12-item version (the B-SIT), can be self-administered in the waiting room. Compared to the three or four-item PST (~$2.00/patient), such tests are more expensive (currently ~$13.00 & $27.00, respectively). Other procedures, which require a test supervisor and cannot be posted, are generally as cost effective as the PST if the expense of the administrator is not taken into account. These include versions of the Sniffin' Sticks and numerous threshold tests (e.g., the Snap & Sniff® and the Sniffin' Sticks threshold tests).

Evaluation of possible malingering can be made with longer assessments but if there is a compensation claim then referral to a Smell and Taste unit is advisable, as discussed in detail in Chapter 7. For both SST and UPSIT it is advisable to obtain local population normative data for comparison with the planned research sample. Use of historical norms is not recommended in

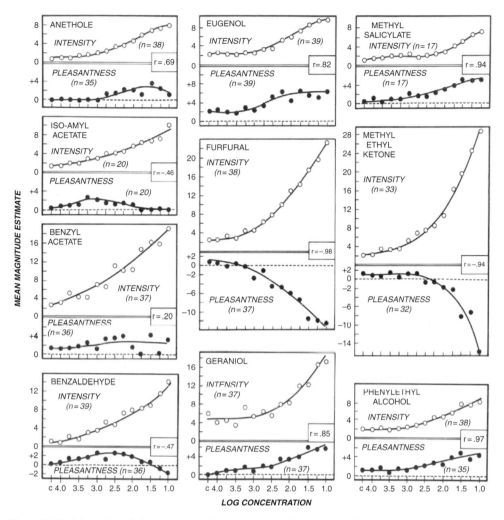

Figure 3.13 Relationship of pleasantness and intensity magnitude estimates to log volume concentration in propylene glycol diluent for 10 compounds. r = Pearson correlation coefficient between pleasantness and intensity estimates across data points differing significantly in intensity from control (c). Lines fitted to data points by visual inspection. From Doty (1975). Copyright © 1975, Psychonomic Society.

many research settings. While psychophysical testing is reliable in the early stages of cognitive disorders, e.g., Alzheimer's disease, such evaluation is questionable where moderate or advanced dementia precludes an understanding of the test requirements. In these cases, non-olfactory tests such as the Picture Identification Test (Vollmecke & Doty, 1985) can be employed to determine whether patients can be evaluated adequately or, in experimental paradigms, as covariates to minimize or control for the influences of cognitive state on test performance.

Electrophysiological Tests

The Electro-olfactogram. Odorants induce a negative potential within the olfactory neuroepithelium that largely reflects summed neural activity of the receptor cells (Hosoya & Yashida,

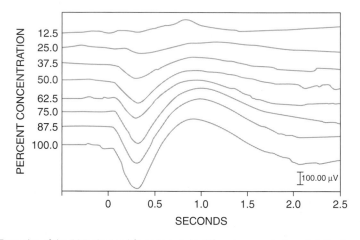

Figure 3.14 Examples of the EOG obtained for H₂S at eight different concentrations (relative to saturation). Note that, in general, the stronger the concentration, the larger the EOG amplitude. Photo courtesy of Bruce Turetsky, University of Pennsylvania.

1937; Ottoson, 1956). This potential, termed the electro-olfactogram (EOG), can be measured by electrodes placed on or near the surface of the epithelium. The size of the this potential varies with stimulus concentration (Figure 3.14) and shows little evidence of adaptation, supporting the notion that adaptation is largely a central phenomenon as reported in 1927 (Zwaardemaker, 1927). While it is possible to measure the EOG extra-nasally with surface electrodes placed on the nasion (the nasal bridge area), the response is relatively small (Wang et al., 2004).

Measurement of the EOG may be useful in some clinical cases with the following provisos: (a) the EOG may be unobtainable in many individuals if, as often happens, the subject is unable to tolerate electrodes placed in the anaesthetized nose; (b) maintaining reliable EOG responses over even brief periods of time can be exacting; (c) there are no published normative data to ascertain whether a given EOG is typical or not; (d) in a study by Turetsky et al. (2009), schizophrenic patients had abnormally large depolarization responses following odor stimulation, implying that compensatory mechanisms may be present. In accord with such findings are reports that long-term unilateral nasal occlusion in mice produces enhanced amplitudes of EOG responses on the occluded side, although the EOGs have slower onset and recovery kinetics (Waggener & Coppola, 2007); (e) the lack of an EOG response can reflect sampling issues, rather than lack of functioning olfactory tissue, since damage to the olfactory epithelium can be patchy; and (f) normal EOGs can be obtained several hours after death in animals, implying that a normal EOG need not always be a reflection of odor perception, per se (Scott et al., 2000).

Olfactory Evoked and Event-Related Potentials. Evoked potentials (EPs), occur during the earliest stages of sensory processing. They are minimally influenced by non-sensory mental events (e.g., attention, ideation). Although such potentials may be obtained from the olfactory bulb and amygdala during surgery, they have not been measured non-invasively (Kobal, 2003). In contrast, olfactory event-related potentials (OERPs) can be measured reliably from the scalp and, for this reason, have some clinical utility. They reflect changes

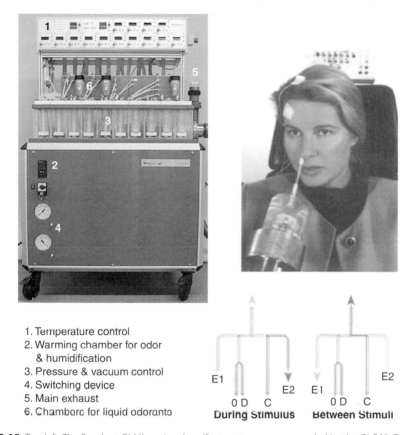

1. Temperature control
2. Warming chamber for odor & humidification
3. Pressure & vacuum control
4. Switching device
5. Main exhaust
6. Chambers for liquid odorants

E1

E2

E I

E2

0 D   C
During Stimulus

0 D   C
Between Stimuli

Figure 3.15 Top left: The Burghart OM6b, a six-odor olfactometer, now superseded by the OLO23. Top right: A recording setup showing a thin piece of Teflon tubing inserted about 1 cm into the nose. Bottom right: Technique of creating an odorant bolus without disturbing the main airflow. The main odorless airstream, C is continually blown into the nose between stimulus presentations. The odor-containing air (O) is sucked away by vacuum E1. During a stimulus presentation, the odorless airstream (C) is vented away by vacuum E2 while E1 is closed simultaneously. This allows the odor-containing gas to reach the nose imperceptibly, without disturbing the main inflow and therefore avoiding trigeminal stimulation. Reproduced with permission from Burghart Messtechnik, Hamburg.

induced in electrical fields generated by large populations of cortical neurons before, during, or after a sensory or internal psychological event (Gevins & Remond, 1987). Unlike pattern-evoked visual potentials, measurement of OERPs is time consuming and exacting. Inter-stimulus intervals are typically 30–60 seconds to minimize adaptation and usually no more than 16 stimuli can be presented per session to avoid subject fatigue. The signals are small (<50 µV) and often difficult to extract by averaging from the background EEG because of the low signal-noise ratio.

A large population of olfactory nerve cells needs to be activated simultaneously to obtain a detectable OERP and to this end, elaborate olfactometers have been developed (Figure 3.15). The technology is upgraded continuously and a small basic machine is available that will handle up to two odors. All olfactometers deliver a well-defined odorant pulse with a rapid rise time (<100 ms) embedded in a fast flowing, heated and humidified airstream delivered to the

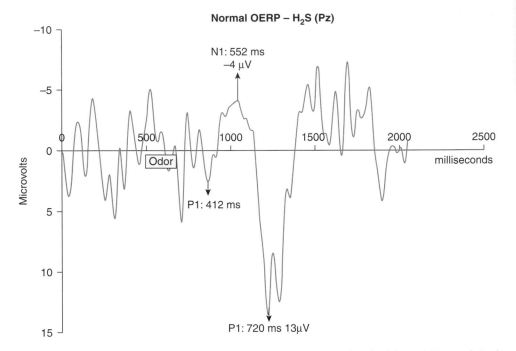

Figure 3.16 Normal olfactory event-related potential evoked by a 200 ms pulse of H_2S (2 ppm). Trace is derived from A1–Pz. Filters are set at 1–50 Hz.

nose at 36°C to simulate imperceptibly the nasal environment, which is about 1°C below body temperature. The continuous airflow (typically 8 liters/min) is calibrated and maintained by mass-flow controllers and the stimulus pulses are computer operated. Care must be taken to select odors with minimal intranasal trigeminal co-stimulation otherwise a trigeminal evoked potential of similar shape but slightly shorter latency will be recorded (Geisler & Murphy, 2000). Suitable stimulants include hydrogen sulfide (bad eggs), vanillin, and phenylethyl alcohol (rose like).

An example of OERP waveforms are shown in Figure 3.16. The shape is a typical triphasic wave similar to the pattern-evoked visual potential. P1, the first positive peak, occurs at latencies around 400 ms which is considerably later than the equivalent peak for visual evoked potentials (about 60ms). The most consistent response, P2, is usually selected for latency measurement while amplitude value is expressed as the difference in microvolts (μV) between N1 and P2. The prolonged latency of OERPs, compared to the visual evoked potentials, presumably reflects absorption and other physiochemical phenomena within the nasal mucosa. Also, the olfactory receptor cell axons are extremely small and slowly conducting. When this delay is taken into account, the OERP N1 and P2 latencies are comparable to the N100 and P200/P300 values seen in other sensory systems. In general, N1 and P2 amplitudes are positively correlated with odorant concentration, i.e., the number of activated neurons, whereas N1 and P2 latencies are negatively correlated with odorant concentration (Tateyama et al., 1998). Thresholds to vanillin are inversely related to latencies, but not amplitudes, for the P1, N1, P2, and P3 components measured at the Cz scalp position (r value ranging from −0.45 to −0.59) (Tateyama et al., 1998). Attempts to relate odorant qualities to differences in the shape of OERPs have not been successful (Kobal & Hummel, 1988). Interestingly, late positive OERP amplitudes and latencies correlate weakly with scores on neuropsychological tests of visual-motor attention (Trail Making Test) and verbal memory (Geisler et al., 1999). Given the relatively high cost (currently $120,000 upwards) and practicality, OERPs are not measured routinely outside of specialized chemosensory clinics and it is uncertain whether OERPs add significantly to basic psychophysical clinical assessment. Even the best commercially available olfactometers are unstable and need daily attention and recalibration, although there is no doubt that with effort a clear olfactory potential can be derived (Figure 3.16). The OERP is of theoretical value in assessment of malingerers, assuming a real cheat can be persuaded to cooperate. Unfortunately, even those with genuine anosmia or hyposmia, especially where large compensation sums are known to be at stake, may become upset with the procedure and this can affect recording quality and its interpretation.

Non-Phase-Locked EEG Responses. Newer, more sensitive measures may overcome some of the problems associated with traditional OERPs. As reviewed in detail by Osman and Silas (2015), traditional EEG and OERP methodology can be combined into discrete and continuous-time frequency analyses. The processing and analysis of *induced* power modulations at any given frequency differs from the processing of OERPs. While a change in the ongoing EEG activity can be *time*-locked to a specific event, it is not necessarily *phase*-locked to that event. Given that phase varies randomly in relation to the event, the process of averaging, as conducted in traditional analysis of OERPs, can eliminate the signal of interest (Pfurtscheller & Lopes da Silva, 1999). For this reason, "continuous time-frequency" measures have been developed that allow for power calculations within both the time and frequency domains. One approach, termed "Continuous Wavelet Transformation" (CWT), passes a series of small frequency windows, or "wavelets," over every sample being subjected to spectral calculation (Schiff et al., 1994). The resulting CWT measurements, in essence, describe the evolution of power for specific frequencies over segments of the time-period of interest. Thus, non-phase-locked information becomes available that is often eradicated in the averaging process of FFT.

Huart et al. (2012) measured the phase-locked component of the EEG (i.e., the event-related potential) in response to olfactory and trigeminal stimulants, as well as non-phase-locked continuous changes in the frequency spectrum. The wavelet analysis assessed the evolution of EEG power across time during the period of odor stimulation for a frequency spectrum ranging from 0.3 to 30 Hz (Figure 3.17). A long-lasting increase in power around the theta frequency range (~5 Hz) was followed by a shorter decrease in alpha power (~10 Hz). Modulations in power were most prominent over the central electrode (Cz) (Figure 3.17). The authors proposed that this common topography indicates that both the ERP and the changes in time-frequency reflect the same stimulus-evoked cortical activity. Importantly, increases in power within the theta frequency range were positively correlated with olfactory function ($r = 0.70$, $p = .02$). This suggests that, in fact, time-frequency EEG modulations in response to olfactory stimulation reflect olfactory related cortical processing of functional relevance.

These more sophisticated measures are now being applied in clinical settings and will undoubtedly change how responses of brain EEG activity to odorants will be measured in future (Figure 3.18). It is yet to be determined how much they will contribute to diagnostic or prognostic aspects of current olfactory evaluations.

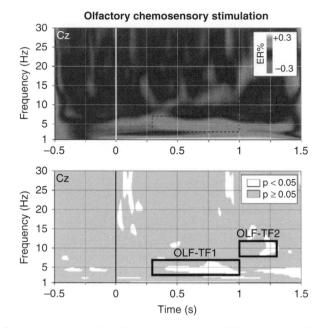

Figure 3.17 Time-frequency representation of the non-phase-locked EEG responses to olfactory chemosensory stimulation. Non-phase-locked EEG responses identified by performing across-trial averaging in the time-frequency domain, a procedure that enhances time-locked EEG responses regardless of whether they are phase-locked to stimulus onset. Upper panel: Group-level average time-frequency maps of oscillation amplitude (group-level average, electrode Cz vs. A1/A2), expressed as percentage increase or decrease relative to baseline (−0.4 to −0.1 sec) Note that olfactory stimulation elicits a long-lasting non-phase-locked increase of signal amplitude around 5 Hz (OLF-TF1; olfactory time frequency domain), possibly followed by event-related desynchronization in the alpha-band (OLF-TF2). Lower panel: Regions of the time-frequency matrix where signal amplitude deviated significantly from baseline (one-sample t-test). Adapted, with permission, from Figure 5 in Huart et al. (2012). (A black and white version of this figure will appear in some formats. For the color version, please refer to the plate section.)

Psychophysiological Tests

Although the term "psychophysiology" can have many meanings, in the present context psychophysiological tests are defined as those tests that rely primarily on reflex or reflex-like physiological responses to the presentation of an odorant. Most such responses are mediated by the autonomic nervous system, e.g., changes in heart rate, respiration rate, sweating, blood pressure, and temperature. Many such responses are highly variable and influenced by stimulation of the trigeminal system. There are few clinically useful psychophysiological tests for assessing olfaction. One test, the Sniff Magnitude Test, measures a reflex-like response to unpleasant odorants.

The Sniff Magnitude Test (SMT) is a computerized test in which odor-containing canisters are presented sequentially to the subject for sniffing (Frank et al., 2003, 2004, 2006) (left side of Figure 3.19). Within milliseconds of sniffing the surface of the canister, its top opens and either air or an unpleasant odor is released e.g., methylthiobutyrate (sulfurous) or ethyl 3-mercaptoproprinate (strong onion-like). Subjects who can smell the bad odor typically inhibit their inhalation irrespective of trigeminal sensory stimulation (Tourbier & Doty, 2007). A piezoelectric pressure transducer senses the negative pressure induced by the

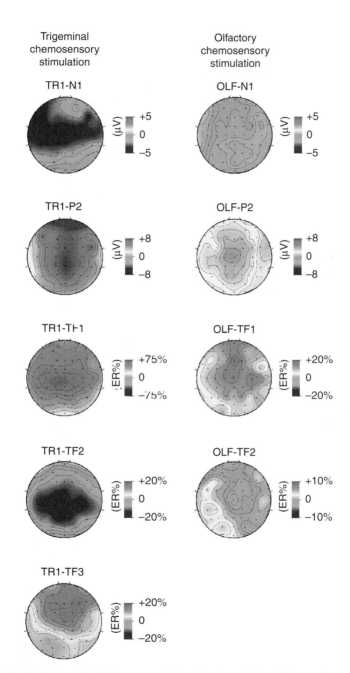

Figure 3.18 Scalp distribution of the EEG responses elicited by trigeminal and olfactory chemosensory stimulation. The scalp distribution of the EEG responses identified using across-trial averaging in the time domain (TRI-N1, TRI-P2, OLF-N1, OLF-P2) are expressed in microvolts, whereas the scalp distribution of the EEG responses identified using across-trial averaging in the time-frequency domain (TRI-TF1, TRI-TF2, TRI-TF3, OLF-TF1, OLF-TF2) are expressed as a percentage increase or decrease relative to baseline. Adapted, with permission, from Figure 2 in Huart et al. (2012). (A black and white version of this figure will appear in some formats. For the color version, please refer to the plate section.)

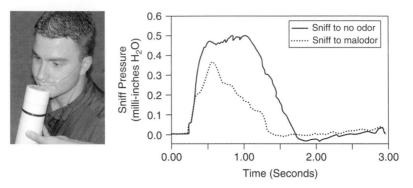

Figure 3.19 Left. Sniff Magnitude Test canister positioned for a sniff. Upon sniffing the top of the canister a bad smelling odor or odorless air is released. The pressure changes during inhalation are sent from the nasal cannula at the base of the nose to a pressure transducer. The digitized signal allows for the dynamics of the entire sniff epoch to be recorded by computer. Right: the top tracing represents a sniff to no odor (air); Bottom tracing represents a sniff to malodor. Note the abrupt attenuation of sniff response upon encountering the unpleasant smell.

subject's sniff via a cannula located just inside the nose and sends a digitized signal to a laptop computer. The sniff pressure measurements are calculated every 10 ms and recording continues until a return to ambient air pressure occurs. Sniff magnitude is a measure of the summated negative pressure values generated during the sniff epoch and it is proportional to the area under the sniff pressure-time curve. The *sniff magnitude ratio* is the ratio of the integrated sniff magnitude value given to an odorant compared to that obtained when sniffing non-odorized air. When suppression occurs more to an odorant than to a non-odorant, then this ratio is less than one. A picture of a subject's sniff tracings is presented on the right in Figure 3.19.

Both odor sniff magnitudes and sniff magnitude ratios correlate moderately with scores obtained from tests of odor identification, phenylethyl alcohol detection, and odor memory (r values range from 0.33 to 0.57) (Tourbier & Doty, 2007). Principal component analyses suggest that the SMT may evaluate aspects of olfactory function somewhat distinct from those measured by tests of odor identification, detection, and short-term memory, probably reflecting suprathreshold hedonics. While this procedure clearly distinguishes those with severe smell loss from normal people, it does not differentiate between mild or moderate degrees of smell loss (Figure 3.20). This happens, in part, because after a few trials some individuals are unwilling to sniff strongly enough those odors that are perceived to be unpleasant, limiting the number of valid trials obtainable. A hood or well-ventilated room is required, given the very unpleasant nature of its stimuli.

The full potential of the SMT has not been explored, but it may have a role in assessing malingerers or those with poor communication skills due to aphasia or dementia. Unfortunately, responses to odors are not purely reflexive, since they can be consciously suppressed. SMT depends critically upon the ability of a subject to perceive the hedonic elements of an odor. Hence, it may be less useful in patients with blunted emotions or those who do not respond normally to unpleasant stimuli, e.g., some patients with schizophrenia.

Psychophysiological responses that have received considerable attention relate to changes in heart rate variations and skin conductance following the presentation of an odorant. Most have recorded extremely variable results, and both of these measures are influenced by stimulus novelty or change. For a review of the earlier skin conductance literature, see Van Toller et al. (1983). Multiple measures of skin conductance have been

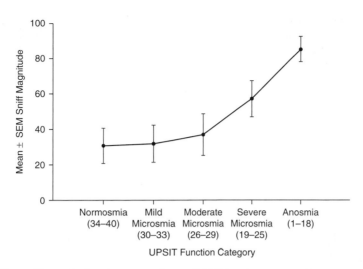

Figure 3.20 Mean sniff magnitude estimates as a factor of UPSIT function category. Means represent average responses across three trials each of six stimuli: 1% methylthiobutyrate; 3% methylthiobutyrate; 1% ethyl 3-mercaptoproprionate (malodors); 3% phenylethyl alcohol; 3% amyl (pentyl) acetate; 3% n-butanol (non-malodors). Sample sizes are as follows: Normosmia (n = 24), Mild Microsmia (n = 22), Moderate Microsmia (n = 17), Severe Microsmia (n = 23), Anosmia (n = 46). From Tourbier & Doty (2007).

assessed (e.g., response latency, amplitude, rise time, and decay times), although no one measure appears to have specific relevance (Van Toller et al., 1983). Importantly, both heart rate changes and skin conductance responses are strongest for stimuli that stimulate the trigeminal nerve, implying that some, if not most, of the effects of odorant stimulation on these autonomic responses are mediated through the trigeminal nerve (Jacquot et al., 2004). Reflecting similar tests on vision, heart rate has been found to correlate inversely with the perceived pleasantness of olfactory test stimuli, again suggesting the possible influence of trigeminal nerve activation (Bensafi et al., 2002).

Nasal Airway Patency and Airflow Measurement

There is little doubt that variation in the internal anatomy of the human nose can influence smell function, presumably by directing more airflow toward or away from the olfactory meatus or epithelium (Frye, 1995; Hornung, 2006). In a classic study, Leopold (1988) obtained CT scans from 34 patients with conductive or idiopathic hyposmia. The volume of nine three-dimensional sections of the nasal cavity above the middle turbinate were defined and entered into a stepwise regression analysis to determine which volumes were related most strongly to odor identification ability. A larger volume in the nasal region 10–15 mm below the cribriform plate and a smaller volume 1–5 mm below and anterior to the cribriform plate were associated with higher odor identification test scores. A higher capacity in the region 10–15 mm below and posterior to the cribriform plate potentiated both effects.

Unfortunately, the translation of such observations to specific clinical cases is difficult, and it is not clear whether they correlate with more practical clinical measures of nasal anatomy and function, such as acoustic rhinometry and rhinomanometry, respectively (see below). Many patients do report "nasal stuffiness" related to smell loss that is associated with

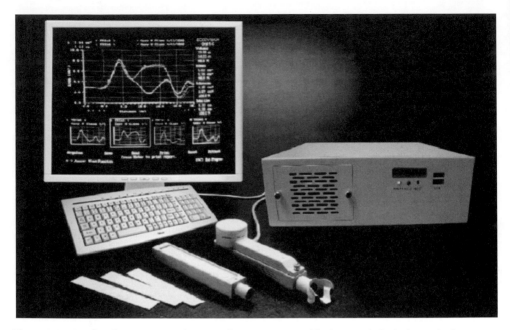

Figure 3.21 Picture of a computerized acoustic rhinometer system. The long vertical tube is attached to one nostril. The sound waves sent into the nose via this tube are reflected back into the same tube and analyzed by computer. Photo courtesy of Hood Laboratories, Penbroke, MA.

nasal congestion, for example, secondary to abnormal engorgement of the nasal turbinates (see Chapter 1). It should be stressed that a patient's perception of nasal blockage may not be consistent with actual airway blockage, given that nerve fibers which mediate sensations of airflow can be damaged even in a patent nose (Eccles et al., 1990). Overzealous removal of the nasal turbinates can result in "empty nose syndrome" where the patient reports a sensation of nasal blockage even though there is no obstruction (Chhabra & Houser, 2009). Similarly, subtle inflammation within the nasal mucosa can influence olfactory function adversely even in the presence of a normally patent and functioning airway (Kern, 2000).

Acoustic Rhinometry

Acoustic rhinometry (Figure 3.21) assesses elements of nasal anatomy. In this procedure, a series of clicks are projected into each nasal chamber and their reflections, detected by a microphone, are analyzed to assess the size of the nasal cavity. This method is analogous to sonar, which is used to identify the distance of objects under water. Volumetric assessment takes only a few minutes and requires minimal patient cooperation. An example of an acoustic rhinometry waveform is shown in Figure 3.22. The smallest cross-sectional area of the nasal cavity is the "nasal valve" (Figure 3.23). It is bounded medially by the nasal septum, inferiorly by the floor of the piriform aperture, and superiorly and laterally by the caudal margin of the upper lateral cartilage and its fibro-adipose attachment to the piriform aperture (Sulsenti & Palma, 1989). The size of the nasal valve can have significant effects on flow rate akin to pinching a garden hose (Figure 3.23).

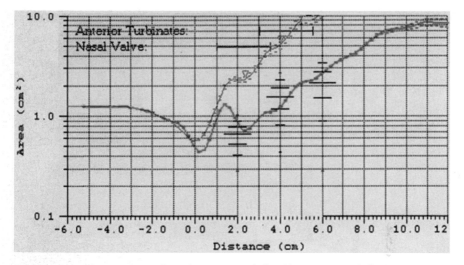

Figure 3.22 Acoustic rhinometry waveforms from a patient before (lower curve) and after (upper curve) nasal decongestion. The second dip in lower curve represents narrowing of the airway at the level of the nasal valve approximately 2.4 cm posterior to the external opening of the nose. The anterior sectors of the turbinates are indicated by the top horizontal line.

Acoustic rhinometry is widely used, in part because of its simplicity. Its usefulness for assessing olfaction has not been explored fully. Nasal volumes do not correlate meaningfully with olfactory thresholds in normal subjects (Nordin et al., 1998) or in patients responding to an acute nasal allergen (Lane et al., 1996), although general associations have been reported when severe congestion is present (Akerlund et al., 1995). The accuracy of this procedure for area and volume measures is less in anterior nasal obstruction compared to more posterior regions.

Rhinomanometry

Rhinomanometry assesses flow and pressure changes during breathing. In *anterior rhinomanometry*, one nostril is occluded with an adhesive patch connected to a small tube to measure pressure changes during inhalation and exhalation. Airflow through the opposite nasal chamber is simultaneously measured using a pneumotachometer (Figure 3.24). Resistance is calculated from a flow/pressure plot (Figure 3.25). In *posterior rhinomanometry*, the pressure-sensing tubing is placed via the mouth near the naso-pharynx. A facemask connected to a pneumotachometer is then employed to measure airflow through both nostrils and the total nasal resistance is calculated from the flow/pressure plot. The pressure tube can easily become clogged with saliva and some individuals do not tolerate the tube near the nasal pharynx, thus some training is required. Unlike anterior rhinomanometry, resistance in each nasal chamber is not assessed.

Although rhinomanometry reflects nasal resistance within the lower regions of the nasal cavity, it is not clear whether this investigation (like acoustic rhinometry) is meaningfully associated with olfactory function. To our knowledge, significant correlations between olfactory and nasal resistance measures have not been demonstrated. Nonetheless,

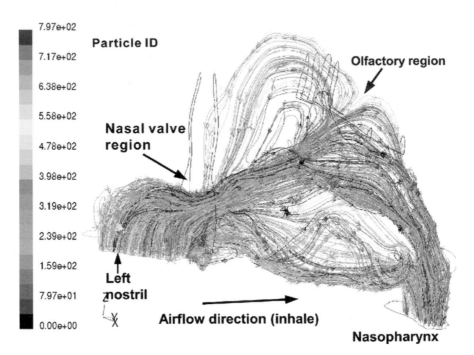

Figure 3.23 Streamline pattern for steady laminar airflow computed in the left nasal cavity. Narrowing the nasal valve airway suppresses the first eddy in the anterior part of the left nasal cavity and enhances the second eddy in the posterior superior part. The very large effect that these small nasal valve anatomical changes can have on streamline patterns is shown. Reproduced with permission from Zhao et al. (2004).

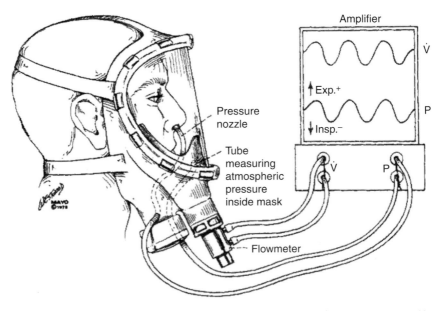

Figure 3.24 Anterior rhinomanometry with mask flow measurement. Transnasal pressure is measured by a pressure catheter occluding one naris. Airflow is measured by a pneumotacho-graph attached to a mask placed over the face. From McCaffrey (1991), © 1991, Raven Press.

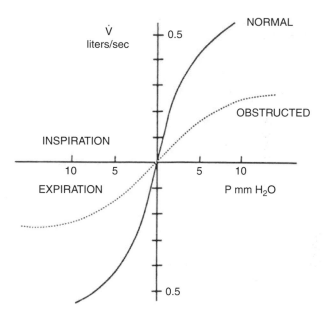

Figure 3.25 Pressure flow curve using rhinomanometry. Since nasal airflow is turbulent, the relationship between pressure and flow as shown by the S-shaped line in this figure is curvilinear. Since there is not a unique value for R = P/V, resistance must be determined at a specific pressure or flow point. The nasal resistance is shown at a pressure of 2 cm H2O (200 Pa). From McCaffrey (1991), © 1991, Raven Press.

septoplasty with partial inferior turbinectomy has been reported to enhance both olfactory function and nasal patency (Damm et al., 2003).

Imaging of Olfactory Structures

Computerized Axial Tomography

Computerized axial tomography (CAT or CT) is an x-ray imaging procedure sensitive to bone changes and to a lesser degree soft tissue inflammation such as rhinosinusitis. CT relies on x-rays passed through the body at multiple angles to construct a set of cross-sectional images. Clinically, such imaging is indicated if nasal obstruction is suspected due to anatomical deformity, polyps, or tumors, and to determine whether a nasal mass has extended intracranially. In patients with chemosensory disturbances associated with nasal disease, the CT evaluation should assess all of the nasal cavity, paranasal sinuses, hard palate, anterior skull base, orbits, and nasopharynx in both axial and coronal planes. Coronal scans are essential to visualize appropriately the anterior naso-ethmoid (ostiomeatal) region. CT scans, however, cannot display the olfactory bulbs or tracts.

Magnetic Resonance Imaging

Magnetic resonance imaging (MRI), like CT, produces multiplanar cross-sectional images using a combination of strong magnetic and radio frequency waves. Unlike CT it does not involve ionizing radiation. The resulting scan is, in essence, a map of water distribution within the brain and surrounding tissues. In T1-weighted images of the brain, fiber tracts are high intensity (white); congregations of neurons are intermediate (gray); and cerebrospinal fluid is low (black). In T2- and T2*-weighted images, cerebrospinal fluid is high intensity (white); fiber tracts low (black), and congregations of neurons intermediate (gray). The resolution of MRI is generally superior to CT. It cannot be used in patients with most varieties of cardiac pacemakers, intracranial magnetizable metallic clips (e.g., from aneurysm surgery), or other potentially mobile metal objects in their bodies. It is the method of choice when CNS lesions are suspected. It is also the preferred examination to display the olfactory bulbs and tracts, skull base (particularly for invasion by tumors), and brain inflammatory lesions associated with smell impairment such as multiple sclerosis or encephalitis. Injection of Gadolinium-DTPA, a paramagnetic contrast agent, is particularly useful for detection of skull base meningeal lesions, differentiating inflamed mucosa within the nose and sinuses from secretions, and separating solidly enhancing tumors from rim-enhancing inflammatory processes. An example of an MRI from a patient with olfactory groove meningioma is shown in Figure 3.26.

In the absence of other clinical signs, brain tumors rarely cause smell loss. A major exception is the olfactory groove meningioma which grows slowly and produces unilateral anosmia in the early stages. This is almost never detected by the patient or clinician as it is largely confined to one side of the nose. Only when anosmia is bilateral is the condition usually detected, assuming the patient is aware of it or the relevant clinician tests for its presence. Conversely, smell distortions, hallucinations, or other features suggestive of

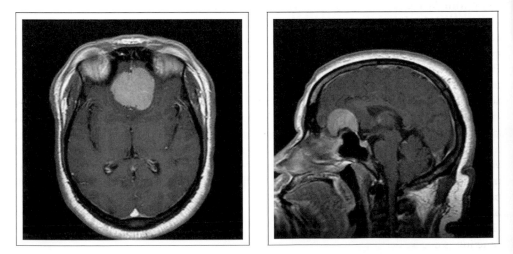

Figure 3.26 Olfactory groove meningioma. Left: Axial T1 MRI with contrast to show a large midline frontal mass with homogeneous enhancement. Right: Sagittal T1 MRI with contrast showing an extra-axial mass which was found to be an olfactory groove meningioma. The patient was anosmic but was not aware of this. Reproduced with permission from Yousem et al. (2001).

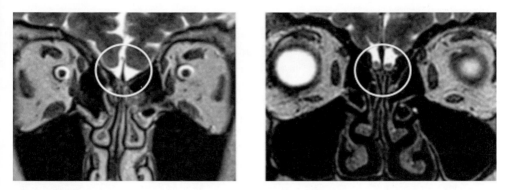

Figure 3.27 Left: MRI of a patient with isolated congenital anosmia. Within the ringed area the olfactory bulbs are missing. Right: healthy control. The olfactory bulbs are clearly visible as gray circular masses in the center of the ringed area. Reproduced with permission from Croy et al. (2012).

complex partial seizures are serious symptoms that merit urgent MRI imaging to detect neoplastic or vascular lesions, most often in the temporal pole. Likewise, those with a history of anosmia secondary to head injury need careful evaluation. Gradient echo (T2 or T2*) MRI sequences are sensitive to hemosiderin deposits, the tell-tale sign of petechial hemorrhages that might otherwise be overlooked by conventional sequences. Such lesions, as well as frank hemorrhage or contusion, are common in the temporal and frontal polar zones in head trauma victims (see Figure 5.3). Defects in either zone may result in central olfactory dysfunction that compounds the more peripheral shearing lesions of the olfactory fibers at the cribriform plate entry zone – a point of medicolegal significance.

In one study, the olfactory bulbs and other olfaction-related structures (Figures 3.27 and 3.28). Reduction in olfactory bulb volume affects older people (Yousem et al., 1998) and those with Alzheimer's disease (Thomann et al., 2009), head trauma (Yousem et al., 1995; Doty et al., 1997; Rombaux et al., 2006a; Collet et al., 2009), idiopathic congenital smell loss (Yousem et al., 1996; Croy et al., 2010), Kallmann syndrome (Bajaj et al., 1993; Yousem et al., 1993; Koenigkam-Santos et al., 2011), multiple sclerosis (Schmidt et al., 2011), Parkinson's disease (Kim et al., 2007; Brodoehl et al., 2012), total laryngectomy (Veyseller et al., 2011), and viral-related smell dysfunction (Rombaux et al., 2006b). Patients with schizophrenia as well as their first-order relatives exhibit decrements in olfactory bulb size (Turetsky et al., 2000; Turetsky et al., 2003; Nguyen et al., 2011). One longitudinal study of patients with hyposmia and anosmia demonstrated that over an average time interval of 15 months, changes in odor detection thresholds correlated with changes in olfactory bulb volume (Haehner et al., 2008). Olfactory bulb volumes of patients with sino-nasal disease increase following successful treatment (Gudziol et al., 2009). One report suggests that people affected by total blindness secondary to bilateral ocular or optic nerve lesions from birth or within two years of birth have larger olfactory bulbs than non-blind persons (Rombaux et al., 2010). However, the degree to which blindness, per se, influences olfactory function is debatable.

In one study of human olfactory bulbs and tracts of *cadavers* were imaged at high-resolution (0.2 mm^3 voxels at 3-Tesla and 0.1 mm^3 voxels at 9.4-Tesla) (Burmeister et al., 2012). The MRI scans were compared to Nissl-stained 20-µm tissue sections from the same

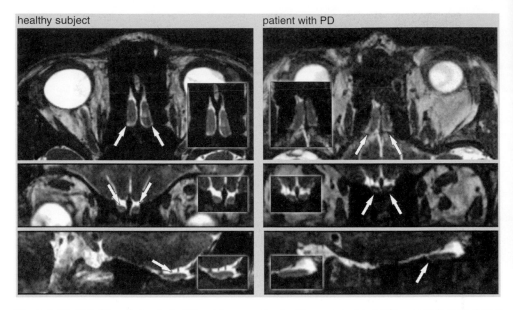

Figure 3.28 MRI of the olfactory bulbs (OBs; white arrows) in a healthy control subject (left) and a Parkinson's disease patient (right). Voxel size: 0.064 mm³. Imaging planes are from top downwards: axial; coronal, and sagittal. Manually traced OBs after segmentation are highlighted in red. Although comparable slices are selected, the OB volumes of the two subjects do not show major visible differences. Reproduced with permission from Brodoehl et al. (2012). (A black and white version of this figure will appear in some formats. For the color version, please refer to the plate section.)

patient donors (Figure 3.29). Four discrete intensity bands were discernible when imaged at 3-Tesla and these corresponded to the bulb's olfactory nerve layer, glomerular layer, external plexiform layer, and sectors of the mitral and granule cell layers. All cytoarchitectonic layers of the bulb were evident at 9-Tesla. Although these data show that MRI can delineate structural details of the olfactory bulb, this experiment was a proof-of-concept study *in vitro*. At present such investigations in living humans cannot be performed given the prolonged scanning time and potential risk of tissue damage, but no doubt these obstacles will be overcome in the future.

The clinical utility of olfactory bulb volume measurements is limited using current technology (typically no greater than 3T) and olfactory bulb volumes are highly variable, not disease specific, and large individual differences in bulb volume are typically present (Yousem et al., 1998; Doty & Kamath, 2014). Moreover, correlations between bulb size and psychophysical test measures are generally only moderate. Despite this, olfactory bulb volume measurement may have prognostic value (Rombaux et al., 2012). Rombaux et al. discovered that no further improvement in olfactory function was likely in post-traumatic anosmia or upper respiratory infection where the olfactory bulb volumes were less than 40 mm³. Such measurement has potential medicolegal relevance where the claimant appears to be anosmic.

Functional Imaging

Functional imaging allows *in vivo* assessment of human brain activity. It is relatively non-invasive, requires no anesthesia, and does not damage brain cells (Sobel et al.,

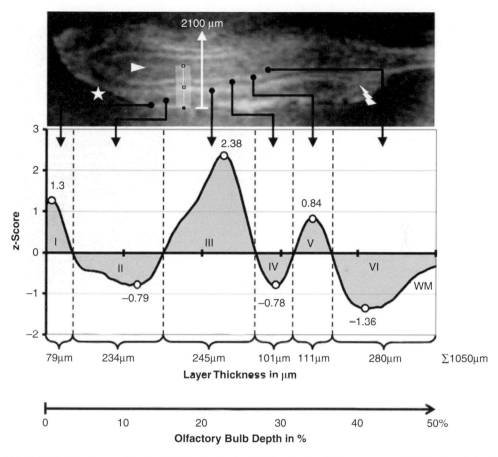

Figure 3.29 MR microscopic analysis of the olfactory bulb (OB) cortical lamination pattern at 9.4 T. Visual analysis of images obtained from MR microscopy at 9.4 T enables a direct identification of all six OB's cortical layers and the central white matter (WM, white arrowhead). This allows an exact assignment with signal intensity profile results obtained from a sagittal T2 w image. The profile line (bright yellow line) expansion of the line width (light yellow semi-transparent band) ranges from the inferior OB's surface (0%) toward the OB center (at 50%) covering the layers I–VI and a part of the WM. Intensity profile analysis (IPA) enables the measurement of intra-individual maximum or minimum z-score values (white dots) as the corresponding layer thickness for each layer. I = olfactory nerve layer (ONL), II = glomerular layer (GL), III = external plexiform layer (EPL), IV = mitral cell layer (MCL), V = internal plexiform layer (IPL), VI = granule cell layer (GCL), white arrow = total OB diameter (=2100 μm), white star/white arrow = regions excluded from evaluation due to structural changes of the lamination pattern. Reproduced with permission from Burmeister et al. (2012).

2003). A considerable amount of new information about the olfactory system has accrued using such procedures. For example, we now know that sectors of the cerebellum, parietal lobe, occipital lobe, and inferior and superior temporal gyri are involved to some degree in higher-order processing of odors as well as sniffing. Functional imaging has been used little in clinical assessment of olfactory disturbances, largely because of practicality, cost, and the fact that most olfactory disorders are easily detected and quantified by less expensive means. While functional imaging has tremendous research potential, its clinical utility for olfaction has yet to be realized. Potentially it may have relevance in the medicolegal domain, especially where there is a question of amplification of symptoms or malingering.

Four types of functional imaging are reviewed in this section; namely, Positron Emission Tomography (PET), functional MRI (fMRI), Single Photon Emission Tomography (SPECT), and magnetoencephalography (MEG).

Positron Emission Tomography

In positron emission tomography (PET), selected radioactive tracers are chosen that identify, indirectly, the level of neural activity in various regions of interest. For example, ^{18}F-2-deoxyglucose (^{18}FDG) is used to investigate cerebral glucose metabolism, whereas $H_2{}^{15}O$ examines cerebral blood flow. In one application of this procedure, specific biologic compounds tagged with a positron emitting radioisotope (tracer) such as ^{15}O, ^{18}F, or ^{11}C are injected intravenously and at a variable period later a sensory stimulus is presented. The brain regions activated by the stimulus increase their glucose metabolism because they emit more positrons than the surrounding brain tissue. This is measured by an array of radiation detectors encircling the head. Since the half-life of most tracers is relatively short (e.g., in the case of ^{15}O, ~2 minutes), the patient's brain can be scanned repeatedly in a single session with relatively minimal radiation exposure, provided there is a continuous supply of ^{15}O from a nearby Cyclotron.

Of particular interest are developments in which specific PET or SPECT tracers target defined neurochemical pathways. For example, ^{18}F-fluoro-L-dopa (^{18}F-FDOPA) is taken up by L-aromatic amino acid decarboxylase (AAAD), converted to ^{18}F-fluorodopamine, packaged in synaptic vesicles, released into the synapse and subsequently degraded. Vesicular monoamine transporter type 2 (VMAT2), which packages monoamines into synaptic vesicles, is labeled by ^{11}C-dihydrotetrabenazine. Dopamine and related membrane transporters can be labeled using ^{11}C, ^{18}F, ^{125}I, or ^{99m}Tc. Interestingly, nigrostriatal dopaminergic denervation, as measured by dopamine transporter tropane PET imaging, is correlated with UPSIT scores in healthy elderly persons who exhibited no evidence of PD-related dopaminergic denervation (Wong et al., 2010).

The first demonstration of the orbitofrontal and piriform cortices by PET scan is shown in Figure 3.30. It suggests that the right orbitofrontal cortex is dominant for higher-level olfactory processing although this may be only partially correct. Figure 3.31 shows PET scan abnormalities in response to phenylethyl alcohol in Alzheimer's disease compared to healthy controls, whereas Figure 3.32 shows decreased PET-related activity in brain regions of PD patients with and without significant hyposmia (SH) at baseline and three years later. Note that the last row illustrates the longitudinal development of hypometabolism, with greater hypometabolism occurring in the patients with SH at baseline.

PET imaging has been a major scientific advance. It displays brain regions activated by odorants or the function of specific neurotransmitter systems, such as dopamine storage capacity (within presynaptic dopaminergic terminals) or dopamine receptor availability. PET has some advantages over fMRI as described in the next section, including the ability to image the whole brain more easily and visualize structures at the skull base that are difficult to identify by fMRI because of "susceptibility artefacts." The injection of radioactive tracers is invasive and PET requires complex, expensive equipment, including a nearby Cyclotron to generate isotopes. With longer-life isotopes such as ^{18}F, the cyclotron does not need to be onsite as in the case of ^{15}O. Relative to the neural events, which occur in milliseconds, PET requires the integration of signals over tens of seconds. PET is time consuming, especially if an MRI scan is required to provide better localization of activated brain structures, although simultaneous

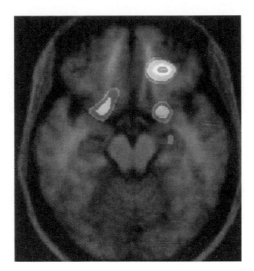

Figure 3.30 PET scan to show odorant-induced activation as indicated by areas of increased blood flow. The activation is seen bilaterally (blue) in the piriform cortex and unilaterally in the right orbitofrontal cortex (red, yellow, & blue). This led to the proposal that the right OFC is dominant for high-level olfactory processing, a concept that is now thought to be only partially correct. Reprinted with permission from Zatorre et al. (1992).

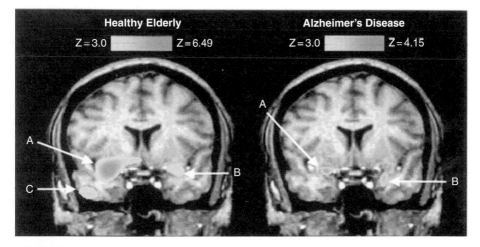

Figure 3.31 PET imaging in Alzheimer's disease. Left: Controls. A: Right frontotemporal junction (piriform area); B: Left piriform area; C: Right anterior ventral temporal lobe (Brodmann area 20). Number of controls: 7; mean UPSIT = 32.4; mean threshold to phenylethyl alcohol: $10^{-5.5}$. Right: Alzheimer's Disease. A: 7 mm anterior to frontotemporal junction; B: left amygdala-uncus. Number of patients: 6. Mean UPSIT = 18.7 (microsmic); mean threshold to phenylethyl alcohol: minus 5.1 (normal). From Kareken et al. (2001). (A black and white version of this figure will appear in some formats. For the color version, please refer to the plate section.)

PET-CT imaging is an alternative approach. The PET signal has a low signal-to-noise ratio, a factor that increases data acquisition time to several minutes. This poor temporal resolution is not appropriate for experiments that involve rapid event-based stimuli. Even under the best of circumstances images are obtained with no greater than ~3mm^3 of spatial resolution.

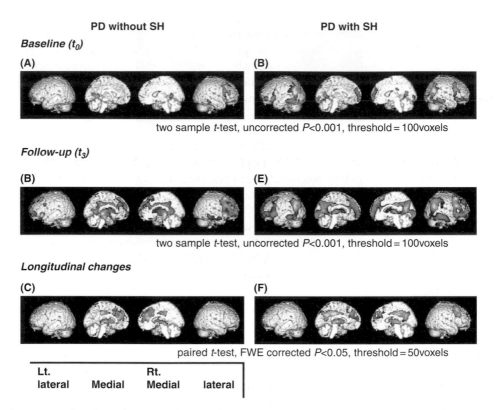

Figure 3.32 Fluorodeoxyglucose-PET data that show the distribution of cortical hypometabolism in the Parkinson's disease (PD) subgroups compared with normal controls. (A) At baseline (t_0), PD patients without severe hyposmia (SH) showed a mild metabolic reduction in the frontal regions and medial occipital cortex. (B) At follow-up (t_3), PD patients without severe hyposmia showed a metabolic reduction in the midbrain and broader frontal regions, medial prefrontal, cingulate, and medial occipital cortices. (C) In PD patients without severe hyposmia, longitudinal metabolic changes (t_0–t_3) were identified in the medial prefrontal and anterior cingulate cortices. (D) At t_0, patients with PD and severe hyposmia showed a metabolic reduction in the bilateral dorsolateral prefrontal, medial prefrontal, and medial occipital cortices and bilateral parieto-occipito-temporal area. (E) At t_3, the metabolic reduction became more prominent, with additional metabolic reduction in the posterior cingulate and precuneus. (F) In PD patients with severe hyposmia, the longitudinal metabolic changes (t_0–t_3) were distributed in the right frontal, medial prefrontal, anterior cingulate, posterior cingulate cortices and precuneus. From Baba et al., 2012. (A black and white version of this figure will appear in some formats. For the color version, please refer to the plate section.)

Functional Magnetic Resonance Imaging (fMRI)

fMRI is the most widely employed functional imaging procedure. Brain oxygen level dependent (BOLD) fMRI, the most popular of the fMRI procedures, capitalizes on the fact that local changes in neural activity produce neighboring changes in the amount of oxygen carried in hemoglobin, i.e., the ratio of oxyhemoglobin to deoxyhemoglobin, and these changes disturb the magnetic field. Thus, T2 relaxation times differ relative to the amount of deoxyhemoglobin in the blood, generating signals that indirectly reflect the amount of neural activity within the more active brain regions. Other fMRI methods increase the signal-to-noise ratio in the target regions by use of contrast agents.

Unlike PET, fMRI is non-invasive, requiring no injection of radioactive materials. It can be performed in most medical centers where MRI machines are available, in contrast to PET imaging, whose isotopes must be generated by a cyclotron which is usually available only in large research units. Since MRI provides detailed neuroanatomy, there is no need for additional scanning as required for PET. Relative to PET, fMRI has the further advantage of high spatial and temporal resolution. However, fMRI can suffer from susceptibility artifacts in areas where bone and brain are adjacent, for example at the skull base.

Although initial studies on olfactory fMRI found it difficult to obtain reliable images of the major cortical olfactory areas, notably the piriform cortex (e.g., Yousem et al., 1997; Zald & Pardo, 1997), this problem has largely been resolved. The earlier studies used block designs where set periods of stimulus presentation (e.g., 30 sec) are alternated with equivalent periods of no stimulus presentation. It was assumed that the odor signal lasted throughout the stimulus block. Subsequent work showed this was not the case, and that the odorant signal rapidly habituated (Sobel et al., 2000). Thus, most paradigms now take this into effect by either analyzing a brief initial segment of the odorant "ON" period or by modeling the habituation with an exponentially decaying signal waveform (Tabert et al., 2007). Substantial improvements in signal recovery from piriform and orbitofrontal cortices followed other improvements, such as shifting the MRI axial acquisition plane by 30°, employment of short stimulus presentations with 10–20 sec interstimulus intervals, and controlling for the influences of sniffing parameters using covariates (Sobel et al., 2000; Deichmann et al., 2003; De & Schwarzbauer, 2005; Hsu & Glover, 2005; Weiskopf et al., 2005; Weiskopf et al., 2006).

Reflecting psychophysical tests, numerous subject variables influence fMRI olfactory images, including sex, age, and various diseases. In general, less activation is seen in older than in younger persons, and in men compared to women. The influences of sex differences are noted in Figure 3.33. Note the greater right- than left-side brain activity.

Single Photon Emission Computerized Tomography (SPECT)

Single photon emission computerized tomography (SPECT) is similar in principle to PET. It is technically simpler, less expensive, and uses radioactive tracers that do not require an on-site cyclotron. SPECT utilizes radionuclides (tracers) that emit a single photon with lower energy (about 140 keV) than those employed in PET. A large sheet of perforated lead known as a collimator allows the radiation to be controlled so that only those photons parallel to the holes can pass through to the crystal to be recorded as an event. The spatial resolution of SPECT is three or four times less than PET, the tracers need to have much greater half-lives, and in many instances long image acquisition periods are required. SPECT is invaluable for assessing cortical responses to odor (Di Nardo et al., 2000). It also detects striatal dopaminergic deficiency by use of a labeled presynaptic dopamine transporter ligand such as [18F]FP–CIT or [99mTc]TRODAT-1. Dopamine transporter imaging is now a major cost effective investigation for many extrapyramidal disorders, in particular Parkinson's disease (PD) and related conditions.

Figure 3.34 depicts a typical SPECT scan from a normal subject and a patient with Parkinson's disease at various stages of disease progression. The brain areas imaged are those known to be the primary regions of motor dysfunction in PD.

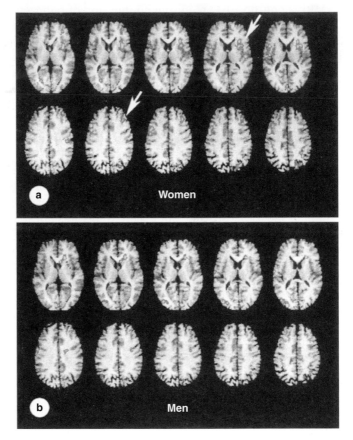

Figure 3.33 fMRI group-averaged activation maps for women and men. The right side of the brain is on the right. Women showed up to eight times more activated voxels than men for specific brain regions, notably in the frontal and perisylvian regions. Note the slightly greater activation on the right compared to the left side of the brain. Odorants were eugenol and phenylethyl alcohol, alternating with hydrogen sulfide. From Yousem et al. (2001). (A black and white version of this figure will appear in some formats. For the color version, please refer to the plate section.)

Magnetoencephalography (MEG)

In addition to detecting and mapping alterations in electric brain currents from the scalp, it is possible to map magnetic fields produced by these currents using magnetoencephalography (MEG). For this procedure, a large array (e.g., >100) of very sensitive magnetometers, usually super conducting quantum interface devices (SQUIDs), are placed over the scalp, much like electrodes for EEG. Many studies have employed MEG in olfaction, beginning with the ground-breaking work of Kettenmann et al. (1996) which showed that three odors, vanillin, phenylethyl alcohol, and hydrogen sulfide, bilaterally activated overlapping regions around the superior temporal sulci. Sakuma et al. (1997) found similar symmetric regional activation for phenylethyl alcohol and pentylacetate. However, Tonoike et al. (1998) reported considerable asymmetry in the MEG responses when stimulating either the right or the left nasal chamber with pentyl acetate. To date, we are unaware of any specific applications of MEG to clinical olfactory disorders.

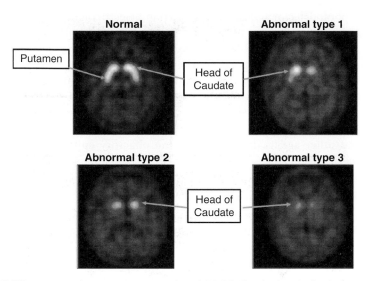

Figure 3.34 DATScan using a dopamine transporter ligand (FP-CIT). This displays the level of presynaptic dopamine transporter, which is highest in the caudate and putamen. Top left: normal pattern of uptake. The abnormal scans are from patients with Parkinson's disease in progressively more severe stages. Note that the first area to show reduced uptake (Type 1) is the putamen (comma-shaped area) which displays reduced uptake on the right side of the scan. As the disease advances the more anterior caudate nucleus becomes deficient (full-stop shaped region) so that in the most advanced stage (Type 3) the caudate is scarcely visible.

Other Measures
Ciliary Motility Tests

The nose, paranasal sinuses, and tracheobronchial tree are lined with ciliated columnar epithelial cells. Their cilia are essential for movement of the mucous blanket, which serves a critical host defense mechanism, trapping and removing particulate matter, bacteria, and other exogenous agents from the region. The top layer of this blanket, termed the gel layer, is derived from mucous glands and goblet cells, whereas the bottom layer, the sol layer, is made up of a water transudate that emanates from the underlying fenestrated capillaries. The cilia move rapidly forward and slowly backward at a beat rate of ~10 Hz. Their motion can be slowed by rhinosinusitis, dehydration, numerous drugs, and irritants, including tobacco smoke, sulfur dioxide, nitrogen dioxide, local anesthetics, neuropeptide Y, $beta_2$-adrenergic antagonists, and the preservative benzalkonium chloride (Doty et al., 2004).

Saccharin Transport Time. A practical, albeit somewhat variable, clinical means to evaluate mucociliary transport utilizes saccharin transport time. A small amount of saccharin is placed on the inferior turbinate, approximately 0.5 cm posterior to its most anterior portion. The transport time is defined as the moment the patient reports sweetness or bitterness of the saccharin. Healthy subjects have a transport time typically less than 15 minutes, while patients with chronic nasal and sinus disease have delay, often longer than 20 minutes.

Ciliary Beat Frequency. This can be measured, *in vivo*, by photoelectric methods and laser light scattering. In the former, changes in light intensity produced by the beating cilia are picked up by a photodetector and converted into photoelectric signals. In rhinoscintigraphy a weak gamma emitting isotope, technetium-99m, is deposited on the floor of the nasal meatus and its transport followed by gamma camera. Such techniques require specialized equipment and are generally not practical in the clinic.

Although ciliary motility tests can provide information about the overall health of the nose, their value in assessing olfactory function is unclear. One exception is ciliary dysfunction disorders, such as cystic fibrosis and the Kartegner and Bardet-Biedl syndromes, which are associated with smell loss, presumably because of poor clearance of bacteria and other agents detrimental to the olfactory epithelium (Weiffenbach & McCarthy, 1984).

The Electronic Nose (E-Nose)

The ability to diagnose illness by the smell of bodily secretions, including breath, is ancient, dating back to Hippocrates and traditional Chinese Medicine over 2,000 years ago. Although not widely employed, the technology to detect multiple odorous volatile substances is now developing rapidly (Wilson 2011; Table 3.2). It is well known, for example, that many micro-organisms produce volatile compounds. These can be identified by expensive and time-consuming techniques such as gas chromatography or mass spectrometry. A breakthrough came in 1982 with the first model of an electronic nose was developed that simulated various stages of the human olfactory system (Figure 3.35; Persaud & Dodd, 1982). Since then, there have been several modifications, but most have three components; namely, a microarray sensor (such as a conducting polymer, metal-oxide, piezo-electric, or optical device), a pre-processor, and a pattern recognition unit using neural networks (Figure 3.35).

It is possible to distinguish *Helicobacter pylori, E Coli, and Enterococcus* species that co-exist in a mixture by estimating the amounts of terpenes (citrus or pine smells), trimethylamine (fishy), and ketones (acetone) that are produced (Pavlou et al., 2000). The E-nose may be used to diagnose tuberculosis in sputum specimens (Fend et al., 2006), ventilator-associated pneumonia (Hockstein et al., 2005), and bacterial sinusitis (Thaler & Hanson, 2006). In a validation study of exhaled air in known active TB patients examined by an E-nose (DiagNose, C-it BV), a sensitivity of 93.5% and a specificity of 85.3% was found for discriminating healthy controls from TB patients, and a sensitivity of 76.5% and specificity of 87.2% when identifying TB patients within the entire test-population (Bruins et al., 2013).

This technology may permit the distinction of serum from cerebrospinal rhinorrhoea (Aronzon et al., 2005) and assist in the diagnosis of metabolic myopathy such as maple syrup urine disease and other metabolic disorders like cystinuria, histidinemia, phenylketonuria, and tyrosinemia (Wilson, 2011; Table 3.2). The E-nose has the potential advantage of providing a rapid and inexpensive diagnosis compared to laboratory cultures. At present, claims for its application are outstripping its practical use in a clinical setting. Issues of specificity and sensitivity need to be fully evaluated and compared to traditional assays before the E-nose may be introduced into, say, a hospital environment. Nonetheless, it is an expanding area of research which in the field of medicine has found most practical value in developing countries for speedy diagnosis of pulmonary tuberculosis.

Table 3.2. Potential electronic-nose applications for human and animal disease diagnoses via detection of volatile biomarker indicator compounds. Modified with permission from Wilson & Baietto (2011).

Disease/disorder/ infection	Aroma sample source	Associated volatile biomarkers
Aerobic gram negative bacteria	Intraperitoneal fluid	Terpenes, ketones
Alcoholic fatty liver disease (AFDL)	Human breath	Acetaldehyde, isoprene, 3 other unidentified VOCs
Alcohol-induced hepatic injury	Human breath	Ethane, pentane (volatile alkanes)
Allograft rejection	Human breath	Carbonyl sulfide
Anaerobic bacterial infections	Intraperitoneal fluid	Acetic acid, butyric acid
	Urine	Isobutylamine, acetic acid, butyric acid
Asthma	Human breath	Pentane, ethane, 8-isoprostane, nitric oxide, leukotriene B4, prostaglandin E2
Bacteremia	Blood cultures	Specific complex mixture of VOCs
	White blood cell cultures	Acetaldehyde, hexanaldehyde
Bacterial infections (local)	Human pus	Isobutyric, isovaleric, & isocaproic acids
Bacterial vaginosis	Vaginal swabs	Specific complex mixture of VOCs
Bacteriuria	Urine	Specific complex mixture of VOCs
Breast cancer	Human breath	C4-C20 alkanes, monomethylated alkanes
Cardiopulmonary disease	Alveolar air	Ethanol, acetone
Cholera	Feces	p-menth-1-en-8-ol, dimethyl disulphide
Chronic hepatitis	Alveolar air	Methyl-mercaptan, dimethyl sulfide
Chronic obstructive pulmonary disease (COPD)	Human breath	NO, H_2O_2, aldehydes, 8-isoprostane, nitrotyrosine, Leukotriene B4, cytokines
Cystic fibrosis	Human breath	Leukotriene B4, interleukin-6, carbonyl sulfide, alkanes
Cystinuria	Human breath	Cadaverine, piperidine, putrescine, pyrrolidine
Diabetes mellitus	Human breath	Acetone, ethanol, methyl nitrate, complex VOCs
Eye infections	Cultures of ocular fluids	Specific complex mixture of VOCs

Table 3.2. (cont.)

Disease/disorder/infection	Aroma sample source	Associated volatile biomarkers
Foetor hepaticus	Human breath	Specific complex mixture of VOCs
Hematuria	Urine	Specific complex mixture of VOCs
Halitosis	Human breath	Hydrogen sulfide, methyl mercaptan, dimethyl sulfide
Hepatic cirrhosis	Alveolar breath	Dimethyl sulfide, hydrogen sulfide, mercaptans, volatile fatty acids
	Alveolar air	Dimethyl sulfide, acetone, 2-pentanone and 2-butanone
	chronic hepatitis	Methyl-mercaptan, dimethyl sulfide
Hepatic coma	Alveolar air	Methyl-mercaptan, dimethyl sulfide
Hepatic encephalopathy	Blood plasma, spinal fluid	3-methylbutanal
Histidinemia	Human breath	2-imidazolepyruvic acid, 2-imidazolelactic acid, 2-imidazoleacetic acid
Hyperglycemia	Human breath	Methyl nitrate, xylene, ethylbenzene
Inflammatory bowel disease (IBD)	Human breath	Pentane, ethane, propane
Ischemic heart disease, angina	Human breath	Alkanes, methylated alkanes
Ketosis	Alveolar air	Acetone
Leg ulcers & wound healing	Contact dressings	Specific complex mixture of VOCs
Liver cancer	Blood	Hexanal, 1-octen-3-ol, octane
Lung cancer	Human breath	Alkanes, monomethylated alkanes
	Human breath	Alkanes, aromatic compounds
	Human breath	Specific complex mixture of VOCs
Maple syrup urine disease	Human breath	2-oxoisocaproic acid
Metabolic disorders	Urine	Isovaleric acid
Necrotizing enterocolitis (NEC)	Feces	2-Ethyl-1-hexanol, fewer esters present in VOCs
Oxidative stress	Human breath	8-isoprostane
Phenylketonuria	Human breath	Phenylpyruvic acid, phenyllactic acid, phenylacetic acid

Table 3.2. (cont.)

Disease/disorder/ infection	Aroma sample source	Associated volatile biomarkers
Renal dysfunction and failure	Urine	Specific complex mixture of VOCs
Respiratory infections	Human breath	Specific complex mixture of VOCs
Rheumatoid arthritis	Alveolar air	Pentane
Tyrosinemia	Human breath	p-hydroxyphenylpyruvic acid
Schizophrenia	Alveolar air	Pentane, carbon disulfide, ethane
Sweaty feet syndrome	Urine, sweat, human breath	Butyric acid, hexanoic acid; trans-3-methyl-2 hexenoic acid
Urinary tract infection	Urine	Isovaleric acid, alkanes

Summary

In this chapter we have provided a relatively comprehensive overview of the means available for quantitatively assessing olfactory function, with an emphasis on procedures applicable in the clinic. Since olfaction is largely a synthetic sense, with considerable spatial intermingling of receptor-related information within the olfactory epithelium, bulb, and cortex, most measures of olfactory function are correlated with one another. This makes it possible to assess a limited number of stimuli to ascertain overall olfactory function.

There are multiple procedures for presenting odorant stimuli to the nose, ranging from simple odor-containing vials to complex computer-controlled olfactometers. In general, most stimulus presentation procedures produce reasonably reliable results, although this depends in part upon the type of olfactory test, its length, and the demands of the involved task. While both sides of the nose are usually tested together, unilateral testing can reveal damage to one side of the nose that is not apparent from bilateral testing. However, persons complaining of olfactory deficits invariably have significant dysfunction on both sides of the nose.

Olfactory tests can be divided into three major classes: psychophysical, electrophysiological, and psychophysiological, with psychophysical tests being the most widely employed. Among nominally disparate psychophysical tests are those of odor detection, identification, discrimination, and memory,

Tests of odor identification have been found to be most reliable and are the most widely employed means for assessing olfactory function. Odor Event-Related Potentials (OERPs), measured from the surface of the scalp, and odor-induced summated receptor potentials, measured from the nasal epithelium, are the most common electrophysiological measures of olfactory function. Psychophysiological tests, i.e., tests that largely measure autonomic nervous system responses to inhaled vapors, are available but have not proven to be as reliable or useful as psychophysical or electrophysiological test measures, largely reflecting hedonic and trigeminal elements of the involved stimuli. Malingering can be detected using forced-choice psychophysical procedures and some electrophysiological responses, although the latter are generally less reliable in this regard.

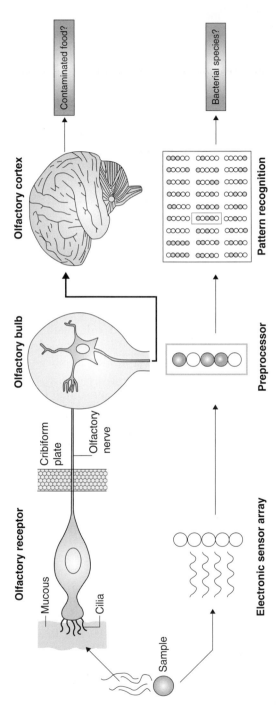

Figure 3.35 Comparison of the elements of the human olfactory system with those of the E-nose. Volatile odor recognition may be achieved using pattern recognition techniques. Reproduced with permission from Turner & Magan (2004).

The integrity and function of the central olfactory system can be measured by imaging procedures, including computerized tomography (CT), magnetic resonance imaging (MRI), positron emission tomography (PET), single photon emission tomography (SPECT), and magneto-encephalography (MEG). Although functional assessments of nasal patency and airflow, such as acoustic rhinometry and anterior rhinomanometry, may be useful in some instances to determine whether odors are actually reaching the olfactory receptors, under most circumstances such measures are not strongly associated with tests of olfactory function.

Many other procedures are associated indirectly with the ability to smell, although in most cases strong associations are not evident. Cilia motility tests can provide information regarding the health of the nasal epithelium and, indirectly, may reflect infectious nasal conditions that, in turn, are associated with damage to the olfactory epithelium.

Various analytical chemical sensors have been developed within the last 30 years that mimic elements of the ways that the olfactory system senses odors. Such devices, many of which have been termed electronic noses, are capable of identifying and discriminating between volatiles associated with various disease states. Although not yet employed in clinical situations, their continued development may result in devices of considerable value for diagnosis of many diseases.

References

Acta Oto-Laryngologica Vol. **120**, Iss. 2, 2000.

Akerlund, A., Bende, M., Murphy, C., 1995. Olfactory threshold and nasal mucosal changes in experimentally induced common cold. *Acta Otolaryngologica (Stockh)***115**, 88–92.

Amoore, J.E., Ollman, B.G., 1983. Practical test kits for quantitatively evaluating the sense of smell. *Rhinology* **21**, 49–54.

Aronzon, A., Hanson, C.W., Thaler, E.R., 2005. Differentiation between cerebrospinal fluid and serum with electronic nose. *Otolaryngology-Head and Neck Surgery.* **133**(1), 16–19.

Baba, T., Kikuchi, A., Hirayama, K., et al. 2012. Severe olfactory dysfunction is a prodromal symptom of dementia associated with Parkinson's disease: A 3 year longitudinal study. *Brain* **135**, 161–169.

Bajaj, S., Ammini, A.C., Marwaha, R., et al. 1993. Magnetic resonance imaging of the brain in idiopathic hypogonadotropic hypogonadism. *Clinical Radiology* **48**, 122–124.

Bensafi, M., Rouby, C., Farget, V., et al. 2002. Autonomic nervous system responses to odours: The role of pleasantness and arousal. *Chemical Senses* **27**, 703–709.

Bonfils, P., Faulcon, P., Avan, P., 2004. Screening of olfactory function using the Biolfa olfactory test: Investigations in patients with dysosmia. *Acta Otolaryngologica (Stockh)* **124**, 1063–1071.

Brodoehl, S., Klingner, C., Volk, G.F., et al. 2012. Decreased olfactory bulb volume in idiopathic Parkinson's disease detected by 3.0-Tesla magnetic resonance imaging. *Movement Disorders* **27**, 1019–1025.

Bromley, S.M., Doty, R.L., 1995. Odor recognition memory is better under bilateral than unilateral test conditions. *Cortex* **31**, 25–40.

Brown, K.S., MacLean, C.M., Robinette, R.R., 1968. The distribution of the sensitivity to chemical odors in man. *Human Biology* **40**, 456–472.

Bruins, M., Rahim, Z., Bos, A., et al. 2013. Diagnosis of active tuberculosis by e-nose analysis of exhaled air. *Tuberculosis.* **93**(2), 232–238.

Burlingame, G.A., Doty, R.L., 2015. The Smell and Taste of Public Drinking Water. Page 1079, Chapter 49 In: Doty RL, editor. *Handbook of Olfaction and Gustation*. New York Wiley-Liss.

Burmeister, H.P., Bitter, T., Heiler, P.M., et al. 2012. Imaging of lamination patterns of the adult human olfactory bulb and tract: In vitro comparison of standard- and high-resolution 3T MRI, and MR microscopy at 9.4 T. *Neuroimage* **60**, 1662–1670.

Cain, W.S., Gent, J., Catalanotto, F.A., Goodspeed, R.B., 1983; Clinical evaluation of olfaction. *American Journal of Otolaryngology* **4**, 252–256.

Cameron, E.L., Doty, R.L., 2013. Odor identification testing in children and young adults using the smell wheel. *International Journal of Pediatric Otorhinolaryngology*. **77**(3), 346–350.

Cardesin, A., Alobid, I., Benitez, P., et al. 2006. Barcelona Smell Test – 24 (BAST-24): Validation and smell characteristics in the healthy Spanish population. *Rhinology* **44**, 83–89.

Carrasco, M., Ridout, J.B., 1993. Olfactory perception and olfactory imagery: A multidimensional analysis. *Journal of Experimental Psychology: Human Perception and Performance* **19**, 287–301.

Chemical Senses 27: A23 (This was an abstract in proceedings)

Chhabra, N., Houser, S.M., 2009. The diagnosis and management of empty nose syndrome. *Otolaryngologic Clinics of North America*. **42**(2), 311–330.

Choudhury, E.S., Moberg, P., Doty, R.L., 2003. Influences of age and sex on a microencapsulated odor memory test. *Chemical Senses* **28**, 799–805.

Christian A. Mueller, Elisabeth, Grassinger, Asami, Naka, Andreas,F.P. Temmel, Thomas Hummel,Gerd Kobal; A Self-administered Odor Identification Test Procedure Using the "Sniffin' Sticks", Chemical Senses, Volume **31**, Issue 6, 1 July 2006, Pages 595–598.

Collet, S., Grulois, V., Bertrand, B., Rombaux, P., 2009. Post-traumatic olfactory dysfunction: A cohort study and update. *B-ENT* **5** Suppl 13, 97–107.

Croy, I., Hummel, T., Pade, A., Pade, J., 2010. Quality of life following nasal surgery. *Laryngoscope* **120**, 826–831.

Croy, I., Negoias, S., Novakova, L., Landis, B.N., Hummel, T., 2012. Learning about the functions of the olfactory system from people without a sense of smell. *PLoS One* e33365.

Damm, M., Eckel, H.E., Jungehulsing, M., Hummel, T., 2003. Olfactory changes at threshold and suprathreshold levels following septoplasty with partial inferior turbinectomy. *Annals of Otology, Rhinology, and Laryngology* **112**, 91–97.

Davidson, T.M., Murphy, C., 1997. Rapid clinical evaluation of anosmia: The alcohol sniff test. *Archives of Otolaryngology - Head and Neck Surgery* **123**, 591–594.

Davidson, T.M., Freed, C., Healy, M.P., Murphy, C., 1998. Rapid clinical evaluation of anosmia in children: The alcohol Sniff Test. *Annals of the New York Academy of Sciences* **855**, 787–792.

De, P.C., Schwarzbauer, C., 2005. Positive or negative blips? The effect of phase encoding scheme on susceptibility-induced signal losses in EPI. *Neuroimage* **25**, 112–121.

Deichmann, R., Gottfried, J.A., Hutton, C., Turner, R., 2003. Optimized EPI for fMRI studies of the orbitofrontal cortex. *Neuroimage* **19**, 430–441.

Di Nardo, W., Di Girolamo, W., Galli, A., et al. 2000. Olfactory function evaluated by SPECT. *American Journal of Rhinology* **14**, 57–61.

Doty, R.L., 1975. An examination of relationships between the pleasantness, intensity, and concentration of 10 odorous stimuli. *Perception and Psychophysics* **17**, 492–496.

Doty, R.L., Deems, D.A., Frye, R.E., Pelberg, R., Shapiro, A., 1988. Olfactory sensitivity, nasal resistance, and autonomic function in patients with multiple chemical sensitivities. *Archives of Otolaryngology - Head and Neck Surgery* **114**, 1422–1427.

Deems, D.A., Doty, R.L., Settle, R.G., et al. 1991. Smell and taste disorders, a study of 750 patients from the University of Pennsylvania Smell and Taste Center. *Archives of Otolaryngology - Head and Neck Surgery* **117**, 519–528.

Doty, R.L., 1976. Reproductive endocrine influences upon human chemoreception: A review. *Mammalian Olfaction, Reproduction, Processes & Behavior*. NY: Academic Press.

Doty, R.L., 1994. Tests of human olfactory function: Principal components analysis suggests that most measure a common source of variance. *Attention, Perception, & Psychophysics* **56**(6), 701–707.

Doty, R.L., 1995 *The Smell Identification Test™ Administration Manual*. 3rd Edition. Haddon Hts., NJ: Sensonics, Inc.

Doty, R.L., Marcus, A., Lee, W.W., 1996. Development of the 12-item cross-cultural smell identification test (CC-SIT). *Laryngoscope* **106**, 353–356.

Doty, R.L., Yousem, D.M., Pham, L.T., et al. 1997. Olfactory dysfunction in patients with head trauma. *Archives of Neurology* **54**, 1131–1140.

Doty, R.L., 2000. *Odor Threshold Test™ Administration Manual*. Haddon Hts., NJ: Sensonics, Inc.

Doty, R.L., 2003.*The Odor Memory Test™ Administration Manual*. Haddon Hts., NJ: Sensonics, Inc.

Doty, R.L., Cometto-Muniz, J.E., Jalowayski, A.A., et al. 2004. Assessment of upper respiratory tract and ocular irritative effects of volatile chemicals in humans. *Critical Reviews in Toxicology* **34**, 85–142.

Doty, R.L., Crastnopol, B., 2010. Correlates of chemosensory malingering. *Laryngoscope* **120**, 707–711.

Doty, R.L., Kamath, V., 2014. The influences of age on olfaction: A review. *Applied Olfactory Cognition* **5**, 213.

Doty, R.L., Shaman, P., Dann, M., 1984. Development of the University of Pennsylvania Smell Identification Test: A standardized microencapsulated test of olfactory function. *Physiology & Behavior* **32**, 489–502.

Doty, R.L., Snyder, P.J., Huggins, G.R., Lowry, L.D., 1981. Endocrine, cardiovascular, and psychological correlates of olfactory sensitivity changes during the human menstrual cycle. *Journal of Comparative and Physiological Physiology* **95**, 45–60.

Doty, R.L., Kerr, K-L., 2005. Episodic odor memory: Influences of handedness, sex, and side of nose. *Neuropsychologia* **43**(12), 1749–1753.

Doty, R.L., Tourbier, I., Ng, V., et al., 2015. Influences of hormone replacement therapy on olfactory and cognitive function in postmenopausal women. *Neurobiol Aging*. **36**(6), 2053–2059.

Drake, B., Johansson, B., von Sydow, D., Doving, K.B., 1969. Quantitative psychophysical and electrophysiological data on some odorous compounds. *Scandinavian Journal of Psychology* **10**, 89–96.

Duchamp-Viret, P., Chaput, M.A., Duchamp, A., 1999. Odor response properties of rat olfactory receptor neurons. *Science* **284**, 2171–2174.

Eccles, R., Jawad, M.S., Morris, S., 1990. The effects of oral administration of (-)-menthol on nasal resistance to airflow and nasal sensation of airflow in subjects suffering from nasal congestion associated with the common cold. *Journal of Pharmacy & Pharmacology* **42**, 652–654.

Engen, T., Kuisma, J.E., Eimas, P.D., 1973, Short-term memory of odors. *Journal of Experimental Psychology* **99**, 222–225.

Engen, T., Ross, B.M., 1973. Long-term memory of odors with and without verbal descriptions. *Journal of Experimental Psychology* **100**, 221–227.

Fend, R., Kolk, A.H., Bessant, C., et al., 2006. Prospects for clinical application of electronic-nose technology to early detection of Mycobacterium tuberculosis in culture and sputum. *Journal of Clinical Microbiology*. 2006; **44**(6): 2039–45.

Fornazieri, M.A., Doty, R.L., Santos, C.A., et al. 2013. A new cultural adaptation of the University of Pennsylvania Smell Identification Test. *Clinics (Sao Paulo)* **68**, 65–68.

Frank, R.A., Dulay, M.F., Gesteland, R.C., 2003. Assessment of the sniff magnitude test as a clinical test of olfactory function. *Physiology & Behavior* **78**, 195–204.

Frank, R.A., Dulay, M.F., Niergarth, K.A., Gesteland, R.C., 2004. A comparison of the sniff magnitude test and the University of Pennsylvania Smell Identification Test in children and nonnative English speakers. *Physiology & Behavior* **81**, 475–480.

Frank, R.A., Gesteland, R.C., Bailie, J., et al. 2006. Characterization of the sniff magnitude test. *Archives of Otolaryngology - Head and Neck Surgery* **132**, 532–536.

Freiherr, J., Gordon, A.R., Alden, E.C. et al. 2012. The 40-item Monell Extended Sniffin' Sticks Identification Test (MONEX-40). *Journal of Neuroscience Methods* **205**, 10–16.

Frijters, J.E., 1980. Three-stimulus procedures in olfactory psychophysics: An experimental comparison of Thurstone-Ura and three-alternative forced-choice models of signal detection theory. *Perception and Psychophysics* **28**, 390–397.

Frye, R.E., 1995. Nasal airway dynamics and olfactory function. In: Doty RL, editor. *Handbook of Olfaction and Gustation.* New York: Marcel Dekker; pp. 471–491.

Gevins, Alan S., and Antoine Rémond, eds. *Methods of Analysis of Brain Electrical and Magnetic Signals.* Vol. **1**. Elsevier Science Limited, 1987.

Geisler, M.W., Morgan, C.D., Covington, J.W., Murphy, C., 1999. Neuropsychological performance and cognitive olfactory event-related brain potentials in young and elderly adults. *Journal of Clinical Experimental Neuropsychology* **21**, 108–126.

Geisler, M.W., Murphy, C., 2000. Event-related brain potentials to attended and ignored olfactory and trigeminal stimuli. *International Journal of Psychophysiology* **37**, 309–315.

Gilbert, A.N., Popper, R., Kroll, J.J., Nicklin, L., Zellner, D.A., 2002. *The Cranial 1 Quick Sniff®: A New Screening Test for Olfactory Function.* Chemical Senses. 27, p. A23.

Green, B.G., Dalton, P., Cowart, B., et al. 1996. Evaluating the "Labeled Magnitude Scale" for measuring sensations of taste and smell. *Chemical Senses* **21**, 323–334.

Green, P., Iverson, G., 1998. Exaggeration of anosmia in 80 litigating head injury cases. *Archives of Clinical Neuropsychology* **13**, 138.

Gudziol, V., Buschhuter, D., Abolmaali, N., et al. 2009. Increasing olfactory bulb volume due to treatment of chronic rhinosinusitis – a longitudinal study. *Brain* **132**, 3096–3101.

Haehner, A., Mayer, A.M., Landis, B.N., et al. 2009. High test-retest reliability of the extended version of the "Sniffin' Sticks" test. *Chemical Senses* **34**, 705–711.

Haehner, A., Rodewald, A., Gerber, J.C., Hummel, T., 2008. Correlation of olfactory function with changes in the volume of the human olfactory bulb. *Archives of Otolaryngology - Head and Neck Surgery* **134**, 621–624.

Hashimoto, Y., Fukazawa, K., Fujii, M., et al. 2004. Usefulness of the odor stick identification test for Japanese patients with olfactory dysfunction. *Chemical Senses.* **29**(7), 565–71.

Hedner, M., Larsson, M., Arnold, N., Zucco, G.M., Hummel, T., 2010. Cognitive factors in odor detection, odor discrimination, and odor identification tasks. *Journal of Clinical Experimental Neuropsychology.* **32** (10), 1062–1067.

Helson, H., 1964. *Adaptation-level theory: an experimental and systematic approach to behavior.* New York: Harper and Row.

Hendriks, A.P., 1988. Olfactory dysfunction. *Rhinology* **26**, 229–251.

Hockstein, N.G., Thaler, E.R., Lin, Y., Lee, D.D., Hanson, C.W., 2005. Correlation of pneumonia score with electronic nose signature: A prospective study. *Annals of Otology, Rhinology, and Laryngology.* **114**(7), 504–508.

Hornung, D.E., 2006. Nasal anatomy and the sense of smell. *Advances in Oto-Rhino-Laryngology* **63**, 1–22.

Hosoya, Y., Yashida, H., 1937. Über die bioelektrische Erscheinungen an der Riechschleimhaut. *Japanese Journal of Medical Science III Biophysics* **5**, 22–23.

Hsu, J.J., Glover, G.H., 2005, Mitigation of susceptibility-induced signal loss in neuroimaging using localized shim coils. *Magnetic Resonance in Medicine* **53**, 243–248.

Huart, C., Legrain, V., Hummel, T., Rombaux, P., Mouraux, A., 2012. Time-frequency analysis of chemosensory event-related potentials to characterize the cortical representation of odors in humans. *PLoS One* **7**, e33221.

Hummel, T., Kobal, G., Gudziol, H., kay-Sim, A., 2007; Normative data for the "Sniffin' Sticks" including tests of odor identification, odor discrimination, and olfactory thresholds: An upgrade based on a group of more than 3,000 subjects. *European Archives of Oto-Rhino-Laryngology* **264**, 237–243.

Hummel, T., Konnerth, C.G., Rosenheim, K., Kobal, G., 2001. Screening of olfactory function with a four-minute odor identification test: reliability, normative data, and investigations in patients with olfactory loss. *Annals of Otology, Rhinology & Laryngology* **110**, 976–981.

Hummel, T., Sekinger, B., Wolf, S.R., Pauli, E., Kobal, G., 1997. "Sniffin' sticks": olfactory performance assessed by the combined testing of odor identification, odor discrimination and olfactory threshold. *Chemical Senses* **22**, 39–52.

Ikeda, K., Tabata, K., Oshima, T., et al. 1999. Unilateral examination of olfactory threshold using the Jet Stream Olfactometer. *Auris Nasus Larynx* **26**, 435–439.

Jackman, A.H., Doty, R.L., 2005. Utility of a three-item smell identification test in detecting olfactory dysfunction. *Laryngoscope* **115**, 2209–2212.

Jacquot, L., Monnin, J., Brand, G., 2004. Unconscious odor detection could not be due to odor itself. *Brain Research* **1002**, 51–54.

Jehl, C., Royet, J.P., Holley, A., 1997. Role of verbal encoding in short- and long-term odor recognition. *Perception & Psychophysics* **59**(1), 100–110.

Jones, F.N., 1955a. Olfactory absolute thresholds and their implications for the nature of the receptor process. *Journal of Psychology* **40**, 223–227.

Jones, F.N., 1955b. The reliability of olfactory thresholds obtained by sniffing. *The American Journal of Psychology* **68**, 289–290.

Kareken, D.A., Doty, R.L., Moberg, P.J., et al. 2001. Olfactory-evoked regional cerebral blood flow in Alzheimer's disease. *Neuropsychology* **15**, 18–29.

Kern, R.C., 2000. Chronic sinusitis and anosmia: Pathologic changes in the olfactory mucosa. *Laryngoscope* **110**, 1071–1077.

Kettenmann, B., Jousmaki, V., Portin, K., et al. 1996. Odorants activate the human superior temporal sulcus. *Neuroscience Letters* **203**, 143–145.

Kim, J.Y., Lee, W.Y., Chung, E.J., Dhong, H.J., 2007. Analysis of olfactory function and the depth of olfactory sulcus in patients with Parkinson's disease. *Movement Disorders* **22**, 1563–1566.

Kobal, G., Hummel, T., Sekinger, B., Barz, S., Roscher, S., and Wolf, S., 1996. "Sniffin' sticks": screening of olfactory performance. *Rhinology* **34**, 222–226.

Kobal, G., Hummel, C., 1988. Cerebral chemosensory evoked potentials elicited by chemical stimulation of the human olfactory and respiratory nasal mucosa. *Electroencephalography and Clinical Neurophysiology* **71**, 241–250.

Kobal, G., 2003. Electrophysiological measurement of olfactory function. *Neurological Disease and Therapy.* **57**, 229–250.

Kobal, G., Plattig, K.H., 1978. Methodische Anmerkungen zur Gewinnung olfaktorischer EEG-Antworten des wachen Menschen (objektive Olfaktometrie). *Zeitschrift fur Elektroenzephalographie Elektromyographie und Verwandte Gebiete* **9**, 135–145.

Koenigkam-Santos, M., Santos, A.C., Versiani, B.R., Diniz, P.R., Junior, J.E., de, C.M., 2011. Quantitative magnetic resonance imaging evaluation of the olfactory system in Kallmann syndrome: Correlation with a clinical smell test. *Neuroendocrinology* **94**, 209–217.

Krantz, E.M., Schubert, C.R., Dalton, D.S., et al. 2009. Test-retest reliability of the San Diego Odor Identification Test and comparison with the brief smell identification test. *Chemical Senses* **34**, 435–440.

Kremer, B., Klimek, L., Mosges, R., 1998. Clinical validation of a new olfactory test. *European Archives of Oto-Rhino-Laryngology* **255**, 355–358.

Kurtz, D.B., White, T.L., Sheehe, P.R., Hornung, D.E., Kent, P.F., 2001. Odorant confusion matrix: The influence of patient history on patterns of odorant identification and misidentification in hyposmia. *Physiology & Behavior* **72**, 595–602.

Laing, D.G., Francis, G.W., 1989. The capacity of humans to identify odors in mixtures. *Physiology & Behavior* **46**, 809–814.

Laing, D.G., Segovia, C., Fark, T., et al. 2008. Tests for screening olfactory and gustatory function in school-age children. *Otolaryngology - Head and Neck Surgery* **139**, 74–82.

Lane, A.P., Zweiman, B., Lanza, D.C., et al. 1996. Acoustic rhinometry in the study of the acute nasal allergic response. *Annals of Otology, Rhinology, and Laryngology* **105**, 811–818.

Lawless, H.T., Malone, G.T. 1986a. A comparison of rating scales: sensitivity, replicates and relative measurement. *Journal of Sensory Studies.* **1**, 155–174.

Lawless, H. T., Malone, G. T. 1986b. The discrimination efficiency of common scaling methods. *Journal of Sensory Studies.* **1**, 85–98.

Lehrner, J., Deecke, L., 2000. The Viennese olfactory test battery – a new method for assessing human olfactory functions. *Aktuelle Neurologie* **27**, 170–177.

Leopold, D.A., 1988. The relationship between nasal anatomy and human olfaction. *Laryngoscope* **98**, 1232–1238.

Linschoten, M.R., Harvey, L.O., Jr., Eller, P.M., Jafek, B.W., 2001. Fast and accurate measurement of taste and smell thresholds using a maximum-likelihood adaptive staircase procedure. *Perception & Psychophysics* **63**, 1330–1347.

Liu, H.C., Wang, S.J., Lin, K.P., et al. 1995. Performance on a smell screening test (the MODSIT): A study of 510 predominantly illiterate Chinese subjects. *Physiology & Behavior* **58**, 1251–1255.

London, B., Nabet, B., Fisher, A.R., et al. 2008. Predictors of prognosis in patients with olfactory disturbance. *Annals of Neurology* **63**, 159–166.

Lorig, T.S., Elmes, D.G., Zald, D.H., Pardo, J.V., 1999. A computer-controlled olfactometer for fMRI and electrophysiological studies of olfaction. *Behavior Research Methods, Instruments, & Computers* **31**, 370–375.

Lötsch, J., Reichmann, H., Hummel, T., 2008. Different odor tests contribute differently to the evaluation of olfactory loss. *Chemical Senses* **3**(1), 17–21.

Maremmani, C., Rossi, G., Tambasco, N., et al. 2012. The validity and reliability of the Italian Olfactory Identification Test (IOIT) in healthy subjects and in Parkinson's disease patients. *Parkinsonism & Related Disorders* **18**, 788–793.

Maruniak, J.A., Silver, W.L., Moulton, D.G., 1983. Olfactory receptors respond to blood-borne odorants. *Brain Research* **265**, 312–316.

McCaffrey, T.V., 1991. Rhinomanometry and vasoactive drugs affecting nasal patency. In: Getchell TV, Doty, R.L., Bartoshuk, L.M., Snow JB, Jr., editors. *Smell and Taste in Health and Disease*. New York: Raven Press pp. 493–502.

McMahon, C., Scadding, G,K., 1996. Le Nez du Vin–a quick test of olfaction. *Clin Otolaryngol Allied Sci* **21**, 278–280.

McReynolds, P., Ludwig, K., 1987. On the history of rating scales. *Personality & Individual Differences* **8**, 281–283.

Mueller, C.A., Grassinger, E., Naka, A., Temmel, A.F., Hummel, T.; Kobal, G. 2006. A self-administered odor identification test procedure

using the "Sniffin' Sticks". *Chemical Senses* **31**, 595–598.

Neely, G., Ljunggren, G., Sylven, C., Borg, G., 1992. Comparison between the Visual Analogue Scale (VAS) and the Category Ratio Scale (CR-10) for the evaluation of leg exertion. *International Journal of Sports Medicine* **13**, 133–136.

Nguyen, A.D., Pelavin, P.E., Shenton, M.E., et al. 2011. Olfactory sulcal depth and olfactory bulb volume in patients with schizophrenia: An MRI study. *Brain Imaging and Behavior* **5**: 252–261.

Nordin, S., Bramerson, A., Liden, E., Bende, M., 1999. The Scandinavian Odor-Identification Test: development, reliability, validity and normative data. *Acta Otolaryngologica* **118**, 226–234.

Nordin, S., Lotsch, J., Kobal, G., Murphy, C., 1998.Effects of nasal-airway volume and body temperature on intranasal chemosensitivity. *Physiology & Behavior* **63**, 463–466.

O'Mahony, M., Gardner, L., Long, D., et al. 1979. Salt taste detection: An R-index approach to signal-detection measurements. *Perception* **8**, 497–506.

Osman, A., Silas, J., 2015. Electrophysiological measurement of olfactory function. In: Doty RL, editor. *Handbook of Olfaction and Gustation*. New York: Wiley-Liss. pp. 263–279.

Ottoson, D., 1956. Analysis of the electrical activity of the olfactory epithelium. *Acta Physiologica Scandinavica* **35**, 1–83.

Patel, S.J., Bollhoefer, A.D., Doty, R.L., 2004. Influences of ethanol ingestion on olfactory function in humans. *Psychopharmacology* **171**, 429–434.

Pavlou, A.K., Magan, N., Sharp, D., et al. 2000. An intelligent rapid odour recognition model in discrimination of Helicobacter pylori and other gastroesophageal isolates in vitro. *Biosensors and Bioelectronics.* **15**(7), 333–342.

Persaud, K., Dodd, G., 1982. Analysis of discrimination mechanisms in the mammalian olfactory system using a model nose. *Nature* **299**(5881), 352–355.

Pfurtscheller, G., Lopes da Silva, F.H., 1999. Event-related EEG/MEG synchronization and desynchronization: Basic principles. *Clinical Neurophysiology* 110, 1842–1857.

Potter, H., Butters, N., 1980. An assessment of olfactory deficits in patients with damage to prefrontal cortex. *Neuropsychologia* 18, 621–628.

Punter, P.H., 1983; Measurement of human olfactory thresholds for several groups of structurally related compounds. *Chemical Senses* 7, 215–235.

Rawal, S., et al. 2015. The taste and smell protocol in the 2011–2014 US National Health and Nutrition Examination Survey (NHANES): Test–retest reliability and validity testing. *Chemosensory Perception* 8(3), 138–148.

Reese, T.S., Stevens, S.S., 1960. Subjective intensity of coffee odor. *The American Journal of Psychology* 73, 424–428.

Richard K. Eyman, P. John Kim, Tom Call. Perceptual and Motor Skills. Volume: **40** issue: 2, page(s): 415–423.

Robson, A.K., Woollons, A.C., Ryan, J., et al. 1996, Validation of the combined olfactory test. *Clinical Otolaryngology* 21, 512–518.

Rombaux, P., Mouraux, A., Bertrand, B., et al. 2006a. Retronasal and orthonasal olfactory function in relation to olfactory bulb volume in patients with post-traumatic loss of smell. *Laryngoscope* 116, 901–905.

Rombaux, P., Mouraux, A., Bertrand, B., et al. 2006b. Olfactory function and olfactory bulb volume in patients with postinfectious olfactory loss. *Laryngoscope* 116, 436–439.

Rombaux, P., Huart, C., De Volder, A.G., et al. 2010. Increased olfactory bulb volume and olfactory function in early blind subjects. *Neuroreport* 21, 1069–1073.

Rombaux, P., Huart, C., Deggouj, N., Duprez, T., Hummel, T., 2012. Prognostic value of olfactory bulb volume measurement for recovery in postinfectious and post-traumatic olfactory loss. *Otolaryngology - Head and Neck Surgery* 147, 1136–1141.

Rovee, C.K., Cohen, R.Y., Shlapack, W., 1975. Life-span stability in olfactory sensitivity. *Developmental Psychology* 11, 311–318.

Saito, S., yabe-Kanamura, S., Takashima, Y., et al. 2006. Development of a smell identification test using a novel stick-type odor presentation kit. *Chemical Senses* 31, 379–391.

Sakuma, K., Kakigi, R., Kaneoke, Y. et al. 1997. Odorant evoked magnetic fields in humans. *Neuroscience Research* 27, 115–122.

Schiff, S.J., Aldroubi, A., Unser, M., Sato, S., 1994. Fast wavelet transformation of EEG. *Electroencephalography and Clinical Neurophysiology* 91, 442–455.

Schiffman, S.S., Reynolds, M.L., Young, F.W., 1981. *Introduction to Multidimensional Scaling: Theory, Methods, and Applications*. Orlando, FL: Academic Press.

Schmidt, F.A., Goktas, O., Harms, L., et al. 2011. Structural correlates of taste and smell loss in encephalitis disseminata. *PLoS One* 6, e19702.

Scott, J.W., Brierley, T., Schmidt, FH., 2000. Chemical determinants of the rat electro-olfactogram. *Journal of Neuroscience* 20, 4721–4731.

Sensors 2011, 11(1), 1105–1176; Advances in Electronic-Nose Technologies Developed for Biomedical Applications Alphus D. Wilson 1,* and Manuela Baietto 2.

Siderowf, A., Jennings, D., Connolly, J., et al. 2007. Risk factors for Parkinson's disease and impaired olfaction in relatives of patients with Parkinson's disease. *Movement Disorders* 22, 2249–2255.

Silveira-Moriyama L, Carvalho Mde J, Katzenschlager R, Petrie A, Ranvaud R, Barbosa ER, Lees AJ. 2008. The use of smell identification tests in the diagnosis of Parkinson's Disease in Brazil. *Movement Disorders*. 23, 2328–2334.

Simmen, D., Briner, H.R., Hess, K., 1999. Screeningtest des Geruchssinnes mit Riechdisketten. *Laryngorhinootologie* 78, 125–130.

Sobel, N., Johnson, B.N., Mainland, J., Yousem, D.M., 2003. Functional neuroimaging of human olfaction. In: Doty RL, editor. *Handbook of Olfaction and Gustation*. New York: Marcel Dekker.

Sobel, N., Prabhakaran, V., Zhao, Z., et al. 2000. Time course of odorant-induced activation in the human primary olfactory cortex. *Journal of Neurophysiology* 83, 537–551.

Stevens, J.C., Cruz, L.A., Marks, L.E., Lakatos, S., 1998. A multimodal assessment of sensory thresholds in aging. *Journals of Gerontology. Series B, Psychological Sciences & Social Sciences*. 53, 263–272.

Stinton, N., Atif, M.A., Barkat, N., Doty, R.L., 2010. Influence of smell loss on taste function. *Behavioral Neuroscience* **124**, 256–264.

Sulsenti, G., Palma, P., 1989. [The nasal valve area: Structure, function, clinical aspects and treatment. Sulsenti's technic for correction of valve deformities]. *Acta Otorhinolaryngologica Italica* **9** Suppl 22, 1–25.

Tabert, M.H., Steffener, J., Albers, M.W. et al. 2007. Validation and optimization of statistical approaches for modeling odorant-induced fMRI signal changes in olfactory-related brain areas. *Neuroimage* **34**, 1375–1390.

Takagi, S.F., 1989. *Human Olfaction*. Tokyo: University of Tokyo Press.

Tanner, W.P., Jr., Swets, J.A., 1954. A decision-making theory of visual detection. *Psychological Review* **61**, 401–409.

Tateyama, T., Hummel, T., Roscher, S., Post, H., Kobal, G., 1998. Relation of olfactory event-related potentials to changes in stimulus concentration. *Electroencephalography and Clinical Neurophysiology* **108**, 449–455.

Thaler, E.R., Hanson, C.W., 2006. Use of an electronic nose to diagnose bacterial sinusitis. *American Journal of Rhinology*. **20**(2), 170–2.

Thomann, P.A., Dos, S.V., Seidl, U., et al. 2009. MRI-derived atrophy of the olfactory bulb and tract in mild cognitive impairment and Alzheimer's disease. *Journal of Alzheimer's Disease* **17**, 213–221.

Thomas-Danguin, T., Rouby, C., Sicard, G., et al. 2003. Development of the ETOC: a European test of olfactory capabilities. *Rhinology* **41**, 142–151.

Tonoike, M., Yamaguchi, M., Kaetsu, I., et al. 1998. Ipsilateral dominance of human olfactory activated centers estimated from event-related magnetic fields measured by 122-channel whole-head neuromagnetometer using odorant stimuli synchronized with respirations. *Annals of the New York Academy of Sciences* **855**, 579–590.

Tourbier, I.A., Doty, R.L., 2007. Sniff magnitude test: Relationship to odor identification, detection, and memory tests in a clinic population. *Chemical Senses* **32**, 515–523.

Turetsky, B.I., Moberg, P.J., Yousem, D.M., Doty, R.L., Arnold, S.E., Gur, R.E., 2000. Reduced olfactory bulb volume in patients with schizophrenia. *American Journal of Psychiatry* **157**, 828–830.

Turetsky, B.I., Moberg, P.J., Arnold, S.E., Doty, R.L., Gur, R.E., 2003. Low olfactory bulb volume in first-degree relatives of patients with schizophrenia. *American Journal of Psychiatry* **160**, 703–708.

Turetsky, B.I., Hahn, C.G., Arnold, S.E., Moberg, P.J., 2009. Olfactory receptor neuron dysfunction in schizophrenia. *Neuropsychopharmacology* **34**, 767–774.

Turner, A.P., Magan, N., 2004. Electronic noses and disease diagnostics. *Nature Reviews Microbiology* **2**(2), 161–166.

Van Toller, C., Kirk-Smith, M., Wood, N., Lombard, J., Dodd, G.H., 1983. Skin conductance and subjective assessments associated with the odour of 5-alpha-androstan-3-one. *Biological Psychology* **16**, 85–107.

Veyseller, B., Aksoy, F., Yildirim, Y.S., et al. 2011. Reduced olfactory bulb volume in total laryngectomy patients: A magnetic resonance imaging study. *Rhinology* **49**, 112–116.

Vollmecke, T., Doty, R. L. 1985. Development of the Picture Identification Test (PIT): A research companion to the University of Pennsylvania Smell Identification Test. *Chemical Senses* **10**, 413–414.

Waggener, C.T., Coppola, D.M., 2007. Naris occlusion alters the electro-olfactogram: Evidence for compensatory plasticity in the olfactory system. *Neuroscience Letters* **427**, 112–116.

Wang, L., Hari, C., Chen, L., Jacob, T., 2004. A new non-invasive method for recording the electro-olfactogram using external electrodes. *Clinical Neurophysiology* **115**, 1631–1640.

Weber, E.H., 1834. *De Pulsu, Resorptione, Auditu et Tactu: Annotationes Anatomicae et Physiologiae*. Leipzig: Koehler.

Weierstall, R., Pause, B.M., 2012. Development of a 15-item odour discrimination test (Dusseldorf Odour Discrimination Test). *Perception* **41**, 193–203.

Weiffenbach, J.M., McCarthy, V.P., 1984. Olfactory deficits in cystic fibrosis: Distribution and severity. *Chemical Senses* **9**, 193–199.

Weiskopf, N., Hutton, C., Josephs, O., Deichmann, R., 2006. Optimal EPI parameters for reduction of susceptibility-induced BOLD sensitivity losses: A whole-brain analysis at 3 T and 1.5 T. *Neuroimage* **33**, 493–504.

Weiskopf, N., Klose, U., Birbaumer, N., Mathiak, K., 2005; Single-shot compensation of image distortions and BOLD contrast optimization using multi-echo EPI for real-time fMRI. *Neuroimage* **24**, 1068–1079.

Wilson, A.D., Baietto, M. 2011. Advances in electronic-nose technologies developed for biomedical applications. *Sensors* (Basel). **11**, 1105–1176.

Wilson, A.D., Baietto, M., 2011. Advances in electronic-nose technologies developed for biomedical applications. *Sensors* **11**(1), 1105–76.

Wilson, D.A., 2001. Receptive fields in the rat piriform cortex. *(Review) (82 refs)*. *Chemical Senses* **26**, 577–584.

Wolfensberger, M., Schnieper, I., Welge Lüssen, A. 2000. Sniffin' Sticks: a new olfactory test battery. *Acta Otolaryngologica*. **120**, 303–306.

Wong, K.K., Muller, M.L., Kuwabara, H., Studenski, S.A., Bohnen, N.I., 2010. Olfactory loss and nigrostriatal dopaminergic denervation in the elderly. *Neuroscience Letters*, **484**(3), 163–167.

Wright, H.N., 1987; Characterization of olfactory dysfunction. *Archives of Otolaryngology - Head and Neck Surgery* **113**, 163–168.

Yoshida, M., 1984. Correlation analysis of detection threshold data for "standard test" odors. *Bulletin of the Faculty of Science and Engineering Chuo University* **27**, 343–353.

Yousem, D.M., Turner, W.J.D., Cheng, L., Snyder, P.J., Doty, R.L., 1993. Kallmann syndrome – Mr evaluation of olfactory system. *American Journal of Neuroradiology* **14**, 839–843.

Yousem, D.M., Geckle, R., Doty, R.L., 1995. MR of patients with post-traumatic olfactory deficits. *Chemical Senses* **20**, 338.

Yousem, D.M., Geckle, R.J., Bilker, W., McKeown, D.A., Doty, R.L., 1996. MR evaluation of patients with congenital hyposmia or anosmia. *American Journal of Roentgenology* **166**, 439–443.

Yousem, D.M., Williams, S.C., Howard, R.O., et al. 1997. Functional MR imaging during odor stimulation: Preliminary data. *Radiology* **204**, 833–838.

Yousem, D.M., Geckle, R.J., Bilker, W.B., Doty, R. L., 1998. Olfactory bulb and tract and temporal lobe volumes. Normative data across decades. *Annals of the New York Academy of Sciences* **855**, 546–555.

Yousem, D.M., Oguz KK, Li C., 2001. Imaging of the olfactory system. *Seminars in Ultrasound, CT and MRI* **22**, 456–472.

Zald, D.H., Pardo, J.V., 1997. Emotion, olfaction, and the human amygdala: Amygdala activation during aversive olfactory stimulation. *Proceedings of the National Academy of Sciences of the United States of America* **94**, 4119–4124.

Zatorre, R.J., Jones-Gotman, M., Evans, A.C., Meyer, E., 1992. Functional localization and lateralization of human olfactory cortex. *Nature* **360**, 339–340.

Zhao, K., Scherer, P.W., Hajiloo, S.A., Dalton, P., 2004. Effect of anatomy on human nasal air flow and odorant transport patterns: Implications for olfaction. *Chemical Senses* **29**, 365–379.

Zwaardemaker, H., 1889. On measurement of the sense of smell in clinical examination. *Lancet* **I**, 1300–1302.

Zwaardemaker, H., 1925. *L'Odorat*. Paris: Doin.

Zwaardemaker, H., 1927. The sense of smell. *Acta Otolaryngologica (Stockh)* **11**, 3–15.

Measurement of Gustation

Chapter 4

Introduction

As noted in Chapter 3, reliable assessment of the chemical senses is essential to determine the extent of dysfunction. In common with the sense of smell, humans are notoriously inaccurate in their self-assessment of less-than-total taste dysfunction (Soter et al., 2008).

This chapter begins with a general review of basic psychophysical, electrophysiological, and imaging procedures to assess taste, including their strengths and weaknesses. In contrast to olfaction, published norms are lacking for most taste investigations and few standardized taste procedures have been developed. One reason is that clinically significant whole-mouth taste deficits are relatively rare in the general population and most of those who present with "taste" dysfunction actually have diminished flavor sensation due to olfactory loss (Deems et al., 1991).

Psychophysical taste tests, by definition, are based upon judgments by human subjects. Most tests assume that taste is composed of a set of independent sensory networks that can be evaluated by separate systems differentially sensitive to sweet, sour, bitter, salt, savory (umami), and possibly other sensations (e.g., "fatty"). Non-psychophysical procedures, such as electroencephalography (EEG), functional magnetic imaging (fMRI), and magneto-encephalography (MEG), are not as dependent upon human judgments and are employed mainly in research. Their clinical applications are limited.

The focus of this chapter is on the major ways in which taste can be assessed by psychophysical, electrophysiological, and various imaging procedures.

Chemical Taste Testing

We first consider the fundamental problems related to taste testing and then discuss various methods of evaluating taste by threshold and suprathreshold procedures.

Basic Considerations

Quantifying taste function is more complicated than measuring olfactory function. This reflects the innervation of taste buds by multiple nerves and the variable distribution of receptors within the oral cavity. Ideally several regions of the tongue, soft palate, and throat should be tested individually since oral taste sensations are dependent upon separate innervations distributed across these areas. As described in Chapter 2, the anterior lingual taste buds, located on the fungiform papillae, are supplied by the chorda tympani division of CN VII, which also innervates the taste buds on the anterior foliate papillae. Taste buds on the anterior soft palate are innervated by the greater (superficial) petrosal nerve, which also

138

accompanies CN VII, whereas those on the posterior soft palate are innervated by phar- yngeal branches of CN IX. The glossopharyngeal nerve supplies taste buds on the posterior tongue, notably those within the vallate (also termed circumvallate) and posterior foliate papillae. Taste buds within the esophagus and on the epiglottal surface are innervated by a branch of CN X, the superior laryngeal nerve. Hence, to apply even a single concentration of a chemical representative of sweet, sour, bitter, salty, and umami (savory) taste qualities to each of these innervated regions on each side of the oral cavity, a total of 50 trials would be required (10 regions × 5 tastants). With rinses, this would result in 100 trials, and with at least 10 trials per tastant – which may be too few for reliable assessment – a total of 1,000 trials would be required! Moreover, multiple tongue regions within the receptive field of each taste nerve should, ideally, be assessed. Obviously, individual testing of all the tongue regions in which taste buds are found is impractical.

Taste buds in the posterior oral cavity and throat are largely inaccessible and attempts to stimulate them without swallowing the taste solutions can induce the gag reflex; thus, compromises must be made. Typically taste is measured by (1) "whole-mouth" procedures in which a solution is sipped and swished within the mouth and expectorated (or in rare cases swallowed) or (2) regional sampling from the left and right anterior (CN VII) and posterior (CN IX) tongue. Although whole-mouth testing is useful for the "gestalt" of a taste experience, it is insensitive to damage involving single taste nerves. Bornstein (1940b) makes the following argument when it comes to clinical taste testing (p. 137):

> To detect pathological alterations of taste, neither the whole-mouth methods nor examina-
> tions of only one area of the tongue are applicable because, in organic lesions, different parts
> of the tongue are usually involved to varying degree. Therefore, separate examinations of
> the several areas of the tongue are necessary. For this purpose, the tongue is divided into
> right and left halves, and each half into three regions, namely, tip, border, and base.

Presentation of tastants may be performed with (a) beakers, flasks, or cups from which whole-mouth "sipping and spitting," or in some cases swallowing, can occur, (b) medicine droppers, syringes, pumps, or micropipettes that permit localized stimulation of the tongue, in some cases with the tastant thickened by cellulose to minimize migration, (c) Q-tips or paint brushes dipped in taste solutions, and (d) small disks or strips made of filter paper or methylcellulose polymers impregnated with tastants. When storing taste stimuli, glass vessels are recommended, as polyethylene-based utensils markedly alter sucrose solutions and their associated threshold values. In the case of sucrose, freshly prepared solutions taste sweeter than those stored for a day or two, reflecting higher α-glucose content (Cameron, 1947). Filter paper disks or strips were first developed in Japan (Hara, 1955), and now used routinely in Japanese hospitals and clinics. They have been developed further and marketed in Europe (Landis et al. 2009). The recent invention of dissolvable disks made from methylcellulose polymers may soon replace such testing, as they can localize the stimulus to the region of interest with essentially no spread to surrounding regions (Smutzer et al., 2008). Electrogustometry (see below) and filter paper disks have provided much of our current psychophysical knowledge about the regional sensitivity of the tongue to tastants (e.g., Collings, 1974).

From a practical point of view some tastants are more amenable to psychophysical testing than others. As pointed out by Holway & Hurvich, (1937), NaCl can be graded over a large range (0 to 5.42 M), in contrast to sour stimuli such as citric acid which produces sharp, astringent sensations at concentrations greater than 0.1 M. Despite the fact that bitter stimuli such as quinine are distasteful and tend to linger and adhere to oral surfaces for several minutes, quinine has been suggested as a substitute for overall taste functioning, as described later in this chapter (Rawal et al., 2015). This proposal is based on a protocol for the 2011–14 US National Health and Nutrition Examination Survey (NHANES). Although sucrose is generally well tolerated, its viscosity changes as a function of concentration, potentially confounding taste with viscosity or "mouth feel" at suprathreshold concentrations.

Threshold Testing

Most psychophysical procedures assess the ability to detect, recognize, or perceive differences in the intensity of taste solutions. Historically, chemical threshold tests have been most widely employed, reflecting, in part, the nineteenth-century development of threshold methodology and the discovery that thresholds are sensitive to subtle changes in the taste system. Unlike some suprathreshold scaling procedures, taste threshold values can be compared directly among subjects. Presentation of electrical stimuli (electrogustometry) for threshold testing is popular clinically, since the stimulus can be confined to small regions of the tongue, and there is no need for rinsing between stimuli or mixing and storage of tastants. Electrical stimuli do not produce any of the classic taste sensations of sweet, sour, bitter, and salty (Murphy et al., 1995), more often a subtle feeling or, in some instances, metallic or bitter sensations. Rarely is salty perceived.

Chemical Threshold Tests

Although numerous psychophysical procedures are available to assess taste threshold, many investigators fail to separate detection from recognition. Recognition threshold requires the subject to report a specific taste *quality* (e.g., sweet) not just the *presence* of something (detection) which may be nondescript. Moreover, forced-choice procedures, where a comparison must be made with a blank or a series of blanks in a counterbalanced order, are often not employed, thus confusing the subjects' tendency to respond with the actual sensitivity of the system (see Doty & Laing, 2015).

The Method of Constant Stimuli. Classically, detection thresholds are determined by the method of constant stimuli. In this method, a tastant such as sucrose, in concentrations ranging from below and above peri-threshold, are presented randomly and repeatedly. This results in a function that relates the percentage of correct responses to tastant concentration. Concentrations are typically based upon logarithmic dilutions, since taste thresholds are log normally distributed. In a non-forced-choice situation, the threshold value is usually defined as the stimulus concentration that is detected 50% of the time, as extrapolated from the stimulus/response function. A 75% percent correct point can also be determined which, theoretically, reflects a point that differs in a reliable fashion from 50% chance performance when two-alternative forced-choice trials are present i.e., blank vs. tastant. The smallest perceived difference in concentrations between two stimulus concentrations is considered a "just noticeable difference" (JND).

Method of Limits and Staircase Procedures. The method of constant stimuli requires many trials. It is liable to subject fatigue and sensory adaptation. Clinically, less time-consuming procedures are more commonly employed, including single series ascending method of limits (AML) and staircase (tracking) procedures. In the simple AML procedure, a stimulus is presented below the threshold and increased in concentration until a sensation (detection threshold) or taste quality (recognition threshold) is perceived. In some instances, as in the ASTM adaptation of this procedure (ASTM, 1997), forced-choice responses are required at each concentration (Jones, 1956). A criterion is adjusted typically to the point at which the threshold value has been reached, e.g., using the concentration a step below that concentration where correct detection occurs repeatedly. Staircase procedures, like the less reliable AML procedure, begin typically at a below-threshold concentration. Once detection occurs, the next lower stimulus is presented. If missed, the next higher concentration is presented. In the adaptation of the two-down, one-up staircase procedure, two correct responses are required before the next lower stimulus concentration is presented (Kunka et al., 1981). If a miss occurs on either of two successive trials, then the next higher stimulus is presented. Following such an algorithm, a series of staircase "reversals" occurs and a number of such reversals are averaged to provide the threshold estimate. Thresholds based upon this procedure reflect 71% correct performance, rather than the 75% correct performance expected in a two-alternative forced-choice method of constant stimuli procedure, i.e., that point between chance performance and perfect performance.

Taste Sorting Procedure. The classic form of this procedure was developed by Harris and Kalmus (see Chapter 2) (Harris & Kalmus, 1949; Barnicot et al., 1951; Harris & Kalmus, 1951). A subject is provided, on a given trial, with eight cups: four contain various concentrations of the tastant dissolved in water and the other four cups, just water alone. The task is to sort the cups correctly into two groups. If correct sorting occurs, then the next lower concentration is presented. The process is continued until accurate sorting is not possible. This approach, which lends itself well to recognition as well as detection thresholds, produces highly reliable threshold estimates. Unfortunately, it is time consuming.

Procedural Issues

There are five major procedural issues associated with taste threshold measurement and the inherent variability associated with them. Although all taste qualities are affected by such problems, the influences on popular NaCl thresholds are particularly germane. This focus on NaCl in many studies underscores the role of salt in maintaining electrolyte balance and the early discovery that adrenalectomized rats and patients with Addison's disease crave salt and salty-tasting foods (Richter, 1936). Particularly in the food industry, it reflects the importance of salt in food flavoring and its critical association with a wide range of diseases, particularly heart disease.

1. Amount and Nature of Saliva in the Mouth. Most thresholds are influenced by the amount and nature of saliva in the mouth, as well as the stimulus concentrations presented on prior trials during a test, i.e., the adaptation level (Hahn, 1934; von Bekesy, 1965). This is particularly evident for NaCl thresholds. Under normal circumstances, taste buds are adapted to 0.9% NaCl, the same level as plasma. For detection, solutions must contain a concentration of NaCl higher than 0.9%. When the saliva is washed away with water, the adapting level of NaCl is no longer present and concentrations of NaCl below 0.9% can be detected. Many procedures fail to take this into account, either by not providing adequate and standard rinses between trials, not counterbalancing the presentation of water only and taste stimuli, or by using interstimulus intervals that are not long enough to remove adequately any residual stimulus from prior tastings. This produces "threshold drift" (O'Mahony & Dunn, 1974; O'Mahony, 1983). The effects of poor technique are clear, as

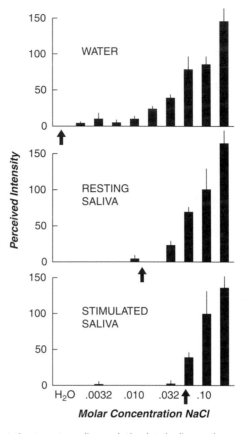

Figure 4.1 Influence of adaptation to water, saliva, and stimulated saliva on the perceived intensity of various concentrations of NaCl. The arrows indicate the concentration at which the stimulus can be perceived. Note that detection of NaCl in the presence of saliva requires higher NaCl concentrations than in the presence of water. From Bartoshuk (1978).

demonstrated in whole-mouth NaCl threshold tests in which the mouth is either exposed to water, resting saliva, or stimulated saliva (Figure 4.1). Importantly, taste sensitivity to NaCl can be influenced by simple chewing movements which, in turn, increases the amount of saliva in the mouth (Delwiche & O'Mahony, 1996). Circadian rhythms in NaCl taste sensitivity are correlated with circadian rhythms in salivary Na^+ content (Dawes, 1974; Ferguson & Botchway, 1979; Fujimura et al., 1990), suggesting that, ideally, tests should be done at the same time of day.

2. Taste Solutions That Are Weaker than the Adapting Solution. These often induce taste sensations that are different from the quality associated with the tastant. For example, Richter and MacLean (1939) noted that NaCl presented at concentrations between the detection and identification thresholds produced a range of taste sensations other than salty in 48 of 122 subjects (39%). The sensations that were most common were sweet (16% of subjects), bitter (6%), sour (5%), alkaline (2%), and bicarbonate (2%). Although the number of subjects reporting the various taste sensations were indicated in a table, it is not clear whether these numbers relate to a total sample size of four studies (n = 122) or only to their last study (n = 53). If they are based on 53 subjects, the percentages change as follows: overall – 91%; sweet – 43%; bitter – 15%; sour – 13%; alkaline – 4%; and bicarbonate – 4%. Some individuals described NaCl as basic, acid slippery, soapy, straw, magnesium, oily, orange juice, woody, potassium chloride, or vanilla. Other investigators have reported similarly that low NaCl concentrations often elicit disparate taste qualities (Bartoshuk et al., 1964; O'Mahony, 1973). Likewise, low concentrations of sucrose, glucose, and citric acid can elicit differing taste sensations (O'Mahony et al., 1976).

It should be emphasized that taste "confusions" occur even at higher tastant concentrations, although such effects are most commonly present in the perithreshold concentration range. Thus, in a recent study of 1000 volunteers that employed differing suprathreshold concentrations of sucrose (sweet), citric acid (sour), caffeine (bitter), and sodium chloride (salty), sour-bitter confusions were relatively common (19.3%) (Doty et al., 2017). This was followed in frequency by bitter-sour (11.4%), salty-bitter (7.3%), salty-sour (7.0%), bitter-salty (3.5%), bitter-sweet (3.4), and sour-salty (2.4%). Age, sex, and smoking habits were among the factors that influenced such confusions.

An interesting example of misidentification of expected taste qualities is the so-called "water taste." Both tap and distilled water often have a weak taste quality for some subjects, which includes bitter, sour, or salty (Bornstein, 1940b). After tasting NaCl, water assumes a bitter-sour taste; after sucrose, water is reported bitter, whereas after urea, water appears salty. Water may be reported sweet after tasting some salts (cynarine) found in the pulp of artichoke leaves. Bartoshuk (1978) points out that low thresholds to a range of tastants in children with cystic fibrosis or in adults with Addison's disease, the thresholds may, in fact, reflect water taste thresholds.

Several factors alter taste quality, although they would be not normally involved in psychophysical studies in Western countries. It has been known since the 1800s, for example, that an agent isolated from the leaves of the Gymnema sylvestre plant, Gymnemic acid, results in a sweet sensation when tastants are administered that are normally sour– an effect that can last more than an hour (Falconer, 1847; Hooper, 1887). Interestingly, Gymnema tea is used to counter diabetes in some Asian communities. Chewing other plants may produce this effect, including *Eriadictyon californicus, Synespalum dulcificum, Sphenacentrum jollyanu, and Thaumatocaccus daniellii* (for review, see Kurihara 1971). Attempts to find similarly effective and safe antagonists to the bitter receptors described in Chapter 2 have yet to be successful.

3. Water Temperature and Threshold. The temperature of the water used in testing influences threshold. In a pioneering study, Hahn and Günther (1932) found that when the temperature of the taste solutions was increased from 19° to 40° C, there was decreased sensitivity to NaCl and quinine sulfate, but not HCl. Thereafter, McBurney et al. (1973) performed a similar study employing a forced-choice staircase procedure that controlled for potential confounds associated with response biases. As shown in Figure 4.2, thresholds for various stimuli were differentially influenced by solution temperatures, but provided test solutions were at room temperature, i.e., 20° to 25° C (68° to 77° F), the temperature effects were relatively minor. It is noteworthy that taste nerve responses from dogs and rats are influenced markedly by tastant temperature (Nakamura & Kurihara, 1991), implying a direct effect on gustatory nerve afferents.

4. Effect of Psychophysical Paradigms. Unsurprisingly, threshold values are very much influenced by the psychophysical paradigms that are employed (O'Mahony, Ivory, & King, 1974). As in olfaction, detection thresholds are generally lower than recognition thresholds.

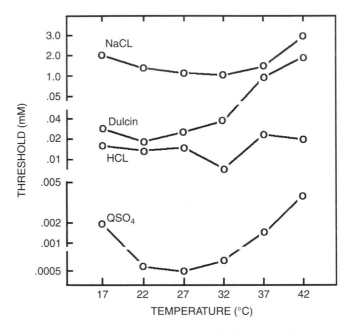

Figure 4.2 Influence of solution temperature on taste thresholds for four tastants. Dulcin is an artificial sweetener reportedly 250 times sweeter than sucrose. Modified from McBurney et al. (1973).

Taste thresholds are influenced by the volume of tastant presented, with larger volumes producing lower thresholds than smaller volumes (Grzegorczyk et al., 1979). The more trials presented at the peri-threshold region, the lower and more reliable the threshold estimate becomes, as in the case of olfaction (Doty et al., 1995).

A good example of the influences of methodology on detection and recognition thresholds is provided by Richter and MacLean (1939). They employed four different psychophysical procedures to establish detection and recognition thresholds for NaCl using an ascending method of limits stimulus presentation. The lowest thresholds were obtained using a method where the taste of NaCl had to be detected but not recognized at each concentration level, relative to a distilled water blank and where multiple sampling was allowed. The NaCl thresholds were computed by different methods: a three-drop procedure, a whole mouth swallowing procedure, a taste detection/recognition procedure without resampling, and a taste detection/recognition procedure with resampling, as shown in Table 4.1. Note that the drop method resulted in higher thresholds and that identification thresholds were consistently higher than detection thresholds.

5. Tongue Region Stimulated. As noted in Chapter 3, threshold measures of taste sensitivity are influenced not only by the presence or type of saliva, but by the location of the tongue that is stimulated and the extent and duration of the stimulus. In general, regions with the highest number of papillae are the most sensitive to tastants and the larger the tongue region stimulated, the lower the threshold (see Chapter 2). The influence of stimulus duration on NaCl thresholds is shown in Figure 4.3 (Bagla et al., 1997). As shown, thresholds are clearly lower, i.e., sensitivity is greater, when stimuli are presented for longer periods, at least within the time range employed in this work. This study employed a

Table 4.1. Detection and recognition thresholds obtained by Richter & MacLean (1939) for NaCl. Values represent percent concentrations in distilled water. D/R: detection, recognition.

	Sample size	Mean salt detection threshold	Range	Mean salt identification threshold	Range
Drop method	17	0.135	0.045–0.225	0.192	0.120–0.350
Swallow method	24	0.047	0.015–0.150	0.167	0.040–0.400
D/R method – no repeats	28	0.037	0.007–0.080	0.080	0.030–0.300
D/R method – repeats	53	0.016	0.007–0.060	0.087	0.020–0.250

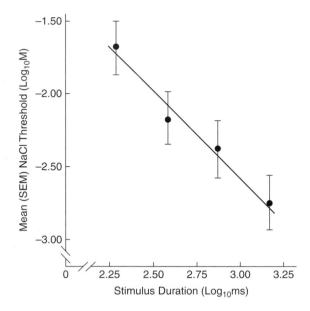

Figure 4.3 Mean NaCl detection thresholds (±SEM) as a function of stimulus duration plotted on log-log axes. The four data points, from left to right, correspond to 200, 400, 750, and 1500 ms. The relationship between threshold and stimulus duration represents a power function. From Bagla et al. (1997), © 1997 Oxford University Press.

computerized stimulus presentation system (Figure 4.4) that allowed presentation of a wide range of discretely timed stimuli to well-defined regions of the tongue via glass pipettes held onto the tongue by a surrounding vacuum (Hebhardt et al., 1999).

The association between NaCl threshold and density of fungiform papillae beneath stimulators of two different areas is shown in Figure 4.5. Note that the threshold scale is inverted, such that greater sensitivity is depicted at the top of the scale. A strong association is present between threshold sensitivity and the number of fungiform papillae (Zuniga et al., 1993; Miller et al., 2002). A robust link between taste sensitivity and lingual tactile perception has also been noted on the anterior tongue, reflecting the density and diameter of the fungiform papillae (Essick et al., 2003) and emphasizing the role of tactile perception/texture in the evaluation of food.

Normative Whole-Mouth Threshold Test Data

A major problem is the widespread lack of normative data. Apart from procedural variables discussed above, both age and gender can alter sensitivity to many tastants. Despite the scarcity of healthy control data, the elderly have higher average taste thresholds than the young, an effect that is most noticeable when small regions of the tongue are tested (Chapter 2).

One set of published threshold norms for whole-mouth NaCl is presented in Table 4.2. In this test, three stimulus drops are presented successively onto the anterior tongue from 60 ml medicine droppers; one contains the tastant and the other two, distilled water. Administration of the three drops is alternated between the left and right sides of the tongue. Initially the participant is given a suprathreshold example of the target stimulus to

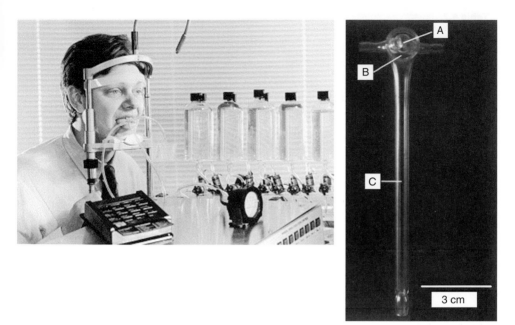

Figure 4.4 Left: University of Pennsylvania Regional Automated Taste Testing System (RATTS). From Doty, Bagla, Morgenson and Mirza (2001); © 2001 Elsevier Science, Inc. Right: Glass stimulation device viewed from below. The stimuli flow through the 25 mm² central chamber (A). A vacuum is present on the annular chamber (B), which holds the device securely to the tongue. The pressure (~40 mmHg) was calibrated with a differential pressure gauge connected to the distal end of the vacuum chamber (C). From Bagla et al. (1997); © 1997 Oxford University Press.

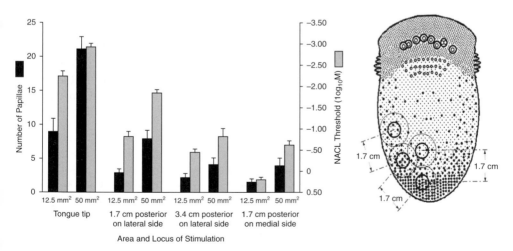

Figure 4.5 Left: Mean (±SEM) threshold values obtained from 8 subjects for NaCl presented to the four tongue regions for two stimulation areas (12.5 and 50 mm²). The number of papillae counted under video-microscopy is indicated by the dark bars, and threshold values by the gray bars. Right: Tongue regions where stimulators were located. From Doty et al (2001); © 2001 Elsevier Science Inc.

Table 4.2. Tastant concentrations employed by Henkin et al. for assessing basic taste qualities. Bottle units greater than four are considered indicative of hypogeusia or ageusia (Sections 5–12). Based on a sample size of 150 controls. From Henkin et al. (1971)

Bottle unit	NaCl (mM/L)	Sucrose (mM/L)	HCl (mM/L)	Urea (mM/L)
1	6	6	0.5	60
2	12	12	0.8	90
3	30	30	3	120
4	60	60	6	150
5	90	90	15	300
6	150	150	30	400
7	300	300	60	500
8	500	500	90	800
9	800	800	150	1000
10	1000	1000	300	2000
11	3000	2000	400	5000
12	Saturation	Saturation	500	8000

make them familiar with the tastant (Henkin & Soloman, 1962), which suggests this is a recognition, rather than detection, threshold procedure. A water rinse is interspersed between each three-drop trial and responses are based on a forced-choice paradigm. To identify the threshold more precisely, they observed the point at which responses changed from consistently correct to incorrect and retested at and around the transition point. Threshold was defined as the lowest concentration of test substance to which the subject gave two successive correct responses while giving two consecutive incorrect responses at the next lower concentration (Henkin et al., 1963). Note that these norms are not adjusted for either gender or age, providing only an absolute rather than relative index of dysfunction.

Another example of NaCl taste norms is presented in Table 4.3 derived from Wen (2010). In his test paradigm, which assesses recognition thresholds in a non-forced-choice context, five drops of the stimulus are presented onto the tip of the tongue. The tongue is then retracted and after a few moments the subject reports whether or not a salty taste is discerned. Hence, this is a whole-mouth recognition threshold procedure. Rinsing with distilled water takes place next. Although Wen did not specifically develop this method for normative purposes, his data set is among the largest from which abnormality can be inferred. In Table 4.3, we have set the cut-off for abnormality at approximately the fifth percentile i.e., steps 8 and 9.

It is noteworthy that in Wen's data, thresholds falling at or above 150 mM/L would be considered abnormal, whereas Henkin et al. defined abnormality as thresholds at or above 90 mM/L. The basis of this disparity is not clear, although several factors may be involved. First, the concentration steps employed are not equivalent between the two studies. Second, Henkin et al. apparently uses the highest range observed for a "normal" threshold in

Table 4.3. NaCl tastant concentrations used by Wen (2010) in a control sample of 600 subjects (428 men; 172 women; mean (SD) age of sample = 57.7 (0.33)). Seventy-three percent of the sample smoked cigarettes. These data are based on a non-forced-choice ascending method of limits procedure. Figures in rows 7–9 are greater than the 5th percentile.

Salt taste sensitivity threshold	NaCl (g/L)	NaCl (mM/L)	Number of subjects	% of subjects
1	0.22	1	12	2
2	0.45	8	48	8
3	0.90	15	108	18
4	1.80	30	174	29
5	3.60	60	132	22
6	7.30	120	60	10
7	14.60	150	42	7
8	29.20	500	18	3
9	58.40	1000	6	1

defining abnormality [see Table III of Henkin et al. 1963), rather than some defined percentile, such as the fifth percentile]. Third, Henkin uses a forced-choice procedure whereas Wen does not. Fourth, Henkin employs a single stimulus drop along with two distilled water drops in various orders whereas Wen uses five drops of the same stimulus. Finally, Wen, unlike Henkin, interspersed a full 30 seconds between trials, possibly minimizing adaption. However, adaptation is likely minimal for peri-threshold concentrations of tastants when water rinses are interspersed between trials.

Landis et al. (2009) developed norms for a taste test in which various concentrations of sweet-, sour-, bitter-, and salty-tasting stimuli are presented to the tongue on dried pieces of filter paper that had been saturated with tastants; namely, sucrose (0.05, 0.1, 0.2, and 0.4 g/ml), citric acid (0.05, 0.09, 0.165, and 0.3 g/ml), sodium chloride (0.016, 0.04, 0.1, 0.25 g/ml), and quinine hydrochloride (0.0004, 0.0009, 0.0024, and 0.006 g/ml). Each stimulus is given once to the left and once to the right side of the anterior tongue, resulting in a total of 32 trials. The stimuli are presented in an ascending series with water rinses between trials. The task is to identify, on each trial, the quality of the stimulus, i.e., sweet, sour, bitter, or salty. Unfortunately, the small number of trials precludes assessment of performance at each concentration level. Moreover, a determination of differences between sweet, sour, bitter, and salty responsiveness is not assessed, since the final test score amalgamates responses across all four tastants (correct responses out of 32). This test does confirm earlier findings of no meaningful differences in the ability to identify tastants between the two sides of the tongue, allowing a combination of responses from left and right sides. As shown in the normative data in Table 4.4, when left- and right-side data are combined, subtle, but significant, influences of sex and age appear which is a strength of this testing method. The normative data would be more useful if fifth percentile scores were reported.

Table 4.4. Normative data (percentiles) for a taste study using filter paper strips for men and women according to three age groups. Data, which were essentially equivalent for the left and right sides of the tongue, represent left and right sides combined. Modified from Landis et al. (2009).

Percentile	Age: 18–40 years		Age: 41–60 years		Age: >60 years	
	Women (n = 141)	Men (n = 84)	Women (n = 122)	Men (n = 84)	Women (n = 55)	Men (n = 51)
10th	19	17	15	9	10.2	9
25th	23	21	19	13	16	13
50th	27	25	24	21	22	19
75th	30	28	27	24.75	26	24
90th	32	30	30	27	28.4	25
Mean & (SD):	26.3 (5.1)	24.3 (5.3)	23.0 (5.7)	19.1 (7.1)	20.6 (6.5)	18.2 (5.9)

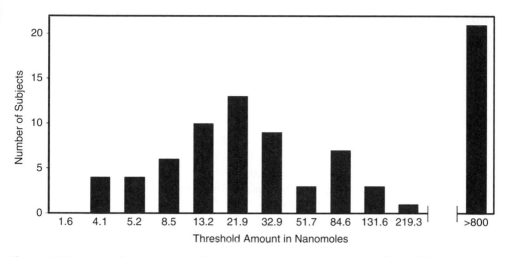

Figure 4.6 Histogram of detection threshold values obtained using taste strips made from pullulan, the polymer hydroxypropyl methyl cellulose and PROP. Tasters are normally distributed around 21.9 nanomoles. Note the large number of non-tasters to PROP with thresholds greater than 800 nanomoles. From Desai et al. (2011).

Desai et al. (2011) validated edible "taste strips" made from pullulan (α-1,4-; α-1,6-glucan) combined with the polymer hydroxypropyl methylcellulose. When placed on the tongue, these strips dissolve and provide a circumscribed taste stimulus. These investigators used both a single ascending method of limits and a staircase procedure to obtain threshold values for the bitter-tasting agent 6-n-propylthiouracil (PROP) and found that both approaches provided essentially equivalent threshold values. A forced-choice procedure was used to establish recognition thresholds, i.e., the lowest value by which a bitter taste was discerned. Water rinses were provided between stimulus presentations. Thirty-nine men and 42 women ranging in age from 18 to 64 years were evaluated. The distribution of test scores is shown in Figure 4.6. Note that a large number of PROP non-tasters was detected; i.e., persons whose threshold values were greater than 800 nanomoles. Once more, had abnormality been assigned at or below the fifth percentile, then concentrations that distinguish PROP tasters from PROP non-tasters would be above 219 nanomoles.

Influence of Taste Sensitivity on Food Acceptance

There is no doubt that acceptability of foods depends upon prior experience and culture. Despite this, associations have been noted between sensitivity to tastants, particularly bitter agents, which are linked to food preference and behavior. In a classic study of 48 college students, Fischer et al. (1961) measured detection thresholds for sucrose, NaCl, HCl, quinine sulfate, and PTC (phenylthiocarbamide; bitter). Each subject filled out a questionnaire that asked which of 118 foods were disliked. There was no association between the number of foods checked as disliked and thresholds for sucrose, NaCl, and HCl. However, thresholds for PTC and quinine, both bitter substances, were significantly correlated with the percentage of food dislikes. In other words, those who were most sensitive to bitter substances disliked a greater number of foods than people who were less sensitive to such agents.

Suprathreshold Testing

By definition, suprathreshold tests are those that measure stimuli above threshold level for most people. The most common procedures document identification, discrimination, memory, and the perception of intensity and pleasantness. Although many such tests have been standardized, normative data are generally lacking.

Whole-Mouth Taste Identification and Attribute Rating Tests

In one whole-mouth test, five concentrations of sucrose (0.08, 0.16, 0.32, 0.64, 1.28 molar [M]), sodium chloride (0.032, 0.064, 0.128, 0.256, 0.512 M), citric acid (0.0026, 0.0051, 0.0102, 0.0205, 0.0410 M), and caffeine (0.0026, 0.0051, 0.0102, 0.0205, 0.0410 M) are presented in 10 mL samples to the patient in a counterbalanced order (Soter et al., 2008). On a given trial, the solution is sipped, swished in the mouth, and spat out. The subject then indicates whether the solution tastes sweet, sour, salty, or bitter, and evaluates its perceived intensity and pleasantness on rating scales. Forty stimuli are administered, i.e., 4 tastants × 5 concentrations × 2 trials. The total possible identification score for a given tastant is 10, with 40 being the maximum for the overall test.

Figure 4.7 is an example of taste identification scores obtained using this test in a study of healthy controls and those with impaired olfaction (Stinton et al., 2010). It clearly shows no effect of impaired olfaction on the ability to taste. Whole-mouth intensity ratings for the same subject group are shown in Figure 4.8 for NaCl, which shows unmistakably that there is no meaningful effect from damage to the olfactory system on suprathreshold intensity perception. It is also apparent that, for the chosen concentrations, sweet (sucrose) and salty (NaCl) tasting stimuli were more readily identified than bitter (caffeine) and sour (citric acid) stimuli (Figure 4.7) and that a log-linear relationship was present for the intensity ratings of NaCl (Figure 4.8). A similar relationship was seen with other tastants.

Magnitude estimation is a popular procedure for assessing differences in perceived intensity of tastant suprathreshold concentration. In the most common adaptation, subjects assign numbers in relative proportion to the perceived intensity of various concentrations of a tastant. A large literature shows that the slope relating stimulus concentration to perceived intensity, as measured by this procedure, is linear on log concentration/log magnitude estimation plots, reflecting a good fit to a power function. Unlike category scales, the unit of measurement is considered to be more-or-less on a ratio scale, i.e., a taste intensity score of 8 reflects a concentration perceived as twice as strong as a score of 4. Note that, in a category scale such as that used in the study above by Stinton et al., a value of 8 need not reflect an intensity that is twice as strong as a value of 4.

Despite the appeal of magnitude estimation, concentration: response functions for taste intensity are variable. In an early review, Meiselman (1971) emphasized that intensity exponents for existing studies of NaCl ranged from 0.41 to 1.59, which is a large variation in values. A similar array was noted for sucrose, whose exponents varied from 0.46 to 1.80, and quinine sulfate, whose exponents ranged from 0.30 to 1.00. Meiselman demonstrated that sip-and-spit procedures result in much larger exponents than procedures in which tastants are flowed over the tongue.

The ratio aspect of magnitude estimation is a difficult concept and the choice of numbers is frequently not standardized across subjects, resulting in difficulty making comparisons of magnitude estimates between subjects. Accordingly, investigators have sought more

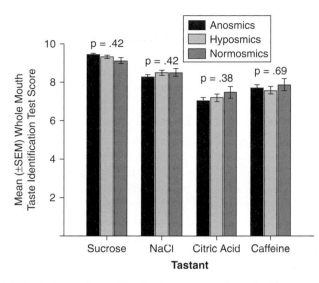

Figure 4.7 Mean (±SEM) whole-mouth taste identification test scores for each of four tastants in anosmics, hyposmics, and normosmics. Smell function is defined according to established norms. P values are for olfactory function group main effects from ANOVAs performed within each stimulus category. There is clearly no effect of impaired olfaction on the ability to identify basic taste qualities. From Figure 1 in Stinton et al. (2010).

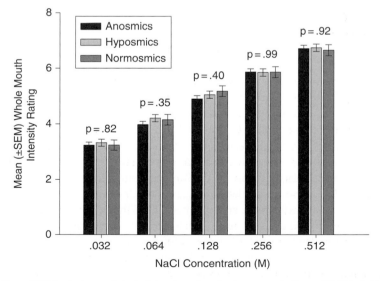

Figure 4.8 Mean (±SEM) whole-mouth taste intensity ratings for five concentrations of NaCl (salty) in anosmics, hyposmics, and normosmics. P values are for olfactory function group main effects from ANOVAs performed on data from each stimulus concentration. This shows no effect of smell impairment on NaCl intensity ratings. From Figure 4 in Stinton et al. (2010).

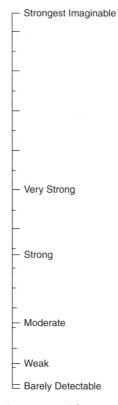

Figure 4.9 The oral label magnitude scale constructed from geometric means of magnitude estimates of the six semantic descriptors. Note the logarithmic-like nature of label distribution. Modified from Green et al. (1993).

practical means of assessing suprathreshold intensities that incorporate the advantages of magnitude estimation and simple rating scales. Green et al. (1993) developed a rating scale (Figure 4.9) for the measurement of oral sensations that provided data comparable to magnitude estimations. This scale, termed the Labeled Magnitude Scale (LMS), was slightly modified by Bartoshuk and colleagues, who changed the label of the extreme end of the scale from "strongest imaginable sensation" to the "strongest imaginable sensation of any kind" (Bartoshuk et al 2001) and called the new scale the "General Labeled Magnitude Scale" (gLMS). Subsequently, Bartoshuk's group noted that "the term 'imaginable' is open to various interpretations and can add noise to the data; thus we no longer use it" (Bartoshuk et al., 2012). Such scales have the advantage of spreading out taste intensity scores in a logarithmic-like manner, minimizing the tendency to clumping of responses at the extreme ends of the scale.

An example of an advantage of this type of scale over a classic category scale shown in Figure 4.10 is that the gLMS is more sensitive to the density of fungiform papillae, and hence the number of activated taste buds. The gLMS overcomes to a large degree the fact that concepts such as "strong" have diverse meanings to different people. As noted by Snyder et al. (2004),

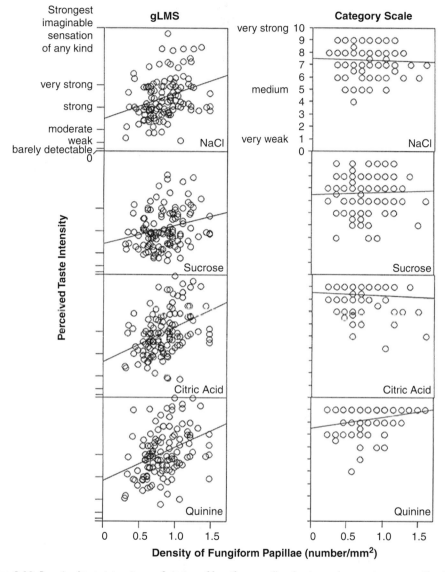

Figure 4.10 Perceived taste intensity as a function of fungiform papillae density on the anterior tongue. Graphs on the left were obtained with the gLMS (General Labeled Magnitude Scale); graphs on the right were obtained with a nine-point category scale. All correlations between perceived intensity and fungiform papilla density using the gLMS on the left were statistically significant ($p < 0.05$), but only the correlation for quinine was significant on the right using a standard category scale. From Snyder et al. (2004).

Imagine a woman who has just given birth. When you ask her about the pain of childbirth, she may describe it as "very strong," but when you present the bouquet of roses you brought to celebrate the arrival of her child, she may describe the floral odor as "very strong" too. Despite using the same words to describe these sensations, there is no implication that the rose odor intensity matched the pain of the "very strong" pain.

Adding a descriptor such as "strongest imaginable sensation of any kind" is an attempt by psychophysicists to stretch out the scale of intensity to a more common metric in an effort to homogenize suprathreshold responses better among individuals.

Based on the gLMS protocol, a clinically useful brief taste test was developed to be part of the US National Health and Nutrition Examination Survey (NHANES) (Rawal et al., 2015). This test is reliable and can be administered in less than five minutes. In the initial proof-of-concept research, 73 adults were evaluated on three occasions: baseline, two weeks later, and six months later. The subjects rated the intensities of 1 M NaCl and 1 mM quinine solutions presented both in a whole-mouth swish and spit and in a regional test of the anterior tongue in which the solution was applied using a Q-tip. A 0.32 M NaCl solution was also evaluated using the whole-mouth procedure. Intraclass reliability correlations ranged from 0.42 to 0.71. Since the whole-mouth quinine intensity ratings were highly correlated with the other measures, the study investigators concluded (p. 138) that that this single whole-mouth taste measure had "utility as a marker for overall taste functioning." Recent analysis of NHANES data based on this test has found that a significant number of people in the general population exhibit taste deficits (Liu et al., 2016).

Influences of Metabolic Processes on Taste Preferences

As noted by Fischer et al. (1961), threshold taste sensitivity to bitter can influence preferences, which in turn are influenced by bodily state. An early study clearly demonstrates how hypoglycemia is associated with pleasantness ratings for sucrose. Mayer-Gross & Walker (1946) presented five glasses of colorless liquid to each of 100 healthy subjects aged 17 to 45 years. The five glasses contained water, 5% sucrose, 30% sucrose, 0.5% NaCl, and saccharine (concentration not specified). Each subject was asked to describe the taste of every liquid and which one would be preferred for a long drink. A total of 202 measurements were made; some people were tested more than once. The patients were undergoing Sakel's classic insulin therapy for early schizophrenia, although only those who were fully alert were tested and the results were viewed as equivalent to those obtained from normal subjects. Blood glucose was determined at the time of testing. As shown in Figure 4.11, the rather sweet 30% sucrose solution was preferred over the other solutions when blood glucose level was below 50 mg/ 100 mg, whereas other solutions were preferred when the glucose level was above this value.

Regional Taste Identification and Attribute Rating Tests

Most regional taste identification procedures measure function on the left and right sides of the anterior tongue, although some test the posterior third, which is innervated by CN IX. Commonly the selected anterior regions are near the lateral margins of the tongue, whereas the posterior regions are on or near the filiform papillae and/or lateral-most vallate papillae. In one clinical test, 15 μL of sucrose (0.49 M), sodium chloride (0.31 M), citric acid (0.015 M), and caffeine (0.04 M), equated for kinematic viscosity using cellulose (~1.53 mm^2/s), was presented to selected tongue regions in a counterbalanced order using a micropipette (Stinton et al., 2010). On each trial, the patient reported whether a given solution tasted sweet, sour, salty, or bitter before retracting the tongue and rinsing with deionized water. A total of 96 forced-choice trials (4 tastants × 4 lingual regions × 6 repetitions) was presented. The maximum score a subject can attain across all segments of the tongue for a given tastant was 24.

Using this technique, gustation was evaluated in six patients with taste impairment associated with Terbinafine (Lamisil®), a widely prescribed oral antifungal agent. They

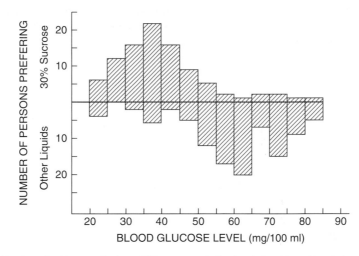

Figure 4.11 Number of subjects preferring a 30% sucrose solution in relationship to blood glucose levels. From Mayer-Gross & Walker (1946).

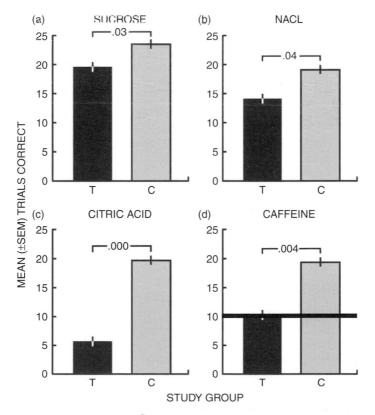

Figure 4.12 Influence of Terbinafine (Lamisil®) on taste identification test scores for stimuli representing the four major taste qualities. The agents were presented to the left and right anterior and posterior regions of the tongue using micropipettes. The test scores represent the summation of scores across all four lingual regions. T = Terbinafine patients; C = Controls (see text for details). From Doty & Haxel (2005).

were compared to six age-, sex-, and race-matched controls (Doty & Haxel, 2005). Despite the small samples, the mean taste scores were significantly lower in the Terbinafine group than in the controls for all stimuli, particularly for citric acid (sour) and caffeine (bitter) (Figure 4.12). In the case of NaCl, the Terbinafine-related deficit was largely confined to the posterior sectors of the tongue.

Normative Data for Regional Taste Testing

Like whole-mouth testing, few normative data are available for assessing regional taste dysfunction relative to healthy controls. An exception is a study by Pingel et al. (2010): no right-left side differences were apparent in their control sample, in keeping with other normative data. They used four concentrations of sucrose (0.03, 0.1, 0.4, 2.0 g/mL), citric acid (0.01, 0.05, 0.1, 0.15 g/mL), NaCl (0.025, 0.075, 0.15, 0.36 g/mL), and quinine HCl (0.0002, 0.0005, 0.001, 0.01 g/mL). Stimuli were administered using an 18 cm long, 0.4 cm diameter "glass probe". As noted by these investigators,

> A drop (approximately 20 μL) of liquid sweet, sour or salty tastant was applied on both sides of the anterior third of the extended tongue (sweet on the tongue tip; sour and salty on the tongue edge). The bitter tastants were presented on both sides of the posterior third of the extended tongue. The tastants were applied in a pseudo-randomized order starting with the lowest concentration, ending with the highest quinine hydrochloride solution and alternating the side of stimulation. In a multiple-alternative procedure, taste stimuli were presented at intervals of about 30 s. After presentation of the stimulus and with their tongue still extended, subjects were asked to pick one of the five descriptors ("sweet", "sour", "bitter", or "water/no taste").

The test score was the sum of correct responses on each side of the tongue (total possible = 16). Given that no left-right side differences were found, the normative data are presented in Table 4.5 for both sides combined. The scores when each side of the tongue is tested can be halved. It is apparent from this table that scores at or below ~23 infer gustatory dysfunction regardless of age. The lack of a sex difference and the very weak effect of age is apparent. It might have been preferable to have subdivided the >55 age category, since the most severe taste deficits occur after the age of 60.

It is unfortunate that there are few published normative data available for threshold or suprathreshold testing. For routine clinical work borrowed controls may suffice, but for most research purposes it is recommended that investigators obtain control data from the local population to avoid confounding from, e.g., social, ethnic, linguistic, and occupational influences.

Electrogustometry

Basic Considerations

As mentioned earlier in this chapter, electrical, rather than chemical, stimulation of the taste system has numerous practical advantages. The duration and extent of electrical stimulus can be controlled without difficulty, rinsing between stimulus presentations is not necessary, areas of the palate can be tested easily, and mixing and storage of tastants is not required. The device is portable, making it amenable to bedside and other out-of-laboratory applications.

Table 4.5. Normative data (percentiles) for a taste study in men (top) and women (bottom) that combine responses to sweet-, sour-, bitter-, and salty-tasting agents presented to the anterior tongue using glass probes. Note minimal influences of both age and sex on the test scores. Modified from Pingel et al. (2010).

MEN				
	AGE GROUP (Years)			
	5–15	**16–35**	**36–55**	**>55**
95th Percentile	32	32	32	32
90th Percentile	32	32	32	32
75th Percentile	32	32	32	32
50th Percentile	32	30	30	30
25th Percentile	30	28	26	28
10th Percentile	27	24	24	24
5th Percentile	25	24	22	23
Mean (SD)	30.7 (2.1)	29.7 (2.9)	28.6 (3.6)	29.1 (3.3)
N:	31	99	177	139

WOMEN				
	AGE GROUP (Years)			
	5–15	**16–35**	**36–55**	**>55**
95th Percentile	32	32	32	32
90th Percentile	32	32	32	32
75th Percentile	32	32	32	32
50th Percentile	30	32	30	30
25th Percentile	29	30	27	28
10th Percentile	28	28	24	24
5th Percentile	24	26	22	23
Mean (SD)	30.3 (2.0)	30.7 (2.1)	28.7 (2.8)	29.9 (2.8)
N:	20	121	193	164

In the most common electrogustometry paradigm, low microampere currents, usually of half-second duration, are applied to selected regions of the tongue via a stainless steel electrode, typically the anode. The cathode is attached elsewhere, e.g., the nape of the neck or on the hand. The electrogustometer (EGM) takes into account resistance differences among people, i.e., it is a constant current generator, thus eliminating any issues associated with different resistances due to body size, composition, or distance between the anode and cathode. Nevertheless, the physiologic basis for the production of electrical sensations remains controversial and electrogustometry rarely produces classic taste sensations (Murphy et al., 1995). In fact, sweet responses are never observed, in accord with observations of rat studies that anodal current does not activate sucrose sensitive fibers (Ninomiya & Funakoshi, 1981). Nonetheless, functional imaging studies demonstrate that electrical

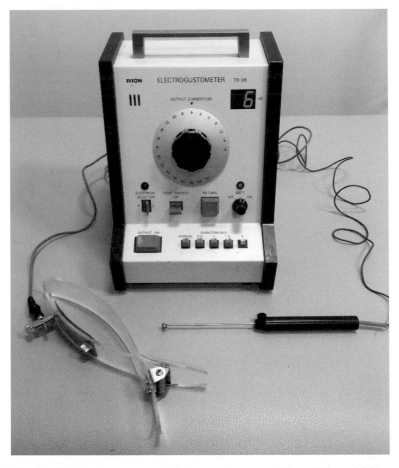

Figure 4.13 The Rion TR06 Electrogustometer. This is a popular commercially available model. Discrete stimulus pulses can be presented at durations varying from 0.5 to 2 sec duration and currents adjustable from −6 dB (4μA) to 34 dB (400μA) in 21 steps. From left to right: earth strip which is placed around the neck; gustometer with stimulating electrode below. Also supplied is a foot pedal and remote stimulator switch (not shown).

stimulation of the tongue activates essentially the same taste-related brain regions as chemical stimulation (Barry et al., 2001), as explained later in this chapter.

Electrogustometric Threshold Testing

Several psychophysical procedures that employ low electrical currents have been used to activate taste afferents on the tongue or palate. The more prevalent methods are staircase procedures. The Rion TR06 (Figure 4.13) is popular partly because it can deliver the lowest current discernable by most healthy people (−4 μA). This is of particular relevance when examining tongue regions such as the tongue tip that are densely packed with papillae. Despite this, "basement" or "floor" effects are often seen in threshold experiments, particularly when forced-choice procedures are involved (Loucks & Doty, 2004). Clinically this is not a major problem, since basement effects signify normal function, but it does reduce the ability to establish a participant's specific threshold values over regions densely populated with papillae. This might become an issue when subtle effects of medication and other interventions, such as surgery, need to be assessed.

Although chemical thresholds decrease monotonically, i.e., in the same orderly direction, as stimuli increase up to 1.5 sec (Bagla et al., 1997), thresholds based upon electrical stimulation are different. For example, one study found that, as expected, electrical thresholds were lower for stimuli of 1.0 sec duration compared to 0.5 sec, but remarkably, thresholds for longer stimuli, lasting 1.5 sec, were equivalent to those of 0.5 sec duration (Loucks & Doty, 2004). Thus, electrical threshold values behaved in a U-shaped curve and were raised if the stimulus duration exceeded one second, unlike chemical thresholds that continue to decline (i.e., show better sensitivity) with increasing stimulus duration. A source of confusion in the literature is the fact that not all studies employ the same stimulus durations, with values ranging from 0.25 sec to 2.0 sec. It is also important to recognize that EGM thresholds obtained on tongue regions where papillae are less dense are lower and more reliable for larger ($125 \ mm^2$) than smaller ($25 \ mm^2$) electrodes, presumably reflecting the number of taste afferents that are activated (Nicolaescu et al., 2005). This becomes important because electrode sizes vary among studies [e.g., 12.5 and 50 mm^2 electrodes by Miller et al. (2002) and Loucks & Doty (2004), 20 mm^2 electrodes by Krarup (1958) and Lobb et al. (2000), 60 mm^2 electrodes by Grant et al. (1987), and 234 mm^2 electrodes by Coates (1974)], making difficult any comparisons across laboratories. Although EGM thresholds correlate well with regional taste tests, often they do not correlate well with whole-mouth taste tests. This would be expected, since they stimulate only small lingual sectors that need not be representative of the taste bud distribution of the entire tongue.

Normative Data for Electrogustometric Thresholds

Like chemical taste testing, reports of "normal" electrical thresholds differ markedly from one study to the next and normative data are rare. Reflecting other taste measures, EGM thresholds are influenced by age and, in some studies, gender, although large individual differences mask such effects frequently. A major issue is how to determine the cut-off for abnormality. In this section, abnormality is defined as thresholds that fall around or below the fifth percentile, as in Tables 4.3 and 4.5.

The distribution of EGM thresholds obtained in 460 subjects aged 15 to 94 years is presented in Figure 4.14 (Nakazato et al., 2002). Two lingual regions on each side of the tongue were evaluated (Figure 4.15), namely an area on the anterolateral tongue 2 cm from the midline and a region on the foliate papillae. Palatal regions innervated by the greater (superficial) petrosal nerve (CN VII) located 1 cm posterior to the uvula and 1 cm to the left and right of the midline were also assessed (not shown).

In a recent study, EGM thresholds were determined for 74 men and 82 women, all non-smokers, aged 10 to 80 years (Pavlidis et al., 2012). They examined six regions of the tongue and palate as shown in Figure 4.16. Stimulus duration was 1 second and a non-forced-choice staircase threshold test was employed. Subjects were instructed to be certain they experienced a metallic rather than electrical sensation, under their assumption that the former was induced by the gustatory system and the latter by the trigeminal system. The right side was tested first. On the basis of learning or other testing order effects, it would be predicted that test performance might be higher on the left than on the right, but the opposite was found. Most thresholds were lower on the right than on the left side at all

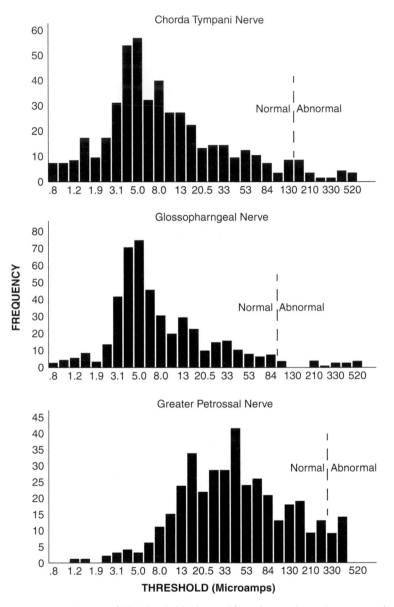

Figure 4.14 Frequency distribution of EGM thresholds obtained from three regions using an ascending single-series non-forced-choice threshold measure. Cut-off for abnormality is at ~5th percentile in each case. Note similarities in the distributions between the chorda tympani (CN VII) and glossopharyngeal (CN IX) responses, and the higher thresholds for the greater petrosal nerve (CN VII). Modified from Nakazato et al. (2002).

the target sites for both sexes. Since counterbalancing of test order was not done, it is not known if this was a true effect or due to some confound, such as adaptation or subject fatigue.

The average test results are presented for each tongue region, sex, and age group in Table 4.5. Pavlidis et al. (2012) reported that thresholds of the subjects older than 65

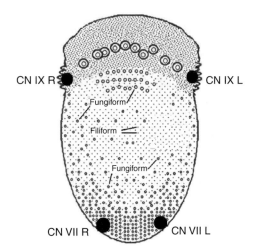

Figure 4.15 Lingual regions tested for EGM thresholds shown in Figure 4.14. Anterior points were 2 cm from the midline at the margin of the tongue.

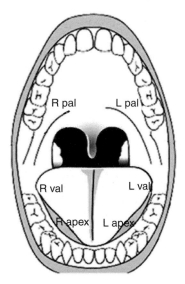

Figure 4.16 Oral sites for electrical threshold determinations described by Pavlidis et al. (2012). Pal = soft palate; Val = vallate papillae; A = apex of tongue. The goal was to evaluate the function of the chorda tympani, glossopharyngeal, and greater petrosal nerves. Actual distances from the midline or other markers were not given.

years were significantly higher than those of younger age groups. No statistically significant sex differences were found in this study. Table 4.5 shows that, in agreement with Nakazato et al. (2002), thresholds were generally higher over the soft palate than on the tongue, and that the lowest thresholds occurred typically on the two anterior

Table 4.6. Electrogustometric thresholds calculated in decades for men and women at six different oral sites shown in Figure 4.16. Data recalculated as µA from dB values reported by Pavlidis et al. (2012). Means (SD) are represented. L&R represents geometric mean of the left and right sides for each age group providing a better indication of overall age effects.

Anterior tongue

Age		Men				Women		
	N	Left	Right	L&R	N	Left	Right	L&R
10–14	8	5.6 (8.8)	5.9 (8.5)	5.7	9	6.1 (9.1)	5.1 (8.6)	5.6
15–19	9	5.2 (9.2)	6.3 (8.1)	5.7	12	5.3 (9.1)	6.4 (8.0)	5.8
20–29	10	10.5 (9.1)	8.3 (8.0)	9.3	11	11.1 (9.3)	8.1 (8.1)	9.5
30–39	10	15.5 (10.2)	12.7 (8.1)	14.0	12	10.6 (9.8)	13.0 (9.1)	11.7
40–49	11	20.1 (9.3)	23.8 (9.3)	21.9	12	20.9 (10.0)	25.7 (9.8)	23.2
50–59	11	31.4 (9.8)	29.1 (10.0)	30.2	11	33.5 (10.4)	54.6 (10.2)	42.8
60–69	10	49.8 (11.2)	43.3 (10.0)	46.4	10	52.4 (11.0)	49.2 (10.3)	50.8
>70	5	51.8 (10.4)	42.2 (9.6)	46.8	5	54.6 (10.3)	40.6 (9.8)	47.1

Posterior (vallate) tongue

Age		Men				Women		
	N	Left	Right	L&R	N	Left	Right	L&R
10–14	8	10.6 (8.8)	13.0 (9.2)	11.7	9	13.0 (9.1)	12.1 (9.1)	12.5
15–19	9	12.2 (8.8)	12.7 (9.1)	12.4	12	13.0 (9.2)	12.9 (9.2)	12.9
20–29	10	15.2 (10.0)	14.0 (9.3)	14.6	11	16.5 (9.6)	15.6 (9.4)	16.0
30–39	10	19.9 (9.8)	19.6 (9.2)	19.7	12	20.9 (9.8)	20.4 (9.6)	20.6
40–49	11	26.6 (10.0)	26.1 (9.8)	26.3	12	33.1 (9.8)	28.8 (10.0)	30.9

	Men					Women		
50–59	11	31.8 (9.8)	32.0 (10.0)	31.9	11	37.9 (10.2)	33.0 (10.2)	35.4
60–69	10	40.7 (10.2)	34.3 (10.4)	37.4	10	42.6 (10.0)	38.5 (10.3)	40.5
>70	5	69.5 (10.4)	58.6 (9.8)	63.8	5	72.1 (10.2)	144.8 10.2)	102.2

Palate

Age	Men				N	Women		
	N	Left	Right	L&R		Left	Right	L&R
10–14	8	22.8 (9.8)	18.6 (9.8)	20.6	9	25.92 (9.8)	20.1 (9.8)	22.8
15–19	9	30.2 (9.4)	33.0 (10.2)	31.6	12	32.3 (9.5)	23.4 (9.8)	27.5
20–29	10	32.1 (9.8)	25.4 (9.6)	28.6	1˙	32.9 (9.6)	31.7 (9.8)	32.3
30–39	10	53.0 (9.8)	40.2 (10.2)	46.2	12	51.7 (10.0)	50.6 (10.0)	51.1
40–49	11	62.0 (10.2)	51.8 (10.3)	56.7	12	67.4 (10.3)	65.2 (10.2)	66.3
50–59	11	93.6 (10.0)	92.8 (8.1)	93.2	11	105.4 (10.2)	102.4 (10.3)	104.4
60–69	10	132.0 (10.3)	116.0 (10.3)	123.7	10	128.8 (10.4)	124.0 (10.0)	126.4
>70	5	146.4 (10.4)	162.4 (10.6)	154.2	5	171.2 (10.0)	162.4 (10.8)	166.7

tongue sites. The posterior tongue was less sensitive than the anterior tongue, unlike the finding of Nakazato et al. (2002), perhaps because the latter investigators tested foliate rather than vallate papillae. The large standard deviations indicated in Table 4.5 illustrate that, with this particular test paradigm, there is considerable individual variation in threshold measures. It is not clear to what degree such disparity is dependent upon the test procedure itself or the large inter-personal variation of taste bud distribution in the human oral cavity.

EGM Suprathreshold Testing

Few investigators have assessed electrical sensitivity at suprathreshold levels. An exception is the study by Salata et al. (1991). These investigators employed a cross-modal matching procedure that allowed for assessment of both the slope and absolute magnitude (position) of the suprathreshold stimulus:response function in college-age subjects. In this paradigm, each subject provided magnitude estimates of stimulus intensity for two sensory continua, namely electric taste and hearing, during the same test session. Assuming that subjects experienced tone loudness in a similar manner, differences between subjects in the derived scale that related loudness to physical stimulus intensity should reflect differences in number usage rather than sensory sensitivity. Operationally, the magnitude estimates given to each electric stimulus are mapped to equivalent points on the function relating tone stimuli to their perceived intensity. The corresponding hearing level value, in decibels, is then plotted for each subject against the subject's electric taste magnitude estimates and a regression line is established. This matching function corrects for the subject's idiosyncratic use of numbers. Stevens and Marks (1980) have shown that such matching functions show far less variability in absolute magnitude, conform better to power functions, and often show less variation in slope than traditional magnitude estimation functions.

As shown in Figure 4.17, the NaCl magnitude estimate function at the tip of the tongue was both larger in absolute magnitude and 69 percent steeper in slope than the functions obtained for the other tongue regions – values that did not differ statistically from one another. This research indicates that the tip of the tongue is more sensitive than other tongue regions to suprathreshold electrical taste stimulation, adding to the observation that the tip exhibits lower thresholds to both electrical and some chemical stimuli such as NaCl (see Figure 4.3).

Gustatory Event-Related Potentials (GEPs)

The pioneering study on GEPs was that of Plattig (1969), who used electrical stimuli. Devices for presenting chemicals to the tongue were developed subsequently, because of concerns that the taste buds, per se, were likely bypassed by electrical stimulation, Among the pioneers in liquid-based GEP studies were Gerull et al. (1984) and Plattig and Haußner (1985). The more refined system developed by Plattig et al. (1988) for measuring GEPs is shown in Figure 4.18, and examples of GEPs for NaCl using this system are presented in Figure 4.19.

Subsequently Kobal (1985) delivered gaseous acetic acid to the tongue of five subjects via an olfactometer in which potential temperature, humidity, and stimulus onset confounds were controlled (see Chapter 2). GEPs were recorded from standard 10/20 scalp positions referred to A1. The vertex was site of the largest GEPs. As acetic acid concentration was

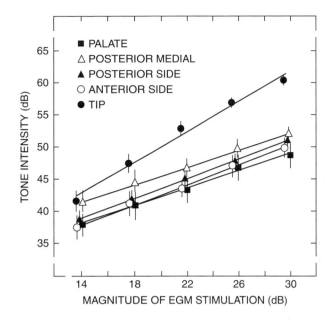

Figure 4.17 Perceived magnitude of electrical taste (converted to a tone level) as a function of electrical stimulus intensity in dB using an electrogustometer. N − 12. From Salata et al. (1991).

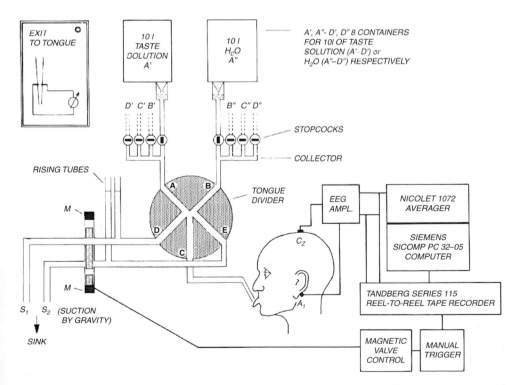

Figure 4.18 Diagram of an early gustometer used to measure gustatory evoked potentials. Tastants are contained in reservoirs (top center box) and water (top right box). Tastants flow through a series of valves and can be diverted to the tongue. For details, see Plattig et al. (1988).

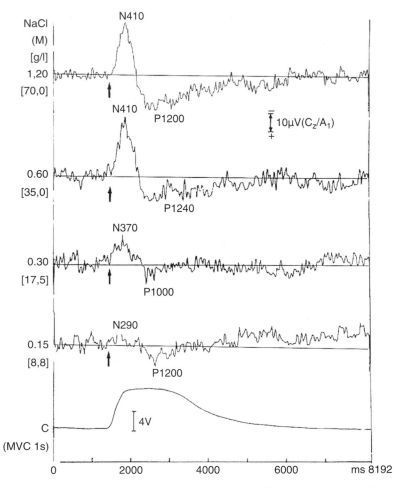

Figure 4.19 Gustatory event-related potentials to four concentrations of NaCl: 1.2 M (top), 0.6 M, 0.3 M, and 0.15 M (bottom). Arrows indicate stimulus onset, which occurs ~1500 ms after the beginning of recording. From Plattig et al. (1988).

increased, GEP latencies decreased and amplitudes increased. Replication and extension of this work was performed by Hummel et al. (2010) in a study of 17 healthy subjects, once more implementing acetic acid vapors at 70% and 100% saturation in air. The stimuli were directed toward the lateral aspects of the anterior tongue using a tube with multiple openings (Figure 4.20). In one patient with hemiageusia, as measured psychophysically, GEPs were absent on the abnormal side. Interestingly, unlike the gustatory psychophysical thresholds, it was found that women displayed larger amplitudes and shorter latencies than men.

Imaging Studies

Location of the Secondary Taste Center. It was widely believed until the mid-twentieth century that the cortical brain regions associated with taste were the same as those for smell,

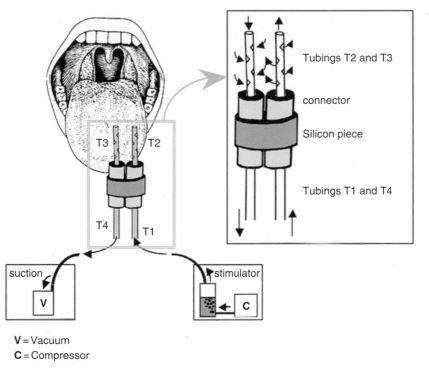

V = Vacuum
C = Compressor

Figure 4.20 Drawing of mouthpiece for presentation of acetic acid vapors to the tongue. During stimulation, subjects kept the mouth closed and used a breathing technique that separated the oral from the nasal cavity. Acetic acid vapor was blown onto the tongue through tubes T1 and T2, and sucked away from the oral cavity through Tubes T3 and T4. The apparatus, which lateralized the side of stimulation, was held in place by the subject who bit onto the connector. Modified from Hummel et al. (2010).

being located together within the temporal lobe. As pointed out by Bornstein (1940a), this belief was confounded, mainly by the investigators' misinterpretation of smell sensations as "taste" sensations. Bornstein (p. 735) states,

> It is this close functional and psychological interrelation which has led to the belief that the two "chemical senses" form basically one morphological and psychological unit, that they are merely divisions of a single chemical sense. Olfaction and gustation differ, according to Nagel (Nagel, 1894) and more recent authors, only in that the sense of smell is stimulated by gases and the sense of taste by fluids. It is, therefore, understandable that the cortical taste center has been placed in the immediate neighborhood of the centers of smell, that is, in the temporal lobe.

Bornstein reviewed anatomical and physiological data that led him to conclude that the cortical taste center was, in fact, within the "inferior part of the parietal lobe." He further noted (p. 726) that "there are many reasons for believing that the cortical taste center is localized in the neighborhood of the cortical tactile representation of the parts carrying taste buds, i.e., tongue, soft palate, pharynx, and epiglottis," and reviewed numerous lines of evidence in support of this concept.

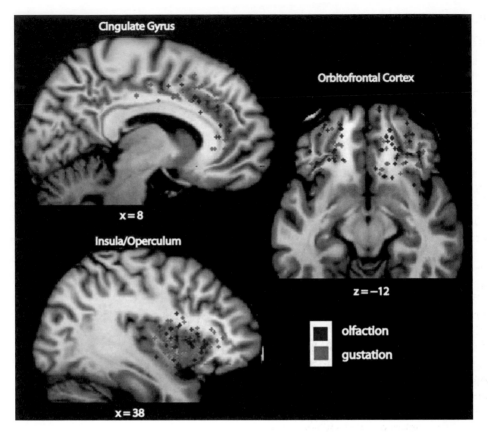

Figure 4.21 Images showing activation foci (peaks) reported in studies of gustatory (red) and olfactory (blue) stimulation in the anterior cingulate cortex (top left sagittal section), insula/operculum (bottom left sagittal section), and orbitofrontal cortex (right axial section). The three plots clearly show that chemosensory stimuli activate a variety of regions within the insula, anterior cingulate, and orbitofrontal cortex and that many of these regions are responsive to both gustatory and olfactory stimulation. Visual inspection of the plots suggests that taste stimuli tend to activate the caudal and lateral orbitofrontal cortex, whereas olfactory stimuli do not (especially in the right hemisphere). In contrast, olfactory stimuli tend to activate the ventral most insular region, which is continuous with primary olfactory cortex; whereas gustatory stimuli do not. Reproduced with permission from Small and Prescott (2005). (A black and white version of this figure will appear in some formats. For the color version, please refer to the plate section Figure 2.10.)

Studies that applied electric current directly to the exposed surface of human brain have since shown that Bornstein's general conclusion is only partially correct and not supported by anatomical studies (see Chapter 2). The thalamic taste relay (VPMpc) projects primarily to the granular regions of the rostral insula that constitute the primary taste cortex (see Figure 4.21). This area connects to the nearby dysgranular and agranular regions of the insula (anterior operculum), which comprise the secondary gustatory cortices. Projections from the secondary taste cortex travel to the caudolateral orbitofrontal cortex for integration with other sensory modalities. Foerster, who stimulated the parietal operculum during human intracranial operations (Foerster, 1936), obtained taste responses but this was likely due to stimulus spread to the nearby primary gustatory areas.

Early Primate Electrophysiological and Human Functional Imaging Studies

The advent of positron emission tomography (PET) and functional magnetic imaging (fMRI) subsequently allowed more global *in vivo* assessment of human gustatory brain activity. The limited resolution of the first PET scanners made it difficult to identify the primary gustatory cortex specifically (Kinomura et al., 1994). A pioneering study by Kobayakawa et al. (1996) that used magneto-encephalography (MEG) found dipoles within the transition area between the insula and inner face of the operculum. Although subsequent PET and fMRI investigators identified taste-related activation in the parietal operculum, insula, cingulate cortex, and orbitofrontal cortex (OFC), the data were pooled without time-locked epochs (Small & Prescott, 2005) The OFC is now considered to be a multisensory association area (Frey & Petrides, 1999; de Araujo et al., 2003; Small et al., 2004; Ogawa et al., 2005; Veldhuizen et al., 2011; Nakamura et al., 2012). Figure 4.21 shows the areas activated by tastes and smells in the primary and secondary olfactory cortical structures.

Influences of Expectation, Motivation, or Bodily Need on Cortical Taste-Related Activity

Expectation is now known to influence the responses of cells within the insula to taste stimulation. According to Woods et al. (2011), when subjects were expecting a very sweet drink but received one that was less sweet, activity within the insula was higher than the expectation for the less sweet drink. Nitschke et al. (2006) found a similar phenomenon for bitter stimulants. In other words, insula activity is modulated by top-down neural processes associated with expectation. Cells that modulate such activity include those within the ventral striatum, the inferior ventral striatum and intraparietal sulcus (Veldhuizen et al., 2011).

In electrophysiological studies of non-human primates, cells within the caudolateral orbitofrontal cortex respond to the sight and taste of food when the animal is hungry, but not when it is sated. This is generally not the case in the nucleus of the solitary tract, where the first brain stem taste relay takes place, nor in the insula cells (Rolls et al., 1989). Interestingly, the responses of orbitofrontal cortex (OFC) cells are tuned specifically to those stimuli to which the animal becomes satisfied. For example, cells sensitive to glucose in this brain region largely stop firing once the animals become replete with glucose but continue to discharge normally to other tastants to which they have not been sated, such as blackcurrant juice. The reverse occurs when satiation is to blackcurrant juice; i.e., responses are suppressed to blackcurrant juice but remain normal to glucose.

When humans are replete with food they find it less appealing or even repugnant, yet not necessarily less intense (Rolls et al., 1983), suggesting that the aforementioned changes in a cell's firing patterns within the OFC are not critical for signaling intensity. Rather, these cells are involved in evaluative processes intimately linked to bodily state or need, along with other brain centers such as the hypothalamus. Such observations support the concept that pleasantness of a taste is represented in the brain separate from its identity and intensity, making it possible to learn about a taste whether or not hunger is felt (Rolls, 2005).

It should be emphasized that the caudolateral OFC is a brain region where cells become conditioned to stimulation from combinations of sensory inputs, including olfactory, gustatory, tactile, and visual modalities. In one primate study of 112 single neurons within the OFC, 34% responded only to taste, 13% just to odorants, and 13% only to visual stimuli

(Rolls & Baylis, 1994). Thirteen percent responded to taste *and* odor stimuli, 13% to taste *and* visual stimuli, and 5% to odor *and* visual stimuli. Interestingly, specific congruence was present in some instances between the multiple inputs. For example, a cell that fired to both glucose and a visual stimulus preferentially fired to a visual stimulus signifying a sweet taste over one associated with water or some other taste quality. These findings suggest that such cells become "conditioned" to a set of previously paired stimuli (Rolls, 2001), although some sensory pairings appear to be more robust than others (Critchley & Rolls, 1996; Rolls et al., 1996).

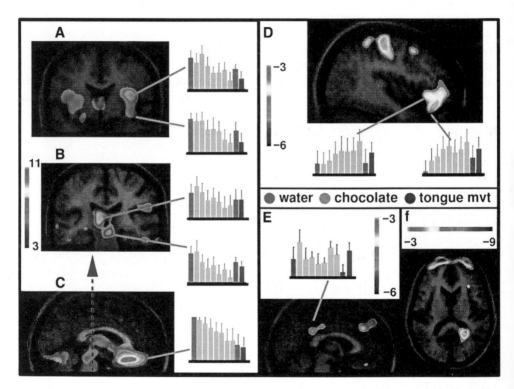

Figure 4.22 Cortical regions demonstrating significant rCBF correlations with pleasantness/unpleasantness ratings following ingestion of chocolate. Correlations are shown as *t* statistic images superimposed on corresponding averaged MRI scans. The *t* statistic ranges for each set of images are coded by color bars, one in each box. Bar graphs represent normalized CBF in an 8 mm radius surrounding the peak. The *y*-axis corresponds to normalized activity and the bars along the *x*-axis represent scans. The three colors represent scan type (purple = water only trials, light blue = chocolate trials, dark blue = tongue movement trials). Each bar graph corresponds to activations indicated by a turquoise line. A. Coronal section taken at *y* = 1 showing the decrease in rCBF in the primary gustatory area (bilaterally in the anterior insula/frontal operculum and in the right ventral insula). B. Coronal section taken at *y* = –26 showing decreases in rCBF in the left thalamus and medial midbrain (possibly corresponding to the ventral tegmental area). C. Sagittal section taken at *x* = –1 showing decreases in rCBF in the subcallosal region, thalamus, and midbrain. D. Sagittal section taken at *x* = 42 showing the increase in rCBF in the right caudolateral orbitofrontal cortex. Activation is also evident in the motor and premotor areas. E. Sagittal section taken at *x* = 8 showing an increase in rCBF in the posterior cingulate gyrus (peak at 8, –30, 45) in subtraction analysis Choc 1 – water-post. This was the only region where CBF was consistently greater in affective scans regardless of valence, compared with the neutral chocolate scan (Choc 4) and the two water baseline scans (water-pre and water-post). F. Horizontal section at *z* = 12 showing an increase in rCBF in the retrosplenial cortex (area 30) that correlated with affective rating (ii) but not the affective rating (i) when scan order was covaried out of the regression. Reproduced with permission from Small et al. (2001). (A black and white version of this figure will appear in some formats. For the colour version, please refer to the plate section.)

Modulation of the OFC and its close association with brain regions associated with reward and punishment are well illustrated by a PET study in which successive scans were obtained from volunteers while they ate chocolate to satiety and beyond (Small et al., 2001). After eating each piece of chocolate, which induces multimodal input from taste, smell, and somatosensation, the subjects rated how pleasant/unpleasant the chocolate experience was to them and how much they wanted or did not want another piece. While they still retained the desire to eat chocolate and found it tasted pleasant, enhanced brain activity was found within the subcallosal region, caudomedial OFC, insula/operculum zone, striatum, and midbrain. When they were sated, without any desire to eat more chocolate, further consumption resulted in greater brain activity within the parahippocampal gyrus, caudolateral OFC, and prefrontal brain regions. These findings, which are illustrated in Figure 4.22, led the authors to suggest that there may be a functional disassociation of the neural representation of reward and punishment within the OFC.

It is important to recognize that the influences on OFC activity, including those of reward and punishment, are quite general. Thus, Plassmann et al. (2008) assessed blood-oxygen-level-dependent (BOLD) fMRI activity in subjects who tasted wines that they were led to believe were different from one another and were sold at different prices. A correlation was present between the believed price of the wine samples, their rated pleasantness, and the amount of brain activity emanating from the medial OFC. This study concludes that marketing-based manipulations can alter not only subject's ratings of how pleasant wines taste, but also the neural correlates of perceived pleasantness within the OFC.

Many Brain Regions Become Activated During Tasting

Although the primary and secondary taste cortices play a significant role in taste perception, many other brain regions are involved. These include the hippocampus, thalamus, anterior cingulate gyrus, parahippocampal gyrus, lingual gyrus, caudate nucleus, temporal gyri, and amygdala (e.g., Kinomura et al., 1994). In the case of the amygdala it was noted that mid-insular activation occurred over a range of aqueous concentrations for sucrose and NaCl (Spetter et al., 2010). Only NaCl showed concentration-related increases in activation of the amygdala. This implies that higher levels of NaCl are perceived as more unpleasant than higher concentrations of sucrose, and that the amygdala is coding for hedonic elements of sensation. In the absence of formal taste stimulation, a wide variety of words activate the left inferior frontal, posterior, middle, and superior temporal gyri. Taste-related words produce stronger activation than other words in the anterior insula, frontal operculum, lateral orbitofrontal gyrus, and thalamus. This suggests that the meaning of taste words is based on distributed cortical circuits extending into brain regions that process taste sensations (Barros-Loscertales et al., 2012). Similar brain areas are activated when subjects simply imagine taste sensations (Levy et al., 1999).

Electrical Stimulation of Lingual Taste Afferents Activate the Same Regions as Chemical Stimuli

Low current (≤50 µA) electrical stimulation of each side of the anterior tongue results in fMRI activations which mimic, in most ways, what is seen using chemical taste stimulation. This was confirmed in a study of 11 right-handed subjects aged 22 to 45 years, where such stimulation activated the primary gustatory cortex, as defined in humans and other primates (Barry et al., 2001). Specifically, the following regions were activated *bilaterally* by electrical stimulation of

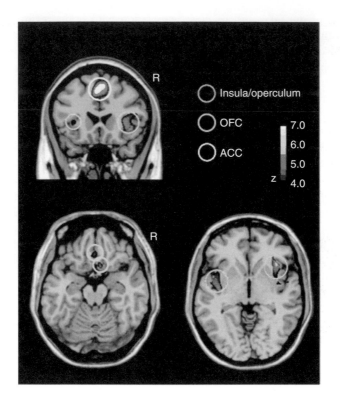

Figure 4.23 fMRI image of brain regions activated by mineral (Evian) water (i.e., water – control water comparison). Statistically significant activations were observed in the insular/opercular cortex, the orbitofrontal cortex (OFC), and the anterior cingulate cortex (ACC). Values > 4.54 on the vertical scale are significant at p < 0.05. From de Araujo et al. (2003), with permission. (A black and white version of this figure will appear in some formats. For the color version, please refer to the plate section.)

either side of the tongue: (a) superior temporal lobe, (b) inferior frontal lobe (including premotor regions), and (c) inferior sectors of the postcentral gyrus. The superior insula was activated bilaterally but uptake was more conspicuous in the right than in the left hemisphere. Activation of the central (inferior) elements of the insula were generally symmetric.

Water Alone Activates the Same Brain Regions as Tastants

Surprisingly, water alone can increase fMRI signals in areas that are also activated by tastants such as NaCl and glucose, namely the frontal operculum/anterior insular region and caudal OFC (Figure 4.23) (Zald & Pardo, 2000; de Araujo et al., 2003). De-ionized distilled water was used by Zald and Pardo (2000), which has no taste, whereas the other group (de Araujo et al., 2003) implemented mineral water (Evian water) which arguably has a distinct flavor. While thirst or water-related satiety had little influence on the magnitude of signal in the aforementioned insular regions, this was not the case for the caudal OFC. No signal change was noted in this area after mineral water had been drunk to satiety. Importantly, ratings of water pleasantness correlated with activations of the caudal and anterior OFC and the anterior cingulate cortex (Figure 4.24). The reason for this apparent anomaly is not clear. According to de Araujo et al. (2003), one possibility is that water acts

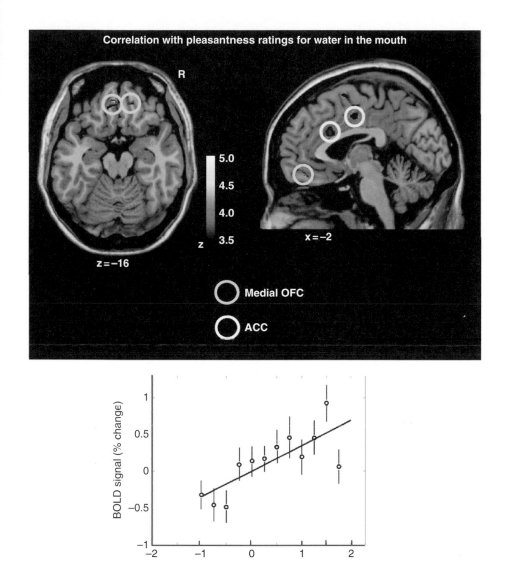

Figure 4.24 fMRI image of brain regions activated by mineral (Evian) water. Top left: regions of the medial caudal orbitofrontal cortex where activation was correlated with perceived pleasantness ratings of water. Bottom: a scatter plot and regression line showing the signal values in the medial orbitofrontal cortex (points represent mean ± SEM values across subjects). From de Araujo et al. (2003), with permission. (A black and white version of this figure will appear in some formats. For the color version, please refer to the plate section.)

through a taste-sensitive system. In particular, salt-best neurons might decrease their firing rate below the spontaneous level when water is placed on the tongue. Such salt-best neurons may be sufficiently sensitive to respond to the decrease of a few micromoles in Na^+ concentration (and other cations) when the saliva in the mouth is replaced by water. Another possibility is that water-best neurons in the cortex respond to a combination of fluid of a low viscosity in the mouth and the lack of taste neurons firing.

Applications of Functional Imaging in Assessing Taste Dysfunction

There are relatively few studies of fMRI in patients with gustatory dysfunction, likely reflecting the difficulties in defining clearly those patients who are appropriate for testing. Henkin et al. (2000) assessed fMRI responses in two patients who had previously experienced obnoxious taste and smell sensations in the absence of sensory stimulation, i.e., phantogeusias and phantosmias, respectively. When the patients were asked to remember the distorted sensations, the brain regions associated with central processing within the relevant sensory systems were activated more than when real sensory stimuli were presented.

In a more recent study, 13 women engaged in binge eating (bulimia nervosa) and 13 healthy female controls underwent fMRI assessment during receipt or anticipated receipt of a chocolate milkshake as well as a tasteless solution (Bohon & Stice, 2012). Affect ratings were obtained just prior to the scan using the Positive and Negative Affect Schedule (PANAS) (Watson et al., 1988). In women with bulimia nervosa, a positive association was found between negative affect and fMRI activity in the putamen, caudate, and pallidum during anticipated receipt of milkshake (versus tasteless solution). There were no significant relations between negative mood and receipt of the milkshake. Connectivity analysis found that amygdala activity was more strongly related to activation in the left putamen and insula in the bulimia group than in the control group during *anticipated* receipt of a milkshake. The opposite was true for the *actual taste* of the milkshake; i.e., the control group showed a greater relation of amygdala activity to activation in the left putamen and insula in response to receiving the milkshake. The authors concluded that negative mood may increase the reward value of food for individuals with bulimia. Alternatively, negative affect may be a conditioned cue, reflecting a history of binge eating while in a negative mood.

Practical Applications

Someone new to this field may be confused with the vast number of procedures available and the pitfalls waiting to trap the unwary. No matter how "perfect" is a given procedure, if it takes hours to evaluate just one subject it is unlikely to be used in any context, clinical or even research. The utility of any test is frequently compromised by a patient's physical and mental health. Thus, more time has to be allocated for someone with Parkinson's disease or Alzheimer's disease. For the busy but enthusiastic clinician with just a few minutes to spare, the number of commercially available tests is severely limited. Electrogustometry is very practical because it does not require mixing or storage of chemicals. If just a basic threshold measure is all that is needed, both sides of the anterior tongue may be assessed in about 10 minutes. Ideally a single staircase approach should be used, and that, in some cases, may require up to 30 minutes. Alternatively, the commercial choice rests between taste sprays or taste filter strips (bundled with the screening version of Sniffin' sticks). For each filter strip tastant a suprathreshold measurement could be used and that would have to be determined by establishing a local aged-based control group. Where time is not so restricted, one might consider single solution" as "One might also consider single solution assessments such as that developed for NHANES or, if more time is available, dissolvable taste strips made from the polymer, hydroxypropyl methyl cellulose. Whole-mouth procedures reflect a patient's general perception and are less time consuming than regional taste tests, although they can overlook unilateral or regional damage to localized taste bud fields of CN VII and CN IX. Hence, whenever possible, testing of at least the left and right sides of the anterior tongue is generally recommended.

Summary

In this chapter we stress that patients are notoriously inaccurate in assessing their own taste abilities, a situation that necessitates quantitative evaluation. Various procedures for understanding or quantifying human taste function are reviewed. These include threshold and suprathreshold psychophysical tests, electrophysiological tests, and sophisticated imaging techniques such as fMRI, PET, and MEG. Although their clinical utility is limited, these imaging procedures have proven extremely valuable in localizing brain areas involved in taste perception. We review important influences on taste function including subject variables (gender, age, mouth movements, and circadian rhythms), procedural factors (taste stimulus temperature, tongue area evaluated, extent and duration of stimulus presentations) and psychophysical procedures employed. We present published normative data for some test measures. It is noted that normative data will be forthcoming from the recent application of a relatively simple suprathreshold intensity rating test based on thousands of volunteers as part of the 2011–14 US National Health and Nutrition Examination Survey.

References

ASTM, 1997. *Standard Practice for Determination of Odor and Taste Thresholds by a Forced-chocie Ascending Concentration Series Method of Limits (E679-97 & E679-04).* Philadelphia: American Society for Testing and Materials.

Bagla, R., Klasky, B., Doty, R.L., 1997. Influence of stimulus duration on a regional measure of NaCl taste sensitivity. *Chemical Senses* **22**(2), 171–175.

Barnicot, N.A., Harris, H., Kalmus, H., 1951. Taste thresholds of further eighteen compounds and their correlation with P.T.C thresholds. *Annals of Eugenics* **16**, 119–128.

Barros-Loscertales, A., Gonzalez, J., Pulvermuller, F., et al. 2012. Reading salt activates gustatory brain regions: FMRI evidence for semantic grounding in a novel sensory modality. *Cerebral Cortex* **22**, 2554–2563.

Barry, M.A., Gatenby, J.C., Zeiger, J.D., Gore, J.C., 2001. Hemispheric dominance of cortical activity evoked by focal electrogustatory stimuli. *Chemical Senses* **26**, 471–482.

Bartoshuk, L.M., Pfaffmann, C., McBurney, D.H., 1964. Taste of sodium chloride solutions after adaptation to sodium chloride – implications for the "Water Taste." *Science* **143** (3609), 967–968.

Bartoshuk, L.M., 1978. The psychophysics of taste. *American Journal of Clinical Nutrition*, **31** 1068–1077.

Bartoshuk, L.M., Duffy, V.B., Fast, K., Green, B.G., Snyder, D.J., 2001. The General Labeled Magnitude Scale provides valid measures of genetic variation in taste and may be a universal psychophysical ruler. *Appetite* **37**, 126.

Bartoshuk, L.M., Catalanotto, F., Hoffman, H., Logan, H., Snyder, D.J., 2012. Taste damage (otitis media, tonsillectomy and head and neck cancer), oral sensations and BMI. *Physiology & Behavior* **107**(4), 516–526.

Bohon, C., Stice, E., 2012. Negative affect and neural response to palatable food intake in bulimia nervosa. *Appetite* **58**, 964–970.

Bornstein, W.S., 1940a. Cortical representation of taste in man and monkey. I. Functional and antaomical relations of taste, olfaction and somatic sensibility. *Yale Journal of Biology and Medicine* **12**, 719–736.

Bornstein, W.S., 1940b. Cortical representation of taste in man and monkey. II. The localization of the cortical taste area in man, a method of measuring impairment of taste in man. *Yale Journal of Biology and Medicine* **13**, 133–156.

Cameron, A.T., 1947. The taste sense and the relative sweetness of sugars and other sweet substances. *Scientific Report Series* **9**, Sugar Research Foundation, 74.

Coates, A.C., 1974. Effects of age, sex, and smoking on electrical taste threshold. *Annals of Otology, Rhinology & Laryngology* **83**, 365–369.

Collings, V.B., 1974. Human taste response as a function of locus of stimulation on the tongue and soft palate. *Perception & Psychophysics* **16**, 169–174.

Critchley, H.D., Rolls, E.T., 1996. Olfactory neuronal responses in the primate orbitofrontal cortex: Analysis in an olfactory discrimination task. *Journal of Neurophysiology* 75 1659–1672.

Dawes, C., 1974. Rhythms in salivary flow rate and composition. *International Journal of Chronobiology* 2, 253–279.

de Araujo, I.E., Kringelbach, M.L., Rolls, E.T., McGlone, F., 2003. Human cortical responses to water in the mouth, and the effects of thirst. *Journal of Neurophysiology* 90, 1865–1876.

Deems, D.A., Doty, R.L., Settle, R.G., et al. 1991. Smell and taste disorders, a study of 750 patients from the University of Pennsylvania Smell and Taste Center. *Archives of Otolaryngology – Head & Neck Surgery*, 117, 519–528.

Delwiche, J., O'Mahony, M., 1996. Changes in secreted salivary sodium are sufficient to alter salt taste sensitivity: Use of signal detection measures with continuous monitoring of the oral environment. *Physiology & Behavior* 59, 605–611.

Desai, H., Smutzer, G., Coldwell, S.E., Griffith, J.W., 2011. Validation of edible taste strips for identifying PROP taste recognition thresholds. *Laryngoscope* 121, 1177–1183.

Doty, R.L., McKeown, D.A., Lee, W.W., Shaman, P., 1995. A study of the test-retest reliability of ten olfactory tests. *Chemical Senses* 20, 645–656.

Doty, R.L., Bagla, R., Morgenson, M., Mirza, N., 2001. NaCl thresholds: Relationship to anterior tongue locus, area of stimulation, and number of fungiform papillae. *Physiology & Behavior* 72, 373–378.

Doty, R.L., Laing, D.G., 2015. Psychophysical measurement of human olfactory function. In: R.L. Doty (Ed.), *Handbook of Olfaction and Gustation* (3rd Edition). Hoboken, N.J.: John Wiley & Sons, pp. 229–261.

Doty, R.L., Haxel, B.R., 2005. Objective assessment of terbinafine-induced taste loss. *Laryngoscope* 115, 2035–2037.

Doty, R.L., Chen, J.H., Overend, J., 2017. Taste quality confusions: Influences of age, smoking, PTC taster status, and other subject characteristics. *Perception* 46, 257–267.

Essick, G.K., Chopra, A., Guest, S., McGlone, F., 2003. Lingual tactile acuity, taste perception, and the density and diameter of fungiform papillae

in female subjects. *Physiology & Behavior.*, **80**, 289–302.

Falconer, A., 1847. Über eine merkwürdige Eigenschaft einer indischen Pflanze (*Gymnema sylvestre*). *Pharmaceutical Journal and Transactions* 7, 551.

Ferguson, D.B., Botchway, C.A., 1979. Circadian variations in the flow rate and composition of whole saliva stimulated by mastication. *Archives of Oral Biology* 24, 877–881.

Fischer, R., Griffin, F., England, S., Garn, S.M., 1961. Taste thresholds and food dislikes. *Nature* 191, 1328.

Foerster, O., 1936. Sensible corticale Felder. *Bumke und Foersters Handb.Neurol.*, 6, 358–448.

Frey, S., Petrides, M., 1999. Re-examination of the human taste region: A positron emission tomography study. *European Journal of Neuroscience* 11, 2985–2988.

Fujimura, A., Kajiyama, H., Tateishi, T., Ebihara, A., 1990. Circadian rhythm in recognition threshold of salt taste in healthy subjects. *The American Journal of Physiology* 259, R931–R935.

Gerull, G., Mrowinski, D., Schilling, V., 1984. [Objective gustometry with adequate stimulation by registration of contingent negative variation]. *EEG.EMG.Z. Elektroenzephalogr.Elektromyogr. Verwandte. Geb.* 15, 121–26.

Grant, R., Ferguson, M.M., Strang, R., Turner, J.W., Bone, I., 1987. Evoked taste thresholds in a normal population and the application of electrogustometry to trigeminal nerve disease. *Journal of Neurology, Neurosurgery & Psychiatry* 50, 12–21.

Green, B.G., Shaffer, G.S., Gilmore, M.M., 1993. Derivation and evaluation of a semantic scale of oral sensation magnitude with apparent ratio properties. *Chemical Senses* 18(6), 683–702.

Grzegorczyk, P.B., Jones, S.W., Mistretta, C.M., 1979. Age-related differences in salt taste acuity. *Journal of Gerontology* 34, 834–840.

Hahn, H., 1934. Die Adaptation des Geschmackssinnes. *Zeitschrift fur Sinnesphysiologie* 65, 1051–45.

Hahn, H., Günther, H., 1932. Uber die Reize und die Reizbedingungen des Geschmackssinnes. *Pflügers Arch.ges.Physiol.*, **231**, 48–67.

Hara, S., 1955. Interrelationship among stimulus intensity, stimulated area and reaction time in the human gustatory sensation. *Bulletin of Tokyo Medical and Dental University* **2**, 147–157.

Harris, H., Kalmus, H., 1949. The measurement of taste sensitivity to phenylthiourea (P.T.C.). *Annals of Eugenics* **15**, 24–31.

Harris, H., Kalmus, H., 1951. The distribution of taste thresholds for phenylthiourea of 384 sib pairs. *Annals of Eugenics* **16**, 226–230.

Hebhardt, P., Bagla, R., Doty, R.L., 1999. An automated regional taste-testing system. *Behavior Research Methods, Instruments, & Computers* **31**, 464–469.

Henkin, R.I., Solomon, D.H., 1962. Salt-taste threshold in adrenal insufficiency in man. *The Journal of Clinical Endocrinology and Metabolism* **22**, 856–858.

Henkin, R.I., Gill, J.R., Bartter, F.C., 1963. Studies on taste thresholds in normal man and in patients with adrenal cortical insufficiency: The role of adrenal cortical steroids and of serum sodium concentration. *Journal of Clinical Investigation* **42**, 727–735.

Henkin, R.I., Schechter, P.J., Hoye, R., Mattern, C.F., 1971. Idiopathic hypogeusia with dysgeusia, hyposmia, and dysosmia. A new syndrome. *JAMA* **217**, 434–440.

Henkin, R.I., Levy, L.M. Lin, C.S., 2000. Taste and smell phantoms revealed by brain functional MRI (fMRI). *Journal of Computer Assisted Tomography* **24**, 106–123.

Holway, A.H., Hurvich, L.M., 1937. Differential gustatory sensitivity to salt. *American Journal of Psychology* **49**, 37–48.

Hooper, D., 1887. An examination of the leaves of Gymnema sylvestre. *Nature (London)* **35**, 565–567.

Hummel, T., Genow, A., Landis, B.N., 2010. Clinical assessment of human gustatory function using event related potentials. *Journal of Neurology, Neurosurgery, & Psychiatry* **81**, 459–464.

Jones, F.N., 1956. A forced-choice method of limits. *The American Journal of Psychology* **69**, 672–673.

Kinomura, S., Kawashima, R., Yamada, K., et al. 1994. Functional anatomy of taste perception in the human brain studied with positron emission tomography. *Brain Research* **659**, 263–266.

Kobal, G., 1985. Gustatory evoked potentials in man. *Electroencephalography and Clinical Neurophysiology* **62**, 449–454.

Kobayakawa, T., Endo, H., Ayabe-Kanamura, S., et al. 1996. The primary gustatory area in human cerebral cortex studied by magnetoencephalography. *Neuroscience Letters* **212**, 155–158.

Krarup, B., 1958. Electro-gustometry: A method for clinical taste examination. *Acta Otolaryngologica* **49**, 294–305.

Kunka, M., Doty, R.L., Settle, R.G., 1981. An examination of intertrial interval and gender influences on sucrose detection thresholds established by a modified staircase procedure. *Perception* **10**, 35–38.

Kurihara, K., 1971. Taste modifiers. In L.M. Beidler (Ed.), *Handbook of Sensory Physiology. Vol. IV. Chemical Senses 2. Taste* (pp. 363–378). Berlin-Heidelberg: Springer-Verlag.

Landis, B.N., Welge-Luessen, A., Bramerson, A., et al. 2009. "Taste Strips" – a rapid, lateralized, gustatory bedside identification test based on impregnated filter papers. *Journal of Neurology* **256**, 242–248.

Liu, G., Zong, G., Doty, R.L., Sun, Q., 2016. Prevalence and risk factors of taste and smell impairment in a nationwide representative sample of the US population: A cross-sectional study. *BMJ Open.* Nov 9; 6(11);e013246. doi:10.1136/bmjopen-2016-013246.

Levy, L.M., Henkin, R.I., Lin, C.S., Finley, A., Schellinger, D., 1999. Taste memory induces brain activation as revealed by functional MRI. *Journal of Computer Assisted Tomography* **23**, 499–505.

Lobb, B., Elliffe, D.M., Stillman, J.A., 2000. Reliability of electrogustometry for the estimation of taste thresholds. *Clinical Otolaryngology & Allied Sciences 2000 December;* **25**, 531–534.

Loucks, C.A., Doty, R.L., 2004. Effects of stimulation duration on EGM thresholds. *Physiology & Behavior* **81**, 1–4.

Mayer-Gross, W., Walker, J.W., 1946. Taste and selection of food in hypoglycaemia. *British Journal of Experimental Pathology* **27**, 297–305.

McBurney, D.H., Collings, V.B., Glanz, L.M., 1973. Temperature dependence of human taste responses. *Physiology & Behavior* **11**, 89–94.

Meiselman, H.L., 1971. Effect of presentation procedure on taste intensity functions. *Perception & Psychophysics* **10**, 15–18.

Miller, S.L., Mirza, N., Doty, R.L., 2002. EGM thresholds: relationship to anterior tongue locus, area of stimulation, and number of fungiform papillae. *Physiology & Behavior* **75**, 753–757.

Murphy, C., Quinonez, C., Nordin, S., 1995. Reliability and validity of electrogustometry and its application to young and elderly persons. *Chemical Senses* **20**, 499–503.

Nagel, W., 1894. Vergleichend physiologische und anatomische Untersuchungen über den Geruchs- and Geschmackssin und ihre Organe. *Bibliotheca Zoologica* **7**, 1–207.

Nakamura, M., Kurihara, K., 1991. Differential temperature dependence of taste nerve responses to various taste stimuli in dogs and rats. *The American Journal of Physiology* **261**, R1402–R1408.

Nakamura, Y., Goto, T.K., Tokumori, K., et al. 2012. The temporal change in the cortical activations due to salty and sweet tastes in humans: fMRI and time-intensity sensory evaluation. *Neuroreport* **23**, 400–404.

Nakazato, M., Endo, S., Yoshimura, I., Tomita, H., 2002. Influence of aging on electrogustometry thresholds. *Acta Oto-Laryngologica* **122**, 16–26.

Nicolaescu, S.A., Wertheimer, J.M., Barbash, S. E., et al. 2005. Electrical taste thresholds established on the medial tongue using two sizes of electrodes. *Laryngoscope*, **115**, 1509–1511.

Ninomiya, Y., Funakoshi, M., 1981. Responses of rat chorda tympani fibers to electrical stimulation of the tongue. *Japanese Journal of Physiology* **31**, 559–570.

Nitschke, J.B., Dixon, G.E., Sarinopoulos, I., et al. 2006. Altering expectancy dampens neural response to aversive taste in primary taste cortex. *Nature Neuroscience* **9**, 435–442.

O'Mahony, M., 1973. Qualitative description of low concentration sodium chloride solutions. *British Journal of Psychology* **64**, 601–606.

O'Mahony, M., Dunn, M., 1974. Do sensitivity drifts occur for stimuli other than sodium chloride? A preliminary investigation. *Perception* **3**, 213–220.

O'Mahony, M., Ivory, H., King, E., 1974. Pair comparison and ascending series NaCl threshold: Criterion and residual effects. *Perception* **3**, 185–192.

O'Mahony, M., Hobson, A., Garvey, J., Davies, M., Birt, C., 1976. How many tastes are there for low concentration "sweet" and "sour" stimuli? – Threshold implications. *Perception* **5**, 147–154.

O'Mahony, M., 1983. Gustatory responses to nongustatory stimuli. *Perception* **12**, 627–633.

Ogawa, H., Wakita, M., Hasegawa, K., et al. 2005. Functional MRI detection of activation in the primary gustatory cortices in humans. *Chemical Senses* **30**, 583–592.

Pavlidis, P., Gouveris, H., Antonia, A., et al. 2012. Age-related changes in electrogustometry thresholds, tongue tip vascularization, density, and form of the fungiform papillae in humans. *Chemical Senses* **38**(1), 35–43.

Pingel, J., Ostwald, J., Pau, H.W., Hummel, T., Just, T., 2010. Normative data for a solution-based taste test. *European Archives of Oto-Rhino-Laryngology* **267**, 1911–1917.

Plassmann, H., O'Doherty, J., Shiv, B., Rangel, A., 2008. Marketing actions can modulate neural representations of experienced pleasantness. *Proceedings of the National Academy of Sciences of the United States of America* **105**, 1050–1054.

Plattig, K.H., 1969. [Electric taste. Stimulus intensity dependent evoked brain potentials following electric stimulation of the tongue in humans]. *Zeitschrift Fur Biologie* **116**, 161–211.

Plattig, K.H., Haußner, C., 1985. A new gustometer system enabling proper computer evaluation of human taste responses. *Medical & Biological Engineering & Computing* **23** (Suppl. Pt 2), 1026–1027.

Plattig, K.H., Dazert, S., Maeyama, T., 1988. A new gustometer for computer evaluation of taste responses in men and animals. *Acta Otolaryngologica Suppl* **458**, 123–128.

Rawal, S., Hoffman, H.J., Honda, M., Huedo-Medina, T.B., Duffy, V.B., 2015. The taste and smell protocol in the 2011–2014 US National Health and Nutrition Survey (NHANES): Test-retest reliability and validity testing. *Chemosensory Perception* **8**, 138–148.

Richter, C.P., 1936. Increased salt appetite in adrenalectomized rats. *American Journal of Physiology* **115**, 155–161.

Richter, C.P., MacLean, A., 1939. Salt taste threshold of humans. *The American Journal of Physiology* **126**, 1–6.

Rolls, E.T., Baylis, L.L., 1994. Gustatory, olfactory, and visual convergence within the primate orbitofrontal cortex. *Journal of Neuroscience* **14**, 5437–5452.

Rolls, E.T., Critchley, H.D., Treves, A., 1996. Representation of olfactory information in the primate orbitofrontal cortex. *Journal of Neurophysiology* **75**, 1982–1996.

Rolls, E.T., Rolls, B.J., Rowe, E.A., 1983. Sensory-specific and motivation-specific satiety for the sight and taste of food and water in man. *Physiology & Behavior* **30**, 185–192.

Rolls, E.T., Sienkiewicz, Z.J., Yaxley, S., 1989. Hunger modulates the responses to gustatory stimuli of single neurons in the caudolateral orbitofrontal cortex of the macaque monkey. *European Journal of Neuroscience* **1**, 53–60.

Rolls, E.T., 2001. The rules of formation of the olfactory representations found in the orbitofrontal cortex olfactory areas in primates. *Chemical Senses* **26**, 595–604.

Rolls, E.T., 2005. Taste, olfactory, and food texture processing in the brain, and the control of food intake. *Physiology & Behavior* **85**, 45–56.

Salata, J.A., Raj, J.M., Doty, R.L., 1991. Differential sensitivity of tongue areas and palate to electrical stimulation: A suprathreshold cross-modal matching study. *Chemical Senses* **16**, 483–489.

Small, D.M., Zatorre, R.J., Dagher, A., Evans, A. C., Jones-Gotman, M., 2001. Changes in brain activity related to eating chocolate: From pleasure to aversion. *Brain*, **124**, 1720–1733.

Small, D.M., Voss, J., Mak, Y.E., et al. 2004. Experience-dependent neural integration of taste and smell in the human brain. *Journal of Neurophysiology* **92**, 1892–1903.

Small, D.M., Prescott, J., 2005.Odor/taste integration and the perception of flavor. *Experimental Brain Research* **166** (3–4), 345–357.

Smutzer, G., Lam, S., Hastings, L., et al. 2008. A test for measuring gustatory function. *The Laryngoscope* **118**(8), 1411–1416.

Snyder, D., Fast, K., Bartoshuk, L.M., 2004. Valid comparisons of suprathreshold sensations. *Journal of Consciousness Studies* **11** (7–8), 96–112.

Soter, A., Kim, J., Jackman, A., et al. 2008. Accuracy of self-report in detecting taste dysfunction. *Laryngoscope* **118**, 611–617.

Spetter, M.S., Smeets, P.A., De, G.C., Viergever, M. A., 2010. Representation of sweet and salty taste intensity in the brain. *Chemical Senses* **35**, 831–840.

Stevens, J.C., Marks, L.E., 1980. Cross-modality matching functions generated by magnitude estimation. *Perception & Psychophysics* **27**, 379–389.

Stinton, N., Atif, M.A., Barkat, N., Doty, R.L., 2010. Influence of smell loss on taste function. *Behavioral Neuroscience* **124**, 256–264.

Veldhuizen, M.G., Albrecht, J., Zelano, C., et al. 2011. Identification of human gustatory cortex by activation likelihood estimation. *Human Brain Mapping* **32**, 2256–2266.

Veldhuizen, M.G., Douglas, D., Aschenbrenner, K., Gitelman, D.R., Small, D.M., 2011. The anterior insular cortex represents breaches of taste identity expectation. *Journal of Neuroscience* **31**, 14735–14744.

von Bekesy, G., 1965. The effect of adaptation on the taste threshold observed with a semiautomatic gustometer. *Journal of General Physiology* **48**, 481–488.

Watson, D., Clark, L.A., Tellegen, A., 1988. Development and validation of brief measures of positive and negative affect: The PANAS scales. *Journal of Personality and Social Psychology* **54**, 1063–1070.

Wen, X.Y., 2010. Salt taste sensitivity, physical activity and gastric cancer. *Asian Pacific Journal of Cancer Prevention* **11**, 1473–1477.

Woods, A.T., Lloyd, D.M., Kuenzel, J., et al. 2011. Expected taste intensity affects response to sweet drinks in primary taste cortex. *Neuroreport* **22**, 365–369.

Zald, D.H., Pardo, J.V., 2000. Cortical activation induced by intraoral stimulation with water in humans. *Chemical Senses* **25**, 267–275.

Zuniga, J.R., Davis, S.H., Englehardt, R.A., et al. 1993. Taste performance on the anterior human tongue varies with fungiform taste bud density. *Chemical Senses* **18**, 449–460.

Non-neurodegenerative Disorders of Olfaction

Chemosensory disorders are common in the general population. Olfactory impairment, which is more prevalent than taste dysfunction, affects 1–2% of people below the age of 65 years and more than 50% in those above this age (Doty et al., 1984; Hoffman et al., 1998; Murphy et al., 2002). Of 750 consecutive patients presenting to the University of Pennsylvania Smell and Taste Center with chemosensory complaints, 68% reported decreased quality of life, 46% changes in appetite or body weight, and 56% adverse influences on daily living or psychological well-being (Deems et al., 1991). In another study of 445 such patients, at least one significant hazardous event (e.g., food poisoning or failure to detect fire or leaking natural gas) was reported by 45.2% of those with anosmia (total loss of smell ability), 34.1% of those with severe hyposmia (lowered smell function), 32.8% of those with moderate hyposmia, 24.2% of those with mild hyposmia, and 19.0% of those with normal olfactory function. It is particularly noteworthy that a number of longitudinal studies have found mortality risk to be much higher in older non-demented persons with smell identification deficits than in those with a normal sense of smell (Wilson et al., 2010; Gopinath et al., 2012; Pinto et al., 2014; Devanand et al., 2015). In the most definitive of these studies, the increased risk of death progressively increased as olfactory dysfunction increased over a four-year period (Devanand et al., 2015). Participants with the lowest UPSIT scores had a 45% mortality rate over this time, as compared to an 18% mortality rate in those with the highest UPSIT scores.

A recurrent confusion in the minds of patients and many of their medical advisors is the fact that individuals with smell impairment complain regularly of loss of taste. This can lead to unnecessary evaluations such as extensive gastrointestinal investigations, and reflects a lack of understanding of the important role olfaction plays in producing food flavor. When we ingest food, there is taste appreciation from taste buds over the tongue and pharynx but, simultaneously, odorants released from food escape into the retropharyngeal space and enter the nasal cavity where they stimulate the olfactory receptor cells (Burdach & Doty, 1987). Thus, any food entering the mouth will evoke a sensation of both taste and smell, unless it is an odorless tastant that evokes only sweet, sour, salt, bitter, or umami taste perceptions. Sensations such as chocolate, meat sauce, strawberry, cola, lime, walnut, and lemon are mediated principally by smell, not taste. Only on rare occasions will a patient suffer impairment of both smell and taste. Gustatory problems, per se, can be ascertained in many cases by asking patients if they can still detect the sweetness of sugar, the sourness of grapefruit, or the saltiness of potato chips, although these questions are surprisingly insensitive when compared to objective testing (Soter et al., 2008).

This chapter deals with smell problems of relevance to the clinician and describes, from the chemosensory perspective, the major non-neurodegenerative diseases influenced by such disorders, including head injury, tumor, infection and inflammation, endocrine disease, epilepsy, and multiple sclerosis. Non-neurodegenerative taste disorders are similarly reviewed in Chapter 6, and neurodegenerative diseases, such as Alzheimer's, Parkinson's disease, and related syndromes, are discussed in Chapter 7.

Classification of Types of Olfactory Disorders

Olfactory disorders can be classified according to their behavioral or psychological manifestations. The most common terms used in such classification are defined and described as follows:

Anosmia

Anosmia has two meanings; some use it literally to describe total loss of smell, others just to describe some impairment which may be complete or partial or related to just one odor. Similar confusion is mirrored by other neurological words, such as aphasia and dysphasia, alexia and dyslexia, etc. *Specific anosmia* refers to the inability to detect one or a few related odorants while still being able to detect other odors in a normal fashion. Patients with specific anosmias generally do not recognize their problem and do not present clinically with concerns, unlike patients with general anosmia. Most specific anosmics actually can smell the substance to which they are anosmic if it is presented at high enough concentrations; in such cases the term *specific hyposmia* is preferred.

Agnosia

Olfactory agnosia occurs when a cognitively normal individual loses the ability to recognize an odor, yet maintains the ability to perceive and distinguish it from other odors in a normal fashion. Extremely few cases of olfactory agnosia have been identified, which is surprising in view of the well-recognized forms of agnosia in the visual and auditory spheres. In one case report, agnosia was described in a 53-year-old male patient with predominantly right inferior temporal lobe atrophy (presumably degenerative) in association with prosopagnosia, i.e., agnosia for familiar faces. This results usually from disorder of the fusiform gyrus which is also located on the undersurface of the temporal lobe (Mendez & Ghajarnia, 2001). Also described in another case report is a patient with ipsilateral olfactory agnosia (with normal olfactory thresholds) associated with complex partial seizures localized to the right medial temporal lobe (Lehrner et al., 1997). The prediction that patients with semantic dementia (SD) would have difficulty in naming smells in the presence of normal discrimination was confirmed in a study of eight patients with SD, as described in more detail in Chapter 7 (Luzzi et al., 2007).

Hyposmia

Hyposmia refers to decreased sensitivity to odors. Like anosmia, such decrements can exist on one or both sides of the nose. Since hyposmia is classically associated with a raised threshold, the term *microsmia* has been introduced to denote decreased function as measured by odor identification tests, although odor identification and threshold tests are, in general, highly correlated (Doty, 1995). Unilateral microsmia is regularly overlooked in clinical practice – a point of considerable relevance, for example, in diagnosis of an olfactory groove meningioma (which is often one-sided). Temporary hyposmia can occur as a result of accelerated or prolonged adaptation, as in cases of chronic exposure to some workplace chemicals like acrylates or hydrogen sulfide (Schwartz et al., 1989).

Hyperosmia

This is defined as enhanced sensitivity to one or more odors. Although hyperosmia is usually assumed to reflect atypically low olfactory thresholds, many who report this condition show no such alterations. In some cases, hyperosmia is associated with *hyper-reactivity* rather than a true change in sensitivity. Hyper-reactivity can reflect a liberal response criterion, i.e., greater willingness to report the presence of an odor or simply an emotional response to a smell in the absence of any change in sensitivity to that odor. Although rarely reported in humans, the concept of hyperosmia now has a more scientific footing as a result of gene knockout experiments. Mice with gene-targeted deletion of the Kv 1.3 channel had a 1,000- to 10,000-fold lower threshold for detection of odors, and increased ability to discriminate between odorants in comparison with their normal littermates, earning the title of "supersmeller" mice (Fadool et al., 2004). According to Menashe et al. (2007), hypersensitivity to the odor isovaleric acid (sweaty socks smell) may relate to polymorphisms in the human olfactory receptor gene, OR11H7P.

Dysosmia

This refers to any form of distorted smell perception, sometimes termed *parosmia* and, when it has a fetid character, *cacosmia*. Dysosmias can be either stimulated or unstimulated, i.e., appear in the presence or the absence of an identifiable odor. The latter type of dysosmia is often termed *phantosmia* or olfactory hallucination. Phantosmias can be experienced by both healthy and sick people. Thus, medical students who spend long periods in the dissecting room may continue to experience the smell of formalin or phenol several hours after they have left the area and may have temporary decrements in olfactory function (Hisamitsu et al., 2011). Traditional teaching holds that most hallucinations, including the olfactory variety, indicate organic disease within the uncinate region that make up the aura of a complex partial epileptic attack. In fact, most dysosmias reflect degeneration or attempts at regeneration in the olfactory neuroepithelium. Moreover, lesions of the orbito-frontal cortex, an olfactory association area, may also produce olfactory illusions, hallucinations, autonomic signs, or gestural automatisms as part of a seizure complex (Chabolla, 2002). Phantosmias that decrease in frequency or intensity over time probably indicate changes within the olfactory epithelium, whereas those that progressively increase in frequency or intensity likely reflect central nervous system (CNS) anomalies similar to the kindling phenomenon induced in animals. In the latter context, anticonvulsant medication (e.g., phenytoin, gabapentin, pregabalin) may minimize progressive neural damage associated with some centrally mediated dysosmic sensations, although good evidence for this is presently lacking.

Conditions Affecting Olfactory Function

As indicated in Table 5.1 and Figure 5.1, numerous relatively common diseases may compromise the sense of smell, sometimes permanently. These range from the simple cold to extremely debilitating neurodegenerative diseases. Such disturbances may reflect peripheral influences, such as blockage of airflow to the receptors or damage to the olfactory epithelium, whereas others involve central mechanisms, e.g., tumors that compromise the olfactory bulbs or higher-order structures. Systemic factors, such as metabolic changes that generally influence olfactory functioning, can also be involved.

Table 5.1. List of main categories of disease associated with smell disturbance with typical examples.

Neurodegenerative causes are given separately in Chapter 7	
Disease	**Examples**
Local nasal	Polyps; allergic rhinitis; sinus disease
Infection	Common cold; influenza; herpes encephalitis; leprosy; AIDS. Prion disease. Fungi, e.g., aspergillosis, mucormycosis; Paget's disease
Head injury	Usually severe posterior or lateral impact; superficial siderosis
Epilepsy	Olfactory aura. Complex partial seizure
Migraine	Before, during, or after an attack
Immunologic diseases	Multiple sclerosis; Narcolepsy; Sjögren's syndrome; Myasthenia gravis; Wegener's granulomatosis, Churg-Strauss syndrome
Tumors and inflammatory disease	Nasopharyngeal carcinoma; olfactory groove meningioma or neuroblastoma; Paraneoplastic, e.g., small cell lung carcinoma
Endocrine and metabolic	Diabetes; Cushing & Klinefelter's syndromes; Kallman's syndrome; septo-optic dysplasia; Addison's disease; hypoparathyroidism; pseudohypoparathyroidism. Wilson's disease; liver and kidney disease
Rare genetic disorders	Refsum's syndrome; Bardet-Biedel syndrome; Aniridia type 2; Kartagener syndrome; DiGeorge syndrome; Wolfram syndrome
Psychiatric	Depression; Korsakoff syndrome; malingering; hysteria; olfactory reference syndrome
Miscellaneous	Radiotherapy; pregnancy; medication; toxins; idiopathic intracranial hypertension
Neurodegenerative	See Chapter 7

Unfortunately, a given disturbance cannot always be connected with a peripheral, central, or systemic cause. Although total loss of smell is classically associated with peripheral causes, it can result from damage anywhere in the olfactory pathway. Thus, in addition to damage to the olfactory epithelium (as in toxic exposures, chronic rhinosinusitis, or upper respiratory infections), a disturbance can reflect injury to axons of the receptor cells or sectors of the olfactory bulb (as in head trauma-related shearing of the olfactory filaments), or disorders of the olfactory cortex (as in multiple sclerosis). Similarly, dysosmia can be attributed to peripheral, central, systemic, or a combination of these causes. Usually dysosmia is accompanied by lessening of olfaction, regardless of its locus. As mentioned earlier, threshold disorders that are characteristically attributed to peripheral sectors of the olfactory pathway may, in fact, signify central dysfunction; conversely, problems with smell identification do not automatically indicate a more centrally mediated etiology. With these caveats, and purely as a general rule, complete lack of smell early in the course of disease is more likely to be caused by a peripheral than central lesion due, in part, to the direct exposure of the olfactory epithelium to the environment and to the considerable redundancy in central olfactory areas. Impairment of smell that is continuous is more likely to be neurogenic in origin, whereas fluctuating microsmia with intermittent recovery often points to inflammatory pathology/obstruction within the nose or sinuses.

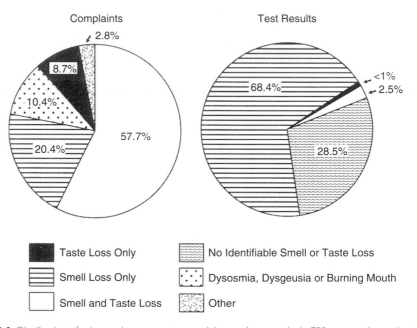

Figure 5.1 Distribution of primary chemosensory complaints and test results in 750 consecutive patients presenting to the University of Pennsylvania Smell and Taste Center. Note that complaint categories of smell loss, taste loss, and smell and taste loss include some patients with secondary complaints of chemosensory distortion and burning mouth. From Deems et al. (1991).

Non-neurodegenerative disorders known to cause olfactory dysfunction are described below, beginning with those that are most frequent (i.e., local nasal disease, upper respiratory infections, and head trauma). A sizeable percentage of all causes is unknown, e.g., 22% in Deems et al. (1991), and many of these are likely due to unrecognized viruses. During seasonal epidemics, the number of serologically documented influenza or arboviral encephalitis infections exceeds the number of acute cases by several hundred-fold (Stroop, 1995) and cases of influenza-related smell dysfunction are much higher during the winter months (Konstantinidis et al., 2006). Although many are presumed to represent unnoticed upper respiratory infections, there is increasing interest in the possibility that some patients with idiopathic anosmia may be in the prodromal phase of Alzheimer's or Parkinson's disease. This concept is discussed in detail in Chapter 7.

Nasal Disease

This is one of the most frequent causes of olfactory disturbance. Nasal disease can prevent air from reaching the olfactory neuroepithelium (conductive problem), as well as inducing nasal inflammation, which inhibits function. Any obstructive or inflammatory process can be responsible for decreased smell ability, including seasonal/allergic rhinitis, polyposis (particularly in the nasal vault), inflammatory disease of the ethmoid or maxillary sinuses, and malignant disease of the nose, paranasal sinuses, or nasopharynx. The point where the frontal and maxillary sinuses drain jointly into the nasal cavity (ostiomeatal complex) may become deformed due to trauma. If there is chronic nasal sinus infection, the mucus clearance rate may be reduced because of disordered ciliary motility. This, along with inflammation, contributes to smell loss and, if left unchecked, can ultimately result in permanent damage to the olfactory receptors. In general, polyps cause anosmia more frequently than allergic rhinitis (Litvack et al., 2008) but exceptions may be found. Experimental studies of allergic rhinitis in mice have noted significant hypertrophy of Bowman's glands, thinning of the olfactory epithelium, and decreased numbers of olfactory receptor cells (Carr et al., 2012).

There is evidence that the nasal airway remains patent in up to 70 percent of those with olfactory disturbance due to local nasal disease. In such instances, the loss is attributed to micro-inflammatory changes within the olfactory mucosa (Kern, 2000). Oddly enough, mild or moderate congestion of the turbinates in the absence of disease does not necessarily cause impairment of smell function and may actually enhance it, perhaps by shunting more air up into the olfactory cleft (Doty & Frye, 1989; Zhao & Frye, 2015). In general, the variation of nasal resistance across the two sides of the nose (i.e., the so-called nasal cycle) does not result in noticeable microsmia on the less patent side, except in cases where the nasal septum is extremely deformed or when adhesions occur between the turbinates and the septum. Although there are reciprocal and cyclic fluctuations in relative airflow in the left and right nasal chambers, they are less common than believed previously (Gilbert, 1989; Mirza et al., 1997). Olfactory sensitivity does appear to be greater when the right side of the nose is relatively more engorged than the left, presumably reflecting greater relative sympathetic activity (Frye & Doty, 1992). Moreover, subtle influences on odor quality, based upon differential absorption patterns, may occur when testing is confined to a single nasal chamber (Sobel et al., 1999). Nasal dryness, which can develop after repeated surgery, atrophic rhinitis, or Sjögren's syndrome, has been associated with microsmia or anosmia since smell – like taste – is believed to require a moist receptor area for optimal function.

Spontaneous improvement in function over time was reported in patients with smell loss secondary to chronic rhinosinusitis. For example, in a longitudinal study of 542 patients presenting to the University of Pennsylvania Smell and Taste Center who were retested, on average, three years after initial presentation, nearly half of those with dysfunction secondary to chronic rhinosinusitis showed statistically significant improvement (i.e., an increase of ≥ 4 in UPSIT score) on the second test occasion. Nearly 25 percent of those who were not initially anosmic improved into the age-adjusted normal range (London et al., 2008), although a significant decline in function occurred in 20 percent of the microsmic individuals

Upper Respiratory System Viral Infections. Olfactory receptor cells are regularly targeted by viruses. Reduction or inhibition of mucociliary transport by disease, drugs, or genetic factors markedly increases susceptibility to viral infection (Bang et al., 1966; Brownstein, 1987). Viruses that gain access to the respiratory tract usually do so in the form of aerosolized droplets. In general, non-enveloped viruses (e.g., adenovirus, rhinovirus, enteroviruses, and poliovirus) survive better than enveloped viruses (e.g., influenza, parainfluenza, respiratory syncytial, mumps, measles, rubella, and herpes simplex). Interestingly, anosmia or hyposmia may be linked in rare instances to trivalent influenza vaccine (Fiser & Borotski, 1978; Doty et al., 2014), analogous to vaccine-associated Guillain–Barre syndrome and Bell's palsy.

It is underappreciated that some viruses not only damage the olfactory mucosa, but may also enter the brain via this route and cause CNS damage. Damage can be (a) indirect, e.g., by anterograde degeneration of the affected primary receptors whose axons project into the bulb, or (b) direct, e.g., by invasion of the bulb through intracellular transport by means of the olfactory receptor cells, through lymphatic or via perineural penetration. Importantly, some viruses that are not ordinarily neurotropic can become so on entering the nose. For example, when the NWS strain of influenza virus is inoculated into the nose of mice, it becomes neurotropic, spreading through the olfactory and trigeminal nerves and may even invade brainstem nuclei. When injected intraperitoneally, neurons within the brain parenchyma are unaffected and the viral antigen is restricted to the meninges, choroid plexus, ependymal cells, and perivascular locations (Reinacher et al., 1983).

In light of such observations, it is not surprising that upper respiratory infections, usually viral in nature, are the primary cause of chronic microsmia or anosmia (Deems et al., 1991; Doty, 2015). Even the common cold may damage olfaction permanently, and this has been attributed chiefly to parainfluenza type 3 virus – at least in Japan (Sugiura, 1998). Hepatitis, flu-like infections, herpes simplex encephalitis, and variant Creutzfeld–Jacob disease are rare causes of olfactory dysfunction and presumably relate to direct viral or prion damage of the olfactory pathways, either peripherally in the olfactory epithelium or more centrally in the olfactory bulb and temporal lobes. Among viruses known to be neurotropic for peripheral olfactory structures in primates or other animals when inhaled or inoculated into the nose are polio, the Indiana strain of wild-type vesicular stomatitis, rabies, herpes simplex types 1 and 2, mouse hepatitis, herpes suis, Borna disease, and canine distemper. Smell loss secondary to viral infection typically does not fluctuate, in contrast to smell loss due to conductive or intranasal inflammatory processes. Patients with the commoner forms of post-viral microsmia may also experience dysosmia or phantosmia – phenomena that usually regress with time.

Case Report 5.1: **Post-Viral Anosmia with Parosmia.** A 54-year-old engineer was in excellent health until he caught a bad cold two years previously. As expected, his ability to smell was poor when the nose was blocked but after the cold cleared, his smell ability was notably diminished, and there was marked distortion (parosmia) of several odors. Although there were no phantosmias, i.e., he did not experience odors which were not present in the external environment, he became nauseous when exposed to most common smells, especially food. He could no longer visit a restaurant and elected to eat alone and consume only food that had no or minimal odor such as rice, potato, and salads. Nasal endoscopy was normal and so was a CT scan of the sinuses. His UPSIT score was 11/40, reflecting chance performance and the inability to identify common odors. Threshold testing to increasing concentrations of phenylethyl alcohol was moderately impaired. Taste identification using impregnated filter strips was within normal limits. *Comment:* The diagnosis was therefore post-viral anosmia with parosmia. Parosmia in this instance may be due to faulty re-wiring or ephaptic (short-circuiting) transmission in the centripetal olfactory neurons, a condition that may be helped by anticonvulsant medication. However, a trial of the antiepileptic agent sodium valproate was not beneficial. He was advised to commence olfactory retraining at home to help re-learn signals from the misdirected olfactory fibers. Some lucky patients experience significant resolution of their parosmia without loss of function. This process may depend on survival of adequate numbers of olfactory receptors or it could reflect a process of central adaptation. Less fortunate patients find that when the parasomnia resolves they are left with no useful sense of smell.

Case Report 5.2: **Post-Viral Anosmia in a Previously Healthy Elderly Woman.** An 84-year-old woman presented with loss of smell for the preceding six months. The loss was first observed while attending a church social function, when it was noted that her sense of smell seemingly disappeared overnight. She remembers distinctly having contracted a severe upper respiratory infection of three weeks' duration just prior to the smell problem. General health was excellent and the only prescription medication was for esophageal reflux. The UPSIT score was within the anosmic range (15/40). Performance on the 12-item Odor Memory Test was at chance level (left: 4/12; 10-s delay: 1/4; 30-s delay: 1/4; 60-s delay: 2/4; right: 5/12; 10-s delay: 0/4; 30-s delay: 3/4; 60-s delay: 2/4). Interestingly, the detection threshold values for the rose-like odorant phenylethyl alcohol were within normal limits (L: –6.58; R: –6.36; B: –6.75; all values log vol/vol in USP grade light mineral oil). Nasal cross-sectional area, as measured by acoustic rhinometry, and nasal resistance, assessed by anterior rhinomanometry, were normal. The percent correct identification of whole-mouth suprathreshold sweet, sour, bitter, and salty tastant concentrations (sucrose, citric acid, caffeine, and NaCl) was low, reflecting difficulties in identifying non-sweet stimuli (21/40; 53%), a phenomenon not uncommon for healthy persons of her age. Intensity and pleasantness ratings assigned to the five concentrations of each of the test stimuli (citric acid, sodium chloride, sucrose, caffeine) were generally monotonic and unremarkable. Anterior (chorda tympani) and posterior (glossopharyngeal) regional tongue tests revealed no marked L-R asymmetries, although performance was depressed for citric acid and caffeine in most tongue regions assessed. Electrogustometric thresholds on the anterior left and right sides of the tongue were normal. At the time of testing, cognitive function was excellent (Mini-Mental State Examination: 30/30) and she exhibited no significant depression (Beck Depression Inventory Score: 8). *Comment:* This woman had experienced considerable loss of smell function, most likely secondary to viral infection, presumably superimposed upon a subclinically compromised olfactory epithelium from prior exposures to viruses and other xenobiotics. The normal olfactory threshold values are atypical, suggesting that some ability to detect low concentrations of the target stimulus remained, or that the trigeminal nerve was sensitized to detecting this agent. The UPSIT score of 15/40 in a female of 84 years could represent severe microsmia rather than a chance result. The decrease in taste largely reflected alterations in the ability to clearly differentiate salty, sour, and bitter substances, a common finding in many otherwise healthy older people. The prospects of regaining useful smell function in this patient are poor because of her age and the severity of loss when tested six months after its appearance.

Upper Respiratory System Bacterial Infections. Like viruses, bacteria can damage the olfactory system, in most cases intranasally. Chronic rhinosinusitis is associated with a predominance of anaerobes, mainly *Prevotella, Fusobacterium,* and *Peptostreptococcus,* whereas aerobic bacteria predominate in acute rhinosinusitis, e.g., *Streptococcus pneumoniae, Haemophilus influenzae,* and *Moraxella catarrhalis* (Hamilos, 2000). Although hundreds of bacterial species can inhabit the oral and nasal passages, to our knowledge no systematic study has sought to identify those forms most likely to damage the olfactory system. Hence, the little we know about bacterial influences on olfaction comes from clinical cases in which smell loss occurs during specific bacterial disorders.

There have been major advances in understanding factors that predispose to upper respiratory tract infections and presumably olfactory epithelial damage from bacteria. For example, the bitter taste receptor T2R38 regulates mucosal innate defense mechanisms within the human upper airway (Lee et al., 2012). These chemoreceptors were discovered first in the oral cavity and were found to transduce bitter tastes, hence their name. However, we now know that they are located in the respiratory and alimentary tracts. In the upper airway, they are activated by secretions from various microbes, including acyl-homoserine lactone quorum-sensing molecules (a signaling system between bacteria) secreted by *Pseudomonas aeruginosa* and other gram-negative bacteria. T2R38 regulates calcium-dependent nitric oxide (NO) production that encompasses direct antibacterial effects within the nasal epithelium and the stimulation of mucociliary clearance. Blunted NO and ciliary responses to gram-negative quorum-sensing molecules occur in upper airway epithelial cells from people with one or two non-functional T2R38 alleles. This results in greater susceptibility to *P. aeruginosa* and other gram-negative bacteria than those with two functional receptor alleles. Such observations may explain why individuals who can taste phenyl thiocarbamide (bitter) are less prone to infection (Lee et al., 2012).

Leprosy (Hansen's Disease). Although rare in Europe and North America, leprosy provides a good example of a bacterial-induced chemosensory disturbance. The disease is a chronic granulomatous infection caused by *Mycobacterium leprae*, which is related to mycobacterium tuberculosis. Leprosy-related olfactory disorder is near universal. In a comprehensive study of 77 patients with mild (tuberculoid, n = 9) to severe (borderline, n = 42; lepromatous, n = 6) forms, *all* patients exhibited some degree of olfactory dysfunction when tested quantitatively (Mishra et al., 2006). It is unclear how this bacterium alters smell function, although the organism is known to have a predilection for cooler facial areas and the nasal cavity is characteristically 1°C below body temperature. Damage to the olfactory receptor membrane is a likely mechanism and as the disease advances, intranasal swelling, ulceration, perforation, and cartilaginous collapse occurs. This concept is supported by a study of 15 leprosy patients and 15 controls (Veyseller 2012). Not only were all leprosy patients anosmic or hyposmic, but MRI imaging showed that their olfactory bulbs were smaller, a phenomenon known to occur when olfactory receptor cells are damaged.

Granulomatous Disease. Congenital syphilis may be responsible for anosmia because it damages the nasal septum, resulting in the characteristic "saddle-nose" deformity (see examples in Figure 5.2). However, this deformity is not specific for syphilis and may result from tuberculosis, sarcoidosis, Wegner's granulomatosis, systemic lupus erythematosis, or cocaine abuse (Alobid et al., 2004).

Head Trauma

Head trauma (HT) is a relatively frequent cause of smell dysfunction, especially in men, although prevalence rates vary, no doubt influenced by the variability of quantitative testing and the populations from which cases are derived. For example, the rate of smell loss in HT

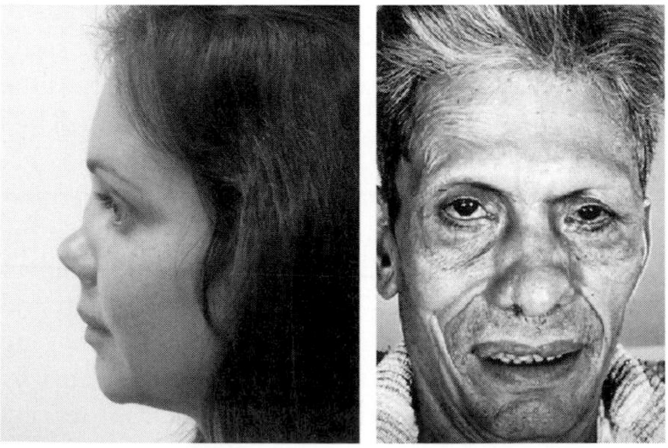

Figure 5.2 Left: Saddle nose deformity in a 30-year-old female, secondary to Wegener's granulomatosis. Right: the characteristic deformed nose in a patient with leprosy. Courtesy of Dr. Thomas Swift, Medical College of Georgia, Augusta.

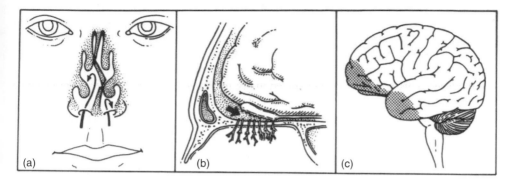

Figure 5.3 Mechanisms of traumatic olfactory dysfunction. A. injury to sinonasal tract. B. tearing of the olfactory nerves. C. cortical contusions and haemorrhage. Reproduced with permission from Costanzo et al. (1995).

patients who present to smell and taste clinics is high and clearly not representative of the prevalence in the population at large. Examples of various sites of peripheral and central damage are shown in Figure 5.3.

In a study of 1,000 consecutive cases admitted to a World War II military hospital for head injuries, 72 patients with impaired smell function (7.2%) were identified, of which 41 were said to have complete anosmia (4.1%) (Leigh, 1943). Blows to the front and the back of the head were most common (30 frontal; 18 occipital). Nearly all cases in which smell loss was evident had severe trauma. Only six regained smell function (8%) over the course of a year and the time to recovery varied from 20 days to 12 months (median = 3 months). Interestingly, half of the recovering patients went through a period of dysosmia. Unfortunately, quantitative olfactory testing was not performed.

Two decades later, Sumner observed a similar prevalence (7.1%) of smell loss in 1,167 unselected HT cases (Sumner, 1967). In those whose HT was relatively minor, i.e., no amnesia or memory loss shorter than one hour, frontal blows were more likely to result in smell deficits than vertex or occipital blows. However, anosmia was five times more likely to occur from occipital than frontal blows. More improved within 10 weeks than beyond 10 weeks, implying that the earlier improvement was due to resolution of compression, edema, and blood clot formation, whereas the later and slower improvement reflected neural recovery. No meaningful association was found between head trauma severity and the time required for anosmia to resolve. This study differed from earlier ones in that (a) anosmia was sought out in patients soon after their trauma, (b) the sample contained many patients with minor HT, and (c) patients were followed for a relatively long time after injury (up to five years). Once more, quantitative olfactory testing was not performed.

In 1982, Zusho published data on 5,000 patients who presented after head and face injuries (Zusho, 1982). There were 212 (4.2%) who complained of an olfactory disorder, of whom 73% were anosmic, and the rest were hyposmic. Blows to the face and occipital and frontal regions of the skull were more frequent (25.9%, 29.6%, and 18.5%, respectively), with fewer injuries involving the temporal (9.1%) and parietal (6.2%) regions. Quantitative testing was employed with the T&T olfactometer (Chapter 2) but only those with olfactory symptoms were tested. Many with smell impairment may have been unaware of their problem or did not report it because of more severe co-existing symptoms such as deafness and vertigo. Thus, their figures likely under estimate the true prevalence of trauma-related olfactory disorder.

Higher estimates of HT-related smell loss have been noted. Rutka (1999) reported a prevalence of 13.7 percent in 355 consecutive head injured patients who attended a clinic that focused on post-traumatic vertigo. Significant ascertainment bias may have been present given that the majority were referred from a Worker's Compensation Board. The average time from accident to evaluation was 40 months. Olfactory testing was crude and comprised a few strong odorants, many of which may have also stimulated intranasal elements of the trigeminal nerve, e.g., essence of cloves, camphor, peppermint, and wintergreen. That same year, Callahan & Hinkebein (1999) administered the UPSIT to 68 patients recruited from consecutive admissions to the inpatient and outpatient brain injury rehabilitation programs of a Midwestern Medical Center in the United States. While only 13 (30%) acknowledged that they had smell dysfunction, 44 were in fact anosmic (65%). Anosmia was associated with longer periods of unconsciousness or coma. Psychological testing revealed greater functional impairment in the anosmics, with more marked deficits in attention, memory, and problem solving (Callahan & Hinkebein, 1999).

Participants in contact sports, such as football and boxing, are exposed to recurrent head injuries. Apart from potential cognitive change, there is significant risk of olfactory impairment. In boxing, damage to the nasal septum is frequent and when severe, results in variable degrees of conductive anosmia. One study addressed olfaction in a sample of 50 male boxers, mean age 26.4 years and mean weight 74.1 kg, who trained on average four times per week. The majority had performed at least 500 rounds in training fights and averaged 40 official matches during which 24 percent had at least one knockout (Vent et al., 2010). Nasal conductive defects were excluded by endoscopy. A slight but significant reduction of olfactory function was observed. Fourteen (28%) were classed as hyposmic but none was anosmic. Although there was no connection between smell impairment and number of fights, knockouts, or nasal fractures, an inverse relationship between olfactory impairment and degree of cushioning of the boxing gloves was noted. Softer gloves were used in sparring and harder gloves in actual fights, thus confounding the cushioning measure with the severity of facial injuries and number of knockouts, for example.

The most recent study enrolled, prospectively, 231 polytrauma in-patients who were acutely injured from explosions during combat operations in either Afghanistan or Iraq (Xydakis et al., 2015). Olfaction was measured by the UPSIT and correlated with brain imaging (CT and MRI). All troops with mild traumatic brain injury (TBI) had normal olfactory scores. Those with radiographic evidence of frontal lobe injuries were three times more likely to have olfactory impairment than troops with injuries to other brain regions (Figure 5.4). It was suggested that olfactory dysfunction helps to identify soldiers with TBI who will have intracranial radiographic abnormalities with a sensitivity of 35% (95% CI 20.6%–51.7%) and specificity of 100% (95% CI 97.7%–100.0%).

Mechanism. Smell loss is usually attributed to shearing of the olfactory nerve fibers ("fila") as they emerge from the cribriform plate to enter the overlying olfactory bulb (Jafek et al., 1989). In some cases structural damage to the nose is evident, as well as damage to central structures (Figure 5.3). Indirect evidence for shearing of the olfactory fila comes from the study of the olfactory epithelium of patients with HT-related olfactory dysfunction. In such cases, the orderly arrangement of supporting, receptor, and basal cells, including the relative positions of their nuclei, was markedly disrupted, and there were increased numbers of degenerating cells (Moran et al., 1992). The dendrites of the bipolar receptor neurons were less numerous,

Location of brain injury	Normal olfactory function (n = 26)	Olfactory impairment (n = 14)	p value
Frontal	11 (42.3%)	11 (78.6%)	0.046
Parietal	11 (42.3%)	5 (35.7%)	0.746
Temporal	5 (19.2%)	6 (42.9%)	0.147
Occipital	2 (7.7%)	2 (14.3%)	0.602
Multifocal	6 (23.1%)	6 (42.9%)	0.281
Frontal OR temporal	13 (50.0%)	12 (85.7%)	0.040
Frontal AND temporal	3 (11.5%)	5 (35.7%)	0.102

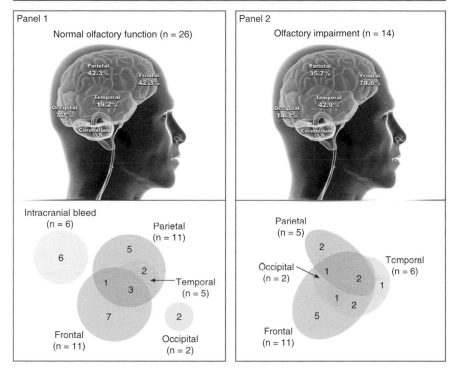

Figure 5.4 Troops with abnormal neuroimaging: Location of injury and its association with olfactory performance and multifocality (n = 40). Reproduced with permission from Xydakis et al. (2015). (A black and white version of this figure will appear in some formats. For the color version, please refer to the plate section.)

thicker, and shorter than normal. The few that reached the epithelial surface often lacked cilia. As shown in an autopsy-based study of 26 head-injured patients (Delank & Fechner, 1996), there may be an additional contribution from hemorrhage within the olfactory bulb or tracts in the absence of other intracranial lesions. Diffuse axonal injury, which interrupts axonal transport within the olfactory tracts, may also account for some HT-related olfactory changes independent of whether or not the fila are sheared (Johnson et al., 2013).

It is important to realize that the skull need not be fractured to produce post-traumatic olfactory disorder (Delank & Fechner, 1996); a simple blow to the head or strong acceleration forces may be sufficient. Additionally, the smell loss may occur gradually over time and may not be noticed by the patient for months. These points are of considerable relevance in medicolegal work. There are very few reports of smell disorder following whiplash injury, e.g., Kramer (1983), but most clinicians involved with chemosensory disorders accept this association. As mentioned above, anosmia is thought more likely to ensue if the front or back or the head is struck rather than the sides (Leigh, 1943b; Sumner, 1975; Zusho, 1982) because the opportunity for shearing forces on the frontal lobes is greater with antero-posterior injury. This may not be correct: detailed study of 179 head-injured patients concluded that occipital and side impact caused most damage and frontal the least (Doty et al., 1997). Often the relevant area of impact can be ascertained from the site of visible superficial trauma or reports from onlookers, although assessment of the most relevant area of impact can be difficult, given the variable context of trauma (e.g., civilian vs. military), inconstant patterns of referral, and assessment. These findings are at odds with those discussed above by Xydakis et al. (2015), who documented more frequent olfactory impairment with frontal injury. The disparate findings likely relate to the different populations examined, i.e., the Xydakis study only addressed TBI in blast-injured combat troops.

It should be emphasized that the olfactory receptor neurons have trophic influences on the olfactory bulb, thus, shearing of the fila will result in gradual bulbar atrophy (Yousem et al., 1996b) and measurement of their volume may give substance to a patient's account, particularly where there is litigation. Unfortunately, there is considerable variation in normal bulb volume and many factors can reduce its size, including airway blockage. The time course of such changes is not well documented.

Investigations. Routine computed tomography (CT) or magnetic resonance imaging (MRI) may identify medium to large areas of intracerebral hemorrhage (Figure 5.5 A–C), but both may fail to detect small post-traumatic petechial lesions that typically involve the frontal or temporal poles such as those as shown in Figure 5.5 (right). Those petechial lesions are identified best by gradient echo sequencing, which is sensitive to hemosiderin, the break-down product of blood. The orbitofrontal cortex, which is a tertiary olfactory area, may be under-perfused, as witnessed by single photon emission computed tomography (SPECT) and positron emission tomography (PET) studies under non-stimulation conditions (Abdel-Dayem et al., 1998). These observations confirm that frontal or temporal lobe lesions commonly underlie post-traumatic olfactory disorders. Damage to the frontal lobes, apart from resulting in centrally based olfactory deficits, may also cause a dysexecutive syndrome characterized by problems with motivation, planning and social behavior (Varney & Bushnelt, 1998; Varney et al., 2001). Thorough imaging of patients with post-traumatic anosmia, particularly with gradient echo MRI, is therefore advisable given the poorer prognosis when there is frontal lobe involvement.

Prognosis. The prospect of recovery from post-traumatic anosmia is a function of multiple variables, including age at the time of the insult, severity of trauma, and the elapsed time since injury (see Table 3.2). Poor recuperation may also relate to development of scar tissue at the level of the cribriform plate, thereby blocking entry of any regenerating olfactory receptor axons into the olfactory bulb (Jafek et al., 1989). When the loss is solely caused by nasal swelling, function would be expected to return within a few months. According to Sumner (1975), patients amnesic for more than seven days have the poorest outlook. In another detailed study of initial features in 268 head trauma patients presenting to a smell and taste center, 67% had anosmia, 20% microsmia, and only 13% were normal (Doty et al., 1997). Recovery was poor: Of 66 patients who could be contacted for retesting, 36% improved slightly, 45% were unchanged, and 18% had worsened. The prevalence of parosmia was 41%, but it decreased to 15% over eight years, implying that it may be a good prognostic indicator. Only three (5%) recovered to normal from initial anosmia. Since this

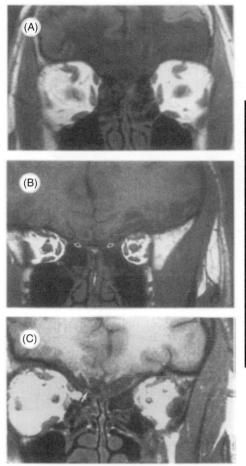

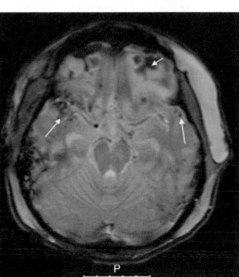

Figure 5.5 Left: MRI images of post-traumatic injury to the olfactory apparatus. Coronal T1-weighted images in three cases of varying degrees of severity. A. This shows complete destruction of the inferior frontal lobes that resulted from a major road traffic accident and was associated with anosmia. B. This shows inferior frontal encephalomalacia, and the patient was microsmic, although the olfactory tracts are visible (arrows). C. This patient had post-traumatic anosmia with no visible olfactory bulb or tract on the left and just a fragment of a tract on the right (arrowed). Both frontal lobes were sheared. Reproduced with permission from Correia et al. (2001), Yousem et al. (2001). Right: Gradient Echo Axial MRI images from another case of severe head injury that shows multiple areas of petechial hemorrhage (small round black areas), mainly in the frontal and temporal poles (long white arrows). The short white arrow in the left frontal region indicates traumatic hemorrhagic contusion in the orbitofrontal cortex, which would have damaged the tertiary (orbito-frontal) olfactory cortex.

study concerned patients in a specialized referral center, there would be over-representation of more severe cases and the outlook might be worse than a population-based sample. According to a later study that examined patients with a wide range of chemosensory disorders (London et al., 2008), the prognosis in anosmia depends more on the severity than the type of initial injury, as long as there is no damage to the frontal or temporal lobes. According to Martzke et al. (1991) and Varney (1988), who studied patients with anosmia but no skull fracture (closed head injury), up to 93% may be vocationally dysfunctional from orbitofrontal damage. Their patients were referred for cognitive, not olfactory problems,

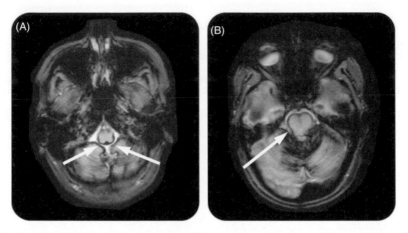

Figure 5.6 Superficial Siderosis. Axial gradient echo MRI showing low signal around the cerebellum, medulla (A) and pons (B). Findings of both T2 and gradient echo sequences consistent with hemosiderin deposition. Reproduced with permission from Ellis et al. (2012).

and quantitative olfactory testing was not performed. A different result was obtained in 15 patients with documented post-traumatic smell loss secondary to mild–moderate closed head injury (Correia et al., 2001). Although about half were upset by the impact of microsmia on their quality of life, only one had difficulty resuming his former occupation. Thus, smell loss, when taken in isolation, does not appear to be a good predictor of vocational disability.

Case Report 5.3: **Post-Traumatic Anosmia from a Fall on Ice.** A 56-year-old woman fell on ice in her driveway, striking the back of her head on the ground and suffering brief disorientation but no amnesia. A few days later she discovered smell impairment, and soon thereafter experienced distortions of smell and taste. Routine CT and MRI assessments proved negative. She received a course of systemic steroids without benefit. The UPSIT score was 17/40; bilateral, left, and right detection threshold scores on the phenylethyl alcohol detection threshold test indicated anosmia or severe microsmia. There was chance-level performance on the 12-item Odor Discrimination/Memory Test. Nasal airway patency assessed by anterior rhinomanometry and nasal airflow resistance measured by acoustic rhinometry were normal. Scores on a series of taste tests were normal, and so were values on the Mini-Mental State Examination and the Beck Depression Inventory II. *Comment:* This is a classic case of trauma-induced bilateral anosmia, unaccompanied by true taste loss. The dysfunction likely reflects movement of the brain and the resulting shearing of olfactory fila at the level of the cribriform plate. The smell and taste "distortions" probably relate to decreased flavor sensations secondary to lack of retronasal olfactory stimulation and the possible presence of a few aberrant olfactory nerve fibers that are still active.

Case Report 5.4: **Post-Traumatic Anosmia in a Chef after Being Hit by a Van.** A 38-year-old chef reported that six months previously he had been knocked to the ground by a van, hitting the back of his head. He was unconscious for one hour, amnesic for two hours, and took one week off work. During this first week he developed headache, positional vertigo, and reduced ability to smell. The smell defect was continuous, with no improvement at any time of the day. On testing, the Mini-Mental State Examination score was normal at 30/30, but the UPSIT score was in the severe microsmic range (21/40). The olfactory event-related potential (OERP) to 2 ppm H2S was delayed significantly at 1200 ms (position Pz). *Comment:* The diagnosis was severe post-traumatic microsmia. The delay on OERP confirmed both the patient's report and identification test findings, and would provide useful evidence if there were a court hearing. Given that he worked as a chef, there would be litigation and a high compensation fee, depending on the degree of recovery and difficulty at work. Although some return of function may occur over time, it is unlikely that normal smell function would be regained.

Superficial Siderosis of the Central Nervous System. This is a chronic basal meningitic process caused by recurrent, usually small, hemorrhages into the subarachnoid space of the brain or spinal cord that develop after head injury, aneurysms, or vascular anomalies (Fearnley et al., 1995). Deposition of hemosiderin in the basal meninges damages the auditory nerves, olfactory tracts, and cerebellum, resulting in ataxia, perceptive deafness, myelopathy and olfactory impairment. The combination of deafness and ataxia may be confused with spino-cerebellar ataxias or mitochondrial diseases. Limited data suggest the onset of smell loss may be relatively sudden (Vadala et al., 2013), although quantitative measurement is rarely performed. The prevalence of "anosmia" appears to range from 20% to 50% (Fearnley et al., 1995; Anderson et al., 1999; Kale et al., 2003).

Tumors

Tumors within the nasal or cranial cavity can damage smell function. Intranasal tumors may block airflow to the nasal olfactory receptor region, facilitate bacterial overgrowth secondary to reduction of mucociliary clearance, or impair the olfactory epithelium and its emerging fila by pressure. Nasopharyngeal carcinoma (NPC) and adenocystcarcinoma are the most frequent epithelial nasal neoplasms. Lymphomas, as well as malignant tumors involving the ethmoid or sphenoid sinuses, often invade the nasal cavity. One extremely rare malignant tumor that arises from the nasal neuroepithelium is the esthesio-neuroblastoma; inevitably smell function is compromised.

Much current knowledge about the influence of intracranial tumors on olfaction dates back to the classic observations of Elsberg (1935a), who stated:

> The olfactory bulbs and tracts lie in a situation in which they can and must be affected by changes in intracranial pressure. Their function must be disturbed early by tumors in their neighborhood. Thus the meningioma which arises from the dura of the cribriform plate and the parts adjacent to it, pituitary growths if they extend above the diaphragm of the sella turcica, and tumors on the floor of or inside the third ventricle must interfere to a greater or less extent with the afferent impulses which pass through the bulbs and tracts. If sufficiently sensitive tests of olfaction were devised, slight disturbances of the functions of the olfactory bulbs and tracts should be recognizable.

In fact, Elsberg found that subfrontal meningiomas could be diagnosed relatively early by raised identification thresholds, using the blast injection test method. This involved quantification of the amount of odorized air needed to be injected to produce a smell sensation, a procedure little used nowadays, chiefly because of co-stimulation of the trigeminal nerves.

The olfactory groove meningioma is the most common benign intracranial tumor that affects the ability to smell . This tumor exerts pressure on the olfactory bulb or tract (Figure 5.7) and, in theory, can damage the overlying orbitofrontal cortex to produce an additional central olfactory defect. In the early phase of tumor growth, anosmia, if present,

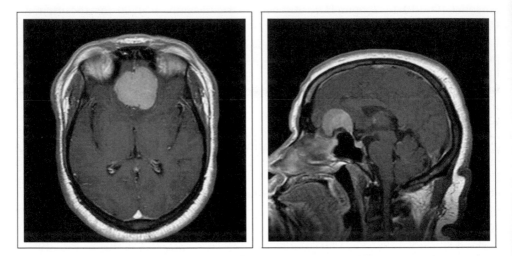

Figure 5.7 Olfactory groove meningioma. Left figure: Axial T1 MRI with contrast to show a large midline frontal mass with homogeneous enhancement. Right figure: Sagittal T1 MRI with contrast showing an extra-axial mass which was found to be an olfactory groove meningioma. The patient was anosmic but was not aware of this. Reproduced with permission from Yousem et al. (2001).

is seldom detected as the patient rarely notices unilateral deficits and the clinician, if he tests olfaction at all, is unlikely to examine each nostril individually. Smell impairment is also associated with parasellar aneurysms arising, for example, from the internal carotid and anterior communicating arteries . Other causes include downward expansion of the third ventricle due to hydrocephalus, and meningiomas arising from the anterior clinoid process, sphenoid ridge, or suprasellar region (Doty, 2015). Rarely, inferior frontal malignant tumors produce anosmia from pressure on the bulb or tracts, although such growths may result in prolonged adaptation on the side of the tumor (Elsberg, 1935b). Classically, the Foster Kennedy syndrome is characterized by an ipsilateral central scotoma, optic atrophy, and anosmia with contralateral papilledema. If there is a structural cause, it is typically a large frontal neoplasm, but other lesions include meningiomas involving the olfactory groove or medial third of the sphenoid wing or frontal lobe abscess. In practice, the Foster Kennedy syndrome is rare. It is mimicked by longstanding anterior ischemic optic atrophy on one side and more recent ischemia on the contralateral side, causing disk swelling suggestive of raised intracranial pressure – the pseudo-Foster Kennedy syndrome.

It is well established that ~20 percent of temporal lobe tumors or lesions of the uncinate gyrus produce some form of olfactory disturbance, most often phantosmias (Furstenberg et al., 1943). The usual cause is a temporal lobe glioma, which is also responsible for uncinate fits (Figure 5.8). The tumor is unilateral and because many temporal lobe functions are duplicated contralaterally, it may achieve a large size before clinical presentation, particularly if it involves the side non-dominant for language. Ablation of the right temporal lobe is associated with impaired olfactory discrimination (Zatorre & Jones-Gotman, 1991), and defects in olfactory discrimination occur in subjects with right (smell-dominant) temporal lobe tumors. Such effects are reportedly less obvious in tumors confined to the left temporal lobe (Daniels et al., 2001).

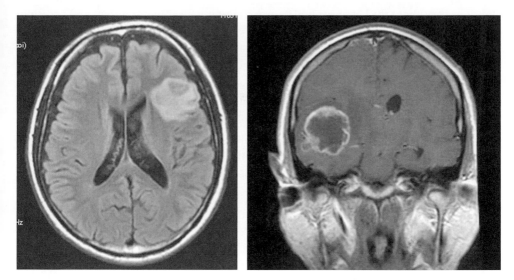

Figure 5.8 Left: Axial T1-weighted enhanced MRI scan that shows an oligodendroglioma in the left frontotemporal area deep in the white matter. Right: MRI T1 enhanced coronal section that shows a large infiltrating glioblastoma multiforme occupying much of the right temporal lobe. Both of these lesions would cause olfactory hallucinations and complex partial seizures from surrounding edema.

Pituitary Tumors. Small pituitary tumors (microadenomas), defined as those under 10 mm diameter, remain within the sella and produce endocrine effects but do not cause pressure on surrounding structures. Pituitary macroadenomas have a diameter of 10 mm or more and they are usually treated by surgical decompression. Olfactory changes from mass effects of the tumor itself are rare but in some patients with a pituitary tumor, as documented by Sherman, Amoore, and Weigel (1979), there was reportedly a 100,000-fold improvement of detection threshold sensitivity to pyridine. This observation begs replication. Surgical intervention carries some risk of damage to the nasal olfactory neuroepithelium. The standard incisions are made through the upper nasal septum, then through the sphenoid sinus which lies directly below the pituitary gland. The main approaches are (1) under direct vision using a microscope (microscopic transsphenoidal surgery; MTSS), or (2) the same route, but using an endoscope (endoscopic trans-sphenoidal surgery; ETSS). Some damage to the olfactory neuroepithelium is inevitable, either transiently from local swelling or possibly permanently from injury to the neuroepithelium. Symptomatic reports suggest there may be smell impairment after surgery for acromegaly, particularly with ETSS (Starke et al., 2013). Hart, Theodosopoulos, and Zimmer (2010) used ETSS and measured smell function by the UPSIT pre-operatively and then one and three months post-operatively. They documented a slight reduction in mean identification score at one month but not at three months, implying that any reduction on olfaction was due to immediate post-operative effects. Kahilogullari et al. (2013) described 25 patients treated by ETSS compared to 25 managed by MTSS. The Smell Diskettes Olfaction Test was used during the pre-operative period, then one month and six months after the operation. In the ETSS group, there were two hyposmic patients and no anosmic patients while in the MTSS group, there were 13 hyposmic patients and five anosmic patients, thus favoring the superiority of ETSS.

Opinions vary about the better surgical approach but it is clear that transient and occasionally permanent smell impairment may take place after transphenoidal pituitary surgery.

Disordered Intracranial Pressure (ICP)

The olfactory bulbs and tracts, like the optic nerves, are covered by a meningeal sheath that encloses the subarachnoid space. In theory, raised ICP from virtually any cause might compress the olfactory tract or bulb and compromise their function.

Classic Hydrocephalus. Experimental hydrocephalus in the dog produces distension of the olfactory bulb cavity and possible impairment of olfaction (Kim et al., 2009). Despite this knowledge, there are no reports of olfactory disorder in classic hydrocephalus. This area clearly merits further investigation, particularly given the frequency of hydrocephalus that affects infants and children.

Normal Pressure Hydrocephalus (NPH). This is a poorly understood condition that results in a triad of dementia, gait ataxia, and bladder problems. Imaging reveals large lateral ventricles but comparatively little atrophy of the cortical ribbon. Contrary to expectation, the spinal fluid pressure is normal, although some patients improve after lumbar puncture or permanent shunting, suggesting that there may be transient elevations of pressure. The disorder may be confused with progressive supranuclear palsy where olfaction is altered very little (see Chapter 7). If olfaction is impaired in NPH, then testing might help to distinguish the two conditions. Two studies have found that NPH is, in fact, associated with decreased olfactory function (Podlesek et al., 2012; Passier et al., 2017). In both studies, olfactory function was impaired at baseline. However, no improvement in either study was found after extended lumbar drainage and, in one study, lack of improvement was still present six months after surgical implantation of a ventriculoperitoneal shunt (Passier et al., 2017). Olfactory bulb volume as measured by MRI (Podlesek et al 2012), was significantly smaller in the NPH group but its size did not change after surgery. Several issues are raised by this observation. If the ICP is in fact normal, then there should be no pressure on the olfactory nerves or bulb and there should be no change in OB size. Some suggest that ICP is raised when the subject is recumbent, i.e., during sleep, but then returns to normal during the day when the subject is upright. These preliminary findings clearly need further exploration.

Idiopathic Intracranial Hypertension (IIH; Pseudotumor Cerebri; Benign Intracranial Hypertension). Typically, this is a disorder of overweight adult females. The etiology of IIH is poorly understood, but most consider it relates to disturbed cerebrospinal fluid (CSF) dynamics, probably affecting absorption. There is usually prior exposure to hormonal contraceptives, steroids, and particularly minocycline, the antibiotic prescribed for facial acne. Two possible mechanisms are proposed for potential olfactory damage, both related to elevated ICP (Kunte et al., 2013). The first is pressure on the subarachnoid space that surrounds the olfactory pathway, given that the olfactory bulb and the olfactory nerve fibers that cross the cribriform plate are covered by a meningeal sheath that encloses the subarachnoid space. The second is impaired passage of CSF as it attempts to drain via lymphatics into the nose in the olfactory nerve perineurial sheath (Johnston et al., 2004); see Chapter 1, Figure 1.5.

Most patients complain of tinnitus (sometimes pulsatile) with morning headaches secondary to raised intracranial pressure. Fundoscopy shows papilledema – the cardinal sign of raised ICP. All require a brain scan to exclude the possibility of a brain tumor – hence the alternate name "pseudotumor cerebri." One questionnaire study found that patients with this disorder report olfactory or taste problems more often than normal controls matched on the basis of age and sex (Giuseffi et al., 1991). They proposed that patients with IIH might suffer from smell impairment as suggested later by Kapoor (2008). These observations prompted a pilot MRI-based survey of 23 subjects with IIH. It was found that olfactory bulb volume, as measured by high resolution MRI, was indeed reduced, particularly in those with short duration of disease (Schmidt et al., 2012). The sense of smell was not measured clinically, but the imaging changes infer that some impairment would be likely. This contention was borne out in a subsequent study of olfaction in 17 patients with IIH (Kunte et al., 2013). There was a significant reduction in the composite threshold-discrimination-identification (TDI) score on the extended Sniffin' Sticks test. Overall threshold was affected least, but in the acute cases all aspects of the TDI score were significantly reduced.

The most recent investigation (Bershad et al., 2014) was prompted in part by the observation that astronauts exposed to long duration flights in space may develop signs of elevated intracranial pressure comparable to IIH, as well as nasal congestion and subjective olfactory impairment. The authors tested 19 patients with IIH and 19 controls to examine the effect on olfactory identification and threshold of 6° head-down tilt, which simulates the rostral fluid shift in microgravity, as in spaceflight. It was found that IIH patients had significant impairment of olfactory threshold that was out of proportion to impaired smell identification, which would suggest, according to some researchers, a peripheral disorder (i.e., olfactory bulb) rather than a more central (cognitive) problem. In the head-down tilt, compared with upright positioning, there was also impairment of olfactory threshold but not identification. The basis for this effect is not entirely clear, since previous studies reported an inverse relationship between odor identification test scores and nasal airflow resistance at varying degrees of tilt (Mester et al., 1988).

Serial olfactory testing to indirectly measure changes in ICP will probably not replace conventional assessments (visual fields, optic disk fluctuations, MRI, lumbar puncture) because of the lag between olfactory change and alteration of ICP.

Radiotherapy

It has been recognized for many years that radiotherapy (RT) can impair the ability to smell. For example, increased Elsberg blast injection thresholds were reported in five patients during and after RT – thresholds that reportedly returned to normal within two months (Schaupp & Krull, 1975). In a more substantive study, Hua et al. (1999) administered an olfactory test battery to 25 patients with nasopharyngeal carcinoma (NPC) who were receiving RT, 24 NPC patients awaiting to receive such therapy, and 36 normal controls. The groups were matched on the basis of age, education, and IQ. Relative to the other groups, those receiving RT had significant deficits on a range of olfactory tests, including threshold, recognition, identification, and memory.

Evidence that RT has long-lasting effects on olfactory function was first presented by Carmichael, Jennings, and Doty (1984). These investigators found that anosmia was evident in a 60-year-old woman after receiving 10 of 26 courses of radiotherapy for the treatment of a pituitary adenoma (UPSIT score = 10). Approximately one year after treatment, smell function seemed to be gradually returning, as witnessed by an UPSIT score of 27 (14th percentile for someone of her age and gender). When tested a further five months later her UPSIT score was of the same magnitude (score = 28), suggesting that some smell dysfunction was present two years after completion of radiotherapy. Similarly, Bramerson et al. (2013) noted in their 71 patients that even after 20 months of RT cessation, smell dysfunction, as measured by identification and threshold tests, was evident. Olfactory deficits were related to radiation dose and proximity of the beam to the olfactory region, but not to age, sex, or concurrent chemotherapy. Holscher et al. (2005) studied olfactory function in six patients with NPC, 15 patients with paranasal sinus tumors, 10 patients with oropharyngeal tumors, and other cancers, all of whom received RT that included the olfactory neuroepithelium. Impaired odor discrimination, but not identification or threshold, was decreased two to six weeks after RT. Despite the apparent unanimity of the above studies, Ho et al. (2002) found no olfactory deficits in 48 NPC patients during or immediately after completion of RT. One year later, threshold scores were affected, but not discrimination or identification scores.

In a prospective study, 24 patients with NPC were assessed by olfactory bulb MRI volumetrics and the Connecticut Chemosensory Clinical Research Center (CCCRC) smell test (Veyseller et al., 2014a). The CCCRC measures threshold to n-butanol and odor identification. Compared to healthy controls, there was significant lowering of CCCRC score in the NPC group, in whom about half displayed varying olfactory deficits. Some patients were receiving chemotherapy, notably cisplatin or docetaxel, but it was considered that neither affected their olfactory test scores. Bulb volume, as expected, was smaller in the NPC group.

In summary, it is likely that radiotherapy for nasopharyngeal or pituitary tumors may impair olfactory performance but the onset of its harmful effects may be delayed by as much as one year.

Psychiatric Disorders

Smell dysfunction has been implicated in range of psychiatric disorders including Korsakoff psychosis, seasonal affective disorder, schizophrenia, the olfactory reference syndrome, and chronic hallucinatory psychoses. Although some studies suggest that major affective disorder or depression is associated with smell loss, this is controversial, as described below.

Korsakoff Psychosis (KS). This is caused by vitamin B1 (thiamine) deficiency, usually secondary to chronic alcoholism or malnutrition. The main characteristics are amnesia and confabulation. There is difficulty in identifying, discriminating, and remembering odors (Gregson et al., 1981; Jones et al., 1975a, 1975b, 1978; Mair et al., 1980, 1986). In one study, UPSIT scores were markedly impaired relative to controls (respective means = 16.57 & 32.86), whereas Picture Identification Test scores were normal (Mair et al., 1986). Although olfactory thresholds, extrapolated from suprathreshold measures, are reportedly altered in this disease (Jones et al., 1978), others have not observed defects in signal detection analysis (Mair et al., 1980). In the 1980 study by Mair et al., KS patients exhibited a more conservative response criterion than that shown by the controls. These investigators also pointed out that the olfactory deficit in KS could reflect (a) damage to the peripheral olfactory system, (b) memory impairment, (c) a generalized perceptual deficit, and/or (d) damage to higher order olfactory structures, most notably the magnocellular layer of the mediodorsal thalamic nuclei. It was concluded that option (d) was the most likely explanation.

A further study examined odor discrimination in 6 patients with frontal lobe damage, 7 with KS, and 16 healthy controls (Pol et al., 2002). Assessment was made by odor detection and odor discrimination tasks. In those with frontal lobe disorder related to pain relief surgery or frontal tumor, there was impaired discrimination, whereas in those with KS,

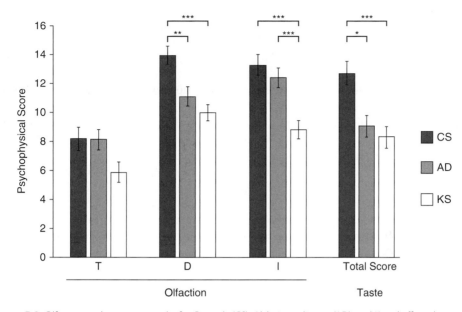

Figure 5.9 Olfactory and gustatory results for Controls (CS), Alzheimer disease (AD), and Korsakoff syndrome (KS) participants. The scores presented for each olfactory subscale (threshold, discrimination, identification) and total taste score are corrected for depression, state anxiety, trait anxiety, education level, and nicotine dependence using covariance analyses. This shows that discrimination and identification are affected in KS patients but not threshold. Reproduced with permission from Brion et al. (2015).

discrimination was decreased only marginally and neither group showed impairment of odor detection. This study differs substantially from those cited above, possibly because of the small number of patients tested (6) and the older age of their sample. When their data were adjusted for age the apparent reduction in discrimination was not sustained.

In a more recent study, Brion et al. (2015) investigated smell and taste in alcohol dependence (AD) and KS. Chemosensory measurements were obtained from 20 KS, 20 AD, and 20 control participants. The extended Sniffin' Sticks test was used to measure threshold, discrimination, and identification. Taste was also assessed and described in Chapter 6. After controlling for psychopathological comorbidities, it was found that those with KS had significant impairment of odor discrimination and identification but not threshold sensitivity (Figure 5.9).

Schizophrenia. Olfactory dysfunction is common in schizophrenia (SZ), although considerable heterogeneity is present and the magnitude of the olfactory deficit is relatively small compared to AD and PD (for review, see Doty et al., 2015). Olfactory hallucinations, which are typically unpleasant, are common (11–34%) (Meats, 1988; Stevenson et al., 2011). Such hallucinations are predictive of poorer prognosis (Kwapil et al., 1996) and earlier age of disease onset (Lewandowski et al., 2009).

Although the olfactory deficit of SZ is typically bilateral, it can be asymmetrical. It occurs early in the illness and relates to disease duration (Moberg et al., 1997). Odor identification test scores correlate with frontal or temporal lobe dysfunction in patients with schizophrenia (Turetsky et al., 2003; Moberg et al., 2006). Like olfactory hallucinations, decreased UPSIT scores may be a marker for poorer outcomes in patients with schizophrenia (Good et al.,

2010). Such scores not only correlate with disease duration (Moberg et al., 1997), but are associated with negative disease symptoms (Brewer et al., 2001; Corcoran et al., 2005; Good et al., 2010), verbal memory (Compton et al., 2006), social drive, and intelligence (Malaspina & Coleman, 2003). In patients with deficit syndrome SZ, odor identification tests correlate with the quality of ocular smooth pursuit (Malaspina et al., 2002). There is some evidence that the impairment in olfaction observed in schizophrenia may be greater for pleasant than for unpleasant odors (Kamath et al., 2011). The olfactory deficit appears to be unrelated to smoking history (Kopala et al., 1993), cannabis use (Brewer et al., 1996), antipsychotic medications (Szeszko et al., 2004), and age of symptom onset (Corcoran et al., 2005).

Anatomical and physiologic changes within the olfactory system of SZ patients are well documented. Smaller nasal cavity volumes (Moberg et al., 2004) and cell loss consistent with the interruption of the rostral migratory stream regeneration have been noted (Chazal et al., 2000). Reduced olfactory bulb volumes of about 23 percent (Chazal et al., 2000; Turetsky et al., 2000) and shallow olfactory, but not orbital, sulci have been found in patients and in some apparently healthy first-degree relatives (Turetsky et al., 2009; Takahashi et al., 2014). The olfactory sulci develop in the first trimester of pregnancy, and the orbital sulci in the last trimester, implying that there may be toxic damage to the olfactory sulci in the early months of pregnancy. In a mouse model of SZ, secretion of reelin, a glycoprotein likely involved in neuronal migration, appears to be compromised in the olfactory bulb (Pappas et al., 2003). Reelin expression is significantly reduced in patients with psychotic disorders (Pantazopoulos et al., 2010) and may be involved in olfactory processing.

Several abnormalities of the SZ olfactory neuroepithelium have been described such as increased olfactory cell proliferation, lower density of basal cells, and increased stability of microtubules (Feron et al., 1999; Arnold et al., 2001; McCurdy et al., 2006; Brown et al., 2014). The electro-olfactogram (EOG; see Chapter 1), which is a summated electrical potential measured at the surface of the epithelium, is larger than normal in SZ, possibly reflecting disorder of the olfactory receptor cells, periglomerular cells, or the olfactory epithelium. EOGs may also be influenced by altered cAMP-mediated signal transduction, since patients with schizophrenia are hyposmic to lyral, a weak stimulator of adenyl cyclase, but not to citralva, which is a strong stimulator of adenyl cyclase (Turetsky & Moberg, 2009). Interestingly, increased P2 latencies and reduced N1 and P2 amplitude odor event-related potentials have been documented in schizophrenics and unaffected first-degree relatives (Turetsky et al., 2008).

Olfactory testing of people at genetic or clinical high risk for schizophrenia may help identify those who are likely to convert to frank psychosis in future (Brewer et al., 2003). Reduced olfactory identification is found in unaffected first-degree relatives of patients with psychotic disorders (Kopala et al., 2001; Keshavan et al., 2009) and in non-psychotic co-twins of monozygotic twin pairs discordant for SZ (Kopala et al., 1998; Ugur et al., 2005). It is recognized that patients with the DiGeorge syndrome (22q11 deletion syndrome) have increased risk of SZ in adulthood, thus raising the prospect of predictive olfactory testing. It was found that 27 of 39 patients with the DiGeorge syndrome had impaired UPSIT scores whether or not there was velopharyngeal insufficiency (Sobin et al., 2006). Clearly this interesting finding might identify those at future risk of SZ.

In summary, there is evidence of mild to moderately severe olfactory dysfunction in schizophrenia. The deficit may extend from the olfactory receptor cells to the temporal and frontal cortices. Abnormalities in some first-degree relatives suggest that smell impairment may be a biomarker of future disease. The recent finding of shallow olfactory sulci in SZ infers that the illness may start in early intrauterine life. Whether this phenomenon is primarily a genetic or intrauterine environmental effect or a combination of such factors has yet to be determined.

Depression-Related Disorders. Depression-related disorders are typified by feelings of sadness, hopelessness, severe despondency, and difficulty in concentrating or maintaining a mental focus. The standard metric is the questionnaire-based Hospital Anxiety and Depression Scale (HADS), which measures these two modalities on a numeric scale from 0–21. A score greater than 8/21 suggests the presence of anxiety and depression. Sometimes those with severe depression are misdiagnosed with dementia, thus a recurrent clinical problem is to decide whether difficulty with short-term memory represents an organic dementia, anxiety-depressive disorder, or both. There is sparse evidence that major affective disorder or related diseases are accompanied by changes in smell function. Since alterations in smell can lead to depression, cause and effect associations are often clouded. Moreover, some diseases, such as Parkinson's disease, are associated with both smell loss and depression, although the smell loss is clearly not caused by depression.

In the first large study on the influences of depression, per se, on the ability to smell, Amsterdam et al. (1987) administered the UPSIT to 51 patients who met DSM-III criteria for major depressive disorder, with or without melancholic features or atypical (bipolar II) depressive disorder. The patients had moderate to severe depression, as indicated by Hamilton Depression Rating Scale scores ranging from 18 to 37. No significant differences were present between the two groups ($p = 0.41$) and no dissimilarities were evident between the melancholic and non-melancholic depression subtypes ($p = 0.85$). Similarly, Pentzek, Grass-Kapanke, & Ihl (2007) found no differences in olfactory identification or detection threshold test scores for 20 elderly people with depression compared to 30 people without. Both groups outperformed those with Alzheimer's disease significantly. An analogous finding was observed by these authors for an odor identification test employing 11 odors (sensitivity: 100%; specificity: 95%) (Pentzek et al., 2007). Two studies have demonstrated that a simple three-item odor identification test distinguished between major depression and Alzheimer's with a sensitivity of 95% and specificity of 100%, and 80% and 100%, respectively – performance exceeding that of the Mini-Mental State Examination (MMSE) (Solomon et al., 1998; McCaffrey et al., 2000).

Other investigators report that depression may influence olfaction, although the direction of the results is not clear. Some report elevated odor detection thresholds (Pause, Raack et al., 2001; Pause, Miranda et al., 2001; Lombion-Pouthier et al., 2006), while others describe decreased odor detection thresholds (Gross-Isseroff et al., 1994; Postolache et al., 2002). Negoias et al. (2010) found that patients with acute major depressive disorder had elevated olfactory thresholds and smaller olfactory bulb volumes and noted a significant negative correlation between olfactory bulb volume and depression scores. Despite this, the effects were weak. Had the authors corrected for the effects of inflated α due to the application of multiple t-tests, it is unlikely that any of their p values would have reached the 0.05 α level of significance. Subsequently, Croy et al. (2014) described 27 depressed inpatients that exhibited impaired olfactory discrimination, prolonged latencies on olfactory event-related potentials, and reduced fMRI activation in the thalamus, insula, and left middle orbitofrontal cortex. Following psychotherapy, they reported improvement in all measures relative to controls.

Hardy et al. (2012) reported no overall differences in UPSIT scores or in PEA detection thresholds between 20 patients with DSM-IV bipolar disorder and 44 controls. However, odor detection thresholds were associated with clinical ratings of depression and mania on the Positive and Negative Syndrome Scale (PANSS; Kay et al. 1987). Depressive symptoms on this scale were correlated with higher olfactory threshold sensitivity, whereas the reverse was the case with manic symptoms. Krugerm et al. (2006) compared bipolar disorder euthymic patients with (n = 7) and without (n = 9) histories of event-triggered episodes. Those with event-triggered episodes exhibited lower PEA thresholds and short latency event-related potentials, although tests of odor identification and detection were not altered. No comparison against controls was made.

There are reports that seasonal affective disorder may be associated with lower PEA detection thresholds (i.e., greater sensitivity) relative to controls (Postolache et al., 1999; Postolache et al., 2002). A similar, albeit borderline, enhancement of PEA detection threshold was discovered in a small group of bipolar affective disorder patients with depression (Fedoroff et al., 1995; Roessner et al., 2005; Aschenbrenner et al., 2008; Rapps et al., 2010).

In summary, depression, per se, appears to have relatively little or no influence on most measures of olfactory function. Unfortunately, inconsistent findings abound. Thus, there are reports of both heightened and lowered thresholds in patients with depressive symptoms. Observations of smaller olfactory bulbs in depressed patients, if replicated, would suggest that at on occasion, decrements on some measures of olfactory function may be present.

Olfactory Reference Syndrome (ORS). An interesting psychiatric disorder is the olfactory reference syndrome, a condition generally viewed as distinct from schizophrenia or affective disorders (Pryse-Phillips, 1971, 1975; Bishop, Jr., 1980; Begum & McKenna, 2010). In ORS, the patient believes that smells emanate either from themselves (intrinsic hallucinations) or from elements of the environment (extrinsic hallucinations). Those with affective disorders such as endogenous depression usually experience intrinsic hallucinations, whereas the hallucinations of schizophrenia were usually extrinsic, sometimes believed to be induced by others who were trying to upset the patient.

Patients' responses may be "minimal," where the odor is complained about but no steps are taken to remove it, or "reasonable," where the subject tries to eliminate the odor by, e.g., complaining to the authorities, visiting a dermatologist, or plugging the chimney with newspapers. Those with intrinsic hallucinations often display compulsive washing behavior, changing clothes, and restriction of social activity. In many instances, ORS is linked closely with an obsessive-compulsive disorder and may be treated with serotonin-uptake inhibitors (Dominguez & Puig, 1997; Stein et al., 1998; O'Sullivan et al., 2000). It is conceivable that some patients with ORS actually have genuine phantosmias, but because of their personality, fail to recognize the true source of the problem. So far, it is not known whether patients with this syndrome exhibit measurable olfactory deficits.

Case Report 5.5: **Olfactory Reference Syndrome.** A 64-year-old warehouseman complained that for the previous two months he had been aware of a continual odor which he likened to the smell of sugar beet, musk, or body odor, present throughout the day. It was more noticeable after a shower but family members could not detect any unusual smell at all. He thought the malodor was coming from his own person. His sleep pattern was abnormal with significant delay in sleep onset and early morning wakening with intrusive dreams. Some 30 years previously he had suffered a bout of severe depression treated by electro-convulsive therapy and antidepressant tablets, long since discontinued. As a child he was affected by Tourette syndrome which had largely subsided. Examination showed normal nasal passages with an UPSIT score of 29/40, which is indicative of mild microsmia but it is at the lower end of the normal distribution for a man of his age (29th percentile). MRI imaging and nasal endoscopy showed no evidence of sino-nasal disorder. *Comment.* The continuous olfactory hallucination, thought to emanate from the patient, rather than outside the body, is characteristic of an intrinsic hallucination and suggests he may be suffering from the olfactory reference syndrome as described by Pryse-Phillips (1971, 1975). Most likely it indicates a recurrence of depression in this patient. Reintroduction of antidepressant medication relieved his phantosmic symptoms.

Endocrine Disorders and Pregnancy

Endocrine disorders account for a small percentage of olfactory disorders. Changes have been reported in the following disorders, which will be discussed below: (a) diabetes, (b) hypothyroidism, (c) Turner's syndrome, (d) Addison's disease, (e) Kallman's syndrome, and (f) pseudohypoparathyroidism. Although pregnancy is not an endocrine disorder, it is associated with major endocrine changes and pregnancy-related alterations in smell function are recognized. Thus, it is included in this section. There is minimal literature on olfaction in Cushing syndrome and hypoparathyroidism.

Diabetes. Given the high frequency of diabetes and its capacity for impairing neural function, it is surprising how few studies of olfaction have been undertaken. This is all the more remarkable given that insulin receptors are prevalent throughout the brain, with their highest concentration in the olfactory bulb (Hill et al., 1986; Baskin et al., 1987). Insulin alters the responsiveness of around a quarter of olfactory bulb mitral cells to some odorants (Cain, 1975). A potential mechanism for diabetes-related olfactory function was identified by Guthoff et al. (2009). They found significant olfactory impairment in 94 outwardly healthy male diabetic homozygous carriers of the polymorphism (normal variant) rs2821557 for the voltage-gated potassium channel Kv1.3. This channel is regulated by insulin and highly expressed in the olfactory bulb. They also found a significant correlation of olfactory dysfunction with higher glycosylated hemoglobin (HbA1c) and fasting plasma glucose, implying that olfaction, glucose metabolism, and genetic variation in Kv1.3 are all associated.

Several investigators have documented changes in diabetic chemoreception. Weinstock et al. (1993) found significant impairment of odor identification in 111 diabetics. UPSIT scores correlated with macrovascular disease but not glycemic control, retinopathy, or polyneuropathy. Use of insulin had no effect on the test results. In the same year, Le Floch et al. (1993) reported on the ability of 68 diabetics (type 1 and type 2) to identify 20 different odors. They demonstrated significant impairment of smell identification that was associated with disease duration, microalbuminuria, peripheral neuropathy, and particularly taste threshold. There was no correlation with blood glucose, glycosylated hemoglobin (HbA1c), or diabetic retinopathy, and there was no difference between olfactory scores for type 1 (insulin dependent) and type 2 diabetes (non-insulin dependent).

Gouveri et al. (2014) tested 119 patients with type 2 diabetes using the extended version of Sniffin' Sticks to obtain a threshold-discrimination-identification (TDI) index. There was an independent association of low TDI score, hypertension, and type 2 diabetes and the total olfactory score was lower in those with peripheral neuropathy or retinopathy.

Despite such observations, other investigators have found no olfactory deficits in diabetic patients. Thus, an early investigation by Patterson, Turner, and Smart (1966) found no change in threshold to an air-coffee mixture in 56 cases of undefined diabetes type and 56 controls. Naka et al. (2010) found no difference in smell or taste between controls (n = 29) and either patients with uncomplicated diabetes (n = 29) or those with diabetic microangiopathy and/or macroangiopathy (n = 24). Relative to the controls, a significant decrement in olfaction was found in 23 diabetics but only when accompanied by disorders that might independently alter smell function, e.g., hypothyroidism, medication for depression, hypertension or rheumatoid arthritis, liver, kidney, or neurological disease. In keeping with the findings of Le Floch et al. (1993), there was no correlation of smell function with level of HbA1c. Unlike Le Floch et al., they found no association with disease duration. Subsequently, Gascon et al. (2013) tested 61 diabetic patients with the Barcelona Smell-Taste Test 24 (BAST-24), a procedure that measures smell and taste detection and recognition. There was no association between HbA1c and olfaction, but lower olfactory scores were significantly associated with albuminuria and glomerular filtration rate.

In summary, the evidence supports impairment of smell sense in diabetes but chiefly when associated with complications such as peripheral neuropathy, retinopathy, hypertension, and renal disorder. It is not established whether the olfactory changes are more severe (as one might expect) in those with insulin dependent disease. Larger, more rigorous studies are required to address these issues and to determine whether olfactory impairment might be able to predict the onset of complications as claimed for taste (see Chapter 6).

Hypothyroidism. Acquired hypothyroidism, if untreated, is associated with multiple sensory disorders. Around 25–45% report auditory or visual problems, particularly night blindness, and 36–83% report somesthetic disturbances (Mattes, Heller, & Rivlin, 1986). Chemosensory disturbances may be no exception.

As early as 1918, McCarrison noted that, in the typical hypothyroid patient, the "sense of taste and smell may be disturbed, although this is difficult to determine" (McCarrison, 1918). Lewitt et al. (1989) found that 11 of 16 (69%) hypothyroid patients complained of altered smell and taste perception. McConnell et al. (1975) reported that 7 of 18 (39%) patients with untreated hypothyroidism believed they had some alteration in their sense of smell, with 3 (17%) reporting dysosmia.

In general, empirical studies have been contradictory. One group reported that odor detection thresholds for pyridine, nitrobenzene, sodium chloride, sucrose, hydrochloric acid, and urea were strikingly elevated in those with untreated hypothyroidism – a problem that resolved after thyroxin treatment (McConnell et al., 1975). Conversely, another group found no detection threshold differences between 16 patients and 17 controls for PEA and only slight but statistically significant differences on a suprathreshold test of odor identification (Lewitt et al., 1989). Various measures of suprathreshold taste ability as well as auditory and visual evoked potentials did not differ between patients and controls, and no pre-/post-thyroxine differences were observed for any measure. Subsequently, Deems et al. (1991) found no UPSIT or PEA threshold differences between patients not taking and those taking thyroxine, although recipients of this medication were more likely to report burning mouth sensations (23.1% vs. 8.4%), identifiable phantosmias (20.5% vs. 9.4%), and dysosmias (82.1% vs. 65.6%). Surprisingly, the thyroxine group scored significantly higher on the taste identification test (89.7% vs. 82.6%) and rated the low concentration of caffeine more intense than did the other participants.

The basis of these discrepancies is not clear, although different odorants and test procedures were employed and the patients may not have been well matched for the nature, duration, and severity of their hypothyroid problems. Importantly, comparing treated to non-treated patients is likely problematic, particularly in patients presenting with a range of chemosensory complaints as in the Deems et al. study (1991). In contrast, animal studies suggest that thyroid problems alter at least some aspects of chemosensation. Thus, hypothyroidism impaired development of the mouse olfactory neuroepithelium and reduced the amount of time spent sniffing food vs. water odors – a decrease that was interpreted as anosmia (Mackay-Sim & Beard, 1987). Anosmia, per se, need not be the basis for poor performance on such a task, because distortions or other alterations in perception could also lead to such decrements. Sophisticated operant conditioning tests specifically designed to assess sensitivity demonstrated no effect of hypothyroidism on the ability of rats to detect low concentrations of tastants or odorants, although odor preferences were impacted (Brosvic et al., 1992, 1996)

In summary, there is limited evidence that thyroid deficiency has some impact on both the senses of taste and smell, although frank deficits in sensitivity are probably not present and the magnitude of the thyroid-related problems does not appear to be large.

Turner's Syndrome (TS). Turner's syndrome is a form of gonadal dysgenesis resulting from a 45, X karyotype (X-chromosomal monosomy). It is characterized by a female phenotype, shield-like chest, reduced height, short and sometimes webbed neck, low-set ears, small mandible, high-arched palate, and sexual infantilism. In a pioneering study, nine TS patients displayed elevated detection and recognition thresholds to pyridine, thiophene, and nitrobenzene (Henkin, 1967). Gonadal hormone therapy reversed the chemosensory deficits. Interestingly, the mothers of the patients exhibited similar olfactory abnormalities. More recent research suggests that TS has an adverse effect on odor identification and odor memory (Ros et al., 2012).

Addison's Disease (Adrenocortical Insufficiency). According to Henkin & Bartter (1966), hyperosmia occurs in Addison's disease. In patients with a pituitary tumor (Sherman et al., 1979), there was reportedly a 100,000-fold increase (i.e., improvement) of detection threshold sensitivity to pyridine in some patients. These findings beg replication, since empirical documentation of chemical hypersensitivity is rare, and numerous tests of auditory, gustatory, and olfactory function in rats before and after adrenalectomy have found no evidence of hypersensitivity. Indeed, available data suggest that adrenalectomy may, in fact, produce not only altered odor preferences, but *decrements* in general sensory function (Conn & Mast, 1973; Kosten & Contreras, 1985; Doty et al., 1991; Brosvic et al., 1989; Weigel et al., 1989).

Kallmann Syndrome (KS). Kallmann syndrome is a congenital form of idiopathic hypo-gonadotropic hypogonadism (IHH). By definition, it is the form of IHH associated with anosmia (Kallmann et al., 1944). KS is more prevalent in males and may be associated with midline craniofacial abnormalities, tooth agenesis, deafness, and renal anomalies. Although bilateral agenesis of the olfactory bulbs and tracts is most frequent (Bajaj et al., 1993; Klingmuller et al., 1987; Yousem et al., 1996a), there is one report of a KS patient with aplasia of the left, but not the right, olfactory tract and bulb (Wustenberg et al., 2001). Interestingly, CT-based measurements of height, width, and surface area of the olfactory fossa in the ethmoid bone were smaller in KS patients compared to normosmic congenital hypogonadotropic hypogonadism subjects (Maione et al., 2013).

Large-scale studies show that IHH is consists of a heterogeneous group of disorders characterized by hypogonadism due to deficient release of gonadotropin releasing hormone (GnRH) from the hypothalamus. There is a spectrum of olfactory deficits ranging from total anosmia (KS) to normosmia (nIHH) (Lewkowitz-Shpuntoff et al., 2012). The main known mutation affects KAL1, the gene that encodes an extracellular glycoprotein, anosmin-1, which is responsible for the X-linked recessive form of the disease (KAL1). Other mutations affect fibroblast growth factor receptor-1 (FGFR1) or fibroblast growth factor-8 (FGF8) and underlie the less frequent autosomal dominant form (KAL2). There are several rarer mutations and it is estimated that in 70% of patients with the KS phenotype, no mutation can be found.

The olfactory epithelia of patients with KS look similar to those of mammals whose olfactory receptor cell axons have been severed. Thus, they exhibit morphologically immature receptor neurons lacking cilia, decreased numbers of olfactory receptor cells, and display intraepithelial neuromas (Schwob et al., 1993). Despite this, calcium imaging has identified some mature olfactory receptor cells in nasal biopsies from KS patients (Rawson et al., 1995). The total lack of an olfactory epithelium was noted in one biopsy study of a KS subject (Jafek et al., 1990), although this observation requires verification in view of sampling problems in the nasal neuroepithelium (Paik et al., 1992).

Anosmia is an important biomarker for KS, since the GnRH deficiency can be treated successfully (Sparkes et al., 1968). It is unfortunate that pediatric examinations rarely involve olfactory testing and many patients do not recognize the deficit or they are too shy to mention it and do not seek help. A delay in diagnosis can have significant psychological and physiological consequences, as described in a report of the suffering of a 22-year-old man before receiving a proper diagnosis of KS (Smith & Quinton, 2012).

Pseudohypoparathyroidism. This is characterized by parathyroid hormone resistance, a high blood parathyroid hormone level and low blood calcium. Typical features are short stature, obesity, subcutaneous ossification, and brachydactyly (Spiegel & Weinstein, 2004). It was initially believed that the olfactory dysfunction of pseudohypoparathyroidism was secondary to deficiency in the stimulatory guanine nucleotide-binding protein (Gs-alpha) of adenylcyclase, an enzyme that plays an important role in olfactory transduction (Weinstock et al., 1986). This deficiency is present in the type 1 variety, along with Albright hereditary osteodystrophy, where there is an unusual constellation of skeletal and developmental deficits. However, smell dysfunction was later found in all types of pseudohypoparathyroidism, including those not associated with Gs-alpha deficiency or Albright hereditary osteodystrophy (Doty et al., 1997).

Pregnancy. Pregnancy, which is accompanied by high circulating levels of hypophyseal and gonadal hormones, is associated with altered olfactory function and therefore included here. During the early months of pregnancy some women report general hypersensitivity to odors, although reliable psychophysical documentation is lacking (Cameron, 2007). Some investigators claim that such hypersensitivity is the basis of hyperemesis gravidarum, and estrogen excess has been suggested as a unifying factor for some types of hyperosmia (Heinrichs, 2002). Although numerous studies have reported cyclic fluctuations in olfactory sensitivity across the phases of the menstrual cycle (Doty et al., 1981), such changes are not large and at no point is there significant hypersensitivity. Moreover, the role of gonadal hormones in the production of such fluctuations is enigmatic (Doty & Cameron, 2009). In a scholarly review, Cameron (2014) evaluated the literature on olfaction in pregnancy up to 2014. It was concluded that although many women report heightened sense of smell during pregnancy, such findings have been difficult to quantify using the available psychophysical procedures.

Menopause. It is not clear whether the menopause induces olfactory dysfunction beyond that of normal aging. It is also uncertain whether hormone replacement therapy (HRT), including estrogen replacement therapy (ERT), influences olfactory function in the menopause. Most studies have found that such treatment does not change UPSIT scores or olfactory threshold values (Hughes et al., 2002; Robinson et al., 2007; Doty et al., 2015). Conversely, Sundermann, Gilbert, & Murphy (2006) noted that ERT improved performance on an odor memory task in 24 postmenopausal women with Alzheimer's disease (AD) and that subsequently improvement occurred on a detection threshold test. This improvement occurred only in carriers of the ApoE-ε4 allele, a known risk factor for AD (Sundermann et al., 2008). More recently, Doty et al. (2015) administered 3 olfactory tests and 12 cognitive tests to 432 healthy postmenopausal women with varied HRT histories. Odor Memory/Discrimination Test scores and values on the National Adult Reading Test were positively influenced by HRT, although the effects were small. Both odor identification and odor memory/discrimination test results were lower in women who scored poorly on a delayed recall test, a surrogate for mild cognitive impairment. The olfactory test scores were unrelated to plasma levels of estrone, estradiol, testosterone, progesterone, follicle stimulating hormone, cortisol, or dehyroepiandrosterone sulfate.

Metabolic Disorders

Wilson's Disease (WD) is a rare inherited disorder of copper metabolism that results in liver failure and a variety of movement disorders if untreated. One group examined 24 patients with WD, all receiving treatment, who were troubled with either liver disorder alone or neurologic complications. Based on the extended Sniffin' Sticks test there was significant impairment of olfaction in the neurologic patients but not in the liver group (Mueller et al., 2006). Long term treatment with penicillamine did not affect the olfactory findings. There is a single case report from Japan that described a patient with an olfactory paranoid syndrome that was improved by such treatment (Sagawa et al., 2003).

Liver Disease. Over 60 years ago it was reported that smokers with early acute viral hepatitis experience a strong dislike for cigarettes (Leibowitz, 1949). Subsequently it was discovered that an initial symptom of hepatitis may be aversion to cooking odors, particularly the smell of fried food (Henkin & Smith, 1971). An extensive study of 88 patients with liver disease found that 33% experienced recent food aversions, many of which presumably had olfactory involvement, although the percentage varied according to etiology (Deems et al., 1993). For example, only 12.5% of patients with primary sclerosing cholangitis experienced such aversions, in contrast to 55% suffering from acute or chronic hepatitis. Up to 75% of the latter patients also described food cravings, particularly for sweet food, including fruits and fruit juices such as grapefruit. In fact, grapefruit was actually preferred by most of these patients, compared to meat and fried food, which were generally avoided.

In addition to the marked changes in hedonic ratings to food and drink, there is considerable evidence that people with chronic or acute liver disease have decreased taste and smell function (findings for taste are reported in Chapter 6). The olfactory deficit includes reduced threshold sensitivity to several odorants (Henkin & Smith, 1971; Burch et al., 1978; Garrett-Laster et al., 1984; Bloomfeld et al., 1999; Temmel et al., 2005), as well as decreased ability to identify odors (Temmel et al., 2005; Zucco et al., 2006) and discriminate among them (Temmel et al., 2005). Temmel's group also found that the degree of liver cirrhosis correlated inversely with both a psychological measure of frontal cortex function and odor identification, but not odor discrimination or threshold. They proposed that this could reflect a central rather than a peripheral process, although some threshold deficits were also detected. As noted later in this chapter, a raised threshold may reflect a central disorder such as epilepsy, thus weakening one aspect of their argument.

In the related condition, hepatic encephalopathy, Zucco and co-workers studied 12 individuals with minimal hepatic encephalopathy and noted impaired olfactory identification and recognition based on their in-house procedure that implemented 40 olfactory stimuli (Zucco et al., 2006).

Kidney Disease. In common with liver disorders, the smell of food is rated less pleasant by patients with kidney disease, than by healthy controls (Lee et al., 2015). Those receiving maintenance hemodialysis often complain about the taste and smell of food and have poor appetite (Schiffman et al., 1978; Vreman et al., 1980). It is now recognized that people with severe kidney disease exhibit deficits on several olfactory tests, namely those of hedonic evaluation (Schiffman et al., 1978), detection threshold sensitivity (Korytowska & Szmeja, 1993; Griep et al., 1997; Landis et al., 2011), identification (Conrad et al., 1987; Corwin, 1989; Frasnelli et al., 2002; Grapsa et al., 2010), and discrimination (Schiffman et al., 1978; Frasnelli et al., 2002). Such deficits may relate to the degree of renal impairment and accumulation of uremic toxins (Griep et al., 1997). Interestingly, one study found that odor identification was normal in children with chronic kidney disease, although a positive relationship with body mass index was found (r = 0.427, p = 0.006) (Correa et al., 2015).

The few studies that have addressed the effect of hemodialysis on olfactory function are conflicting. With regard to odor detection, Korytowska & Szmeja (1993) reported improvement in coffee and lemon odor identification thresholds after hemodialysis, although the method used is one known to confound air pressure with the sensitivity measure (Wenzel, 1948). Landis et al. (2011) found modest improvements in detection thresholds to acetic acid, but not n-butanol. Since acetic acid is a known trigeminal stimulant, their findings need to be interpreted with caution. Griep et al. (1997) discovered no effect of hemodialysis on amyl acetate detection thresholds, as measured in an ascending forced-choice method of limits procedure. Modest amelioration of odor identification was noted by Landis et al. (2011) after hemodialysis, whereas another group (Conrad et al., 1987; Corwin, 1989), in two separate studies, found no such improvement in odor recognition. They employed a yes/no signal detection paradigm whose sensitivity measure is less likely to be confounded by memory or attentional issues. It is well known that fatigue, irritability, and other psychological factors may develop within the first few hours of dialysis, highlighting the need for systematic testing at different time points after commencement of dialysis.

Epilepsy

Olfactory Hallucinations (OHs) can occur at the onset of an epileptic seizure, i.e., as an aura, or during the attack itself. Such hallucinations are relatively uncommon, with a prevalence rate of ~10 percent in cases where the seizure arises from the temporal lobe (Velakoulis, 2006). In the syndrome of Transient Epileptic Amnesia, subjects typically wake in the morning with impaired recent memory for up to one hour. They also experience olfactory hallucinations usually unpleasant in nature, linked to automatisms and brief loss of awareness. Sleep EEG recordings typically show epileptic discharges arising from either temporal lobe (Zeman et al., 1998). OHs are reported occasionally in patients with Parkinson's disease (see Chapter 7).

In rare instances, strong odors can evoke epileptic attacks (olfactory reflex epilepsy). Such odors may induce spike and wave activity in those with absences or tonic-clinic seizures (Stevens, 1962; Takahashi, 1975). Conversely, odor stimulation may have an inhibitory effect on seizure activity in the cat (Ebert & Loscher, 2000) and aromatherapy is claimed to help intractable forms of epilepsy (Betts, 2003). Conversely, Indian folk-lore holds that the smell from the sole of a shoe can terminate an epileptic attack (Jaseja, 2008)!

One of the earliest descriptions of an OH during an epileptic attack, which would now be termed a complex partial seizure (CPS), was documented by Jackson and Beevor (1890). These authors wrote (p. 346):

> In the paroxysm the first thing was tremor of the hands and arms; she saw a little black woman who was always very actively engaged in cooking; the spectre did not speak. The patient had a very horrible smell (so-called subjective sensation of smell) which she could not describe. She had a feeling as if she was shut up in a box with a limited quantity of air . . . she would stand with her eyes fixed . . . and then say "what a horrible smell!" . . . After leaving her kitchen work she had paroxysms with the smell sensation but no spectre.

At autopsy Jackson found a large anterior temporal lobe tumor. Clearly, this growth was irritating the antero-medial temporal lobe and causing the now well-recognized variety of seizure – uncinate epilepsy. In most instances, OHs linked to this condition are unpleasant and difficult to remember or describe in detail. It is not clear why this happens. As explained below, most such hallucinations probably originate in the amygdala rather than hippocampus (Chen et al., 2014) and that the cause of memory impairment most likely results from concurrent disturbance in the nearby hippocampus (Halgren, 1981). Importantly, it is now recognized that the orbitofrontal cortex, an olfactory association area, can also be responsible for seizures that include olfactory illusions, hallucinations, and other autonomic signs or gestural automatisms (Chabolla, 2002).

Probably the best-known olfactory disorder for clinicians is the uncinate aura (West & Doty, 1995). This is an under-reported epileptic phenomenon, as patients commonly fail to mention it unless specifically asked, and the nature of the smell is nearly always unpleasant, in keeping with the concept that it is a positive phenomenon resulting from abnormal neuronal discharge. In one large series of 1,423 patients with intractable seizures emanating from the temporal lobe, there were 14 with olfactory auras lasting 5–30 seconds (Acharya, Acharya, & Luders, 1998). Five patients had an isolated olfactory aura that did not progress to complex partial seizures (CPS) or generalized attack. The electroencephalogram (EEG) focus was localized to the medial temporal zone in all participants. The focus was lateralized to the left in nine and to the right in four subjects; a non-significant difference. Nine patients described the odors as familiar, reporting qualitative sensations of burning, sulfur, alcohol, gas, barbecue, peanut butter, toothpaste, or flowers; five could not identify the smell. Seven thought the odor unpleasant, five were neutral, and two found the smell pleasant and flowerlike. Most OHs were associated with other hallucinations: gustatory, epigastric, visual, or psychic (fear; Deja vu). Ten had a medial temporal lobe tumor, of which six involved the amygdala rather than the uncus, making the term "uncinate attack" a misnomer.

Bilateral amygdala damage results in severe impairment in odor–name matching and odor–odor recognition memory in the absence of impaired auditory verbal learning (Buchanan et al., 2003), confirming that the amygdala plays an important role in odor memory. Irritating processes in this zone would therefore cause OHs and this notion is borne out by many reports of such hallucinations from patients with tumors in this area. Conversely, stereotactic lesions of the amygdala alleviate OHs and the accompanying psychiatric disorder (Chitanondh, 1966). Despite this, none of 1,132 subjects stimulated by Penfield & Perot (1963), and only one of 75 patients with deep brain electrodes implanted in the temporal or frontal lobes, reported olfactory sensations and that instance followed left amygdala stimulation (Fish et al., 1993). In general, OHs have good localizing value (to the amygdala), but they are not specific to any particular brain pathology, having been described in medial temporal sclerosis, malignant glioma, and metastatic deposits (Chen et al., 2003). Glioma is probably the most common cause (see Figure 5.7).

Until recently the influence of temporal lobe epilepsy (TLE) on olfactory function was not clear, largely reflecting small sample sizes, unorthodox testing methods, absence of age- and sex-matched controls, etc. In the case of threshold measures, some studies have noted enhanced threshold sensitivity, whereas others have found no such effects (for review, see Doty et al., 2017). In the largest and most definitive study on this topic, staircase detection thresholds for phenylethyl alcohol were measured on each side of the nose of 71 TLE patients (35 with left foci and 36 with right foci) and 71 age- and gender-matched normal controls (Doty et al., 2017). Independent of the foci side and which nostril was tested, the mean thresholds of the epilepsy patients were higher than those of the controls. In patients who underwent temporal lobe resection, the operation elevated further the olfactory thresholds mainly on the operated side; i.e., left-side operations resulted in elevated thresholds on the left side of the nose and vice versa.

Variable findings about the influence of TLE on suprathreshold olfactory function are also evident in the literature. For example, one group reported that patients with left-side foci performed less well than those with right-side foci on a bilateral delayed multi-odor matching task (Hudry et al., 2003). In contrast, others found that patients with right, but not left, foci are more impaired on bilateral odor matching or discrimination tests (Abraham & Mathai, 1983; Rausch, Serafetinides, & Crandall, 1977), as well as an odor memory test for nameable or non-nameable, common odorants (e.g., coconut, coffee, nail varnish, and garlic) (Carroll, Richardson, & Thompson, 1993). Some investigators report no differences between left- and right-sided foci on tests of odor memory, identification, or discrimination (Eskenazi et al., 1983, 1986; Jones-Gotman & Zatorre, 1988; Zatorre & Jones-Gotman, 1991; Doty et al., 2016). In the large study by Doty and colleagues (2017), bilateral epilepsy-related decrements in UPSIT scores were observed that were unrelated to the side of the epileptic focus. Men showed a larger odor identification deficit than did women. Reflecting olfactory thresholds, this study found that UPSIT and odor discrimination/memory scores were negatively influenced by temporal lobectomy on the side of the nose ipsilateral to the operation.

Case Report 5.6: **Complex Partial Seizures with Olfactory Aura.** A 59-year-old unemployed man went out drinking heavily one Saturday evening. The next morning, while lying in bed, he experienced a strange smell, like burnt toast. When he looked at the clock, it appeared brighter than normal, he felt slightly dreamy, and his right arm began to jerk for a few minutes. There was no loss of consciousness or urinary incontinence. On direct questioning, he recalled there were several isolated episodes of olfactory aura over the preceding six months, but no jerking or loss of consciousness. There were other periods suggestive of Deja vu. He was a nonsmoker but known to abuse alcohol. Physical examination was normal. The UPSIT score was 27/40 (in microsmic range); an MRI brain scan (which included hippocampal views) was unremarkable but the EEG showed intermittent sharp waves and occasional spikes from the left temporal electrodes. *Comment:* This history is typical of a CPS with olfactory aura and an epileptic focus in the left temporal zone. It is possible that the main episode was provoked by alcohol withdrawal. The unpleasant smell, which is a positive phenomenon (like the visual enhancement here also), is typical of uncinate attacks – which should be renamed

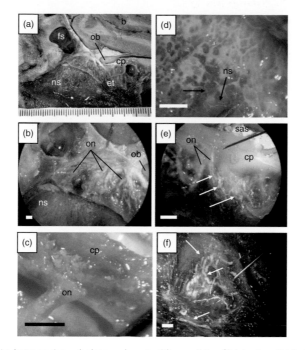

Figure 1.5 Lymphatic drainage through the nasal cavity. Silicone (Microfil) injection distribution patterns in the head of a human (a-f). All images are presented in sagittal plane with gradual magnification of the olfactory area adjacent to the cribriform plate. Reference scales are provided either as a ruler in the image (mm) or as a longitudinal bar (1 mm). Microfil introduced into the subarachnoid space was observed around the olfactory bulb (a), in the perineurial spaces of the olfactory nerves (b, c), and in the lymphatics of the nasal septum (d), ethmoid labyrinth (e), and superior turbinate (f). Some lymphatic vessels ruptured and Microfil was noted in the interstitium of the submucosa of the nasal septum (d). In (e), Microfil is observed in the subarachnoid space and the perineurial space of olfactory nerves. The perineurial Microfil is continuous with that in lymphatic vessels (arrows). Intact lymphatic vessels containing Microfil are outlined with arrows (d-f). Key to abbreviations: b – brain; fs – frontal sinus; cp – cribriform plate; et – ethmoid turbinates; ob – olfactory bulbs; on – olfactory nerves; ns – nasal septum; sas – subarachnoid space. Reproduced with permission from Johnston, Zakharov, et al. (2005).

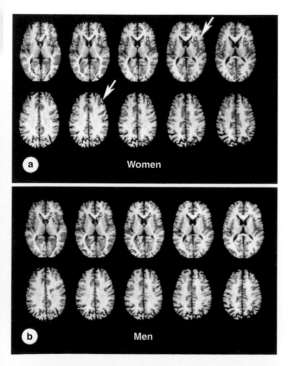

Figure 3.33 fMRI group-averaged activation maps for women and men. The right side of the brain is on the right. Women showed up to eight times more activated voxels than men for specific brain regions, notably in the frontal and perisylvian regions. Note the slightly greater activation on the right compared to the left side of the brain. Odorants were eugenol and phenylethyl alcohol, alternating with hydrogen sulfide. From Yousem et al. (2001).

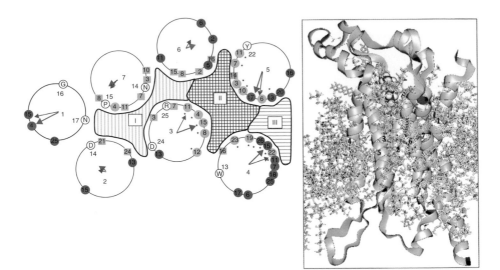

Figure 1.9 Left: Presumed odorant-binding pockets of an odor receptor protein. Overhead view of the seven transmembrane-spanning barrels of an odor receptor protein modeled against the rhodopsin G-protein coupled receptor (GPCR). Residues that are conserved among all GPCRs are shown in open circles. Colored squares and circles represent positions of conserved and variable residues, respectively, in OR proteins. Residues that align with ligand contact residues in other GPCRs are colored green and residues that do not align with such residues are colored red. The residues in each helix are numbered separately, according to the predicted transmembrane boundaries. Hypervariable residues (putative odorant-binding residues) are indicated by asterisks. Area II denotes a hypervariable pocket that corresponds to the ligand-binding pocket in other GPCRs. Reproduced from Pilpel & Lancet (1999). Right: Predicted structure for mouse olfactory receptor (OR) S25. Model depicts the putative binding pocket for the hexanol ligand (purple) to the receptor protein (side view). Each transmembrane and inter-transmembrane loop is labeled. The membrane is represented in yellow. This computed model of the S25 odorant receptor protein atoms successfully predicts the relative affinities to a panel of odorants, including hexanol, which is predicted to interact with residues in transmembranes 3, 5, and 6. Reproduced with permission from Floriano et al. (2000).

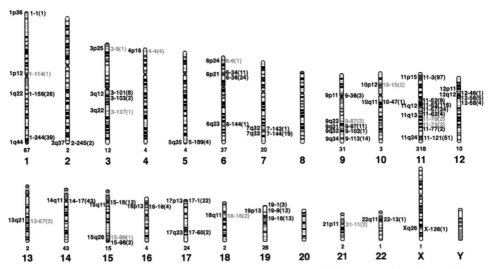

Figure 1.10 Chromosome locations of human OR genes. There were 630 OR genes that localized to 51 different chromosomal loci distributed over 21 human chromosomes. OR loci containing one or more intact OR genes are indicated in red; loci containing only pseudogenes are indicated in green. The cytogenetic position of each locus is shown on the left, and its distance in megabases from the tip of the small arm of the chromosome is shown on the right (chromosome-Mb). The number of OR genes at each locus is indicated in parentheses, and the number of OR genes on each chromosome is indicated below. Most human homologs of rodent ORs for n-aliphatic odorants are found at a single locus, chromosome 11p15. Reproduced with permission from Malnic et al. (2004). Since this map was published OR genes have been found on chromosome 8.

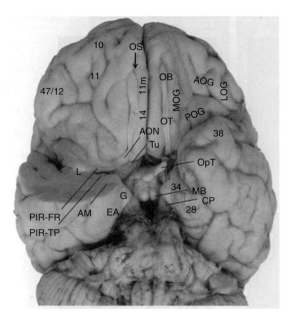

Figure 1.11 Base of human brain showing the ventral forebrain and medial temporal lobes. The blue oval area represents the monkey olfactory region, whereas the pink oval represents the probable site of the human olfactory region as identified by functional imaging studies. Modified from: Gottfried J.A., Small D.M., & Zald D.H. (2006), Chapter 6, Plate 9. Key: numbers refer to the approximate position of Brodmann areas as follows: 10 – fronto-polar area; 11/11 m – orbitofrontal/gyrus rectus region; 28 – posterior entorhinal cortex; 34 – anterior entorhinal cortex; 38 – temporal pole; 47/12 – ventrolateral frontal area. Other abbreviations: AM – amygdala; AOG/POG/LOG/MOG – anterior, posterior, lateral, medial orbital gyri; AON – anterior olfactory nucleus; CP – cerebral peduncle; EA – entorhinal area; G – gyrus ambiens; L – limen insulae; MB – mamillary body; PIR-FR – frontal piriform cortex; PIR-TR – temporal piriform cortex; OpT – optic tract; OS – olfactory sulcus; OT – olfactory tract; Tu – olfactory tubercle.

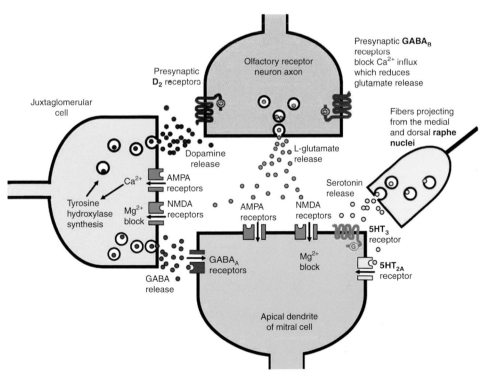

Figure 1.13 Glomerular synapses showing the variety of receptors. The axons from the olfactory receptor neurons (pink) form the olfactory nerve, which synapses on the primary apical dendrites of the mitral cells (green). L-glutamate is the primary excitatory transmitter at this synapse, which binds to AMPA and NMDA receptors on the postsynaptic membrane. Juxtaglomerular cells (blue) are inhibitory GABAergic/dopaminergic interneurons that mediate inhibition between glomeruli. Centrifugal fibers (yellow) project from the raphe nuclei to the glomeruli modulating the mitral cell activity via postsynaptic 5HT (serotonergic) receptors. Reproduced with permission from O'Connor & Jacob (2008).

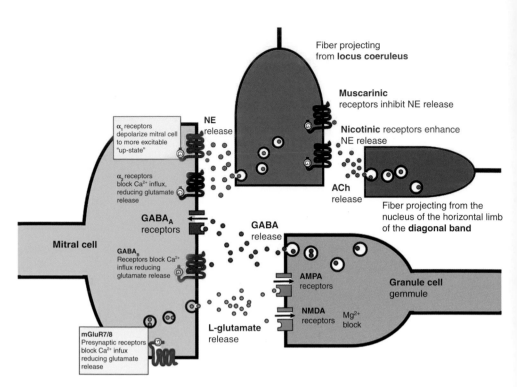

Figure 1.14 Synapses in the external plexiform layer of the olfactory bulb showing the variety of receptors and neurotransmitters. Granule cells (gray) mediate feedback and lateral inhibition between mitral cells (green) with which they form reciprocal dendro-dendritic synapses. Adrenergic and cholinergic efferent fibers project from the diagonal band (pink) and the locus coeruleus (orange), respectively. Reproduced with permission from O'Connor & Jacob (2008).

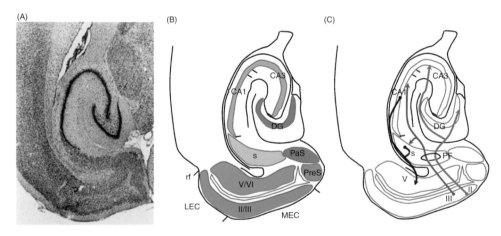

Figure 1.17 (A) Horizontal cresyl-stained section through the hippocampal formation. (B) Cytoarchitectonically defined subfields of the hippocampal formation using the same section as in (A). The rhinal fissure (rf; equivalent to the collateral sulcus in humans) delineates the entorhinal cortex from the peri-rhinal cortex. The hippocampal formation comprises the dentate gyrus (DG), the hippocampal fields CA1 and CA3, the subiculum (S), the Pre- (PreS) and Para (PaS) subiculum, and the lateral (LEC) and medial (MEC) portion of the entorhinal cortex. Within the entorhinal cortex, the deep layers V/VI are separated from the superficial ones II/III by the lamina dissecans. (C) Overall connections between the entorhinal cortex and the hippocampus use the same section as before. Cells in layer II of the EC project to both the DG and CA3 (green arrow). Cells in layer III project to the subiculum and the CA1 (orange arrows). These two groups of fibers form the perforant path. Cells in CA1 and subiculum back project to the deep layer V of the entorhinal cortex (purple arrows). Modified with permission from Coutureau & Di Scala (2009).

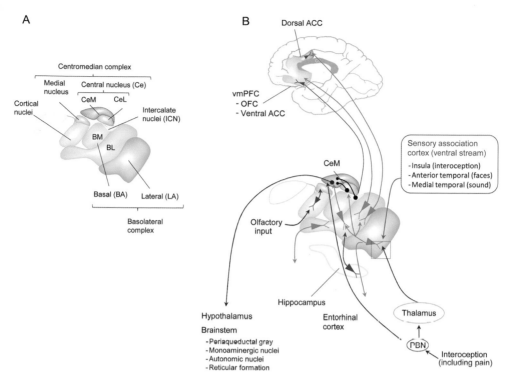

Figure 1.19 Anatomical organization and main connectivity of the amygdala. Left figure (A) shows the nuclei of the amygdala which are divided into: (1) a basolateral complex, including the lateral (LA) and basal (BA) nuclei; (2) the superficial cortex-like laminated region; and (3) the centromedial nuclear group, that includes the central (Ce) and medial nuclei plus the intercalate cell mass (IC). The BA consists of the basolateral (BL) and basomedial (BM) nuclei; the Ce comprises lateral (CeL) and medial (CeM) subdivisions. The basolateral complex and cortical nuclei resemble the cerebral cortex and contain primarily pyramidal-like projection neurons and receive inputs from unimodal cortical association areas and the thalamus; the centromedial nuclear extended amygdala resembles the striatum or globus pallidus and contains GABAergic neurons. Right figure (B). Inputs from cortical sensory areas and thalamus terminate primarily in the LA; the LA projects to the BA; the BA is interconnected with the ventromedial prefrontal cortex (vmPFC) including the orbitofrontal cortex (OFC) and ventral anterior cingulate cortex (ACC) as well as the dorsal ACC, hippocampal formation, and striatum (not shown) and projects to the CeM, which provides the main output of the amygdala to the hypothalamus and brainstem, including the parabrachial nucleus. The CeM also receives interoceptive inputs directly from the parabrachial nucleus (PBN). Reproduced and modified with permission from Benarroch (2015).

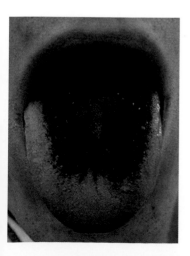

Figure 2.3 Black hairy tongue. This is due to hypertrophy of the centrally located filiform papillae which become yellow or black from contact with food or tobacco. Note the filiform papillae are not involved with taste; they help move and abrade food. From Wikipedia.

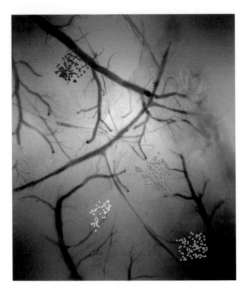

Figure 2.6 "Hot spots" for bitter (red), salty (orange), umami (yellow), and sweet (green) taste in the mouse gustatory cortex. Fluorescent dyes were used to visualize intracellular waves of calcium in active neurons in the gustatory cortex of anesthetized mice. Note that no hot spot for sour was detected. Adapted with permission from Chen et al. (2011).

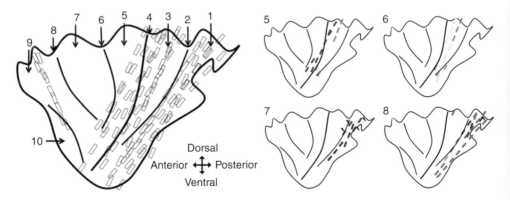

Figure 2.8 Localizations of those electrode contacts that evoked clinical responses with electrocortical stimulation. Left: Anatomical landmarks of the insula are indicated by numbers: 1 posterior long gyrus of the insula, 2 postcentral insular sulcus, 3 anterior long gyrus of the insula, 4 central insular sulcus, 5 Posterior short gyrus of the insula, 6 precentral insular sulcus, 7 middle short gyrus of the insula, 8 short insular sulcus, 9 anterior short gyrus of the insula, 10 accessory gyrus of the insula. Right: responses were grouped into gustatory (figure 5, blue): viscerosensory (figure 6, yellow), warmth or pain (figure 7, red) and general somatosensory (figure 8, green). Composite color bars indicate qualitatively inconsistent or ambiguous symptoms after stimulation. Reproduced with permission from Figures 4–8 in Stephani et al. (2011).

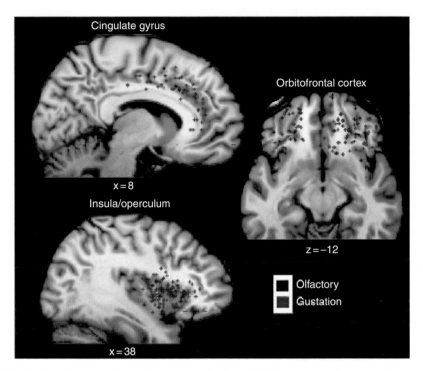

Figure 2.10 PET and fMRI plots from multiple sources to show that chemosensory stimuli activate a variety of regions within the insula, anterior cingulate, and orbitofrontal cortex, and that most respond to both gustatory and olfactory stimulation. Taste stimuli tend to activate the caudal and lateral orbitofrontal cortex; whereas olfactory stimuli do not (especially in the right hemisphere). In contrast, olfactory stimuli activate the most ventral insular region, which is continuous with the primary olfactory cortex; whereas gustatory stimuli do not. Reproduced with permission from Small & Prescott (2005).

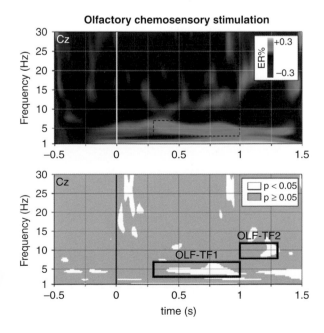

Figure 3.17 Time-frequency representation of the non-phase-locked EEG responses to olfactory chemosensory stimulation. Non-phase-locked EEG responses identified by performing across-trial averaging in the time-frequency domain, a procedure that enhances time-locked EEG responses regardless of whether they are phase-locked to stimulus onset. Upper panel: Group-level average time-frequency maps of oscillation amplitude (group-level average, electrode Cz vs. A1/A2), expressed as percentage increase or decrease relative to baseline (−0.4 to −0.1 sec) Note that olfactory stimulation elicits a long-lasting non-phase-locked increase of signal amplitude around 5 Hz (OLF-TF1; olfactory time frequency domain), possibly followed by event-related desynchronization in the alpha-band (OLF-TF2). Lower panel: Regions of the time-frequency matrix where signal amplitude deviated significantly from baseline (one-sample t-test). Adapted, with permission, from Figure 5 in Huart et al. (2012).

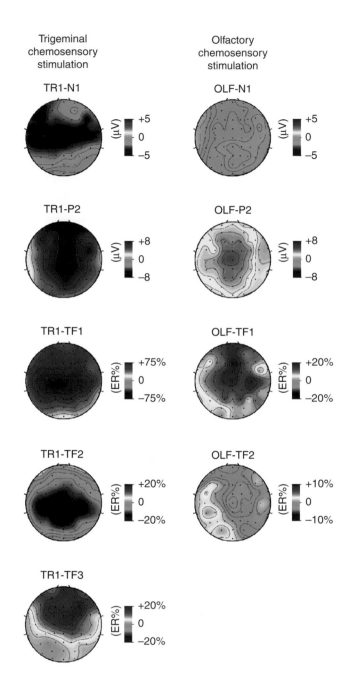

Figure 3.18 Scalp distribution of the EEG responses elicited by trigeminal and olfactory chemosensory stimulation. The scalp distribution of the EEG responses identified using across-trial averaging in the time domain (TRI-N1, TRI-P2, OLF-N1, OLF-P2) are expressed in microvolts, whereas the scalp distribution of the EEG responses identified using across-trial averaging in the time-frequency domain (TRI-TF1, TRI-TF2, TRI-TF3, OLF-TF1, OLF-TF2) are expressed as a percentage increase or decrease relative to baseline. Adapted, with permission, from Figure 2 in Huart et al. (2012).

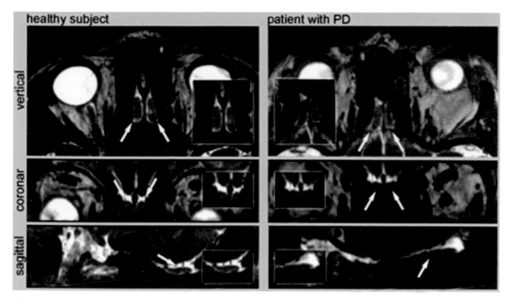

Figure 3.28 MRI of the olfactory bulbs (OBs; white arrows) in a healthy control subject (left) and a Parkinson's disease patient (right). Voxel size: 0.064 mm³. Imaging planes are from top downwards: axial; coronal, and sagittal. Manually traced OBs after segmentation are highlighted in red. Although comparable slices are selected, the OB volumes of the two subjects do not show major visible differences. Reproduced with permission from Brodoehl et al. (2012).

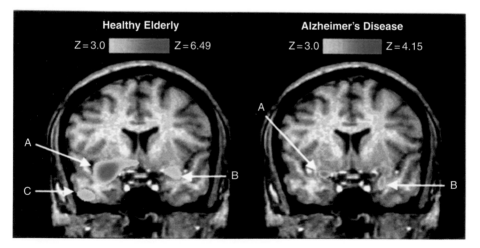

Figure 3.31 PET imaging in Alzheimer's disease. Left: Controls. A: Right frontotemporal junction (piriform area); B: Left piriform area; C: Right anterior ventral temporal lobe (Brodmann area 20). Number of controls: 7; mean UPSIT = 32.4; mean threshold to phenylethyl alcohol: $10^{-5.5}$. Right: Alzheimer's Disease. A: 7 mm anterior to frontotemporal junction; B: left amygdala-uncus. Number of patients: 6. Mean UPSIT = 18.7 (microsmic); mean threshold to phenyl ethyl alcohol: minus 5.1 (normal). From Kareken et al. (2001).

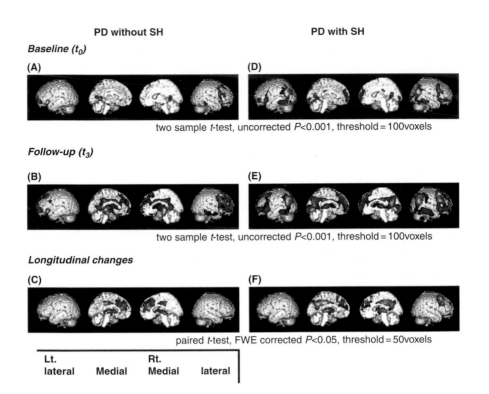

PD without SH   **PD with SH**

Baseline (t₀)

(A)   (D)

two sample *t*-test, uncorrected *P*<0.001, threshold = 100voxels

Follow-up (t₃)

(B)   (E)

two sample *t*-test, uncorrected *P*<0.001, threshold = 100voxels

Longitudinal changes

(C)   (F)

paired *t*-test, FWE corrected *P*<0.05, threshold = 50voxels

| Lt. lateral | Medial | Rt. Medial | lateral |

Figure 3.32 Fluorodeoxyglucose-PET data that show the distribution of cortical hypometabolism in the Parkinson's disease (PD) subgroups compared with normal controls. (A) At baseline (t_0), PD patients without severe hyposmia (SH) showed a mild metabolic reduction in the frontal regions and medial occipital cortex. (B) At follow-up (t_3), PD patients without severe hyposmia showed a metabolic reduction in the midbrain and broader frontal regions, medial prefrontal, cingulate, and medial occipital cortices. (C) In PD patients without severe hyposmia, longitudinal metabolic changes (t_0-t_3) were identified in the medial prefrontal and anterior cingulate cortices. (D) At t_0, patients with PD and severe hyposmia showed a metabolic reduction in the bilateral dorsolateral prefrontal, medial prefrontal, and medial occipital cortices and bilateral parieto-occipito-temporal area. (E) At t_3, the metabolic reduction became more prominent, with additional metabolic reduction in the posterior cingulate and precuneus. (F) In PD patients with severe hyposmia, the longitudinal metabolic changes (t_0-t_3) were distributed in the right frontal, medial prefrontal, anterior cingulate, posterior cingulate cortices and precuneus. From Baba et al., 2012.

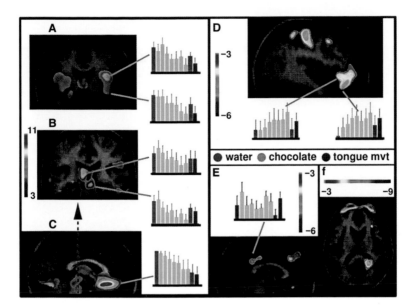

Figure 4.22 Cortical regions demonstrating significant rCBF correlations with pleasantness/unpleasantness ratings following ingestion of chocolate. Correlations are shown as *t* statistic images superimposed on corresponding averaged MRI scans. The *t* statistic ranges for each set of images are coded by color bars, one in each box. Bar graphs represent normalized CBF in an 8 mm radius surrounding the peak. The *y* axis corresponds to normalized activity and the bars along the *x*-axis represent scans. The three colors represent scan type (purple = water only trials, light blue = chocolate trials, dark blue = tongue movement trials). Each bar graph corresponds to activations indicated by a turquoise line. A. Coronal section taken at *y* = 1 showing the decrease in rCBF in the primary gustatory area (bilaterally in the anterior insula/frontal operculum and in the right ventral insula). B. Coronal section taken at *y* = −26 showing decreases in rCBF in the left thalamus and medial midbrain (possibly corresponding to the ventral tegmental area). C. Sagittal section taken at *x* = −1 showing decreases in rCBF in the subcallosal region, thalamus, and midbrain. D. Sagittal section taken at *x* = 42 showing the increase in rCBF in the right caudolateral orbitofrontal cortex. Activation is also evident in the motor and premotor areas. E. Sagittal section taken at *x* = 8 showing an increase in rCBF in the posterior cingulate gyrus (peak at 8, −30, 45) in subtraction analysis Choc 1 − water-post. This was the only region where CBF was consistently greater in affective scans regardless of valence, compared with the neutral chocolate scan (Choc 4) and the two water baseline scans (water-pre and water-post). F. Horizontal section at *z* = 12 showing an increase in rCBF in the retrosplenial cortex (area 30) that correlated with affective rating (ii) but not the affective rating (i) when scan order was covaried out of the regression. Reproduced with permission from Small et al. (2001).

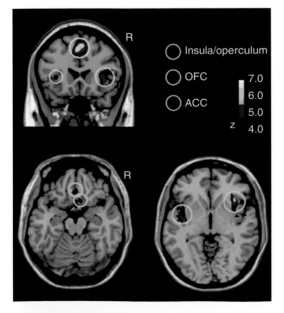

Figure 4.23 fMRI image of brain regions activated by mineral (Evian) water (i.e., water − control water comparison). Statistically significant activations were observed in the insular/opercular cortex, the orbitofrontal cortex (OFC), and the anterior cingulate cortex (ACC). Values > 4.54 on the vertical scale are significant at p < 0.05. From de Araujo et al. (2003), with permission.

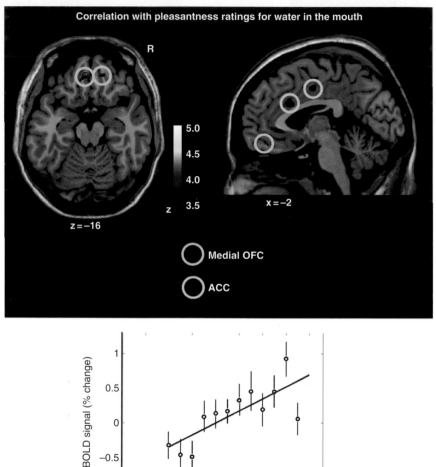

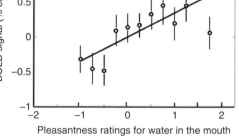

Figure 4.24 fMRI image of brain regions activated by mineral (Evian) water. Top left: regions of the medial caudal orbitofrontal cortex where activation was correlated with perceived pleasantness ratings of water. Bottom: a scatter plot and regression line showing the signal values in the medial orbitofrontal cortex (points represent mean ± SEM values across subjects). From de Araujo et al. (2003), with permission.

Location of brain injury	Normal olfactory function (n = 26)	Olfactory impairment (n = 14)	p value
Frontal	11 (42.3%)	11 (78.6%)	0.046
Parietal	11 (42.3%)	5 (35.7%)	0.746
Temporal	5 (19.2%)	6 (42.9%)	0.147
Occipital	2 (7.7%)	2 (14.3%)	0.602
Multifocal	6 (23.1%)	6 (42.9%)	0.281
Frontal OR temporal	13 (50.0%)	12 (85.7%)	0.040
Frontal AND temporal	3 (11.5%)	5 (35.7%)	0.102

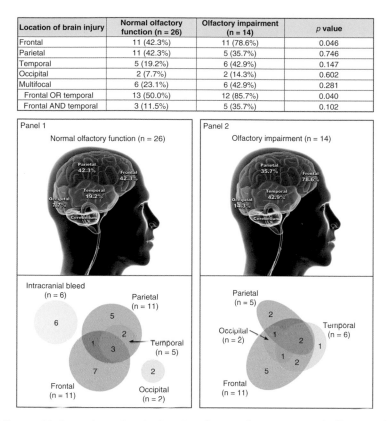

Figure 5.4 Troops with abnormal neuroimaging: Location of injury and its association with olfactory performance and multifocality (n = 40). Reproduced with permission from Xydakis et al. (2015).

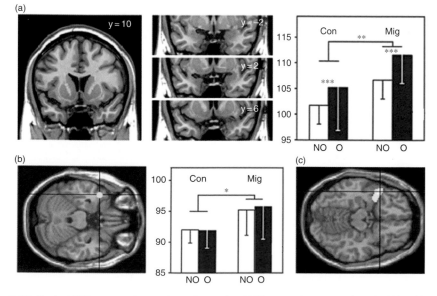

Figure 5.10 Cerebral PET scan superimposed on a T1 weighted MRI scan to show regional cerebral blood flow (rCBF) differences found in the odor–no odor (O–NO) contrast between controls (Con) and migraineurs (Mig) in (A) the left piriform cortex (red) and (B) the left anterior superior temporal gyrus (yellow). (C) High rCBF observed in the baseline condition with the Mig–Con contrast. Statistical Parametric Mappings are superimposed on axial sections of a T1-weighted MRI scan. Vertical axis on graphs represents cerebral blood flow (ml/minute). Reproduced with permission from Demarquay et al. (2008).

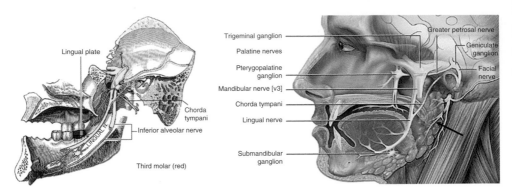

Figure 6.2 Left: The position of the lingual nerve in relation to the third-molar tooth, shown in red. The lingual nerve carries taste afferents from the anterior two-thirds of the tongue in the chorda tympani. Right: The course of the lingual nerve and chorda tympani. It passes deep to the temporo-mandibular joint and attaches to the lingual nerve at an oblique angle. The greater petrosal nerve, which supplies taste buds in the soft palate, is labeled. The glossopharyngeal nerve innervates the posterior foliate and circumvallate papillae in the posterior two-thirds of the tongue (black arrow). In the tonsillar bed it may be damaged during tonsillectomy. Reproduced with permission from the Yale Center for Advanced Instructional Media, figure 6.16b. The relations of the chorda tympani to the ear drum are shown in Figure 6.1.

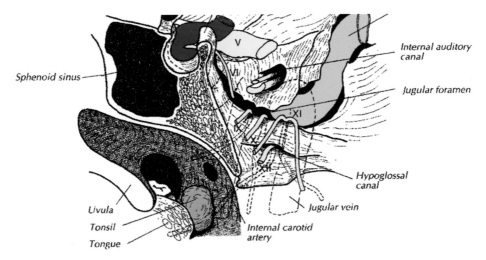

Figure 6.3 The jugular foramen seen from inside the skull in sagittal section with the midbrain, pons, medulla, and cerebellum removed. Anterior is on the left; posterior on the right. Note CN IX, X, and XI colored yellow having emerged from the medulla disappearing through the jugular foramen close to the jugular vein and lateral (transverse) sinus that drains into the sigmoid sinus (blue). Their subsequent course is shown as dotted lines. Note CN IX as it approaches the tongue, soft palate, and tonsil just above the Eustachian tube (black). Reproduced and modified with permission from Neurological Differential Diagnosis. Author, John Patten, Second edition. Figure 6.14. Springer-Verlag 1995. Patten J Neurological Differential Diagnosis.

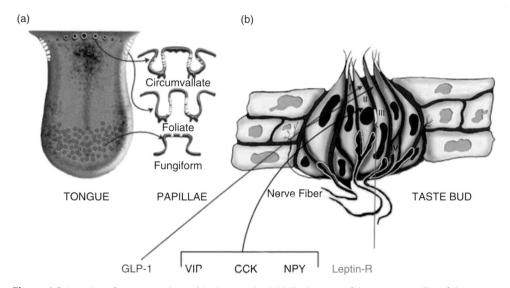

(a)

Circumvallate

Foliate

Fungiform

TONGUE PAPILLAE Nerve Fiber TASTE BUD

(b)

GLP-1 VIP CCK NPY Leptin-R

Figure 6.5 Location of neuropeptides within the taste bud. (a) The location of the various papillae of the tongue are shown. (b) The type of taste cell within the taste buds of the tongue and the corresponding hormones. The arrows demarcate the location of each hormone within taste cell types 2, 2, 3, and 4. Abbreviations. GLP-1, glucagon-like peptide 1; VIP, vasoactive intestinal peptide; CCK, cholecystokinin; NPY, neuropeptide Y; leptin-R, leptin receptor. Modified with permission from Martin, Maudsley et al. (2009).

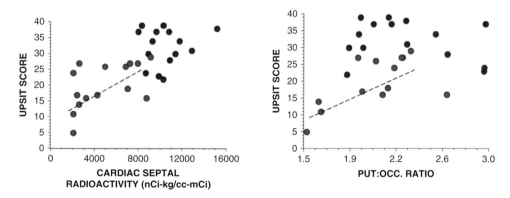

CARDIAC SEPTAL
RADIOACTIVITY (nCi-kg/cc-mCi)

PUT:OCC. RATIO

Figure 7.12 University of Pennsylvania Smell Identification Test (UPSIT) results in patients with Parkinson disease (red) or Multiple System Atrophy (blue). Left graph: this shows individual UPSIT scores, expressed as a function of septal myocardial fluorodopamine derived radioactivity. Right graph. This shows individual UPSIT scores, expressed as a function of the putamen: occipital cortex ratio of fluorodopa-derived radioactivity. Dashed lines indicate line of best fit among PD patients. Reproduced with permission from Goldstein, Holmes et al. (2008).

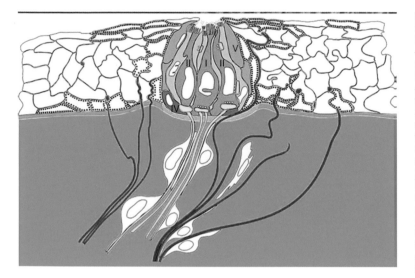

Figure 7.17 Brain-Derived Neurotrophic Factor (BDNF) -expressing taste cells (brown) are innervated by gustatory chorda tympani axons (yellow). Many of the cells surrounding the taste bud are innervated by somatosensory lingual nerve axons (light blue) and express neurotrophin-3 (NT3; light blue) and p75 Nerve Growth Factor Receptor (NGFR; dots). Types of taste bud cells (I-V) according to Reutter and Witt. Adapted with permission from Oakley & Witt (2004).

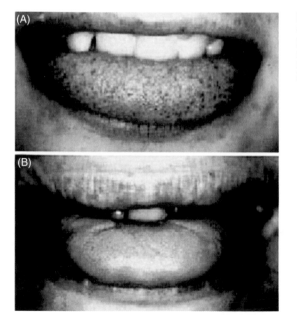

Figure 7.18 Images of normal (A) and familial dysautonomic (B) tongues. Red fungiform papillae are obvious on the normal tongue and missing on the familial dysautonomic tongue. Images courtesy of Professor Felicia Axelrod MD, New York University.

amygdala attacks, as explained above. Many patients presenting with a history similar to the above are found to have a temporal lobe glioma or metastasis.

Migraine

Occasionally, sufferers of migraine report that an attack is provoked by exposure to unpleasant odors such as gasoline, acetone, or strong perfume (Kelman, 2004b). Apart from precipitating migraine, smells may aggravate the headache, a finding that led to the suggestion that odors might be used to distinguish tension from migraine headache in adults (Spierings et al., 2001) and children (Corletto et al., 2008).

Before or during migraine attacks, there may be temporary heightened and unpleasant smell perception (osmophobia) in a manner comparable to photophobia and phonophobia (Kelman, 2004a; Kelman, 2004b). Osmophobia is common, affecting 25–50% subjects according to some (Kelman, 2004a; Saisu et al., 2011). Another group found osmophobia in 172/200 (86%) migraineurs but only 12/200 (6%) of those with tension headache, a point that might allow distinction of the two varieties of headache (Silva-Neto et al., 2014). Migraine auras have been associated with olfactory hallucinations and these are nearly always disagreeable, e.g., decaying animals, burning cookies, cigars, peanut butter, and cigarette smoke (Fuller & Guiloff, 1987). Olfactory hallucinations (phantosmias) are rare, affecting, fewer than 1% of migraineurs (Kelman, 2004b; Coleman et al., 2011).

During headache-free periods, several studies that employed quantitative olfactory tests found no evidence of altered olfactory function (Marmura et al., 2014; Saisu et al., 2011). In contrast, one study that lacked a control group reported that 18% were *hyposensitive* to pyridine (Hirsch, 1992), a stimulus known to have trigeminal nerve reactivity, whereas another group found that thresholds for vanillin were lower (i.e., better) in migraine sufferers than in controls (Saisu et al., 2011). The latter study employed a single series ascending threshold procedure that likely confounds the sensitivity measure with the response criterion (see Chapter 3). More recently, Marmura et al. (2014) quantified olfactory identification ability in 50 migraine sufferers over three phases: baseline (no headache), during migraine episodes, and after a treated attack. Their test scores were compared to those of sex- and age-matched controls. Of the migraineurs, 19 percent had microsmia during their migraine attack, as defined by UPSIT scores 4 points or more below those at baseline. UPSIT scores were normal at baseline and after treated attacks. It is not known whether the test scores were compromised by testing during a migraine attack and its associated symptoms such as nausea, pain, visual defects, etc.

In a $H_2^{15}O$ PET study of 11 migraineurs with olfactory hypersensitivity and 12 healthy controls, Demarquay et al. (2008) found heightened regional cerebral blood flow (rCBF) in the left piriform cortex and antero-superior temporal gyrus in the migraineurs, whether or not odor stimulation was present. During odor stimulation, migraineurs showed significantly greater activation than controls in the left temporal pole and lower activation in the frontal and temporo-parietal regions, posterior cingulate gyrus, and right locus coeruleus (Figure 5.10). They proposed a key role for the piriform cortex/antero-superior temporal gyrus in olfactory hallucinations and odor-triggered migraine, but were unsure whether the rCBF changes were a cause or effect of odor-triggered migraines and interictal hallucinations.

Olfactory hallucinations were recorded in one case of cluster headache (Silberstein et al., 2000). The patient complained of a bad citrus fruit odor, which preceded the headache by three–four minutes.

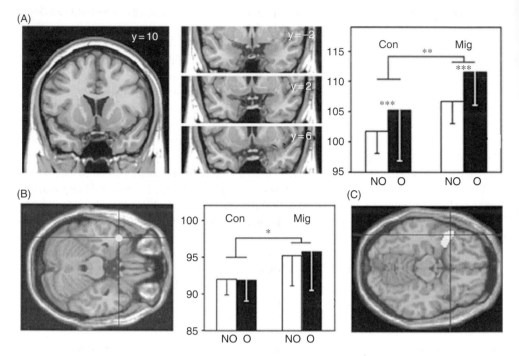

Figure 5.10 Cerebral PET scan superimposed on a T1 weighted MRI scan to show regional cerebral blood flow (rCBF) differences found in the odor–no odor (O–NO) contrast between controls (Con) and migraineurs (Mig) in (A) the left piriform cortex (red) and (B) the left anterior superior temporal gyrus (yellow). (C) High rCBF observed in the baseline condition with the Mig–Con contrast. Statistical Parametric Mappings are superimposed on axial sections of a T1-weighted MRI scan. Vertical axis on graphs represents cerebral blood flow (ml/minute). Reproduced with permission from Demarquay et al. (2008). (A black and white version of this figure will appear in some formats. For the color version, please refer to the plate section.)

Immune-Related Diseases

The prevalence of immune-related olfactory disturbances is probably underestimated simply because so few bother to test it. This section focuses on disorders of presumed autoimmune origin where there are reasonable case numbers, namely multiple sclerosis (MS), myasthenia gravis (MG), Sjögren's syndrome, narcolepsy/cataplexy syndrome, Human Immunodeficiency Virus (HIV), CADASIL, and paraneoplastic disorder. Where there is limited information this is described under "miscellany."

Multiple Sclerosis (MS). Initial pathologic reports suggested that the olfactory tracts and bulbs were spared in multiple sclerosis, and that this might relate to the anatomical properties of myelin basic protein (Lumsden, 1983). Indeed, early workers were unable to find any plaques in the olfactory tract of MS patients (Zimmerman & Netsky, 1950), but subsequently others have shown convincing evidence of demyelination in the tract (Peters, 1958; McDonald, 1986). The most definitive study on this topic explored olfactory pathology in three demyelinating diseases, namely MS, neuromyelitis optica, acute disseminated encephalomyelitis, and compared these to herpes simplex virus encephalitis, Alzheimer's disease, and non-neurologic controls (DeLuca et al., 2014). Olfactory bulb/tract demyelination was frequent in all three demyelinating diseases but it was absent in the other groups.

The highest prevalence of olfactory bulb/tract axonal loss was found for MS (12/17; 71%) and its presence correlated with the extent of demyelination in the brain, particularly the inferior frontal cortex, but not the hippocampus.

The first quantitative clinical investigation of smell function in multiple sclerosis (MS) compared amyl acetate and nitrobenzene recognition thresholds of 40 MS patients to those of 24 controls. No differences were noted, suggesting that smell function was spared (Ansari, 1976). Subsequent investigators observed MS-related deficits for both threshold and supra-threshold measures. Pinching (1977) asked 22 MS patients to smell and identify a set of above-threshold odorants. Ten (45%) exhibited anosmia or microsmia. An additional five (23%) had difficulty in describing the odor sensations. A more recent study by Doty, Shaman, and Dann (1984) used the UPSIT and found microsmia in 7 of 31 (23%) MS patients. This ratio was not too dissimilar to those reported later by Hawkes, Shephard, and Kobal (1997), who described abnormal UPSIT scores in 11/72 (15%) MS patients, and by Zivadinov et al. (1999), who documented abnormal B-SIT scores in 5 of 40 (12.5%) MS patients.

It is noteworthy that the study by Hawkes et al. (1997) found significant correlations between UPSIT scores and measures of anxiety, depression, and severity of neurological impairment, but only two (5%) of the patients were aware of their smell problem prior to testing, presumably reflecting microsmia rather than anosmia. Changes were also demonstrated in the olfactory event-related potential (OERP) induced by H_2S in a subgroup of MS patients. Six of 26 patients (23%) had a delayed N1 response and 3 of 26 (12%) had a delay in the latency of the P2 response. When the trigeminal stimulant CO_2 was employed, 5 of 26 patients (19%) exhibited latency delays, two for the N1 and three for the P2 responses. Patients with more disability, as measured by the Kurtzke Expanded Disability Status Score, had longer OERP latencies, as well as lower UPSIT scores. These findings were confirmed and expanded in a further study that applied H_2S/CO_2 OERP and MRI volumetrics to the olfactory bulb and "olfactory brain" (Holinski et al., 2014). Hyposmia was found in 5/20 patients; the volume of the olfactory bulb was smaller and lesion load of the olfactory brain was higher. Increased latencies to H_2S and CO_2 as well as reduced olfactory bulb volume correlated with lesion load in the olfactory brain in all patients.

Among the few negative studies was that by Kesslak et al. (1988). These investigators reported that scores on both the UPSIT and a match-to-sample discrimination test did not differ significantly between a group of 14 MS patients and 14 controls. The lack of an effect in their small sample may have related to the average age of the MS patients which was significantly less than that of controls (47 versus 63 years) and the preponderance of females in the MS sample. As noted above, all other studies using quantitative test procedures have found abnormalities in a small proportion of patients with MS. Indeed, on rare occasion, acute loss of smell function may be a presenting feature of MS (Constantinescu et al., 1994).

UPSIT scores are reported to fluctuate according to MS plaque activity (Doty et al., 1998, 1999). This group found an inverse correlation between UPSIT score and plaque number within the frontal and temporal lobes, but not in other brain regions, thus providing a physiologic basis for the varying UPSIT scores (see also Zorzon et al., 2000). More recent work indicates that detection thresholds are bilaterally elevated in MS patients and that the threshold scores are correlated with UPSIT scores (Good et al., 2017).

According to one publication, so far not replicated, olfactory thresholds are elevated in MS before detectable changes in identification can be discerned (Lutterotti et al., 2011). A further study using MRI volumetry showed that reduction of olfactory bulb volume correlates with olfactory function (Goektas et al., 2011). The frequency of olfactory impairment is reported to be higher in patients with secondary progressive MS than in those with the relapsing-remitting variety (Silva et al., 2012).

The sub-ventricular zone (SVZ) is a region that provides neuroblasts (at least in the non-human brain; see Chapter 1) via the sub-ventricular migratory stream for the genesis of periglomerular and granule cell neurons within the bulb (Belvindrah et al., 2009). Interestingly, in the mouse experimental allergic encephalomyelitis model of MS, decrements in neurogenesis were evident within the SVZ (Tepavcevic et al., 2011). It was also found that neurogenesis was reduced in the SVZ of MS patients compared to controls. This interesting finding at face value suggests a possible migratory problem in MS – assuming the rostral migratory stream is functional in adult humans.

Neuromyelitis Optica (NMO, Devic's Disease). This is another demyelinating disorder that simulates MS but is found principally in Asian and Oriental populations. The optic nerve, brain stem, hypothalamus, and spinal cord are the main sites of attack. In the olfactory pathology study mentioned above (DeLuca et al., 2014), demyelination was found in the olfactory bulb/tract in two of their three NMO cases. In the only published clinical study, 10 patients with NMO were compared to healthy controls using the extended Sniffin' Sticks test (Schmidt et al., 2013). They found significant impairment of the mean threshold-discrimination-identification score in 5 of their 10 patients.

Myasthenia Gravis. Myasthenia gravis (MG) is a presumed autoimmune disease that results from reduced sensitivity of the post-synaptic muscle receptor zone in the presence of normal amounts of secreted acetylcholine. Although at least 10 studies claim chemosensory alterations in MG, in most instances neither taste nor smell were assessed quantitatively (Leon-Sarmiento et al., 2013). Recently, Leon-Sarmiento et al. (2012) demonstrated that MG is accompanied by smell loss of severity similar to that seen in neurodegenerative diseases such as AD and PD. Their observation was based on the UPSIT which was administered to 27 medicated MG patients, 27 matched healthy controls, and 11 patients with polymyositis (PM). PM is an inflammatory muscle disease that affects bulbar and proximal limb muscles, but has no known central nervous system involvement. The UPSIT scores of the MG patients (mean (SD) = 20.15 (6.40)) were much lower (p < 0.0001) than those of the PM group {mean (SD) = 33.30 (1.42)} and age- and sex-matched normal controls {mean (SD) = 35.67 (4.95)}. No correlations were found between (1) olfactory test scores and thymectomy, (2) time since diagnosis, (3) type of treatment regimen, or (4) the presence or absence of serum nicotinic or muscarinic antibodies. These findings imply that there may be a CNS cholinergic defect in MG or a deficit within the nasal epithelium. The concept of a CNS deficit has received indirect support from a meta-analysis of 300 adult MG subjects who were evaluated neuropsychologically (Mao et al., 2015). Verbal learning and memory were most significantly affected whereas attention, response fluency, visual learning/memory were preserved. Verbal learning and memory are dependent on cholinergic function; thus abnormalities in these measures would be in keeping with a central cholinergic defect in MG and the concept that that MG is not purely a disease of the neuromuscular junction.

Sjögren's Syndrome. Primary Sjögren's syndrome (pSS) is associated with excessive dryness of the mouth, nose, and eyes, as well as a peripheral neuropathy in some cases. Decreased olfactory function, as measured by threshold and odor identification tests, has been reported (Henkin et al., 1972; Weiffenbach & Fox, 1993; Kamel et al., 2009). In the

Weiffenbach and Fox study, 30 patients who met strict criteria for Sjögren's syndrome and 60 matched normal controls were evaluated by the UPSIT. Some olfactory impairment was found in 30% of the patients and 10% of the controls. Although the median score of the patients fell within normal limits (36.5), considerable variation was present and the median was significantly lower (p < 0.02) than that of the controls (38.0). Only one of the Sjögren's syndrome patients scored normally on the UPSIT (3%), in contrast to 19 (32%) of the controls (p < 0.001). In a recent small study from China, Su et al. (2016) measured identification with the SST in 15 subjects with Sjögren's syndrome (presumably of the primary variety) and compared them to 32 patients with the burning mouth syndrome (BMS). Although there was no significant difference between the two groups, 6/15 (40%) of the SS group scored below their normal values. In the BMS group, 9/32 (28%) were abnormal suggesting that those with BMS may also have olfactory impairment. Kamel et al. (2009) present evidence that the chemosensory dysfunction of pSS significantly impacts quality of life. In this study, olfactory threshold test scores were found to correlate with the physical health component of the 12-item Short-Form Healthy Survey Questionnaire (Ware et al., 1996).

Narcolepsy and Cataplexy. Narcolepsy is a possible autoimmune disorder associated with compulsive and inappropriate daytime sleepiness. It is often combined with cataplexy, where there are sudden, disabling attacks of falling. Those with simple narcolepsy have impaired smell sense and so do subjects with narcolepsy and cataplexy (Bayard et al., 2010). It is not yet known whether individuals with pure cataplexy are affected. Patients with idiopathic rapid eye movement sleep behavior disorder (RBD) experience decreased smell function and some develop parkinsonism after a variable interval, sometimes several decades later (see Chapter 7). This association led Stiasny-Kolster and colleagues (2007) to explore whether subjects with RBD and narcolepsy had smell impairment. They found that narcolepsy with or without RBD was associated with olfactory dysfunction, but this was not a predictor of future parkinsonism. Narcolepsy is linked to deficiency in Orexin A (hypocretin-1), an important neurotransmitter throughout the olfactory pathways. This deficiency was found in patients who suffered from narcolepsy and cataplexy, some of whom reportedly experienced improvement in their sense of smell following intranasal Orexin A (Baier et al., 2008).

Human Immunodeficiency Virus (HIV). Odor identification and threshold deficits are reported in patients with the human immunodeficiency virus (Graham et al., 1995; Razani et al., 1996; Hornung et al., 1998; Westervelt et al., 1997; Mueller et al., 2002). The odor identification deficits are relatively mild. For example, Brody et al. (1991) administered the UPSIT to 42 HIV-infected patients and 37 age- and sex-matched normal controls. Ten of the patients were HIV-seropositive but lacked clinical symptoms, 24 were clinically immunocompromised, and 8 had HIV dementia. The UPSIT scores in the asymptomatic and non-demented group were mildly but significantly lowered (respective means (SDs) = 34.9 (5.1) & 34.6 (4.5)) relative to controls (mean (SD) = 38.3 (1.8)). The UPSIT values of the HIV dementia patients were significantly lower than those of the other groups (mean (SD) = 28.1 (5.1)). Similar findings have been noted by others, where demented patients underperformed other groups and the degree of deficit correlated with the number of circulating CD4+ lymphocytes (Zucco & Ingegneri, 2004) and symptoms (Westervelt et al., 1997).

CADASIL (Cerebral Autosomal Dominant Arteriopathy with Subcortical Infarcts and Leukoencephalopathy). This is an inherited angiopathy caused by various mutations in the Notch 3 gene on chromosome 19. It is included here because it is a leukodystrophy that affects frontal, parietal, and anterior temporal white matter and may be confused with MS. White matter changes are seen consistently on MRI, particularly in the anterior temporal poles. Thus, olfactory impairment would not be surprising. CADASIL results in strokes, transient ischemic attacks, migraine-like headaches, and progressive cognitive impairment. One study found impaired olfactory identification in 25 CADASIL subjects (Lee et al., 2010). They used the 16-item Korean version of Sniffin' Sticks, which screens identification to 16 odors, and found a significantly lower mean score of 9.4 in the CADSIL group compared to their control mean of 11.8. There was a weak negative correlation between olfactory identification scores and anterior temporal white matter lesions. In another study, Vishnevetsky et al. (2017) found, upon initial presentation, UPSIT scores indicative of anosmia in two Peruvian CADASIL patients (13, 15) and severe microsmia in a third (24). Although confounding from cognitive dysfunction is unavoidable, some impairment of olfaction is not surprising given the extent of white matter involvement in this disorder.

Paraneoplastic Disorders. Impaired smell appreciation is rare in these disorders. In 2001, investigators at the Mayo Clinic discovered a novel autoantibody, termed CRMP-5, in 116 patients suspected to have a paraneoplastic disorder (Yu et al., 2001). There were 12 (11%) with chorea and unquantified patient reports of smell or taste disturbance in another 12. Many (29) were demented, thus accurate testing of chemosensory function might have been difficult. Most had an underlying small cell lung cancer and a few had thymoma. There is a single case report of anosmia and sensory ataxic neuropathy as presenting features of a presumed autoimmune process with antibodies to dorsal root ganglia and olfactory cells (Gambelli et al., 2004).

Miscellaneous Immune Disorders. In one study of *systemic lupus erythematosus*, the prevalence of olfactory impairment measured by reduced TDI score (Sniffin' Sticks) was 46 percent and its severity correlated with disease activity (Shoenfeld et al., 2009). The presumed mechanism is ischemia of peripheral olfactory structures, because the vasa nervorum of the olfactory bulb and nasal neuroepithelium derive their blood supply from the anterior and posterior ethmoid arteries, which are tributaries of the ophthalmic branch of the internal carotid artery. There are single-case reports of smell impairment due to *Churg–Strauss syndrome* (Ros et al., 2003; Tallab & Doty, 2014); *giant cell arteritis* (Schon, 1988), and *lymphocytic hypophysitis* (Lee et al., 2004). Theoretically, microsmia in someone suspected to suffer from giant cell arteritis would indicate disease in the ophthalmic artery, and this observation would alert the clinician to pending visual loss – a recognized major complication. Finally, there is some evidence of impaired olfaction in *Behcet's disease*, a disorder of possible immune or infective origin. In the only study on this topic (Veyseller et al., 2014b,) olfaction was measured in 30 patients and 30 controls by n-butanol odor threshold and odor identification tests. Significant impairment in threshold and identification was reported, although the smell test scores did not correlate with observed patients' symptoms or nasal endoscopy findings.

Multiple Chemical Hypersensitivity (MCS)

Some individuals report hypersensitivity to environmental odors, particularly those associated with plastics, household cleaners, solvents, vehicular exhausts, insecticides, preservatives, cigarette smoke, fragrances, perfumes, and colognes. Typically, they claim that such chemicals and their odors induce a wide variety of somatic symptoms, including anxiety, depression, fatigue, general malaise, mental confusion, lightheadedness, headache, insomnia, myalgia, loss of appetite, and numbness. Physiological tests generally fail to correlate with their symptoms (Miller & Mitzel, 1995) and no documentable signs of medical disease are apparent (Ross et al., 1999).

This unorthodox collection of symptoms was termed "environmental illness" or "chemical reactivity" in the 1960s by Randolph (1962). It was later termed "multiple chemical sensitivities" (MCS) (Cullen, 1987), although numerous other descriptors have been used, including ecological illness, multiple chemical hypersensitivity, multiple chemical intolerance, idiopathic environmental intolerance, universal allergy, and, most recently, toxicant-induced loss of tolerance (TILT) (Miller, 2003). Such symptoms have been associated with other syndromes including chronic fatigue syndrome, fibromyalgia, and the sick building syndrome. Whatever its name, numerous attempts have been made to delineate the disorder operationally. Cullen's original criteria were used for a survey of 89 clinicians and scientists familiar with MCS, although they held differing opinions about its origins (Bartha et al., 1999). A list of six "consensus criteria" was derived for the diagnosis of MCS, namely:

1. Chronicity
2. Symptoms present in multiple organ systems
3. Reliably recurring symptoms
4. Induction by low levels of chemical exposures
5. Involvement of multiple chemicals
6. Resolution after removal of the identified incitants.

Several investigators sought to establish whether measurable alterations in smell function are present in MCS. In the first of these studies, PEA and methyl ethyl ketone-detection thresholds were obtained from 18 MCS patients and 18 age- and sex-matched controls (Doty et al., 1988). The MCS group did not have lower thresholds, although they exhibited higher respiratory rates, increased nasal resistance to airflow, and raised Beck Depression Inventory scores (Doty et al., 1988). In the second study, PEA thresholds of 23 MCS subjects did not differ from those of 23 controls (Hummel et al., 1996). Paradoxically, in this study, MCS subjects were less adept than controls at identifying and discriminating suprathreshold odors and exhibited smaller odor event-related potentials, raising the possibility that MCS is associated with decreased suprathreshold olfactory function.

More recently, Ojima et al. (2002) administered the UPSIT and B-SIT to 25 MCS subjects and 50 age- and sex-matched controls. No differences in test scores of the MCS and controls were present for either test, in accord with the aforementioned findings, although the MCS patients reported a larger number of odorants to be unpleasant compared to the controls.

A psychogenic basis for the complaints of several MCS patients is likely. Zucco, Militello, and Doty (2008) administered the UPSIT and other olfactory tests to a 36-year-old-woman who met a strict set of criteria for MCS. No evidence of hypersensitivity was found. Some odorants were then presented along with blanks following two sets of instructions. Under one set of instructions, the patient was led to believe that the presented odors were likely harmful and under the other set, that they were benign. The patient's task was to rate the intensity of the odors and indicate which ones induced MCS-related symptoms. When the odorants were presented as being harmless, they were judged significantly less intense and triggered fewer symptoms than when they were presented as being harmful. The authors suggested that this simple test may help identify patients whose MCS symptoms are psychogenic.

Exposure to High Levels of Air Pollution

If air pollution is high, inhabitants are inevitably vulnerable to mixtures of volatile chemicals and particulate matter. Olfactory dysfunction is found in many people living in highly polluted areas for prolonged periods such as Mexico City (Hudson et al., 2006; Calderon-Garciduenas et al., 2010; Gudziol et al., 2010). Even relatively short-term exposure to extreme air pollution can alter smell function. For example, following the World Trade Center (WTC) collapse on September 11, 2001, more than 40,000 people were exposed to high levels of a complex mixture of airborne pollutants over several weeks. Many developed nasal problems and smell deficits that were present years after the disaster (Dalton et al., 2010; Altman et al., 2011).

In a study by Calderon-Garciduenas et al. (2010), decreased UPSIT scores were evident in 35.5% residents in highly polluted regions of Mexico City but only in 12% controls of similar age and sex who lived in a less polluted control city. Among the Mexico City residents, the ApoE epsilon 4 genotype – a risk factor for AD – exacerbated the dysfunction. Thus, ApoE epsilon 4 carriers on average failed 2.4 of the 10 UPSIT odors that were most strongly associated with AD (Tabert et al., 2005). Conversely, ApoE 2/3 and 3/3 phenotypes failed only 1.36 such items (p = 0.01). Autopsy studies performed on even young Mexico City exposed residents have revealed marked olfactory bulb inflammation and the presence of ultrafine particulate matter <100 nm (nanoparticles) in their olfactory bulbs. Such matter appears to provoke an innate immune response from the brain, i.e., the induction of monocytes that secrete TNF-α, interleukin-6 (IL-6), and IL-1β. In turn, these monocytes recruit and increase the activity of other immune cells (Simard & Rivest, 2006; Calderon-Garciduenas et al., 2012).

Work-Place Exposures to Industrial Toxic Chemicals

Numerous airborne agents involved in manufacturing can influence olfactory function adversely. In many instances the effects are specific to a given chemical or a set of closely related chemicals. This happens in many plastic manufacturing operations that involve styrene, acrylates, and solvents. As described below, the adverse effects of exposure are in some instances reversible, presumably indicating long-term adaptation rather than lasting damage to the olfactory system. In other situations, the damage may reflect permanent injury to the olfactory system, especially when there is longstanding contact with airborne dusts or aerosolized particles from industrial metals such as cadmium, chromium, manganese, and mercury. For reviews, see Amoore (1986), Calderon-Garciduenas (2015), Doty (2015), and Naus (1975).

Toxic Metals. Smell loss caused by heavy metal fume exposure is documented best for *nickel* (Ni) and *cadmium* (Cd). Both are highly toxic agents involved in the production of batteries, paints, plastics, and metal alloys. As early as 1950 it was reported that nearly half of 43 workers employed in an alkaline battery factory complained of smell problems (Friberg, 1950). In this case, high levels of exposure had occurred for periods of 9–34 years to Cd-iron dust ($5–15$ mg/m^3 of air) and Ni graphite dust ($10–150$ mg/m^3 of air). A third of the workers were said to be anosmic. Adams and Crabtree (1961) used an odor threshold test to measure olfaction in 106 workers exposed to nickel-cadmium alkaline batteries. Over a quarter of exposed workers were anosmic, compared to only 5% of 84 matched controls. Other studies have documented similar levels of anosmia affecting workers in contact with relatively high levels and/or long durations of these metals (Yin-Zeng et al., 1985; Rose et al., 1992; Rydzewski et al., 1998; Sulkowski et al., 2000). Even moderate exposure to cadmium, i.e., levels close to or below legal permissible limits, have been associated with smell loss (Mascagni et al., 2003).

Watanabe & Fukuchi (2000) tested odor detection and recognition thresholds of 26 male and 7 female employees of a chromate-producing factory who had a minimum of seven years' contact with *chromium*. Over half (54.5%) had elevated thresholds to the five target odorants: phenylethyl alcohol (rose), cyclopentenolone (caramel), isovaleric acid (sweaty feet), r-undecalactone (fruity), and scatol (fecal). A similar number (51.4%) had perforated nasal septa. Two were anosmic. Duration of employment, but not the presence of septal perforations, correlated with the degree of olfactory dysfunction. Similar changes afflicted 27 male chromate factory workers (mean age 32 years) in Korea (Kitamura et al., 2003).

Olfactory dysfunction is reported in workers in contact with *manganese* (Mn). Manganese can be taken up via the olfactory pathways and passed transneuronally to other parts of the brain (Tjalve & Henriksson, 1999). In one study, a battery of sensory, neuromuscular, and psychological tests was administered to 74 employees of a large Canadian ferromanganese and silico-manganese alloy facility (Mergler et al., 1994). Seventy-four employees with no occupational history of exposure to manganese, matched by age, sex, and education, served as controls. Only the olfactory threshold measure (phenylethyl methyl ethyl carbinol; PEMEC) discriminated between the two groups. Paradoxically, exposed workers were actually *more* sensitive, not less sensitive, to PEMEC, even though they had higher blood levels of manganese at the time of the testing. The investigators suggested this might reflect a dose-related excitatory component of manganese intoxication.

In contrast to the Mergler et al. study, lower UPSIT scores relative to controls were found in a study 43 professional welders who had been exposed for one to two years to airborne Mn-containing fumes while working in confined spaces (Antunes et al., 2007). Most were not wearing respirators. At the time of testing, about half had elevated blood levels of Mn, but not iron, copper, or lead. Although the cumulative time spent in the welding operations correlated with Mn blood levels, workers with the highest Mn blood levels at the time of testing paradoxically had better olfactory function than those with the lowest Mn blood levels. This observation is similar to the finding of Mergler et al.; namely, greater olfactory sensitivity in Mn-exposed employees with the highest Mn blood levels. A similar association with higher urine levels of Mn and better performance on a threshold test was reported earlier by Lucchini et al. (1997).

Although exposure to *lead* can produce transient or possibly permanent psychological deficits, occupational contact appears to have, at most, only minor effects on the sense of smell. Schwartz et al. (1993) administered the UPSIT and a battery of neuropsychological tests to 222 employees of a tetraethyl lead manufacturing plant. Differences in test scores were estimated by comparing the average scores of the moderate, high, and highest exposure groups to those of the low exposure (reference) group and by adjusting statistically for the confounding influences of age, intellectual ability, race, and alcohol consumption. No influence of lead on UPSIT scores was found, even though lead exposure-related decrements were documented for several neuropsychological measures. In a subsequent study, UPSIT scores from 190 of the lead-exposed subjects were compared to those from 144 solvent-exposed workers and 52 non-exposed comparison subjects (Bolla et al., 1995). The UPSIT scores of lead-exposed workers did not differ significantly from those of the controls (respective mean scores, 36.4 and 36.9). When lead-exposed workers were divided into three separate exposure durations, namely less than 11 years, 11 to 17 years, and more than 17 years, significantly lower UPSIT scores were noted relative to the controls for the 11 to 17-year exposure group, but not for the other two groups. Despite this observation, the investigators concluded that lead had no meaningful adverse effect on the workers. In contrast, more recent work also using the UPSIT suggests some association between exposure to lead and olfactory test performance. Odor identification was measured in 165 men from the Normative Aging Study (NAS; average age: 80.3 years) who had previously taken part in bone lead measurements using K-X-ray (Grashow et al., 2015). Tibial bone lead was significantly and negatively associated with olfactory identification in models adjusted for smoking and age. This work, along with earlier findings, suggests that lead exposure has a minor harmful effect on the sense of smell.

Another metal linked to smell loss is *mercury* (Hg). Minamata disease (MD) is a serious condition acquired largely from eating Hg-contaminated fish. Several studies report smell loss in patients with MD. In one study, Furuta et al. (1994) administered the B-SIT and a PEA detection threshold test to 19 MD patients in the age bracket 36 to 97 years (mean: 78.8 years), 19 age- and sex-matched controls, and 16 patients with senile dementia. The detection threshold was more than two log units higher in the MD patients than in the controls (p < 0.003) and did not differ from that of the dementia patients. Although inhaled mercury vapor can enter the olfactory bulbs, it is less able than Mn to travel further along the olfactory pathways into the brain (Tjalve & Henriksson, 1999). Mercury encephalopathy ("erythrism") is well recognized and so is a cerebellar tremor, but entry of mercury salts into the brain is likely blood-borne. Strict international controls of mercury handling have reduced the overall risk of Hg exposure and, as a result, the prevalence of mercury poisoning has diminished.

Chemicals Involved in Manufacturing. In an extensive study of occupational exposure to *acrylates* at a chemical manufacturing plant in Texas, Schwartz et al. (1989) administered the UPSIT to 731 workers whose exposure histories were well established. A nested case-control design found odds ratios of 2.0 for all workers and 6.0 for workers who never smoked cigarettes, suggesting a protective effect of smoking. Logistic regression analysis, adjusting for multiple confounders, revealed exposure odds ratios of 2.8 and 13.5, respectively, in these same groups. A dose-response relationship between olfactory dysfunction and cumulative exposure scores was observed. Decreasing exposure odds ratios with increasing duration since last exposure suggested that the effects were, to some extent, reversible. Similar observations were made by the same group in a study of olfactory function among paint-manufacturing workers who were exposed to solvents described below in the Solvents section.

Several studies have examined the effect of *styrene* on olfaction. In the first of two studies, Dalton et al. (2003) tested odor identification performance and detection threshold sensitivity to styrene and phenylethyl alcohol (PEA) in 62 workers who had been in contact with styrene. Sixty-seven age- and sex-matched unexposed controls were also examined. The styrene thresholds were markedly elevated in the exposed workers relative to the non-exposed workers, a difference that was magnified in the older group. No exposure effects were evident for PEA thresholds or the other tests, all of which were within normal limits. This led the authors to conclude that the elevated styrene thresholds most likely reflected long-term adaptation specific to styrene. In the second study, 30 workers in a reinforced-plastics boat manufacturing facility were similarly tested (Dalton et al., 2007). Fifteen held positions where there was relatively high contact with styrene, whereas 15 occupied jobs where exposure was much less. As before, thresholds to styrene, but not to PEA, were elevated in the more exposed workers, but those with high styrene contact performed worse than the less exposed workers on the odor identification test. The investigators concluded that this effect was unlikely caused by styrene contact, since no correlation was present between the identification test scores and either the lifetime exposure profiles of the worker or the exposure levels on either the day of testing or the day before testing.

Cheng et al. (2004) assessed odor identification performance and 1-butanol thresholds in 52 employees involved with injection molding operations in Taiwan. They had been in contact with decomposition products of acrylonitrile butadiene styrene for a minimum of six months. Seventy-two control workers who were not similarly exposed were tested over the same time periods. The detection thresholds were significantly higher in the unprotected workers than the non-exposed employees after, but not before, their work shifts, suggesting this was a case of adaptation rather than sustained neurological damage to the olfactory system.

Solvents. Given their high lipophilic properties, most solvents cross the blood-brain barrier and reach the central nervous system, where they may cause impairment of sensory, motor, and cognitive function, depending on the concentration and exposure time of the solvent in question. In severe cases, such as long-term glue sniffers and chronically exposed painters, a widespread encephalopathy may ensue that most notably damages the basal ganglia, cerebellum, and periventricular white matter (Rosenberg et al., 1988; Tvedt et al., 1989).

Ahlstrom et al. (1986) measured odor thresholds to the vapors of fuel oil, pyridine, dimethyl disulfide, and n-butanol in 20 industrial fuel oil tank cleaners who gave a history of exposure to hydrocarbon solvents. Controls matched for gender, age, and smoking were also tested. No differences in sensitivity to pyridine and dimethyl disulfide were found, but thresholds to n-butanol and fuel oil vapors were elevated, particularly those for fuel oil. Within two days of removal from the exposure environment, the thresholds returned to normal. This finding, along with evidence that pyridine and dimethyl disulfide sensitivities were unaffected, suggested that the elevated thresholds were due to adaptation rather than damage to the olfactory system ("industrial anosmia"). Subsequently, Sandmark et al. (1989) administered the UPSIT to 54 painters who had been exposed on a near-daily basis to organic solvents and to 42 unexposed controls. On average the subjects were in their mid-30s. A multiple regression analysis controlling for the effects of age and smoking found no meaningful difference in UPSIT scores between the two groups.

A series of olfactory function studies were performed on a group of 187 workers in two paint manufacturing groups by Schwartz and his colleagues (Schwartz et al., 1990). The levels of organic solvent exposure were relatively low (2–40% of the existing threshold limit volumes (TLVs)). In the first of these studies, slightly lower (i.e., worse) UPSIT scores were found in non-smoking workers with the longest exposure histories (below the fifth percentile for their age) (Schwartz et al., 1990). This was not true for workers who smoked, suggesting that smoking may be protective (Schwarz et al., 1990) and resonating with classical Parkinson's disease (see Chapter 6). One possible mechanism for the apparent protective effect of smoking is through up-regulation of nasal epithelial cytochromes which constitute a major first line of defense against xenobiotics. Another potential mechanism is through chronic stimulation of cholinergic neurons – a system whose damage is associated with PD and a number of other neurodegenerative diseases (Doty, 2017). In the second study, correlations were determined between the UPSIT scores and measurements on eight neuropsychological tests that explored learning and memory (Schwartz et al., 1991). Although positive correlations were observed between the UPSIT scores and several of the cognitive measures, such associations disappeared after adjustment for the effects of age and vocabulary. There was no evidence that UPSIT scores were predictive of cognitive dysfunction. In the third study, UPSIT scores from 144 of the aforementioned solvent-exposed workers were compared to those from 52 non-exposed controls (Bolla et al., 1995). To minimize age and verbal intelligence differences among groups, they included only workers over 30 years whose vocabulary scores were 25–68 on the vocabulary subtest of the WAIS-R. UPSIT scores were slightly but significantly lower in the exposed than in the non-exposed group, although still within the normal range {respective UPSIT (SD) scores = 34.7 (5.4) & 36.9 (2.2); p = 0.005}.

Case Report 5.7: **Loss of Smell and Taste in an Industrial Painter.** A 48-year-old worker presented with loss and distortion of smell and taste. This problem occurred after transfer to the painting area of an automobile plant, where he had worked for approximately one year. For most of this time appropriate inhalation protection was *not* used, and the patient eventually experienced frequent nosebleeds, long bouts of coughing, and flu-like symptoms. The non-chemosensory symptoms resolved when he stayed at home while receiving disability benefit for a broken leg, but smell function never returned, despite treatment with antibiotics, systemic corticosteroids, and antihistamines. The UPSIT score was at chance level (11/40); likewise, tests of odor detection threshold (bilateral, left, or right >−2.00 log vol/vol) and odor memory (8/24). The taste test scores were also diminished slightly, and he exhibited a low score on the Mini-Mental State Examination (25/30) were indicative of significant dysfunction. Nasal cross-sectional area, assessed by acoustic rhinometry, and nasal resistance, as measured by anterior rhinomanometry, were within normal limits. *Comment:* This patient experienced marked impairment of smell function, and possibly some loss of true taste function, secondary to exposure to paint, solvents, and other volatiles at the workplace. His cognitive function may have been impaired as well, although more sophisticated cognitive testing would be needed to verify this. The complaint of loss and distortion of taste and smell mainly reflects the olfactory deficit, which alters the flavor sensation derived from retronasal stimulation of the olfactory receptors during chewing and swallowing.

Medication

Among the major systemic causes of chemosensory disturbances that should concern the clinician are those associated with medication (Table 5.2; for reviews, see Doty & Bromley, 2004; Doty et al., 2008; Schiffman, 2016). Although some drugs interfere with the ability to smell, taste is affected much more frequently, as described in detail in Chapter 6. Unfortunately, most reports of drug-related disorders are case studies relying on patient self-report with no quantitative testing. Considering how many patients (and clinicians) confuse smell and taste, any alleged association should be viewed with caution. Furthermore, the disease for which a drug is given, e.g., diabetes or hypothyroidism, may be the cause of smell dysfunction, rather than the drug itself. Table 5.2 lists drugs that likely influence chemosensation in some individuals. This listing is largely based on case reports and includes calcium channel blockers, antibiotics, anti-thyroid drugs, opiates, antidepressants, and sympathomimetics. It must be emphasized that very few studies have evaluated quantitatively the influences of medication on olfactory function, per se.

Table 5.2. List of the major drugs that have been reported to be linked to smell impairment.

Drug group	Examples
Calcium channel blocker	Nifedipine; amlodipine; diltiazem
Lipid lowering	Cholestyramine; Clofibrate; Statins
Antibiotic & antifungal	Streptomycin; doxycycline; terbinafine
Anti-thyroid	Carbimazole
Chemotherapy	Taxanes
Opiates	Codeine; morphine; cocaine (snorted)
Antidepressant	Amitriptyline
Sympathomimetic	Dexamphetamine; phenmetrazine
Antiepileptic	Phenytoin
Nasal decongestant	Phenylephrine; pseudoephedrine; oxymetazoline (long term use probably required for damage); intranasal zinc gluconate (e.g., Zicam)
Miscellaneous	Smoking; argyria (from topical application of silver nitrate); cadmium fumes; phenothiazines; pesticides. influenza vaccine; betnesol-N

Chemotherapeutic agents, particularly those used for breast and gynecological cancers, are associated with significant effects on smell (and taste), as shown in one study of 87 patients (Steinbach et al., 2009). The investigators found significant impairment of both modalities during chemotherapy, but there was almost complete recovery three months later. In this series, odor threshold scores were affected more than those of discrimination or identification and Taxane- based agents appeared to cause most dysfunction. These findings underscore previous subjectively based observations that poor appetite and weight loss are connected more to the chemosensory disturbance than the effect of the underlying cancer itself (Wismer, 2008). Although robust data are lacking, there are anecdotal reports that some lipid-lowering drugs (e.g., statins) may cause olfactory disturbances, but not so frequently as taste impairment. Antiviral and antifungal drugs may influence smell also. Again, they are more likely to impair taste than smell (Doty & Haxel, 2005). Sudden withdrawal of benzodiazepines or antidepressants is alleged to cause hyperosmia (Pelissolo & Bisserbe, 1994; Mourad et al., 1997), although this phenomenon has not been verified by olfactory testing.

Several medications produce volatiles that arise from lung air and stimulate olfactory receptors, whereas others influence synaptic transmission. Cocaine, when snorted, may damage the olfactory epithelium and, in extreme cases, erode the septum, presumably from sustained constriction of the nasal vasculature. Addicts report smell impairment, which may in part relate to cocaine-induced nasal stuffiness, but it is likely that the risk of smell dysfunction is small and that permanent smell loss is unusual, according to the only published study of just 11 addicts (Gordon et al., 1990). This information contrasts with an investigation of olfactory event-related potentials in 19 cocaine abusers (Bauer & Mott, 1996). It was noted that the first positive component (P1) was significantly smaller in those who snorted cocaine compared to controls, thus implying that there was some impairment at peripheral or central level. Once more, it is difficult to disentangle this observation from the non-specific effect of nasal stuffiness induced by cocaine.

Intranasal zinc gluconate preparations, namely Zicam, are apparently effective in reducing the symptoms of the common cold (D'Cruze et al., 2009), but they have been reported to cause smell impairment which may be permanent (Jafek et al., 2004; Alexander and Davidson, 2006). Widespread advertising by attorneys identified such cases, thereby alerting anyone who had used this product at the time of a cold, to seek compensation. As a result, many successful high-profile lawsuits have followed in the USA and Zicam nasal spray has since been banned by the FDA. Use of this drug is initiated by early signs of a cold in efforts to avert the severity of infection, but it is not clear in many instances whether the underlying viral infection or the medication itself is responsible. This is especially pertinent, given that the most frequent cause of *chronic* smell impairment is the common cold. The potential for faulty attribution is obvious, since Zicam often causes nasal irritation and burning, mediated by the trigeminal nerve. In addition, it is uncertain whether the Zicam nasal spray actually reaches the olfactory cleft in many individuals. Unfortunately, the sole study on this topic used only one model of the nasal cavity, precluding individual differences in nasal anatomy (Kundoor and Dalby, 2010). Another investigation found that Zicam nasal gel (rather than the spray) does not reach the olfactory receptors (González-Botas & Seara, 2012), suggesting that the gel format cannot produce olfactory damage.

Despite this, it is well known that various forms of zinc can be toxic to the olfactory epithelium. In perhaps the most definitive study relative to Zicam, Lim et al. (2009) examined the electro-olfactogram from the olfactory epithelia of mice three and nine days after intranasal administration of Zicam, Afrin, Nasacort, epinephrine, and lidocaine. Only Zicam induced meaningful decrement in such potentials – reductions that were associated with significant cytotoxity. Human nasal explants treated with Zicam also displayed severe necrosis. The authors concluded (p. 134), "Our results demonstrate that Zicam use could irreversibly damage mouse and human nasal tissue and may lead to significant smell dysfunction." Based on the known olfactotoxicity of zinc ions, the large volume of complaints about this product, and the resulting ruling by the FDA, it would appear that varying degrees of smell impairment may occur in at least some individuals who have administered the spray form of this drug.

Rare Genetically Determined Disorders of Olfaction

Inherited neurodegenerative disorders associated with smell loss are considered in Chapter 7. Apart from these conditions are a variety of rare genetically determined disorders affecting children and young adults associated with olfactory dysfunction. Among these are Bardet–Biedl syndrome, Aniridia type 2 syndrome, Kartagener syndrome, DiGeorge syndrome (22q11.2 deletion syndrome), Refsum's syndrome, Wolfram syndrome, and various forms of congenital anosmia (see Chapter 1).

Bardet–Biedl Syndrome (BBS) is characterized by retinal dystrophy, polydactyly, mental retardation, obesity, and occasionally microsmia. The condition has several postulated genetic loci, but it is similar to the Laurence-Moon-Biedl syndrome. The disorder is classed as a ciliopathy, and the gene BBS4 may play a role in ciliary motility in the olfactory neuroepithelium (Kulaga et al., 2004). Impaired motility may impair smell function, possibly as the result of poor mucociliary clearance and subsequent bacterial accumulation (Kulaga et al., 2004; Blacque & Leroux, 2006). This reasoning has proven to be correct given the demonstration of impaired UPSIT scores in two studies with genetically confirmed BBS where nearly all patients (total of 62) had some degree of olfactory impairment (Brinckman et al., 2013; Braun et al., 2014). Bardet–Biedl syndrome is thought to be related to another suspected ciliopathy, namely juvenile myoclonic epilepsy.

Aniridia Type 2, also a primary visual disorder, is accompanied by underdevelopment of the iris, usually bilaterally, and severe structural abnormalities of the retina. It has a gene locus at 11p13. This condition relates to abnormalities in an organizer gene, PAX6, but there are less severe forms associated with microsmia (Sisodiya et al., 2001).

Kartagener Syndrome comprises bronchiectasis, dextrocardia, infertility, severe headache, and respiratory cilia immotility. Some patients are anosmic, probably because of recurrent sinus infection and olfactory ciliary immotility (Mygind & Pedersen, 1982). The condition is likely to be an incompletely penetrant autosomal recessive disorder. Three loci are known, one of which (9p21-p13) codes for the axonemal dynein complex, a "motor protein" that allows bending movements of cilia.

DiGeorge Syndrome (22q11.2 deletion syndrome) comprises parathyroid and thymic hypoplasia associated with outflow tract defects of the heart, facial dysmorphism, and, in some varieties, velopharyngeal insufficiency. Patients present with neonatal hypocalcemia causing tetany or seizures and susceptibility to infection because of a deficit of T cells. In the only study of smell function in 62 affected children (Sobin et al., 2006), there was a significant impairment of UPSIT scores compared to controls. Those with velopharyngeal insufficiency did not differ from the classical type of disease.

Refsum's Disease. The typical features are short stature, polyneuropathy, ichthyosis, deafness, and retinitis pigmentosa (Wierzbicki et al., 2002). It is less well recognized that most patients with this syndrome are anosmic – thus a patient who presents with impaired vision due to retinitis pigmentosa who is also anosmic most likely has Refsum disease (Gibberd et al., 2004).

Wolfram Syndrome. This is a childhood-onset endocrinopathy with an easily identifiable phenotype comprising diabetes insipidus, diabetes mellitus, optic atrophy and deafness, hence the acronym, DIDMOAD. It is caused by a mutation in the WFS1 gene which encodes the mitochondrial endoplasmic reticulum protein Wolframin. It was observed that 13/18 (72%) displayed significant olfactory defects as measured by the UPSIT (Marshall et al., 2013), making microsmia just as frequent as two of the other cardinal features, namely diabetes insipidus and optic neuropathy. This observation has been substantiated further in 19 patients with Wolfram syndrome (Bischoff et al., 2015). There was a highly significant difference between healthy controls and patients using the UPSIT. The possible confounding from type 1 diabetes was addressed but not found to be relevant.

References

Abdel-Dayem, H.M., Abu-Judeh, H., Kumar, M., et al. 1998. SPECT brain perfusion abnormalities in mild or moderate traumatic brain injury. *Clinical Nuclear Medicine* 23, 309–317.

Abraham, A., Mathai, K.V., 1983. The effect of right temporal lobe lesions on matching of smells. *Neuropsychologia* 21, 277–281.

Acharya, V., Acharya, J., Luders, H., 1998. Olfactory epileptic auras. *Neurology* 51, 56–61.

Adams, R.G., Crabtree, N., 1961. Anosmia in alkaline battery workers. *British Journal of Industrial Medicine* 18, 216–221.

Ahlstrom, R., Berglund, B., Berglund, U., Lindvall, T., Wennberg, A., 1986. Impaired odor perception in tank cleaners. *Scandinavian Journal of Work, Environment & Health* 12, 574–581.

Alobid, I., Guilemany, J.M., Mullol, J., 2004. Nasal manifestations of systemic illnesses. *Current Allergy and Asthma Reports* 4, 208–216.

Alexander, T.H., Davidson, T.M., 2006. Intranasal zinc and anosmia: the zinc-induced anosmia syndrome. *Laryngoscope* **116**, 217–220.

Altman, K.W., Desai, S.C., Moline, J., et al. 2011. Odor identification ability and self-reported upper respiratory symptoms in workers at the post-9/11 World Trade Center site. *International Archives of Occupational and Environmental Health* **84** 131–137.

Amoore, J.E., 1986. Effects of chemical exposure on olfaction in humans. In Barrow, C.S. (ed.), *Toxicology of the Nasal Passages*. New York: Hemisphere Publishing Corporation, pp. 155–190.

Amsterdam, J.D., Settle, R.G., Doty, R.L., Abelman, E., Winokur, A., 1987. Taste and smell perception in depression. *Biological Psychiatry* **22**, 1481–1485.

Anderson, N.E., Sheffield, S., Hope, J.K., 1999. Superficial siderosis of the central nervous system: A late complication of cerebellar tumors. *Neurology* **52**, 163–169.

Ansari, K.A., 1976. Olfaction in multiple sclerosis. With a note on the discrepancy between optic and olfactory involvement. *European Neurology* **14**, 138–145.

Antunes, M.B., Bowler, R., Doty, R.L., 2007. San-Francisco/Oakland Bay Bridge welder study: Olfactory function. *Neurology* **69**, 1278–1284.

Arnold, S.E., Han, L.Y., Moberg, P.J., et al. (2001). Dysregulation of olfactory receptor neuron lineage in schizophrenia. *Archives of General Psychiatry* **58**, 829–835.

Aschenbrenner, K., Scholze, N., Joraschky, P., Hummel, T. (2008). Gustatory and olfactory sensitivity in patients with anorexia and bulimia in the course of treatment. *Journal of Psychiatric Research* **43**, 129–137.

Baier, P.C., Weinhold, S.L., Huth, V., Gottwald, B., Ferstl, R., Hinze-Selch, D., 2008. Olfactory dysfunction in patients with narcolepsy with cataplexy is restored by intranasal Orexin A (Hypocretin-1). *Brain* **131**, 2734–2741.

Bajaj, S., Ammini, A. C., Marwaha, R., et al. 1993. Magnetic resonance imaging of the brain in idiopathic hypogonadotropic hypogonadism. *Clinical Radiology* **48**, 122–124.

Bang, F.B., Bang, B.G., Foard, M.A., 1966. Responses of upper respiratory mucosa to drugs and viral infections 1, 2. *American Review of Respiratory Disease* **93**, 142–149.

Bartha, L., Baumzweiger, W., Buscher, D.S., et al. 1999. Multiple chemical sensitivity: A 1999 consensus. *Archives of Environmental Health* **54**, 147–149.

Baskin, D.G., Figlewicz, D.P., Woods, S.C., Porte, D., Jr., Dorsa, D.M., 1987. Insulin in the brain. *Annual Review of Psychology* **49**, 335–347.

Bauer, L.O., Mott, A.E., 1996. Differential effects of cocaine, alcohol, and nicotine dependence on olfactory evoked potentials. *Drug and Alcohol Dependence* **42**(1), 21–26.

Bayard, S., Plazzi, G., Poli, F., et al. 2010. Olfactory dysfunction in narcolepsy with cataplexy. *Sleep Medicine* **11**, 876–881.

Beard, M.D. Mackay-Sim, A., 1987. Loss of sense of smell in adult, hypothyroid mice. *Brain Research* **433**, 181–189.

Begum, M. McKenna, P.J., 2010. Olfactory reference syndrome: A systematic review of the world literature. *Psychological Medicine* Volume **41**, Issue 3 March 2011, pp. 453–461.

Belvindrah, R., Lazarini, F., Lledo, P.M., 2009. Postnatal neurogenesis: From neuroblast migration to neuronal integration. *Reviews in the Neurosciences* **20**, 331–346.

Bershad, E.M., Urfy, M.Z., Calvillo, E., et al. (2014). Marked olfactory impairment in idiopathic intracranial hypertension. *Journal of Neurology, Neurosurgery, & Psychiatry* **85**(9), 959–964.

Betts, T. (2003). Use of aromatherapy (with or without hypnosis) in the treatment of intractable epilepsyGÇöa two-year follow-up study. *Seizure* **12**, 534–538.

Bischoff, A.N., Reiersen, A.M., Buttlaire, A., et al. (2015). Selective cognitive and psychiatric manifestations in Wolfram Syndrome. *Orphanet Journal of Rare Diseases* **10**(1), 1–11.

Bishop, E.R., Jr. 1980. An olfactory reference syndrome – monosymptomatic hypochondriasis. *Journal of Clinical Psychiatry* 1980 February; **41**, 57–59.

Blacque, O., Leroux, M., 2006. Bardet-Biedl syndrome: an emerging pathomechanism of intracellular transport. *Cellular and Molecular Life Sciences CMLS* **63**(18), 2145–2161.

Bloomfeld, R.S., Graham, B.G., Schiffman, S.S., Killenberg, P.G., 1999. Alterations of chemosensory function in end-stage liver disease. *Physiology & behavior*, **66**, 203–207.

Bolla, K.I., Schwartz, B.S., Stewart, W., et al. 1995. Comparison of neurobehavioral function in workers exposed to a mixture of organic and inorganic lead and in workers exposed to solvents. *American Journal of Industrial Medicine* **27**, 231–246.

Bramerson, A., Nyman, J., Nordin, S., Bende, M. 2013. Olfactory loss after head and neck cancer radiation therapy. *Rhinology* **51** 206–209.

Braun, J.J., Noblet, V., Durand, M., et al. 2014. Olfaction evaluation and correlation with brain atrophy in Bardet-Biedl syndrome. *Clinical Genetics* **86**(6), 521–529.

Brewer, W.J., Edwards, J., Anderson, V., Robinson, T., Pantelis, C., 1996. Neuropsychological, olfactory, and hygiene deficits in men with negative symptom schizophrenia. *Biological Psychiatry* **40**, 1021–1031.

Brewer, W.J., Pantelis, C., Anderson, V., et al. 2001. Stability of olfactory identification deficits in neuroleptic-naive patients with first-episode psychosis. *American Journal of Psychiatry* **158**, 107–115.

Brewer, W.J., Wood, S.J., McGorry, P.D., et al. (2003). Impairment of olfactory identification ability in individuals at ultra-high risk for psychosis who later develop schizophrenia. *American Journal of Psychiatry* **160**, 1790–1794.

Brinckman, D.D., Keppler-Noreuil, K.M., Blumhorst, C., et al. 2013. Cognitive, sensory, and psychosocial characteristics in patients with Bardet–Biedl syndrome. *American Journal of Medical Genetics Part A* **161**(12), 2964–2971.

Brion, M., de Timary, P., Vanderstappen, C., et al. 2015. Chemosensory dysfunction in alcohol-related disorders: A joint exploration of olfaction and taste. *Chemical Senses* **40**(9), 605–608.

Brody, D., Serby, M., Etienne, N., Kalkstein, D.S., 1991. Olfactory identification deficits in HIV infection. *American Journal of Psychiatry* **148**, 248–250.

Brosvic, G.M., Doty, R.L., Rowe, M.M., Harron, A., Kolodiy, N., 1992. Influences of hypothyroidism on the taste detection performance of rats: A signal detection analysis. *Behavioral Neuroscience* **106**, 992–998.

Brosvic, G.M., Risser, J.M., Doty, R.L., 1989. No influence of adrenalectomy on measures of taste sensitivity in the rat. *Physiology & Behavior* **46**, 699–705.

Brosvic, G.M., Risser, J.M., Mackay-Sim, A., Doty, R.L., 1996. Odor detection performance in hypothyroid and euthyroid rats. *Physiology & Behavior* **59**, 117–121.

Brown, A.S., Borgmann-Winter, K., Hahn, C. G., et al. 2014. Increased stability of microtubules in cultured olfactory neuroepithelial cells from individuals with schizophrenia. *Progress in Neuro-Psychopharmacology and Biological Psychiatry* **48**, 252–258.

Brownstein, D.G., 1987. Resistance/susceptibility to lethal Sendai virus infection genetically linked to a mucociliary transport polymorphism. *Journal of Virology*, **61**, 1670–1671.

Buchanan, T.W., Tranel, D., Adolphs, R., 2003. A specific role for the human amygdala in olfactory memory. *Learning & Memory* **10**, 319–325.

Burch, R.E., Sackin, D.A., Ursick, J.A., Jetton, M.M., Sullivan, J.F., 1978. Decreased taste and smell acuity in cirrhosis. *Archives of Internal Medicine* **138**, 743–746.

Burdach, K.J., Doty, R.L., 1987. The effects of mouth movements, swallowing, and spitting on retronasal odor perception. *Physiology & Behavior* **41**, 353–356.

Cain, D.P., 1975. Effects of insulin injection on responses of olfactory bulb and amygdala single units to odors. *Brain Research* **99**, 69–83.

Calderon-Garciduenas, L., 2015. *Influence of Toxins on Olfactory Function and their Potential Association with Neurodegenerative Disease*, Wiley Online Library, pp. 485–510.

Calderon-Garciduenas, L., Franco-Lira, M., Henriquez-Roldan, C., et al. 2010. Urban air pollution: Influences on olfactory function and pathology in exposed children and young adults. *Experimental and Toxicological Pathology* **62**, 91–102.

Calderon-Garciduenas, L., Kavanaugh, M., Block, M., et al. 2012. Neuroinflammation, hyperphosphorylated tau, diffuse amyloid plaques, and down-regulation of the cellular prion protein in air pollution exposed children and young adults. *Journal of Alzheimer's Disease* **28**, 93–107.

Callahan, C.D., Hinkebein, J. 1999. Neuropsychological significance of anosmia following traumatic brain injury. *The Journal of Head Trauma Rehabilitation* **14**, 581–587.

Cameron, E.L., 2007. Measures of human olfactory perception during pregnancy. *Chemical Senses* **32**, 775–782.

Cameron, E.L., 2014. Pregnancy and olfaction: A review. *Frontiers in Psychology* **5**, 67. doi: 10.3389/fpsyg.2014.00067.

Carmichael, K.A., Jennings, A.S., Doty, R.L., 1984. Reversible anosmia after pituitary irradiation. *Annals of Internal Medicine* **100**, 532–533.

Carr, V.M., Robinson, A.M., Kern, R.C., 2012. Tissue-specific effects of allergic rhinitis in mouse nasal epithelia. *Chemical Senses* **37**, 655–668.

Carroll, B., Richardson, J.T., Thompson, P., 1993. Olfactory information processing and temporal lobe epilepsy. *Brain and Cognition* **22**, 230–243.

Chabolla, D.R., 2002. Characteristics of the epilepsies. *Mayo Clinic Proceedings* **77**(9), 981–990.

Chazal, G., Durbec, P., Jankovski, A., Rougon, G., Cremer, H. (2000). Consequences of neural cell adhesion molecule deficiency on cell migration in the rostral migratory stream of the mouse. *The Journal of neuroscience*, **20**, 1446–1457.

Chen, C., Shih, Y., Yen, D., et al. (2003). Olfactory auras in patients with temporal lobe epilepsy. *Epilepsia*, **44**, 257–260.

Chen, S., Tan, H.Y., Wu, Z.H., et al. (2014). Imaging of olfactory bulb and gray matter volumes in brain areas associated with olfactory function in patients with Parkinson's disease and multiple system atrophy. *Eur.J.Radiol.*, **83**, 564–570.

Cheng, S.F., Chen, M.L., Hung, P.C., Chen, C.J., Mao, I.F. (2004). Olfactory loss in poly (acrylonitrile-butadiene-styrene) plastic injection-moulding workers. *Occup.Med.(Lond)*, **54**, 469–474.

Chitanondh, H. (1966). Stereotaxic amygdalotomy in the treatment of olfactory seizures and psychiatric disorders with olfactory hallucination. *Stereotactic and Functional Neurosurgery*, **27**, 181–196.

Coleman, E.R., Grosberg, B.M., Robbins, M.S. (2011). Olfactory hallucinations in primary headache disorders: Case series and literature review. *Cephalalgia*, **31**(14), 1477–1489.

Compton, M.T., Mack, L.M., Esterberg, M.L., et al. (2006). Associations between olfactory identification and verbal memory in patients with schizophrenia, first-degree relatives, and non-psychiatric controls. *Schizophrenia research*, **86**, 154–166.

Conn, F.W., Mast, T.E. (1973). Adrenal insufficiency and electrophysiological measures of auditory sensitivity. *Amer J Physiol*, **225**, 1430–1436.

Conrad, P., Corwin, J., Katz, L., et al. (1987). Olfaction and hemodialysis: baseline and acute treatment decrements. *Nephron*, **47**, 115–118.

Constantinescu, C.S., Raps, E.C., Cohen, J.A., West, S.E., Doty, R.L. (1994). Olfactory disturbances as the initial or most prominent symptom of multiple sclerosis. *Journal of Neurology, Neurosurgery, & Psychiatry* **57**, 1011–1012.

Corcoran, C., Whitaker, A., Coleman, E., et al. (2005). Olfactory deficits, cognition and negative symptoms in early onset psychosis. *Schizophr Res*, **80**, 283–293.

Corletto, E., Dal Zotto, L., Resos, A., et al. (2008). Osmophobia in juvenile primary headaches. *Cephalalgia*, **28**, 825–831.

Correa, M., Laing, D.G., Hutchinson, I., et al. (2015). Reduced taste function and taste papillae density in children with chronic kidney disease. *Pediatr.Nephrol.* **30**, 2003–2010.

Correia, S., Faust, D., Doty, R.L. (2001). A re-examination of the rate of vocational dysfunction among patients with anosmia and mild to moderate closed head injury. *Archives of Clinical Neuropsychology*, **16**, 477–488.

Corwin, J. (1989). Olfactory identification in hemodialysis: acute and chronic effects on discrimination and response bias. *Neuropsychologia*, **27**, 513–522.

Costanzo, M.R., DiNardo, J., Zasler, M.D. (1995). Head injury and olfaction. In: R.L. Doty ed., *Handbook of Olfaction and Gustation*. New York: Marcel Dekker, Inc., pp. 629–638.

Croy, I., Symmank, A., Schellong, J., et al. 2014. Olfaction as a marker for depression in humans. *J.Affect.Disord.* **160**, 80–86.

Cullen, M.R. (1987). Workers with multiple chemical hypersensitivities. *State of the Art Reviews of Occupational Medicine*, **2**, 655–806.

Dalton, P., Cowart, B., Dilks, D., et al. (2003). Olfactory function in workers exposed to styrene in the reinforced-plastics industry. *American Journal of Industrial Medicine* **44**, 1–11.

Dalton, P., Lees, P.S., Gould, M., et al. (2007). Evaluation of long-term occupational exposure to styrene vapor on olfactory function. *Chemical Senses* **32**, 739–747.

Dalton, P.H., Opiekun, R.E., Gould, M., et al. (2010). Chemosensory Loss: Functional Consequences of the World Trade Center Disaster. *Environ.Health Perspect.* **118L**, 1251–2156.

Daniels, C., Gottwald, B., Pause, B.M., et al. (2001). Olfactory event-related potentials in patients with brain tumors. *Clinical Neurophysiology*, **112**, 1523–1530.

D'Cruze, H., Arroll, B., Kenealy, T. (2009) Is intranasal zinc effective and safe for the common cold? A systematic review and meta-analysis. *Journal of Primary Health Care*, **1**(2): 134–139.

Deems, D.A., Doty, R.L., Settle, R.G., et al. (1991). Smell and taste disorders, a study of 750 patients from the University of Pennsylvania Smell and Taste Center. *Archives of Otolaryngology – Head and Neck Surgery*, **117** 519–528.

Deems, R.O., Friedman, M.I., Friedman, L.S., Munoz, S.J., Maddrey, W.C. (1993). Chemosensory function, food preferences and appetite in human liver disease. *Appetite*, **20**, 209–216.

Delank, K.W., Fechner, G. (1996). [Pathophysiology of post-traumatic anosmia]. *Laryngo-rhino-otologie*, **75**, 154–159.

DeLuca, G.C., Joseph, A., George, J., et al. (2014). Olfactory pathology in central nervous system demyelinating diseases. *Brain Pathol.* **25**, 543–551.

Demarquay, G., Royet, J.P., Mick, G., Ryvlin, P. (2008). Olfactory hypersensitivity in migraineurs: A H(2)(15)O-PET study. *Cephalalgia*, **28**, 1069–1080.

Devanand DP, Lee S, Manly J, et al. Olfactory identification deficits and increased mortality in the community. *Annals of Neurology* 2015; **78** (3): 401–11.

Dominguez, R.A. & Puig, A. (1997). Olfactory reference syndrome responds to clomipramine but not fluoxetine: a case report. *Journal of Clinical Psychiatry* Nov; **58**, 497–498.

Doty, R.L. (1995). *The Smell Identification Test™ Administration Manual – 3rd Edition*. Haddon Hts., NJ: Sensonics, Inc.

Doty, R.L. (2014). Neurotoxic exposure and impairment of the chemical senses of taste and smell. *Handbook of Clinical Neurology*, **131**, 299–324.

Doty, R.L. (2015). Clinical disorders of olfaction. In: R.L. Doty (Ed.), *Handbook of Olfaction and Gustation*. 3rd edition. Hoboken, N.J., John Wiley & Sons, pp. 375–402.

Doty, R.L. (2017). Olfactory dysfunction in neurodegenerative diseases: Is there a common pathological substrate? *Lancet Neurology*, **16**, 478–488.

Doty, R.L., Bromley, S.M. (2004). Effects of drugs on olfaction and taste. *Otolaryngologic Clinics of North America*, **37**(6), 1229–1254.

Doty, R.L., Cameron, E.L. (2009). Sex differences and reproductive hormone influences on human odor perception. *Physiology & Behavior* **97**, 213–228.

Doty, R.L., Deems, D.A., Frye, R.E., Pelberg, R., Shapiro, A. (1988). Olfactory sensitivity, nasal resistance, and autonomic function in patients with multiple chemical sensitivities. *Archives of Otolaryngology – Head & Neck Surgery*, **114**, 1422–1427.

Doty, R.L., Haxel, B.R. (2005). Objective Assessment of Terbinafine-Induced Taste Loss. *The Laryngoscope*, **115**(11), 2035–2037.

Doty, R.L., Li, C., Mannon, L.J., Yousem, D.M. (1998). Olfactory dysfunction in multiple sclerosis. Relation to plaque load in inferior frontal and temporal lobes. *Annals of the New York Academy of Sciences* **855**, 781–786.

Doty, R.L., Li, C., Mannon, L.J., Yousem, D. M. (1999). Olfactory dysfunction in multiple sclerosis: relation to longitudinal changes in plaque numbers in central olfactory structures. *Neurology*, **53**, 880–882.

Doty, R.L., Risser, J.M., Brosvic, G.M. (1991). Influence of adrenalectomy on the odor detection performance of rats. *Physiology & Behavior* **49**, 1273–1277.

Doty, R.L., Shah, M., Bromley, S.M. (2008). Drug-induced taste disorders. *Drug Safety*, **31**(3), 199–215.

Doty, R.L., Shaman, P., Applebaum, S.L., et al. (1984). Smell identification ability: changes with age. *Science*, **226**, 1441–1443.

Doty, R.L., Tourbier, I.A., Silas, J., et al. (2017). Influences of temporal lobe epilepsy and temporal lobe resection on olfactory function. *Submitted*.

Doty, R.L., Berman, A.H., Izhar, M., et al. (2014). Influenza vaccinations and chemosensory function. *American Journal of Rhinology & Allergy*, **28**, 50–53.

Doty, R.L., Fernandez, A.D., Levine, M.A., Moses, A., McKeown, D.A. (1997). Olfactory Dysfunction in Type I Pseudohypoparathyroidism: Dissociation from Gs+¦ Protein Deficiency 1. *The Journal of Clinical Endocrinology & Metabolism*, **82**, 247–250.

Doty, R.L., Frye, R. (1989). Influence of nasal obstruction on smell function. *Otolaryngol Clin North Am*, **22**, 397–411.

Doty, R.L., Shaman, P., Dann, M. (1984). Development of the University of Pennsylvania Smell Identification Test: a standardized microencapsulated test of olfactory function. *Physiology & Behavior (Monograph)* **32**, 489–502.

Doty, R.L., Snyder, P.J., Huggins, G.R., Lowry, L.D. (1981). Endocrine, cardiovascular, and psychological correlates of olfactory sensitivity changes during the human menstrual cycle. *Journal of comparative and physiological psychology*, **95**, 45.

Doty, R.L., Tourbier, I., Ng, V., et al. (2015). Influences of hormone replacement therapy on olfactory and cognitive function in postmenopausal women. *Neurobiology of aging*, **36**, 2053–2059.

Doty, R.L., Yousem, D.M., Pham, L.T., et al. (1997). Olfactory dysfunction in patients with head trauma. *Archives of Neurology*, **54**, 1131–1140.

Ebert, U., Loscher, W. (2000). Strong olfactory stimulation reduces seizure susceptibility in amygdala-kindled rats. *Neuroscience Letters*, **287**, 199–202.

Ellis, H., Webb, T., Warren, D., Jung, A. (2012). Teaching NeuroImages: MRI changes in superficial siderosis. *Neurology*, **78**, e116.

Elsberg, C.A. (1935a). The sense of smell. XII. The localization of tumors of the frontal lobe of the brain by quantitative olfactory tests. *Bull. Neurol. Inst. N.Y.*, **4**, 535–543.

Elsberg, C.A. (1935b). The sense of smell XI, the value of quantitative olfactory tests for the localization of supratentorial tumors of the brain: a preliminary report. *Bull Neurol Inst NY*, **4**, 511–522.

Eskenazi, B., Cain, W.S., Novelly, R.A., Friend, K.B. (1983). Olfactory functioning in temporal lobectomy patients. *Neuropsychologia.*, 1983; **21**, 365–374.

Eskenazi, B., Cain, W.S., Novelly, R.A., Mattson, R. (1986). Odor perception in temporal lobe epilepsy patients with and without temporal lobectomy. *Neuropsychologia*, **24**, 553–562.

Fadool, D.A., Tucker, K., Perkins, R., et al. (2004). Kv1. 3 channel gene-targeted deletion produces G Super-Smeller MiceGÇØ with altered glomeruli, interacting scaffolding proteins, and biophysics. *Neuron*, **41**, 389–404.

Feron, F., Perry, C., Hirning, M.H., McGrath, J., & Mackay-Sim, A. (1999). Altered adhesion, proliferation and death in neural cultures from adults with schizophrenia. *Schizophrenia Research*, **40**, 211–218.

Fearnley, J.M., Stevens, J.M., Rudge, P. (1995). Superficial siderosis of the central nervous system. *Brain*, **118**, 1051–1066.

Fedoroff, I.C., Stoner, S.A., Andersen, A.E., Doty, R.L., Rolls, B.J. (1995). Olfactory dysfunction in anorexia and bulimia nervosa. *International Journal of Eating Disorders*, **18**, 71–77.

Fiser, D.J., Borotski, L. (1978). [Anosmia after administration of influenza vaccine]. *Medicinski pregled*, **32**, 455–457.

Fish, D. R., Gloor, P., Quesney, F. L., Oliver, A. (1993). Clinical responses to electrical brain stimulation of the temporal and frontal lobes in patients with epilepsy. *Brain*, **116**, 397–414.

Frasnelli, J.A., Temmel, A.F., Quint, C., Oberbauer, R., Hummel, T. (2002). Olfactory function in chronic renal failure. *American Journal of Rhinology.*, **16**, 275–279.

Friberg, L. (1950). Health hazards in the manufacture of akaline accumulators with special reference to chronic cadmium poisoning. *Acta Med Scand*, **138**, 1–124.

Frye, R.E., Doty, R.L. (1992). The influence of ultradian autonomic rhythms, as indexed by the nasal cycle, on unilateral olfactory thresholds. In Doty, R.L., and Muller-Schwarze, D. *Chemical Signals in Vertebrates VI*. New York: Plenum Press, pp. 595–598.

Fuller, G.N., Guiloff, R.J. (1987). Migrainous olfactory hallucinations. *Journal of Neurology, Neurosurgery, and Psychiatry*, **50**, 1688.

Furstenberg, A.C., Crosby, E., Farrior, B. (1943). Neurologic lesions which influence the sense of smell. *Archives of Otolaryngology*, **48** 529–530.

Furuta, S., Nishimoto, K., Egawa, M., Ohyama, M., Moriyama, H. (1994). Olfactory dysfunction in patients with Minamata disease. *American Journal of Rhinology* **8**, 259–263.

Gambelli, S., Ginanneschi, F., Malandrini, A., et al. (2004). Antibodies to dorsal root ganglia and olfactory cells in a patient with chronic sensory neuropathy and anosmia. *Journal of the Neurological Sciences*, **221**, 105–108.

Garrett-Laster, M., Russell, R.M., Jacques, P.F. (1984). Impairment of taste and olfaction in patients with cirrhosis: The role of vitamin A. *Human Nutrition. Clinical Nutrition*, **38**, 203–214.

Gascon, C., Santaolalla, F., Martinez, A., Sanchez Del, R.A. (2013). Usefulness of the BAST-24 smell and taste test in the study of diabetic patients: a new approach to the determination of renal function. *Acta Otolaryngologica* **133**, 400–404.

Gibberd, F., Feher, M., Sidey, M., Wierzbicki, A. (2004). Smell testing: An additional tool for identification of adult Refsum's disease. Journal of Neurology, *Neurosurgery & Psychiatry*, **75**(9), 1334–1336.

Gilbert, A.N. (1989). Reciprocity versus rhythmicity in spontaneous alternations of nasal airflow. *Chronobiology international*, **6**, 251–257.

Giuseffi, V., Wall, M., Siegel, P.Z., Rojas, P.B. (1991). Symptoms and Disease Associations in Idiopathic Intracranial Hypertension (Pseudotumor Cerebri) – A Case-Control Study. *Neurology*, **41**, 239–244.

Goektas, O., Schmidt, F., Bohner, G., et al. (2011). Olfactory bulb volume and olfactory function in patients with multiple sclerosis. *Rhinology*, **49**, 221–226.

Good, K. P., Tibbo, P., Milliken, H., et al. (2010). An investigation of a possible relationship between olfactory identification deficits at first episode and four-year outcomes in patients with psychosis. *Schizophrenia Research*, **124**, 60–65.

Good, K.P., Tourbier, I.A., Moberg, P., et al. (2017). Unilateral olfactory sensitivity in multiple sclerosis. *Physiology & Behavior*, **168**, 24 30.

Gopinath B, Anstey KJ, Kifley A, Mitchell P. (2012). Olfactory impairment is associated with functional disability and reduced independence among older adults. *Maturitas.*, **72**: 50–5.

Gordon, A.S., Moran, D.T., Jafek, B.W. Eller, P. M., Strahan, R.C. (1990). The effect of chronic cocaine abuse on human olfaction. *Archives of Otolaryngology-Head & Neck Surgery*, **116**(12), 1415–1418.

Gouveri, E., Katotomichelakis, M., Gouveris, H., et al. (2014). Olfactory dysfunction in type 2 diabetes mellitus: an additional manifestation of microvascular disease? *Angiology*, **65**, 869–876.

Graham, C.S., Graham, B.G., Bartlett, J.A., Heald, A.E., Schiffman, S.S. (1995). Taste and smell losses in HIV infected patients. *Physiology & Behavior* **58**, 287–293.

Grashow, R., Sparrow, D., Hu, H., Weisskopf, M.G. (2015). Cumulative lead exposure is associated with reduced olfactory recognition performance in elderly men: The Normative Aging Study. *Neurotoxicology*, **49**, 158–164.

Grapsa, E., Samouilidou, E., Pandelias, K., et al. (2010). Correlation of depressive symptoms and olfactory dysfunction in patients on hemodialysis. *Hippokratia.*, **14**, 189–192.

Gregson, R.A., Free, M.L., Abbott, M.W. (1981). Olfaction in Korsakoffs, alcoholics and normals. *British Journal of Clinical Psychology*, **20**, 3–10.

Griep, M.I., Van, d. N., Sennesael, J.J., Mets, T.F., et al. (1997). Odour perception in chronic renal disease. *Nephrology, Dialysis, Transplantation*, **12**, 2093–2098.

Gross-Isseroff, R., Luca-Haimovici, K., Sasson, Y., et al. 1994. Olfactory sensitivity in major depressive disorder and obsessive compulsive disorder. *Biological Psychiatry* **35**, 798–802.

Gudziol, V., Pietsch, J., Witt, M., Hummel, T. (2010). Theophylline induces changes in the electro-olfactogram of the mouse. *European Archives of Oto-Rhino-Laryngology* **267**, 239–243.

Guthoff, M., Tschritter, O., Berg, D., et al. (2009). Effect of genetic variation in Kv1. 3 on olfactory function. *Diabetes/metabolism research and reviews*, **25**, 523–527.

Halgren, E. (1981). Mental phenomena induced by stimulation in the limbic system. *Human neurobiology*, **1**, 251–260.

Hamilos, D.L. (2000). Chronic sinusitis. *Journal of Allergy and Clinical Immunology*, **106**, 213–227.

Hardy, C., Rosedale, M., Messinger, J.W., et al. (2012). Olfactory acuity is associated with mood and function in a pilot study of stable bipolar disorder patients. *Bipolar. Disord.*, **14**, 109–117.

Hart, C.K., Theodosopoulos, P.V., Zimmer, L.A. (2010). Olfactory changes after endoscopic pituitary tumor resection. *Otolaryngology – Head and Neck Surgery* **142**, 95–97.

Hawkes, C.H., Shephard, B.C., Kobal, G. (1997). Assessment of olfaction in multiple sclerosis: evidence of dysfunction by olfactory evoked response and identification tests. *Journal of Neurology, Neurosurgery, & Psychiatry* **63**, 145–151.

Heinrichs, L. (2002). Linking olfaction with nausea and vomiting of pregnancy, recurrent abortion, hyperemesis gravidarum, and migraine headache. *American journal of obstetrics and gynecology*, **186**, S215–S219.

Henkin, R.I. (1967). Abnormalities of taste and olfaction in patients with chromatin negative gonadal dysgenesis. *Journal of Clinical Endocrinology & Metabolism*, **27**, 1436–1440.

Henkin, R.I., Bartter, F.C. (1966). Studies on olfactory thresholds in normal man and in patients with adrenal cortical insufficiency: the role of adrenal cortical steroids and of serum sodium concentration. *J.Clin.Invest*, **45**, 1631–1639.

Henkin, R.I., Talal, N., Larson, A.L., Mattern, C.F.T. (1972). Abnormalities of taste and smell in Sjogren's syndrome. *Annals of Internal Medicine*, **76**, 375–383.

Henkin, R., Smith, F.R. (1971). Hyposmia in acute viral hepatitis. *The Lancet*, **297**, 823–826.

González-Botas, H., Seara, Padin (2012). Nasal gel and olfactory cleft. *Acta Otorrinolaringol. Esp.* **63**: 370–375.

Hill, J.M., Lesniak, M.A., Pert, C.B., Roth, J. (1986). Autoradiographic Localization of Insulin-Receptors in Rat-Brain – Prominence in Olfactory and Limbic Areas. *Neurosci*, **17**, 1127–1138.

Hirsch, A.R. (1992). Olfaction in migraineurs. *Headache*, **32**, 233–236.

Hisamitsu, M., Okamoto, Y., Chazono, H., et al. (2011). The influence of environmental exposure to formaldehyde in nasal mucosa of medical students during cadaver dissection. *Allergol.Int.*, **60**, 373–379.

Ho, W.K., Kwong, D.L., Wei, W.I., Sham, J.S. (2002). Change in olfaction after radiotherapy for nasopharyngeal cancerGÇöa prospective study. *American journal of otolaryngology*, **23**, 209–214.

Hoffman, H.J., Ishii, E.K., Macturk, R.H. (1998). AgeGÇÉRelated Changes in the Prevalence of Smell/Taste Problems among the United States Adult Population: Results of the 1994 Disability Supplement to the National Health Interview Survey (NHIS). *Annals of the New York Academy of Sciences* **855**, 716–722.

Holinski, F., Schmidt, F., Dahlslett, S.B., et al. (2014). MRI Study: Objective olfactory function and CNS pathologies in patients with multiple sclerosis. *European Neurology*, **72**(3–4), 157–162.

Holscher, T., Seibt, A., Appold, S., et al. (2005). Effects of radiotherapy on olfactory function. *Radiotherapy and Oncology*, **77**, 157–163.

Hornung, D.E., Kurtz, D.B., Bradshaw, C.B., et al. (1998). The olfactory loss that accompanies an HIV infection. *Physiology & Behavior* **64**, 549–556.

Hua, M.S., Chen, S.T., Tang, L.M., Leung, W.M. (1999). Olfactory function in patients with nasopharygeal carcinoma following radiotherapy. *Brain Injury*, **13**, 905–915.

Hudry, J., Perrin, F., Ryvlin, P., Mauguiere, F., Royet, J.P. (2003). Olfactory short-term memory and related amygdala recordings in patients with temporal lobe epilepsy. *Brain.*, **126**, 1851–1863.

Hudson, R., Arriola, A., Martinez-Gomez, M., Distel, H. (2006). Effect of air pollution on olfactory function in residents of Mexico City. *Chemical Senses*, **31**, 79–85.

Hughes, L.F., McAsey, M.E., Donathan, C.L., et al. (2002). Effects of hormone replacement therapy on olfactory sensitivity: cross-sectional and longitudinal studies. *Climacteric.*, **5**, 140–150.

Hummel, T., Roscher, S., Jaumann, M.P., Kobal, G. (1996). Intranasal chemoreception in patients with multiple chemical sensitivities: a double-blind investigation. *Regulatory Toxicology & Pharmacology*, **24**, S79–S86.

Jackson, J.H., and Beever, C.E. (1890). Case of tumor of the right temporo-sphenoidal lobe bearing on the localization of the sense of smell. *Brain*, **12**, 346.

Jafek, B.W., Gordon, A.S., Moran, D.T., Eller, P.M. (1990). Congenital anosmia. *ENT J*, **69**, 331–337.

Jafek, B.W., Eller, P.M., Esses, B.A., Moran, D.T. (1989). Post-traumatic anosmia: Ultrastructural correlates. *Archives of Neurology*, **46**, 300–304.

Jafek, B.W., Linschoten, M.R., Murrow, B.W. (2004). Anosmia after intranasal zinc gluconate use. *American journal of rhinology*, **18**(3), 137–141

Jaseja, H. (2008). Scientific basis behind traditional practice of application of "shoe-smell" in controlling epileptic seizures in the eastern countries. *Clinical Neurology and Neurosurgery*, **110**, 535–538.

Johnson, V.E., Stewart, W., Smith, D.H. (2013). Axonal pathology in traumatic brain injury. *Experimental neurology*, **246**, 35–43.

Johnston, M., Zakharov, A., Papaiconomou, C., Salmasi, G., Armstrong, D. (2004). Evidence of connections between cerebrospinal fluid and nasal lymphatic vessels in humans, non-human primates and other mammalian species. *Cerebrospinal Fluid Res*, **1**, 1–13.

Jones, B.P., Butters, N., Moskowitz, H.R., Montgomery, K. (1978). Olfactory and gustatory capacities of alcoholic Korsakoff patients. *Neuropsychologia.*, **16**, 323–337.

Jones, B.P., Moskowitz, H.R., Butters, N., Glosser, G. (1975). Psychophysical scaling of olfactory, visual, and auditory stimuli by alchoholic Korsakoff patients. *Neuropsychologia*, **13**, 387–393.

Jones, B.P., Moskowitz, H.R., Butters, N. (1975). Olfactory discrimination in alcoholic Korsakoff patients. *Neuropsychologia*, **13**, 173–179.

Jones-Gotman, M., Zatorre, R.J. (1988). Olfactory identification deficits in patients with focal cerebral excision. *Neuropsychologia*, **26**, 387–400.

Kahilogullari, G., Beton, S., Al-Beyati, E.S., et al. (2013). Olfactory functions after transsphenoidal pituitary surgery: endoscopic versus microscopic approach. *Laryngoscope*, **123**, 2112–2119.

Kale, S.U., Donaldson, I., West, R.J., Shehu, A. (2003). Superficial siderosis of the meninges and its otolaryngologic connection: a series of five patients. *Otology & Neurotology*, **24**, 90 95.

Kallmann, F.J., Schoenfeld, W.A., Barrera, S.E. (1944). The genetic aspects of primary eunuchoidism. *Am J Ment Defic*, **48**, 203–236.

Kamath, V., Bedwell, J.S., Compton, M.T. (2011). Is the odour identification deficit in schizophrenia influenced by odour hedonics? *Cogn Neuropsychiatry*, **16**, 448–460.

Kamel, U.F., Maddison, P., Whitaker, R. (2009). Impact of primary Sj+Ägren's syndrome on smell and taste: Effect on quality of life. *Rheumatology*, **48**, 1512–1514.

Kapoor, K.G. (2008). Do patients with idiopathic intracranial hypertension suffer from hyposmia? *Med.Hypotheses*, **71**, 816–817.

Kay, S.R., Fiszbein, A., Opler, L.A. (1987). The positive and negative syndrome scale (PANSS) for schizophrenia. *Schizophr. Bull.*, **13**, 261–276.

Kelman, L. (2004a). Osmophobia and taste abnormality in migraineurs: A tertiary care study. *Headache: The Journal of Head and Face Pain*, **44**, 1019–1023.

Kelman, L. (2004b). The premonitory symptoms (prodrome): A tertiary care study of 893 migraineurs. *Headache: The Journal of Head and Face Pain*, **44**, 865–872.

Kern, R.C. (2000). Chronic sinusitis and snosmia: Pathologic vhanges in the olfactory mucosa. *Laryngoscope*, **110**, 1071–1077.

Keshavan, M.S., Vora, A., Montrose, D., Diwadkar, V.A., Sweeney, J. (2009). Olfactory identification in young relatives at risk for schizophrenia. *Acta Neuropsychiatrica*, **21**, 121–124.

Kesslak, J.P., Cotman, C.W., Chui, H.C., et al. (1988). Olfactory tests as possible probes for detecting and monitoring Alzheimer's disease. *Neurobiol. Aging*, **9**, 399–403.

Kim, J.H., Jeon, H.W., Woo, E.J., Park, H.M. (2009). Dilation of the olfactory bulb cavity concurrent with hydrocephalus in four small breed dogs. *J Vet. Sci.*, **10**, 173–175.

Kitamura, F., Yokoyama, K., Araki, S., et al. (2003). Increase of olfactory threshold in plating factory workers exposed to chromium in Korea. *Ind. Health*, **41**, 279–285.

Klingmuller, D., Dewes, W., Krahe, T., Brecht, G., Schweikert, H.U. (1987). Magnetic resonance imaging of the brain in patients with anosmia and hypothalamic hypogonadism (Kallmann's syndrome). *Journal of Clinical Endocrinology & Metabolism*, September; **65**, 581–584.

Konstantinidis, I., Haehner, A., Frasnelli, J., et al. (2006). Post-infectious olfactory dysfunction exhibits a seasonal pattern. *Rhinology*, **44**, 135–139.

Kopala, L.C., Clark, C., Hurwitz, T. (1993). Olfactory deficits in neuroleptic naive patients with schizophrenia. *Schizophrenia Research*, **8**, 245–250.

Kopala, L.C., Good, K.P., Morrison, K., et al. (2001). Impaired olfactory identification in relatives of patients with familial schizophrenia. *American Journal of Psychiatry*, **158**(8): 1286–1290.

Kopala, L.C., Good, K.P., Torry, E.F., Honer, W.G. (1998). Olfactory function in monozygotic twins discordant for schizophrenia. *American Journal of Psychiatry*, **155**, 134.

Korytowska, A., Szmeja, Z. (1993). [Smell and taste in patients with chronic renal failure treated by hemodialysis]. *Otolaryngologia Polska*, **47**, 144–152.

Kosten, T., Contreras, R.J. (1985). Adrenalectomy reduces peripheral neural responses to gustatory stimuli in the rat. *Behavioral Neuroscience* August; **99**, 734–741.

Kramer, G. (1983). [Diagnosis of neurologic disorders after whiplash injuries of the cervical spine]. *Deutsche medizinische Wochenschrift (1946)*, **108**, 586–588.

Kruger, S., Frasnelli, J., Braunig, P., Hummel, T. (2006). Increased olfactory sensitivity in euthymic patients with bipolar disorder with event-related episodes compared with patients with bipolar disorder without such episodes. *J Psychiat Neurosci*, **31**, 263–270.

Kulaga, H.M., Leitch, C.C., Eichers, E.R., et al. (2004). Loss of BBS proteins causes anosmia in humans and defects in olfactory cilia structure and function in the mouse. *Nature genetics*, **36**(9), 994–998.

Kundoor V, Dalby RN. Assessment of nasal spray deposition pattern in avsilicone human nose model using a color-based method. *Pharm Res*. 2010 **27**(1), 30–36.

Kunte, H., Schmidt, F., Kronenberg, G., et al. (2013). Olfactory dysfunction in patients with idiopathic intracranial hypertension. *Neurology* **81**, 379–382.

Kwapil, T.R., Chapman, J.P., Chapman, L.J., Miller, M.B. (1996). Deviant olfactory experiences as indicators of risk for psychosis. *Schizophr Bull*, **22**, 371–382.

Landis, B.N., Marangon, N., Saudan, P., et al. (2011). Olfactory function improves following hemodialysis. *Kidney Int.*, **80**, 886–893.

Le Floch JP, Le Lièvre G, Labroue M, et al. Smell dysfunction and related factors in diabetic patients. *Diabetes Care*. 1993; **16**(6),934–7.

Lee, J., Tucker, R.M., Tan, S.Y., et al. (2015). Nutritional implications of taste and smell dysfunction. In R.L. Doty (Ed.), *Handbook of Olfaction and Gustation*. New York: John Wiley & Sons, Inc., pp. 833–865.

Lee, J.S., Choi, J.C., Kang, S.Y., et al. (2010). Olfactory identification deficits in cerebral autosomal dominant arteriopathy with subcortical infarcts and leukoencephalopathy. *European Neurology* **64**, 280–285.

Lee, R.J., Xiong, G., Kofonow, J.M., et al. (2012). T2R38 taste receptor polymorphisms underlie susceptibility to upper respiratory infection. *Journal of Clinical investigation*, **122**, 4145–4159.

Lee, S.J., Yoo, H.J., Park, S.W., Choi, M.G. (2004). A case of cystic lymphocytic hypophysitis with cacosmia and hypopituitarism. *Endocrine Journal*, 51, 375–380.

Leibowitz, S. (1949). Distaste for smoking; an early symptom in virus hepatitis. *The Review of Gastroenterology*, 16, 721.

Leigh, A.D. (1943). Defects of smell after head injury. *Lancet*, 1, 38–40.

Leon-Sarmiento, F.E., Bayona, E.A., Bayona-Prieto, J., Osman, A., & Doty, R.L. (2012). Profound olfactory dysfunction in myasthenia gravis. *PLoS One*, 7, e45544.

Leon-Sarmiento, F.E., Leon-Ariza, D.S., Doty, R. L. (2013). Dysfunctional chemosensation in myasthenia gravis: a systematic review. *J.Clin. Neuromuscul. Dis.*, 15, 1–6.

Lehrner, J., Baumgartner, C., Serles, W., Olbrich, A., Pataraia, E., Bacher, J., Aull, S., Deecke, L. (1997). Olfactory prodromal symptoms and unilateral olfactory dysfunction are associated in patients with right mesial temporal lobe epilepsy. *Epilepsia*. 38(9): 1042–1044.

Lewandowski, K.E., DePaola, J., Camsari, G.B., Cohen, B.M., Ongur, D. (2009). Tactile, olfactory, and gustatory hallucinations in psychotic disorders: a descriptive study. *Ann. Acad. Med. Singapore*, 38, 383–385.

Lewitt, M.S., Laing, D.G., Panhuber, H., Corbett, A., Carter, J.N. (1989). Sensory perception and hypothyroidism. *Chemical Senses*, 14, 537–546.

Lewkowitz-Shpuntoff, H.M., Hughes, V.A., Plummer, L., et al. (2012). Olfactory Phenotypic Spectrum in Idiopathic Hypogonadotropic Hypogonadism: Pathophysiological and Genetic Implications. *Journal of Clinical Endocrinology & Metabolism*, 97, E136–E144.

Lim JH, Davis GE, Wang Z, et al. (2009). Zicam-induced damage to mouse and human nasal tissue. *PLoS One*, 4(10): e7647.

Litvack, J.R., Fong, K., Mace, J., James, K.E., Smith, T.L. (2008). Predictors of olfactory dysfunction in patients with chronic rhinosinusitis. *The Laryngoscope*, 118, 2225–2230.

Lombion-Pouthier, S., Vandel, P., Nezelof, S., Haffen, E., Millot, J.L., 2006. Odor perception in patients with mood disorders. *J. Affect. Disord.* 90, 187–191

London, B., Nabet, B., Fisher, A.R., et al. (2008). Predictors of prognosis in patients with olfactory disturbance. *Annals of Neurology*, 63, 159–166.

Lucchini, R., Bergamaschi, E., Smargiassi, A., Festa, D., Apostoli, P. (1997). Motor function, olfactory threshold, and hematological indices in manganese-exposed ferroalloy workers. [erratum appears in Environ Res 1997 Nov;75 (2):187]. *Environmental Research.*, 73, 175–180.

Lumsden, C.E. (1983). The neuropathology of multiple sclerosis. In Vinken PJ and Bruyn GW (eds.), *Handbook of Clinical Neurology*, Amsterdam: Elsevier, 217–309.

Lundstrom, J.N., Hummel, T., Olsson, M.J. (2003). Individual differences in sensitivity to the odor of 4, 16-androstadien-3-one. *Chemical Senses*, 28, 643–650.

Lutterotti, A., Vedovello, M., Reindl, M., et al. (2011). Olfactory threshold is impaired in early, active multiple sclerosis. *Multiple Sclerosis Journal*, 17, 964–969

Luzzi, S., Snowden, J.S., Neary, D., et al. (2007). Distinct patterns of olfactory impairment in Alzheimer's disease, semantic dementia, frontotemporal dementia, and corticobasal degeneration. *Neuropsychologia*, 45, 1823–1831.

Mackay-Sim, A., Beard, M.D. (1987). Hypothyroidism disrupts neural development in the olfactory epithelium of adult mice. *Brain Research* 433, 190–198.

Maione, L., Benadjaoud, S., Eloit, C., et al. (2013). Computed tomography of the anterior skull base in Kallmann syndrome reveals specific ethmoid bone abnormalities associated with olfactory bulb defects. *The Journal of Clinical Endocrinology and Metabolism* 98, E537–E546.

Mair, R., Capra, C., McEntee, W.J., Engen, T. (1980). Odor discrimination and memory in Korsakoff's psychosis. *Journal of Experimental Psychology: Human Perception & Performance*, 6, 445–458.

Mair, R.G., Doty, R.L., Kelly, K.M., et al. (1986). Multimodal sensory discrimination deficits in Korsakoff's psychosis. *Neuropsychologia*, 24, 831–839.

Malaspina, D., Coleman, E. (2003). Olfaction and social drive in schizophrenia. *Archives of General Psychiatry*, 60, 578–584.

Malaspina, D., Coleman, E., Goetz, R.R., et al. (2002). Odor identification, eye tracking and deficit syndrome schizophrenia. *Biological Psychiatry*, **51**, 809–815.

Mao, Z., Yin, J., Lu, Z., Hu, X. (2015). Association between myasthenia gravis and cognitive function: A systematic review and meta-analysis. *Annals of Indian Academy of Neurology*, **18**(2), 131.

Marmura, M.J., Monteith, T.S., Anjum, W., et al. (2014). Olfactory function in migraine both during and between attacks. *Cephalalgia* **34**: 977–985.

Marshall, B.A., Permutt, M.A., Paciorkowski, A.R., et al. (2013). Phenotypic characteristics of early Wolfram syndrome. *Orphanet. J. Rare. Dis.*, **8**, 64.

Martzke, J.S., Swan, C.S., Varney, N.R. (1991). Post-traumatic anosmia and orbital frontal damage: Neuropsychological and Neuropsychiatric correlates. *Neuropsychology*, **5**, 213.

Mascagni, P., Consonni, D., Bregante, G., Chiappino, G., Toffoletto, F. (2003). Olfactory function in workers exposed to moderate airborne cadmium levels. *Neurotoxicology*, **24**, 717–724.

Mattes, R.D., Heller, A.D., Rivlin, R.S. (1986). Abnormalities in suprathreshold taste function in early hypothyroidism in humans. In H.L. Meiselman & R. S. Rivlin (Eds.), *Clinical Measurement of Taste and Smell* (pp. 467–486). New York: Macmillan Publishing Company.

McCaffrey, R.J., Duff, K., Solomon, G.S. (2000). Olfactory dysfunction discriminates probable Alzheimer's dementia from major depression: a cross-validation and extension. *J Neuropsychiat ClinNeurosci*, **12**, 29–33.

McCarrison, R. (1918). The effects of deprivation of "B" accessory food factors. *Indian J. Med. Research*, 19.

McConnell, R.J., Menendez, C.E., Smith, F.R., Henkin, R.I., Rivlin, R.S. (1975). Defects of taste and smell in patients with hypothyroidism. *Am J Med*, **59**, 354–364.

McCurdy, R.D., F+®ron, F., Perry, C., et al. (2006). Cell cycle alterations in biopsied olfactory neuroepithelium in schizophrenia and bipolar I disorder using cell culture and gene expression analyses. *Schizophrenia research*, **82**, 163–173.

McDonald, W.I. (1986). The mystery of the origin of multiple sclerosis. *J Neurol Neurosurg Psych*, **49**, 113–123.

Meats, P. (1988). Olfactory hallucinations. *British medical journal (Clinical research ed.)*, **296**, 645.

Menashe, I., Abaffy, T., Hasin, Y, et al. (2007). Genetic elucidation of human hyperosmia to isovaleric acid. *PLoS Biol*, **5**, e284.

Mendez, M.F., Ghajarnia, M. (2001). Agnosia for familiar faces and odors in a patient with right temporal lobe dysfunction. *Neurology*, **57**, 519–521.

Mergler, D., Huel, G., Bowler, R., et al. (1994). Nervous system dysfunction among workers with long-term exposure to manganese. *Environmental Research*, **64**, 151–180.

Mester, A.F., Doty, R.L., Shapiro, A., Frye, R.E. (1988). Influence of body tilt within the sagittal plane on odor identification performance. *Aviation, Space, and Environmental Medicine.* **59**: 734–737.

Miller, C.S. (2003). Multiple chemical intolerance. In R.L. Doty (Ed.), *Handbook of Olfaction and Gustation*. New York: Marcel Dekker, pp. 525–547.

Miller, C.S. & Mitzel, H.C. (1995). Chemical sensitivity attributed to pesticide exposure versus remodeling. *Archives of Environmental Health* **50**, 119–129.

Mirza, N., Kroger, H., Doty, R.L. (1997). Influence of age on the nasal cycle. *Laryngoscope*, **107**, 62–66.

Mishra, A., Saito, K., Barbash, S.E., Mishra, N., Doty, R.L. (2006). Olfactory dysfunction in leprosy. *Laryngoscope*, **116**, 413–416.

Moberg, P.J., Arnold, S.E., Doty, R.L., et al. (2006). Olfactory functioning in schizophrenia: relationship to clinical, neuropsychological, and volumetric MRI measures. *Journal of Clinical Experimental Neuropsychology* **28**, 1444–1461.

Moberg, P.J., Doty, R.L., Turetsky, B.I., et al. (1997). Olfactory identification deficits in schizophrenia: correlation with duration of illness. *Amer J Psychiat*, **154**, 1016–1018.

Moberg, P.J., Roalf, D., Gur, R.E., Turetsky, B.I. (2004). Smaller nasal volumes as stigmata of aberrant neurodevelopment in schizophrenia. *Am. J. Psychiat.* **161**, 2314–2316.

Moran, D.T., Jafek, B.W., Eller, P.M., Rowley, J.C. (1992). Ultrastructural histopathology of human olfactory dysfunction. *Microsc. Res. Techn.* **23**, 103–110.

Mourad, I., Lejoyeux, M., Ades, J. (1997). [Prospective evaluation of antidepressant discontinuation]. *L'Encephale*, **24**, 215–222.

Mueller, A., Reuner, U., Landis, B., et al. (2006). Extrapyramidal symptoms in Wilson's disease are associated with olfactory dysfunction. *Movement Disorders* **21**, 1311–1316.

Mueller, C., Temmel, A.F.P., Quint, C., Rieger, A., Hummel, T. (2002). Olfactory function in HIV-positive subjects. *Acta Otolaryngologica (Stockh)*, **122**, 67–71.

Murphy, C., Schubert, C.R., Cruickshanks, K.J., et al. (2002). Prevalence of olfactory impairment in older adults. *JAMA*, **288**, 2307–2312.

Mygind, N., Pedersen, M. (1982). Nose-, sinus- and ear-symptoms in 27 patients with primary ciliary dyskinesia. *European Journal of Respiratory Diseases. Supplement*, **127**, 96–101.

Naka, A., Riedl, M., Luger, A., Hummel, T., Mueller, C.A. (2010). Clinical significance of smell and taste disorders in patients with diabetes mellitus. *Eur Arch Oto-Rhino-Laryngology*, **267**, 547–550.

Naus, A. (1975). *Olphactoric properties of industrial matters*. Prague: Charles University.

Negoias, S., Croy, I., Gerber, J., et al. (2010). Reduced olfactory bulb volume and olfactory sensitivity in patients with acute major depression. *Neuroscience*, **169**(1): 415–421.

O'Sullivan, R.L., Mansueto, C.S., Lerner, E.A., Miguel, E.C. (2000). Characterization of trichotillomania. A phenomenological model with clinical relevance to obsessive-compulsive spectrum disorders. *Psychiatric Clinics of North America*, September; **23**, 587–604.

Ojima, M., Tonori, H., Sato, T., et al. (2002). Odor perception in patients with multiple chemical sensitivity. *Tohoku J. Exp. Med.*, **198**, 163–173.

Paik, S.I., Lehman, M.N., Seiden, A.M., Duncan, H.J., Smith, D.V. (1992). Human olfactory biopsy. The influence of age and receptor distribution. *Archives of Otolaryngology – Head and Neck Surgery* **118**, 731–738.

Pantazopoulos, H., Woo, T.U., Lim, M.P., Lange, N., Berretta, S. (2010). Extracellular matrix-glial abnormalities in the amygdala and entorhinal cortex of subjects diagnosed with schizophrenia. *Archives of General Psychiatry*, **67**, 155–166.

Pappas, G.D., Kriho, V., Liu, W.S., et al. (2003). Immunocytochemical localization of reelin in the olfactory bulb of the heterozygous reeler mouse: An animal model for schizophrenia. *Neurological Research*, **25**, 819–830.

Patterson, D.S., Turner, P., Smart, J.V. (1966). Smell threshold in diabetes mellitus. *Nature*, **209**, 625.

Passler, J.S., Doty, R.L., Dolske, M.C., Louis, P.G.S., Basignani, C., Pepe, J.W. and Bushnev, S., 2017. Olfactory ability in normal pressure hydrocephalus as compared to Alzheimer's disease and healthy controls. *Journal of the neurological sciences*, **372**, pp. 217–219.

Pause, B.M., Miranda, A., Goder, R., Aldenhoff, J.B., Ferstl, R., 2001. Reduced olfactory performance in patients with major depression. *J. Psychiatr. Res.* **35**, 271–277.

Pause, B.M., Raack, N., Eggers, U., et al. 2001. Olfaction and affective state: Emotional and odor perception in patients with major depression. *Journal of Psychophysiology* **15**, 54.

Pelissolo, A., Bisserbe, J.C. (1994). Benzodiazepines dependence: Clinical aspects and biological perspectives. *Enc+®phale*, **20**, 147–158.

Penfield, W., Perot, P. (1963). The brain's record of auditory and visual experience. A final summary and discussion. *Brain*, **86**, 595–696.

Pentzek, M., Grass-Kapanke, B., Ihl, R. (2007). Odor identification in Alzheimer's disease and depression. *Aging Clin Exp Res.*, **19**, 255–258.

Peters G (1958). Multiple Sklerose. In O. Lubarsch, F. Henke, & Rossle R (Eds.), *Handbuch der speziellen pathologischen Anatomie und Histologi*. Berlin: Springer.

Pinching, A.J. (1977). Clinical testing of olfaction reassessed. *Brain*, **100**, 377–388.

Pinto J.M., Wroblewski K.E., Kern D.W., Schumm L.P., McClintock M.K. (2014).

Olfactory dysfunction predicts 5-year mortality in older adults. *PLoS One*, **9**(10), e107541.

Pittman, J.A., Beschi, R.J. (1967). Taste thresholds in hyper- and hypothyroidism. *Journal of Clinical Endocrinology & Metabolism*, **27**, 895–896.

Podlesek, D., Leimert, M., Schuster, B., et al. (2012). Olfactory bulb volume in patients with idiopathic normal pressure hydrocephalus. *Neuroradiology*, **54**, 1229–1233.

Pol, H.E.H., Hijman, R., Tulleken, C.A., et al. (2002). Odor discrimination in patients with frontal lobe damage and Korsakoffs syndrome. *Neuropsychologia*, **40**, 888–891.

Postolache, T.T., Doty, R.L., Wehr, T.A., et al. (1999). Monorhinal odor identification and depression scores in patients with seasonal affective disorder. *J.Affect.Disord.*, **56**, 27–35.

Postolache, T.T., Wehr, T.A., Doty, R.L., et al. (2002). Patients with seasonal affective disorder have lower odor detection thresholds than control subjects. *Arch.Gen.Psychiatry*, **59**, 1119–1122.

Pryse-Phillips, W. (1971). An olfactory reference syndrome. *Acta Psychiat Scand*, **47**, 484–509.

Pryse-Phillips, W. (1975). Disturbance in the sense of smell in psychiatric patients. *Proceedings of the Royal Society of Medicine*, **68**, 472.

Randolph, T.G. (1962). *Human Ecology and Susceptibility to the Chemical Environment*. Springfield, IL: Charles C. Thomas.

Rapps, N., Giel, K.E., Âhngen, E., et al. (2010). Olfactory deficits in patients with anorexia nervosa. *European Eating Disorders Review*, **18**, 385–389.

Rausch, R., Serafetinides, E.A., Crandall, P.H. (1977). Olfactory memory in patients with anterior temporal lobectomy. *Cortex*, **13**, 445–452.

Rawson, N.E., Brand, J.G., Cowart, B.J., et al. (1995). Functionally mature olfactory neurons from two anosmic patients with Kallmann syndrome. *Brain Research* **681**, 58–64.

Razani, J., Murphy, C., Davidson, T.M., Grant, I., McCutchan, A. (1996). Odor sensitivity is impaired in HIV-positive cognitively impaired patients. *Physiology & Behavior* **59**, 877–881.

Reinacher, M., Bonin, J., Narayan, O., Scholtissek, C. (1983). Pathogenesis of neurovirulent influenza A virus infection in mice. Route of entry of virus into brain determines infection of different populations of cells. *Laboratory Investigation*, **49**, 686–692.

Robinson, A.M., Philpott, C.M., Gaskin, J.A., Wolstenholme, C.R., Murty, G.E. (2007). The effect of female hormone manipulation on nasal physiology. *American Journal of Rhinology*, **21**, 675–679.

Roessner, V., Bleich, S., Banaschewski, T., Rothenberger, A. (2005). Olfactory deficits in anorexia nervosa. *European Archives of Psychiatry and Clinical Neuroscience*, **255**, 6–9.

Ros, C., Alobid, I., Centellas, S., et al. (2012). Loss of smell but not taste in adult women with Turner's syndrome and other congenital hypogonadisms. *Maturitas*, **73**(3): 244-250.

Ros, R.S., Bernardino, d. l. S. J., Peiteado, L. p. D., & García, P. J. (2003). [Anosmia as presenting symptom of Churg-Strauss syndrome]. *Revista clinica espanola*, **203**, 263–264.

Rose, C.S., Heywood, P.G., Costanzo, R.M. (1992). Olfactory impairment after chronic occupational cadmium exposure. *J Occup Med*, **34**, 600–605.

Rosenberg, N.L., Kleinschmidt-DeMasters, B.K., Davis, K.A., et al. (1988). Toluene abuse causes diffuse central nervous system white matter changes. *Annals of Neurology* **23**, 611–614.

Ross, P.M., Whysner, J., Covello, V.T., et al. (1999). Olfaction and symptoms in the multiple chemical sensitivities syndrome. *Prev.Med.*, **28**, 467–480.

Rutka, T.O. (1999). Olfactory dysfunction in head injured workers. *Acta Oto-laryngologica*, **119**, 50–57.

Rydzewski, B., Sulkowski, W., Miarzynska, M. (1998). Olfactory disorders induced by cadmium exposure: a clinical study. *International Journal of Occupational Medicine & Environmental Health*, **11**, 235–245

Sagawa, M., Takao, M., Nogawa, S., et al. (2003). [Wilson's disease associated with olfactory paranoid syndrome and idiopathic thrombocytopenic purpura]. *No To Shinkei*, **55**, 899–902.

Saisu, A., Tatsumoto, M., Hoshiyama, E., Aiba, S., Hirata, K. (2011). Evaluation of olfaction in patients with migraine using an odour stick identification test. *Cephalalgia*, **31**, 1023–1028.

Sandmark, B., Broms, I., Lofgren, L., Ohlson, C.G. (1989). Olfactory function in painters exposed to organic solvents. *Scandinavian Journal of Work, Environment & Health*, **15**, 60–63.

Santos, D.V., Reiter, E.R., DiNardo, L.J., Costanzo, R.M. (2004). Hazardous events associated with impaired olfactory function. *Archives of Otolaryngol Head & Neck Surgery*, **130**, 317–319.

Schaupp, H., Krull, R. (1975). [Radiogenic disorder in sense of smell (author's transl)]. *Laryngologie, Rhinologie, Otologie*, **54**, 340–343.

Schiffman, S.S. (2016). Influence of drugs on taste function. In R.L. Doty (Ed.), *Handbook of Olfaction and Gustation*. 3rd edition. Hoboken: John Wiley & Sons, pp. 911–926.

Schiffman, S.S., Nash, M.L., Dackis, C. (1978). Reduced olfactory discrimination in patients on chronic hemodialysis. *Physiology & Behavior* **21**, 239–242.

Schmidt, C., Wiener, E., Hoffmann, J., et al. (2012). Structural olfactory nerve changes in patients suffering from idiopathic intracranial hypertension. *PLoS One*, **7**, e35221.

Schmidt, F., Goktas, O., Jarius, S., et al. (2013). Olfactory dysfunction in patients with neuromyelitis optica. *Mult.Scler.Int.*, 654501.

Schon, F. (1988). Involvement of smell and taste in giant cell arteritis. *Journal of Neurology, Neurosurgery, and Psychiatry*, **51**, 1594.

Schwartz, B.S., Bolla, K.I., Stewart, W., et al. (1993). Decrements in neurobehavioral performance associated with mixed exposure to organic and inorganic lead. *Amer J Epidemiol*, **137**, 1006–1021.

Schwartz, B.S., Doty, R.L., Monroe, C., Frye, R., Barker, S. (1989). Olfactory function in chemical workers exposed to acrylate and methacrylate vapors. *Am J Public Health*, **79**(5), 613–618

Schwartz, B.S., Ford, D.P., Bolla, K.I., Agnew, J., Bleecker, M.L. (1991). Solvent-associated olfactory dysfunction: not a predictor of deficits in learning and memory. *Amer J Psychiat*, **148**, 751–756.

Schwartz, B.S., Ford, D.P., Bolla, K.I., et al. (1990). Solvent-associated decrements in olfactory function in paint manufacturing workers. *American Journal of Industrial Medicine* **18**, 697–706.

Schwob, J.E., Szumowski, K.E., Leopold, D.A., Emko, P. (1993). Histopathology of olfactory mucosa in Kallmann's syndrome. *Annals of Otology, Rhinology, and Laryngology* **102**, 117–122.

Sherman, A.H., Amoore, J.E., Weigel, V. (1979). The pyridine scale for clinical measurement of olfactory threshold: a quantitative reevaluation. *Otolaryngology and Head and Neck Surgery*, **87**, 717.

Shoenfeld, N., Agmon-Levin, N., Flitman-Katzevman, I., et al. (2009). The sense of smell in systemic lupus erythematosus. *Arthritis & Rheumatism*, **60**, 1484–1487.

Silberstein, S.D., Niknam, R., Rozen, T.D., Young, W.B. (2000). Cluster headache with aura. *Neurology*, **54**, 219–221.

Silva, A.M., Santos, E., Moreira, I., et al. (2012). Olfactory dysfunction in multiple sclerosis: association with secondary progression. *Mult. Scler.*, **18**, 616–621.

Silva-Neto, R.P., Peres, M.F., Valenca, M.M. (2014). Accuracy of osmophobia in the differential diagnosis between migraine and tension-type headache. *Journal of the Neurological Sciences* **339**(1–2), 118–122.

Simard, A.R., Rivest, S. (2006). Neuroprotective properties of the innate immune system and bone marrow stem cells in Alzheimer's disease. *Mol.Psychiatry*, **11**, 327–335.

Sisodiya, S.M., Free, S.L., Williamson, K.A., et al. (2001). PAX6 haploinsufficiency causes cerebral malformation and olfactory dysfunction in humans. *Nature Genetics*, **28**(3), 214–216.

Sobel N, Khan RM, Saltman A, Sullivan EV, Gabrieli JD. The world smells different to each nostril. *Nature*. 1999; **402**(6757), 35.

Smith, N., Quinton, R. (2012). Kallmann syndrome. *BMJ*, **345**, e6971.

Sobin, C., Kiley-Brabeck, K., Dale, K., et al. (2006). Olfactory disorder in children with 22q11 deletion syndrome. *Pediatrics*, **118**, e697–e703.

Solomon, G.S., Petrie, W.M., Hart, J.R., Brackin, H.B., Jr. (1998). Olfactory dysfunction discriminates Alzheimer's dementia from major depression. *J Neuropsych Clin Neurosci*, **10**, 64–67.

Soter, A., Kim, J., Jackman, A., et al. (2008). Accuracy of self-report in detecting taste dysfunction. *Laryngoscope.*, **118**, 611–617.

Sparkes, R.S., Simpson, R.W., Paulsen, C.A. (1968). Familial hypogonadotropic hypogonadism with anosmia. *Arch Intern Med*, **121**, 534–538.

Spiegel, A.M., Weinstein, L.S. (2004). Inherited Diseases Involving G Proteins and G Protein-Coupled Receptors. *Annu. Rev. Med.*, **55**, 27–39.

Spierings, E.L., Ranke, A.H., Honkoop, P.C. (2001). Precipitating and aggravating factors of migraine versus tension-type headache. *Headache.* **41**, 554–558.

Starke, R.M., Raper, D.M., Payne, S.C., et al. (2013). Endoscopic vs microsurgical transsphenoidal surgery for acromegaly: outcomes in a concurrent series of patients using modern criteria for remission. *The Journal of Clinical Endocrinology and Metabolism* **98**, 3190–3198.

Stein, D.J., Le Roux, L., Bouwer, C., Van Heerden, B. (1998). Is olfactory reference syndrome an obsessive-compulsive spectrum disorder? Two cases and a discussion. *J Neuropsychia. Clin. Neurosci.* **10**, 96–99.

Steinbach, S., Hummel T., Bohner, C., et al. (2009). Qualitative and quantitative assessment of taste and smell changes in patients undergoing chemotherapy for breast cancer or gynecologic malignancies. *Journal of Clinical Oncology*, **27**(11), 1899–1905.

Stevens, J.R. (1962). Central and Peripheral Factors in Epileptic Discharge: Clinical Studies. *Archives of Neurology*, **7**, 330–338.

Stevenson, R.J., Langdon, R., McGuire, J. (2011). Olfactory hallucinations in schizophrenia and schizoaffective disorder: A phenomenological survey. *Psychiatry Research*, **185**, 321–327.

Stiasny-Kolster, K., Clever, S.C., Moller, J.C., Oertel, W.H., Mayer, G. (2007). Olfactory dysfunction in patients with narcolepsy with and without REM sleep behaviour disorder. *Brain*, **130**, 442–449.

Stroop, W.G. (1995). Viruses and the olfactory system. In R.L. Doty (Ed.), *Handbook of Olfaction and Gustation*. New York: Marcel Dekker, pp. 367–393.

Su, N., Poon, R., Grushka, M. (2015). Does Sjogren's syndrome affect odor identification abilities?. *European Archives of Oto-Rhino-Laryngology*, **272**(3), 773–774.

Sugiura, M., Alba, T., Mori, J., Nakai, Y. (1998). An epidemiological study of postviral olfactory disorder. *Acta Ot-laryngologica Suppl*, : 191–196.

Sulkowski, W.J., Rydzewski, B., Miarzynska, M. (2000). Smell impairment in workers occupationally exposed to cadmium. *Acta Oto-Laryngologica.*, **120**, 316–318.

Sumner, D. (1975). Disturbance of the senses of smell and taste after head injuries. In P.J. Vinken and G.W Bruyn, (Eds.), *Handbook of Clinical Neurology*. Amsterdam: North-Holland Publishing Co, pp. 1–25.

Sumner, D (1967). Post-traumatic ageusia. *Brain*, **90**, 187–202.

Sundermann, E., Gilbert, P.E., Murphy, C. (2006). Estrogen and performance in recognition memory for olfactory and visual stimuli in females diagnosed with Alzheimer's disease. *Journal of the International Neuropsychological Society*, **12**, 400–404.

Sundermann, E.E., Gilbert, P.E., Murphy, C. (2008). The effect of hormone therapy on olfactory sensitivity is dependent on apolipoprotein E genotype. *Hormones and Behavior*, **54**, 528–533.

Szeszko, P.R., Bates, J., Robinson, D., Kane, J., Bilder, R.M. (2004). Investigation of unirhinal olfactory identification in antipsychotic-free patients experiencing a first-episode schizophrenia. *Schizophr Res*, **67**, 219–225.

Tabert, M.H., Liu, X., Doty, R.L., et al. (2005). A 10-item smell identification scale related to risk for Alzheimer's disease. *Annals of Neurology* **58**, 155–160.

Takahashi, T. (1975). Seizures induced by odorous stimuli. *Clin EEG (Osaka)*, **17**, 769.

Takahashi, T., Wood, S.J., Yung, A.R., et al. (2014). Altered depth of the olfactory sulcus in ultra high-risk individuals and patients with psychotic disorders. *Schizophrenia Research*, **153**(1), 18–24

Tallab, H.F., Doty, R.L. (2014). Anosmia and hypogeusia in Churg-Strauss syndrome. *BMJ Case Rep.*, May 13, **pii**: bcr2014203959. doi: 10.1136/bcr-2014-203959.

Temmel, A.F., Pabinger, S., Quint, C., et al. (2005). Dysfunction of the liver affects the sense of smell. *Wien.Klin.Wochenschr.*, **117**, 26–30.

Tepavcevic, V., Lazarini, F., Alfaro-Cervello, C., et al. (2011). Inflammation-induced subventricular zone dysfunction leads to olfactory deficits in a targeted mouse model of multiple sclerosis. *J.Clin.Invest*, **121**, 4722–4734.

Tjalve, H., Henriksson, J. (1999). Uptake of metals in the brain via olfactory pathways. *Neurotoxicology*, **20**, 181–195.

Turetsky, B.I., Moberg, P.J., Roalf, D.R., Arnold, S.E., Gur, R.E. (2003). Decrements in volume of anterior ventromedial temporal lobe and olfactory dysfunction in schizophrenia. *Archives of General Psychiatry.*, **60**, 1193–1200.

Turetsky, B.I., Crutchley, P., Walker, J., Gur, R. E., Moberg, P.J. (2009). Depth of the olfactory sulcus: A marker of early embryonic disruption in schizophrenia? *Schizophrenia Research*, **115**, 8–11.

Turetsky, B.I., Kohler, C.G., Gur, R.E., Moberg, P.J. (2008). Olfactory physiological impairment in first-degree relatives of schizophrenia patients. *Schizophrenia Research*, **102**, 220–229.

Turetsky, B.I., Moberg, P.J. (2009). An odor-specific threshold deficit implicates abnormal intracellular cyclic AMP signaling in schizophrenia. *American Journal of Psychiatry*, **166**, 226–233.

Turetsky, B.I., Moberg, P.J., Yousem, D.M., et al. (2000). Reduced olfactory bulb volume in patients with schizophrenia. *American Journal of Psychiatry* **157**, 828–830.

Tvedt, B., Skyberg, K., Berstad, J. (1989). Chronic toxic encephalopathy among house painters with disability pension. *J.Oslo.City Hosp.*, **39**, 74–80.

Ugur, T., Weisbrod, M., Franzek, E., Pfuller, U., Sauer, H. (2005). Olfactory impairment in monozygotic twins discordant for schizophrenia. *Eur Arch Psych Clin Neurosci*, **255**, 94.

Vadala, R., Giugni, E., Pezzella, F.R., Sabatini, U., Bastianello, S. (2013). Progressive sensorineural hearing loss, ataxia and anosmia as manifestation of superficial siderosis in post traumatic brain injury. *Neurol.Sci.*, **34**, 1259–1262.

Varney, N.R. (1988). Prognostic significance of anosmia in patients with closed-head trauma. *Journal of Clinical and Experimental Neuropsychology*, **10**, 250–254.

Varney, N.R., Bushnelt, D. (1998). NeuroSPECT findings in patients with post-traumafic anosmia: A quantitative analysis. *Journal of Head Trauma Rehabilitation*, **13**, 63–72.

Varney, N.R., Pinkston, J.B., Wu, J.C. (2001). Quantitative PET findings in patients with post-traumatic anosmia. *Journal of Head Trauma Rehabilitation*, **16**, 253–259.

Velakoulis, D. (2006). Olfactory hallucinations. In: W. Brewer, D. Castle, and C. Pantelis (Eds.), *Olfaction and the Brain*. Cambridge: Cambridge Univesity Press, pp. 322–333.

Vent, J., Koenig, J., Hellmich, M., Huettenbrink, K.B., Damm, M. (2010). Impact of recurrent head trauma on olfactory function in boxers: A matched pairs analysis. *Brain Research*, **1320**, 1–6.

Veyseller, B., Aksoy, F., Yildirim, Y.S., et al. (2012). Olfactory dysfunction and olfactory bulb volume reduction in patients with leprosy. *Indian J Otolaryngology Head & Neck Surgery*, **64**(3), 261–265.

Veyseller, B., Ozucer, B., Degirmenci, N., et al. (2014a). Olfactory bulb volume and olfactory function after radiotherapy in patients with nasopharyngeal cancer. *Auris Nasus Larynx*, **41**(5), 436–440.

Veyseller, B., Dogan, R., Ozucer, B., et al. (2014b). Olfactory function and nasal manifestations of Behcet's disease. *Auris Nasus Larynx*, **41**, 185–189.

Vishnevetsky, A., Inca-Martinez, M., Milla-Neyra, K., et al. (2016). The first report of CADASIL in Peru: Olfactory dysfunction on initial presentation. *eNeurologicalSci.* **5**: 15–19.

Vreman, H.J., Venter, C., Leegwater, J., Oliver, C., Weiner, M.W. (1980). Taste, smell and zinc metabolism in patients with chronic renal failure. *Nephron*, **26**, 163–170.

Walczak, M., Pruszewicz, A., Lacka, K., Karlik, M. (2002). [Olfaction in congenital hypothyroidism]. *Otolaryngol.Pol.*, **56**, 577–581.

Ware, J., Jr., Kosinski, M., Keller, S.D. (1996). A 12-Item Short-Form Health Survey: construction of scales and preliminary tests of reliability and validity. *Med.Care*, **34**, 220–233.

Watanabe, S., Fukuchi, Y. (2000). Occupational impairment of the olfactory sense of chromate producing workers. *Japanese Journal of Industrial Health*, **23**, 606–611.

Weiffenbach, J.M., Fox, P.C. (1993). Odor identification ability among patients with Sjogren's syndrome. *Arthritis & Rheumatism*, **36**, 1752–1754.

Weigel, M.T., Prazma, G., Pillsbury, H.C. (1989). Auditory acuity in adrenocorticoid insufficiency. *Am.J.Otol.*, July; **10**, 267–271.

Weinstock, R.S., Wright, H.N., Smith, D.U. (1993). Olfactory dysfunction in diabetes mellitus. *Physiology & behavior*, **53**, 17–21.

Weinstock, R.S., Wright, H.N., Spiegel, A. M., Levine, M.A., Moses, A.M. (1986). Olfactory dysfunction in humans with deficient guanine nucleotide-binding protein. *Nature*, **322**(6080), 635–636.

Wenzel, B.M. (1948). Techniques in olfactometry. A critical review of the last one hundred years. *Psychological Bulletin*, **45**, 231–247.

West, S.E., Doty, R.L. (1995). Influence of epilepsy and temporal lobe resection on olfactory function. *Epilepsia*, **36**, 531–542.

Westervelt, H.J., McCaffrey, R.J., Cousins, J.P., Wagle, W.A., Haase, R.F. (1997). Longitudinal analysis of olfactory deficits in HIV infection. *Archives of Clinical Neuropsychology* **12**, 557–565.

Wierzbicki, A.S, Lloyd, M.D., Schofield, C.J., Feher, M.D., Gibberd, F.B. (2002). Refsum's disease: A peroxisomal disorder affecting phytanic acid α-oxidation. *Journal of neurochemistry*, **80**(5), 727–735.

Wilson, R.S., Yu, L., Bennett, D.A. (2011). Odor identification and mortality in old age. *Chemical Senses* **36**, 63–67.

Wismer, W.V. (2008). Assessing alterations in taste and their impact on cancer care. *Current Opinion in Supportive and Palliative Care*, **2**(4), 282–287.

Wustenberg, E.G., Fleischer, A., Gerbert, B., et al. (2001). Lateralized normosmia in a patient with Kallmann's syndrome. *Laryngo-Rhino-Otologie*, **80**, 85–89.

Xydakis, M.S., Mulligan, L.P., Smith, A.B., et al. (2015). Olfactory impairment and traumatic brain injury in blast-injured combat troops: A cohort study. *Neurology*, **84**(15), 1559–1567.

Yin-Zeng, L., Jin-Xiang, H., Cheng-Mo, L., Bo-Hong, X., Cui-Juan, Z. (1985). Effects of cadmium on cadmium smelter workers. *Scand J Work Environ Health*, **11**, 29–32.

Yousem, D.M., Geckle, R.J., Bilker, W., McKeown, D.A., Doty, R.L. (1996a). MR evaluation of patients with congenital hyposmia or anosmia. *American Journal of Roentgenology* **166**, 439–443.

Yousem, D.M., Geckle, R.J., Bilker, W.B., McKeown, D.A., Doty, R.L. (1996b). post-traumatic olfactory dysfunction: MR and clinical evaluation. *American Journal of Neuroradiology*, **17**, 1171–1179.

Yousem, D.M., Oguz, K.K., Li, C. (2001). Imaging of the olfactory system. *Seminars In Ultrasound CT RM*, **22**, 456–472.

Yu, Z., Kryzer, T.J., Griesmann, G.E., et al. (2001). CRMP-5 neuronal autoantibody: marker of lung cancer and thymoma-related autoimmunity. *Annals of Neurology* **49**, 146–154.

Zatorre, R.J., Jones-Gotman, M. (1991). Human olfactory discrimination after unilateral frontal or temporal lobectomy. *Brain*, **114**, 71–84.

Zeman, A.Z., Boniface, S.J., Hodges, J.R. (1998). Transient epileptic amnesia: a description of the clinical and neuropsychological features in 10 cases and a review of the literature. *Journal of Neurology, Neurosurgery & Psychiatry*. **64**(4): 435–443.

Zhao, K., Frye, R.E. (2015). nasal patency and the aerodynamics of nasal airflow in relation to olfactory function. In: R.L. Doty (Ed.), *Handbook of Olfaction and Gustation*. 3rd edition. Hoboken, NJ: John Wiley & Sons, pp. 355–374.

Zhao, K., Cowart, B.J., Rawson, N.E., et al. (2007). Nasal airflow and odorant transport modeling in patients with chronic rhinosinusitis. *Department of*

Otolaryngology - Head and Neck Surgery Faculty Papers, **10**.

Zimmerman, H.M., Netsky, M.G. (1950). The pathology of multiple sclerosis. *Research publications-Association for Research in Nervous and Mental Disease*, **28**, 271.

Zivadinov, R., Zorzon, M., Monti, B.L., Pagliaro, G., Cazzato, G. (1999). Olfactory loss in multiple sclerosis. *Journal of the Neurological Sciences* **168**, 127–130.

Zorzon, M., Ukmar, M., Bragadin, L.M., et al. (2000). Olfactory dysfunction and extent of white matter abnormalities in multiple sclerosis: a clinical and MR study. *Mult.Scler.*, **6**, 386–390.

Zucco, G.M., Amodio, P., Gatta, A. (2006). Olfactory deficits in patients affected by minimal hepatic encephalopathy: A pilot study. *Chemical Senses* **31**, 273–278.

Zucco, G.M., Ingegneri, G. (2004). Olfactory deficits in HIV-infected patients with and without AIDS dementia complex. *Physiology & Behavior* **80**, 669–674.

Zucco, G.M., Militello, C., Doty, R.L. (2008). Discriminating between organic and psychological determinants of multiple chemical sensitivity: A case study. *Neurocase*, **14**, 485–493

Zusho, H. (1982). post-traumatic anosmia. *Archives of Otolaryngology*, **108**, 90–92.

Non-neurodegenerative Disorders of Gustation

Taste disorders are often overlooked by patients or their medical attendants and they are generally more difficult to detect and quantify than smell disorders. In common with olfactory ailments, disorders of taste may reflect peripheral or central pathology but inevitably there is overlap. As described in Chapter 5, patients who complain of impaired taste usually have an olfactory problem which, in turn, influences the flavor of foods. Importantly, the taste system appears more resistant than smell to central and peripheral damage although medication is more likely to induce distortion of taste. One explanation for the resilience of taste lies in the considerable redundancy across several taste-conveying nerves, thus permitting compensation. Moreover, damage to one nerve may release inhibition of other nerves, probably through lowering of threshold. In some instances, this process evokes phantom tastes (Kveton & Bartoshuk, 1994; Lehman et al., 1995).

Given these compensatory processes and the regenerative capacity of taste buds, *whole-mouth* dysfunction is relatively rare and, when present, is usually associated with metabolic conditions, bilateral middle ear infections, or central ischemic lesions such as brain stem infarcts. For example, in one study 433 of 585 patients (74%) with verifiable olfactory loss complained of smell and taste disturbance (Deems et al., 1991), but less than 4% exhibited measurable whole-mouth gustatory impairment. Regional taste dysfunction is more common. Thus, in a recent study of taste sensitivity in 16 different regions of the tongue, sensitivity to all four classic taste qualities, as well as to electric current, decreased markedly with age (Doty et al., 2015). Interestingly, there was significant anterior to posterior, and lateral to medial, age-related gradients of decreasing performance. Such regional deficits contrast with decrements noted in whole-mouth taste testing, where the age-related effects are typically more subtle.

Classification of Types of Gustatory Disorders

In parallel with olfactory disorders described in the previous chapter, taste disorders can be classified in terms of their behavioral or psychological manifestations. The following classifications are most commonly employed.

Ageusia. Ageusia is the lack of ability to taste via taste receptors located mainly on the taste buds. Although some use this term to describe total loss, others use it to describe loss specific to only some substances. In the latter case, the term "specific ageusia" is preferred.

Hypogeusia. Hypogeusia reflects decreased taste function, as manifested, for example, by heightened taste thresholds.

Hypergeusia is enhanced sensitivity to one or more tastants, usually defined by lowered threshold values. In keeping with hyperosmia, hypergeusia can reflect *hyper-reactivity* rather than a true change in sensitivity.

Dysgeusia is any form of distorted taste perception. When a stimulus is needed to induce the distortion, this is often called a stimulated dysgeusia, whereas if the sensation is not provoked, it is called an unstimulated dysgeusia or phantogeusia. Examples of dysgeusias include metallic taste sensations secondary to damage of one or more taste afferents (e.g., the chorda tympani nerve) and chronic salty sensations of unknown origin. Dysgeusia is often present in Burning Mouth Syndrome (glossalgia or glossodynia), a multifactorial disorder probably analogous to the neuropathic pain seen in fine fiber axonal peripheral neuropathy.

In the next section we describe taste disorders according to their main site of pathology, namely peripheral or central, although overlap does exist in some cases. The peripheral conditions include infection, neuropathy, neoplasia, surgery, and trauma. The central processes encompass brain stem, thalamic and cortical disorders, traumatic brain injury, epilepsy, and migraine. Conditions which do not fall easily into either category are then outlined, including immune-related diseases, metabolic and endocrine diseases, and disorders associated with medications, toxins, and pollutants.

The main diseases associated with taste disorder are summarized in Table 6.1.

Peripheral Taste Disorders

Altered peripheral taste perception may reflect impaired transport of tastants to the taste buds, poor oral hygiene, destruction of the taste buds or receptors, as well as damage to the taste nerves themselves. Impaired transport of taste buds can be secondary to chronic oral dryness or taste pore damage from inflammation or burns. Without moisture, taste cannot be appreciated; similarly, a chronically dry nose may cause anosmia. Poor oral hygiene contributes to ageusia or dysgeusia, and may produce phantogeusia. Poor hygiene promotes release of foul-tasting materials from the oral or nasal cavities and facilitates oral infection, such as candida. Thus, enquiry should probe for unhealthy teeth or dentures, gingivitis, oral thrush, cryptic tonsillitis, and chronic salivary gland infection (sialadenitis). Many inhabitants of nursing homes have dry mouth (xerostomia) which may result from medication, mouth breathing, water or dietary insufficiency. Damage to taste buds, taste receptors, and supporting tissue results from several causes, in particular radiotherapy to the head or neck. Such therapy may also damage taste nerves that innervate the taste buds. Specific taste fibers can be damaged also from Bell's palsy, third-molar extraction, and tonsillectomy.

Infections: Viral

Viral infections are a major cause of taste impairment, just like olfactory disorders. It is assumed that the virus enters the taste nerves where it may continue to penetrate into more central structures, depending upon the virus involved. The best documented virus-related deficits are indicated below (Table 6.1).

1. **Bell's Palsy.** Although the etiology of this common facial nerve palsy is often unknown, in many cases viruses are implicated (Adour et al., 1975; Takahashi et al., 2001). For example,

Table 6.1. Summary of main diseases associated with loss of taste with some examples. FOSMN = facial onset sensor-motor neuropathy (see Chapter 7). For causes of medication and toxin-related conditions see Table 6.2.

Disease process	Examples
Infection	Bell's palsy (herpes simplex type 1); Ramsay Hunt syndrome (herpes zoster); HIV/AIDS; Hepatitis C Virus; Upper respiratory viral infections; Oral candida; Viral encephalitis; Influenza; Leprosy; Periodontitis; Glossitis; Streptococcus
Neuropathies	Diabetes; Dysautonomia; Amyloid; Guillain-Barre syndrome; FOSMN, Burning mouth syndrome
Neoplasia	Middle ear (cholesteatoma); Jugular foramen tumor (glomus jugulare); Paraneoplastic; Radiation therapy for neck tumors; Jugular foramen tumors
Surgical procedures	Middle ear surgery; Tonsillectomy; Tracheal intubation; Bilateral thalamotomy; Laryngectomy; Third-lower-molar tooth extraction or local anesthetic for inferior alveolar nerve; Deep brain stimulation
Trauma	Chorda tympani (petrous bone fracture); Lingual or glossopharyngeal nerve (neck injury); Traumatic brain injury affecting insula or orbitofrontal cortex
Allergic disorder	Allergic rhinitis; Pine mouth syndrome
Vascular disorder	Lateral medullary syndrome; pontine hemorrhage; internal carotid artery dissection; Migraine; Hypertension
Epilepsy	Lesion in opercular region or amygdaloid nucleus
Systemic disease	Cystic fibrosis; renal & liver disease; Cushing's disease; hypopituitarism; Addison's disease; Cretinism; cranial arteritis
Immune-related disease	Myasthenia Gravis; Multiple sclerosis; Sjögren's syndrome; Hypothyroidism
Deficiency states	Niacin (B3); Vitamin A; Zinc; B12
Psychiatric	Depression; Schizophrenia
Developmental	Congenital facial hypoplasia
Miscellaneous	Smoking; aging; Parkinson's disease (see Chapter 7); High altitude exposure; Severe blood loss; Turner's syndrome

herpes simplex virus-1 genome has been isolated from the facial nerve endoneural fluid of affected patients (Murakami et al., 1966). This palsy, which affects both sexes and all ages, is associated regularly with unilateral taste impairment over the anterior two-thirds of the tongue, a loss that sometimes goes unnoticed by the patient, probably because it is one-sided. Usually the lesion is in the geniculate ganglion through which the chorda tympani passes, thus impairing *taste input* to the solitary tract in the medulla and damaging *secretomotor output* to the salivary glands. Thus, damage to the chorda tympani affects a major afferent taste pathway and compounds the ability to taste by making the mouth dry.
2. **Ramsay-Hunt Syndrome.** This syndrome is a severe form of facial palsy due to varicella zoster virus (VZV) infection of the geniculate ganglion. The facial weakness is accompanied by pain and vesicles involving the external auditory canal and sometimes the soft palate.

Little is known about the prospects of taste recovery. Bartoshuk and Miller (1991) described the longitudinal changes in taste intensity ratings for nearly two years in a patient with additional infection of the left CN V and CN IX nerves. For three months after the VZV attack, the entire left tongue and palate was devoid of taste. A year later essentially all taste qualities were perceived on the posterior left region of the tongue and the palate (CN IX territory), but only sweetness was perceived on the left anterior tongue (chorda tympani). Even by the end of the study, normal taste in this tongue region had not returned. More recently, Heymans et al. (2011) described a similar taste deficit in two patients with VZV infection of the mandibular nerve, the branch of the trigeminal nerve that transmits the peripheral sector of the chorda tympani. Return of function occurred within two months of the viral attack.

3. **Human Immunodeficiency Virus (HIV).** HIV is associated with decreased taste appreciation, although the site of damage and mechanism are not clear. In one study of 40 HIV patients it was observed that, relative to 40 controls, the HIV group exhibited highly significant threshold elevations to glutamic acid (savory) and quinine hydrochloride (bitter), as well as poorer performance on a taste quality identification task (Graham et al., 1995). A non-significant trend was noted between the test scores and HIV infection stages, which ranged from generalized lymphadenopathy to opportunistic infections and malignancies. The taste deficits may have been medication related, given that all patients were on several drugs, including highly activate antiretroviral therapy (HAART). This problem was addressed in a case-control study of 50 subjects with HIV and 50 healthy controls (Raja et al., 2013). Twenty-four (48%) of the HIV group, but none of the controls, complained of taste perversion. In the HIV group, identification and intensity scores were lower and detection thresholds were higher for the standard four tastants. In patients with taste complaints, 16 were receiving HAART and 8 were not. It was concluded that drug-naïve, HIV-infected subjects experience taste impairment that is compounded further by introduction of HAART.

4. **Hepatitis C Virus (HCV).** Although HCV is a primary liver infection, it is well recognized that peripheral nerves and autonomic pathways may be affected, either of which can involve taste. The likely mechanism is vasculitic, although some argue that deposition of cryoglobulins within the peripheral nerves may contribute, especially where there is a single nerve involved (mononeuritis). Apart from peripheral nerve damage, in rare instances the vasculitic process may affect the CNS, resulting in a variety of ischemic disorders. Despite this uncertain pathologic background, it is well established that patients with acute or chronic HCV exhibit taste dysfunction (for review of the earlier literature, see Deems et al. (1991)). Many are unaware of the gustatory deficit (Smith et al., 1976).

In general, hepatitis patients rate food as less pleasant than do controls (Deems et al., 1993). In one study, detection thresholds for NaCl, sucrose, HCl, and urea were elevated in those with early viral hepatitis compared to healthy controls (Smith et al., 1976). Recognition thresholds were similarly elevated for all stimuli except sucrose. Interestingly, ratings of stimulus intensity were larger in patients than controls, a phenomenon that was also noted for sucrose in a more recent study (Musialik et al., 2012). In the latter study, suprathreshold intensity, hedonic ratings, and taste recognition thresholds were measured for NaCl (salty), sucrose (sweet), monosodium glutamate (umami), citric acid (sour), and quinine hydrochloride (bitter) in 40 chronic HCV patients and 110 matched controls (Musialik et al., 2012). Monosodium glutamate thresholds were significantly elevated in the hepatitis group. In addition to greater ratings of sucrose intensity, evaluations of citric acid intensity were depressed relative to controls. These effects were more marked in those with the most advanced disease, i.e., with stage 3 liver fibrosis and cirrhosis. Such observations, along with reports that (a) the threshold and suprathreshold changes of patients with acute hepatitis wane as the hepatitis resolves (Smith et al., 1976) and (b) chemosensory dysfunction improves after liver transplantation (Bloomfeld et al., 1999), suggest that the HCV-related changes are secondary to liver problems. However, a neuropathy affecting the taste nerves is not excluded and most studies have not allowed for the effect of antiviral therapies.

5. **Upper Respiratory Viral Infections.** Taste dysfunction may follow the common cold or influenza. Typically, there is nearly always simultaneous olfactory impairment (Henkin et al., 1975). Dysgeusia is not unusual and, to a lesser extent, burning sensations within the oral cavity (Deems et al., 1991). Taste is seldom assessed quantitatively, making it difficult to know the prevalence and severity of the defect, although complete loss is unusual. The prospect for recovery is not yet established.

Infections: Bacterial and Fungal

Although it is generally assumed that bacterial and fungal infections alter taste, surprisingly little basic information is available on this topic. One group investigated elderly hospital in-patients with elevated bacterial viability counts ($\geq 10^5$ colony forming units (CFU)/ml) of *Streptococcus mutans* and *Lactobacilli* in their stimulated saliva. They performed less well on a whole-mouth taste identification test that employed paper strips embedded with tastants than patients with $<10^5$ CFU/ml of these bacteria (Solemdal et al., 2012). The taste measurements were inversely related to the number of decayed teeth and indices of poor oral hygiene and dry mouth. Sakashita et al. (2004) used filter-paper-based non-forced-choice threshold tests with ascending concentration series of sucrose, NaCl, tartaric acid, and quinine hydrochloride. They applied this test to a large sample of 200 healthy individuals, of whom 33 were oral carriers of *Candida Albicans*. Disordered taste in the carriers was higher than non-carriers (72.7% vs. 27.5%, p < 0.001), with significantly greater mean threshold values across all modalities in the carrier group. In 18 patients with well-defined lingual candidiasis, ~95% had impairment of taste that for the majority was classed as severe. Of seven patients whose candidiasis had been treated successfully with an anti-fungal agent, three regained normal taste and two showed a degree of recovery. Some were receiving medication that may have affected their findings and there was no healthy control group. Although it is likely that candida infection is associated with impaired taste, controls are needed to eliminate confounders such as medication, age, reduced salivation, and co-existing disease, including diabetes, collagen disease, malignancies, and neurologic disorders.

Neuropathies

Taste disorders are frequent in neuropathy, especially in those with autonomic dysfunction such as diabetes, as described below. Pan-dysautonomia is characterized by a dry mouth, but taste is also impaired, probably because of autonomic neuropathy. In familial dysautonomia (Riley-Day syndrome) there are reduced numbers of fungiform and circumvallate papillae, with impaired perception of sweet and salty flavors, possibly due to deficiency of Brain Derived Neurotropic Factor (BDNF). Ageusia may be the presenting symptom of light-chain (AL) amyloidosis and appears to be an almost universal feature in established cases (Marinone et al., 1994). Taste loss may be a presenting feature of Guillain-Barre syndrome, where the facial nerve is regularly affected on one or both sides. In leprosy, taste impairment is extremely common, particularly in the lepromatous type where over 70% of patients are affected (Rathi et al., 1986).

Burning Mouth Syndrome, sometimes called glossalgia or glossodynia, is a multi-factorial disorder analogous to the neuropathic pain seen in fine fiber axonal peripheral neuropathies. Commonly it affects postmenopausal women and those with diabetes, Sjögren's syndrome, Parkinson's disease, dry mouth, or depression. Some have vitamin deficiencies, typically B12, folate, or iron; others have a cancer phobia which disappears with reassurance. Patients complain of an intense burning pain chiefly in the anterior two-thirds of the tongue, lips, and anterior hard palate. There is persistent dysgeusia and altered taste perception. It is unknown whether the mechanism is mediated peripherally or centrally and some assert it is a psychogenic disorder. Its occurrence in diseases known to cause trigeminal neuropathy such as diabetes or Sjögrens syndrome implies that at least a proportion are physically based. The reader is referred to an extensive review of this poorly understood condition (Klasser et al., 2016).

Neoplasia

A wide variety of oral, pharyngeal, and neck tumors affect taste. These are characterized by decrements in function, dysgeusia, and phantogeusia in varying combinations. The situation is often aggravated by the onset of malnutrition. Paraneoplastic autonomic antibody-mediated neuropathy may impair taste, as in the Lambert Eaton Myasthenic syndrome, where some patients report a persistent metallic taste (Mareska & Gutmann, 2004), or secondary to the neuronal antibody marker, CRMP-5, where subjective reports of "loss of olfaction/taste" in 10% have been noted (Yu et al., 2001). There is one report of dysgeusia associated with inappropriate secretion of antidiuretic hormone (ADH) secondary to oral squamous-cell carcinoma (Danielides et al., 2005). Excess ADH and the consequent lowering of blood sodium level may cause an unpleasant sweet taste that improves once the sodium level returns to normal (Nakazato et al., 2006). Variants (polymorphisms) in the gene for bitter taste (TAS2R38) are associated with slightly increased risk of colorectal cancer (Carrai et al., 2011), suggesting that inadvertent ingestion of unpalatable food may relate to the development of such tumors.

Taste dysfunction can result from intensive immunosuppression secondary to radiation and chemotherapy for numerous types of cancers. Such therapies can induce oral mucositis, xerostomia, tooth loss, chewing difficulties, and neurotoxicity (Caputo et al., 2012). These treatments, including those for tumors of the oral cavity, head, and neck, often produce more debilitating symptoms than the cancers themselves (Xiao et al., 2013). This includes decreased numbers of taste buds (Mirza et al., 2008), losses and distortions of perceived taste qualities (Mossman et al., 1979), xerostomia (Mossman et al., 1981; Salisbury, III, 1997), weight loss (Bolze et al., 1982), nutritional changes (Chencharick & Mossman, 1983), and food aversions (Smith & Blumsack, 1981; Smith et al., 1981; Brewin, 1982; Bernstein, 1985; Carrell et al., 1986; Mattes et al., 1992). A decrease in taste bud number, measured *in vivo* by decrements in lingual taste pores, is well documented (Salisbury, III, 1997), as is damage to salivary glands (e.g., parotid or submandibular). In one longitudinal taste study of patients undergoing head and neck irradiation, decreased ability to identify sour, bitter, and salty tastants was evident *prior to therapy*, which was most marked for bitter (caffeine), followed by salty (NaCl) and sour (citric acid) suprathreshold taste sensations (Mirza et al., 2008). Taste-quality specific influences of radiation therapy were found, particularly for sour. Other researchers have noted taste-specific radiotherapy or chemotherapy changes, with greater decrements for bitter substances (Caputo et al., 2012). While taste bud cell turnover is clearly influenced by radiation therapy, regeneration of such buds usually occurs several months after therapy. Recovery to pre-therapeutic levels is rare (Conger, 1973). Susceptibility to opportunistic infections (e.g., dental caries, candidiasis) invariably increases after therapy, thereby potentially impacting taste function. Arterial chemotherapy is associated with tongue necrosis, altered basal cell and taste receptor production (Duhra & Foulds, 1988; Shih et al., 1999).

A major difficulty in radiotherapy and chemotherapy is the formation of taste aversions during treatment. Medications such as cytotoxic drugs induce bitter sensations and presumably activate taste receptors via saliva, crevicular (gingival sulcus) fluid, and blood (Berteretche et al., 2004). Indeed, over three-quarters of patients undergoing cancer chemotherapy exhibit food avoidance (Holmes, 1993) and more than half develop food aversions (Mattes et al., 1987). This results typically from the pairing of treatment-induced sickness with the taste of foodstuffs. Such conditioning may occur even if the malaise happens hours after eating the food. Conditioned aversions are usually transient, but may be long lasting and lead to generalized anorexia and cachexia. Interestingly, some taste aversions can be eliminated or minimized by having the patient consume a novel food immediately before the initiation of therapy (Mattes, 1994). Subsequent conditioned aversions become focused mainly on the novel food, thus protecting against conditioned aversions to preferred food items. Alternative unconfirmed methods for reducing the side effects of head and neck radiation include administration of zinc (Najafizade et al., 2013) or a protein from the *Synsepalum dulcificum* plant (miracle fruit) (Wilken & Satiroff, 2012).

Surgery and Trauma

The *chorda tympani* (CT) division of CN VII innervates the taste buds on the anterior two-thirds of the tongue. It leaves the tongue with the lingual nerve, a branch of the mandibular division of the trigeminal (CN V). In addition to innervating the taste buds, the CT provides secretomotor supply to the salivary glands. Thus, damage to the CT anywhere along its path can influence taste by altering afferent taste signals and by drying the mouth, thereby preventing tastants from being solubilized and potentially reducing taste pore patency.

1. **Middle Ear Surgery.** The passage of the CT nerve through the middle ear makes it vulnerable to damage from surgery in this area. The degree of damage is influenced by the type of operation, as well as the nature and extent of the problem prior to surgery. The main part of the ear drum that transmits vibration is known as the pars tensa and the upper flaccid region is the pars flaccida (Figure 6.1). Preoperatively, patients with pars tensa retraction-type cholesteatomas exhibit higher electrogustometric thresholds than those with chronic otitis media, pars flaccida retraction-type cholesteatomas, otosclerosis, or ossicular anomalies (Sakaguchi et al., 2012). In many cases, post-operative trigeminal sensations such as tingling and numbness occur in the tongue, although the basis for such phenomena is poorly understood (Sakagami, 2009).

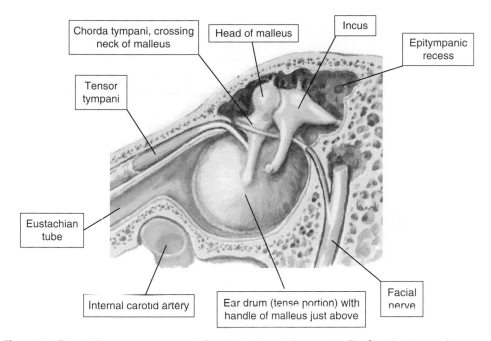

Figure 6.1 The middle ear structures viewed from inside the middle ear cavity. The flaccid portion and tense portion refer to the *pars flaccida* and *pars tensa*, respectively. Note the course of the chorda tympani as it crosses the neck of the malleus and then joins the facial nerve at an acute angle. During middle ear surgery, such as stapedectomy, the chorda tympani may be injured.

In general, 15–30% of patients who undergo middle ear surgery experience postoperative taste change, dry mouth, or both, although typically the symptoms resolve over time (Michael & Raut, 2007; McManus al., 2012). Stretching of the chorda tympani nerve generally produces more symptoms than sectioning the nerve (Michael & Raut, 2007). Inadvertent damage to the CT is not uncommon, and even slight manipulations of the CT can influence taste adversely in a significant number of patients (Guder, Bottcher et al., 2012). In one study of 107 patients undergoing middle ear surgery for chronic otitis media, symptoms arose in 19% (Lloyd et al., 2007). Middle ear surgery in which the chorda tympani is moved slightly, but not severed, results in deficits on multiple lingual regions, including those adjacent to the tongue tip, medial areas of the tongue off the midline, and more posterior portions of the tongue. According to one group (Berteretche et al., 2008), the medial tongue tip and lateral rear sections of the tongue are influenced little by such surgery, suggesting cross-innervation of CN VII in the tongue tip and dual innervation of CN V and CN IX in the rear lateral tongue. This notion has since been rebutted (see Doty et al., 2015, figure 3). There is some evidence that small branches of CN IX may extend beyond the sulcus terminalis on lateral areas of the tongue, although it is unknown whether they innervate taste buds (Doty et al., 2009).

Anatomically, preoperative damage to the CT from chronic suppurative otitis media is evident in histological studies of nerve sections and includes edema, reduced number of unmyelinated nerve fibers, myelin sheath disintegration, Schwann cell nucleus condensation, shrunken electron-dense axoplasm, and an increase in collagen fibers (Teker et al.,

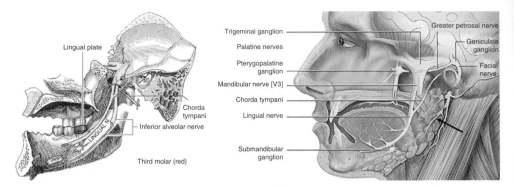

Figure 6.2 Left: The position of the lingual nerve in relation to the third-molar tooth, shown in red. The lingual nerve carries taste afferents from the anterior two-thirds of the tongue in the chorda tympani. Right: The course of the lingual nerve and chorda tympani. It passes deep to the temporo-mandibular joint and attaches to the lingual nerve at an oblique angle. The greater petrosal nerve, which supplies taste buds in the soft palate, is labeled. The glossopharyngeal nerve innervates the posterior foliate and circumvallate papillae in the posterior two-thirds of the tongue (black arrow). In the tonsillar bed it may be damaged during tonsillectomy. Reproduced with permission from the Yale Center for Advanced Instructional Media, figure 6.16b. The relations of the chorda tympani to the ear drum are shown in Figure 6.1. (A black and white version of this figure will appear in some formats. For the color version, please refer to the plate section.)

2010). Postoperatively, the number of taste buds that return after regeneration of a severed CT is inevitably less than before surgery, even when taste appears to have completely recovered (Saito et al., 2011; Saito et al., 2011). Animal studies have demonstrated that after CT resection there is prolonged glial activity and morphological changes within the nucleus tractus solitarius (Bartel, 2012). For example, in the rat, the volume of labeled CT nerve terminals is reduced by 44% at 30 days after CT severance and by 63% at 60 days (Reddaway et al., 2012).

2. **Third-Molar Extraction.** Taste impairment following third-molar extraction is well documented, since the lingual nerve (which contains the CT) is adjacent to the tooth capsule, making it vulnerable to surgical damage (Figure 6.2) (Valmaseda-Castellon et al., 2000). Factors associated with such damage include severity of impaction, variations in anatomy, experience of the surgeon, and the specific surgical techniques employed

Akal et al. (2004) evaluated taste function in 27 patients undergoing third-molar extraction before and at one-month and six-month postoperative intervals and noted that gustation returned to normal after six months. In contrast, Shafer et al. (1999), in a similar study, assessed taste quantitatively in 17 patients at the same time points and observed that some taste deficits were present even six months after surgery. Yung et al. (2008) reported rates of dysgeusia at 39% at three months and 27% at six months. While it has been stated that less than 1% of third-molar extraction-related lingual tactile dysesthesias fail to resolve within six months, such data are not available for taste and it should be questioned whether resolution may, in many cases, simply reflect the patient's ultimate acceptance of their symptoms (Rud, 1984; Mason, 1988).

It should be noted that injection of local anesthesia used for third-molar extractions can itself cause altered taste function, either by direct contact of the needle with the lingual nerve or from neurotoxic effects of the local anesthetic, typically lidocaine and epinephrine

(Nickel, 1993; Shafer et al., 1999). As indicated earlier, anesthetizing one chorda tympani nerve (CN VII), which might be viewed as a surrogate for nerve trauma, may enhance taste perception, particularly to bitter, on the rear of the tongue (CN IX) primarily on the side opposite that of anesthetized nerve (Kveton & Bartoshuk, 1994; Yanagisawa et al., 1998). In one study, a phantom taste was mentioned by ~40 percent of patients in the absence of stimulation, a phenomenon that disappeared when the lingual region of origin was anesthetized (Yanagisawa et al., 1998). Such phantoms may reflect central interactions among the taste nerves (e.g., release of inhibition), since the taste pathways do not cross until they reach the thalamus.

In addition to iatrogenic taste dysfunction from third molar extractions, several other types of dental procedures may influence taste. For example, on rare occasions operations on the temporomandibular joint result in partial taste impairment. The likely cause is damage to the chorda tympani, where it lies medial (deep) to this joint.

3. **Tonsillectomy.** The glossopharyngeal nerve (CN IX) conveys taste from the posterior third of the tongue and lies in the tonsillar bed (Figure 6.2 right), thus making it vulnerable to damage during surgery. In a large series of 3,583 tonsillectomy patients, only 11 complained of a taste disorder. Just three of these complaints were attributed directly to surgery (Tomita & Ohtuka, 2002). A less favorable outcome was documented elsewhere following a questionnaire enquiry (Heiser et al., 2010). Sixty (32%) reported taste disorders two weeks postoperatively and 15 (8%) at six-month follow-up. Metallic and bitter parageusias were the major complaints. A small but more definitive study measured taste by electrogustometry and questionnaire in 35 patients who underwent tonsillectomy by electric coagulator and 35 who received laryngo-microsurgery (Tomofuji et al., 2005). There were 3/35 with taste disturbance in the electric coagulator group and this was attributed to "pressure on the tongue." There was just one instance of taste impairment in the laryngo-microsurgery group and this was confirmed by electrogustometry. Stathas et al. (2010) assessed 60 tonsillectomy patients by regional detection to four tastants in differing concentrations, 15 days and one month after surgery. They found that bitter and sour tastes were affected more than those of sweet and salty, in keeping with the traditional view of a glossopharyngeal nerve lesion (but now challenged, see Chapter 2). Subsequent evaluation showed near normal results for all but two patients. One reverted to normal at one month but was persistently abnormal. A significant problem with all these investigations is the absence of pre-operative measurement and, in some cases, reliance on patients' reports. Given the anatomy of the pharyngeal tonsil it is likely that tonsillectomy carries a small risk of taste impairment from injury to the glossopharyngeal nerve and that this may be permanent on rare occasions. Complete ageusia is very unusual, but it may happen if there is undue pressure or stretching of the lingual nerve either from a mouth or tongue retractor. If the glossopharyngeal nerve is damaged as well, then taste appreciation will be impaired severely. In one personal case, no subjective recovery was noted at two years, although there was some preservation of sweet and salt appreciation, possibly due to preserved chorda tympani function.

4. **Lesions Involving the Jugular Foramen (Figure 6.3).** Three cranial nerves – CN IX, X, and XI – pass through the jugular foramen, where all may be compromised to varying degrees. When this occurs, the disorder is sometimes termed Vernet's syndrome, a relatively rare condition. Causes of the jugular foramen syndrome include neuromas (growing on any of the three nerves), meningiomas, epidermoid, or glomus jugulare tumors, and trauma

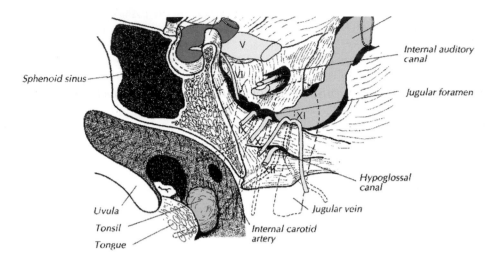

Figure 6.3 The jugular foramen seen from inside the skull in sagittal section with the midbrain, pons, medulla, and cerebellum removed. Anterior is on the left; posterior on the right. Note CN IX, X, and XI colored yellow having emerged from the medulla disappearing through the jugular foramen close to the jugular vein and lateral (transverse) sinus that drains into the sigmoid sinus (blue). Their subsequent course is shown as dotted lines. Note CN IX as it approaches the tongue, soft palate, and tonsil just above the Eustachian tube (black). Reproduced and modified with permission from Neurological Differential Diagnosis. Author, John Patten, Second edition. Figure 6.14. Springer-Verlag 1995. Patten J Neurological Differential Diagnosis. (A black and white version of this figure will appear in some formats. For the color version, please refer to the plate section.)

to the skull base. Typical symptoms consist of a hoarse voice, nasal speech due to palatal weakness, dysphagia, and sternomastoid paresis. The glossopharyngeal nerve is often affected, resulting in taste impairment over the posterior third of the tongue.

Allergic or Allergic-like Reactions

1. **Allergic Rhinitis.** Although olfactory dysfunction is well established in allergic rhinitis, particularly when polyps are involved, studies of the possible associations of allergic rhinitis with alterations in taste bud-mediated processes are few. Rydzewski et al. (2000) reported that 31.2% of 240 patients with hypersensitivity reactions of the respiratory tract had elevated electrogustometric thresholds, as defined by values published earlier by Pruszewicz (1981). In a more recent study of 82 patients with chronic rhinosinusitis (Dzaman et al., 2009), electrical and chemical taste tests were administered before and after steroid therapy. Prior to medication, electrical taste disturbances were, relative to controls, abnormal in 32.26% of their patients. Chemical thresholds varied according to the stimulus, ranging from 19.4 to 51.6%. Those with polyps differed significantly from controls prior to therapy. Steroids improved electrical taste function in 12.9% and chemical taste function in up to 29% of the patients.

2. **Pine Nut Mouth Syndrome.** Several thousand anecdotal reports have described a delayed bitter or metallic taste that begins hours to days after consumption of pine nuts. This may recur with intake of any food or meal (Flesch et al., 2011). In some instances, the dysgeusia lasts several weeks, but eventually resolves without serious health consequences. It is suspected that the cause of the problem is a nut from two particular pine species, *Pinus*

armandii and *Pinus massoniana*, mostly from China. The majority (70%) of 501 separate consumer reports of pine mouth events reported to the FDA between June 2008 and June 2012 were from women (Kwegyir-Afful et al., 2013). Interestingly, nearly all persons (99.6%) registering complaints were not first-time eaters of pine nuts and had eaten such nuts without incident prior to the reported episode. A pesticide screen of 15 samples of pine nuts from various regions was negative. Of the complainants, 40.7% mentioned a history of some type of allergic disorder, including seasonal and perennial rhinitis (21.1%), drug allergies (6.6%), and asthma (1.2%). Only 2.2% of the consumers reported to the FDA comorbid symptoms such as oral itching or swelling, hives, or swollen lymph nodes. The basis of the dysgeusia remains unknown.

Central Taste Disorder

Taste dysfunction from damage to CNS structures is well recognized, although it is reported less frequently than the peripheral varieties. The functional deficit is unilateral when the lesion affects one side the brainstem, as in the lateral medullary syndrome, for example. Some unilateral lesions above the level of the midbrain go unrecognized, given the probable bifurcation of the ascending taste pathways above this level. In this section we describe the gustatory effects of discrete lesions within the brain stem, thalamus, and cerebral hemispheres. This is followed by the influences of traumatic brain injury, epilepsy, and migraine on the ability to taste.

Brain Stem Lesions

Lesions of the brain stem are definitely associated with ageusia or hypogeusia, although documentation in the human literature is sparse and generally lacking in detail. In rats, bilateral lesions of the nucleus tractus solitarius eliminates the concentration-response function for sucrose and NaCl. For citric acid and Polycose, the sensitivity function is shifted to the right, i.e., higher concentrations are needed to produce the same effect (Shimura et al., 1997). Ageusia or hypogeusia has been observed in unilateral medullary vascular lesions where the solitary tract or its nucleus is involved (Shikama al., 1996). In the lateral medullary (Wallenberg) syndrome (Figure 6.4), the solitary tract would be affected, given the usual area of infarction. However, with rare exception (Luker & Scully, 1990), taste is not tested, probably because the loss is unilateral and fails to be recognized or complained of by the patient. Busy clinicians rarely ask and may not have time to perform regional testing as needed to reveal the deficit. Since infarcts associated with this syndrome most likely involve the superior part of the dorsal vagal nucleus, i.e., the salivatory nucleus, ipsilateral impairment of salivation also should be detectable in Wallenberg's syndrome. Taste function in patients with uncomplicated paramedian medullary infarcts (medial medullary syndrome) should be normal, as the lesion is well clear of the dorsolaterally placed solitary tract nucleus. There are sparse reports of ageusia from pontine demyelination in multiple sclerosis (MS; see section below) and a few instances of ageusia due to pontine or midbrain hemorrhage where both central tegmental tracts are damaged (Onoda & Ikeda, 1999).

Thalamic and Cortical Lesions

As noted earlier, unilateral lesions *above* the brainstem do not cause complete loss of taste. This is partly due to bilateral representation of taste above the level of the midbrain. There are scattered reports of vascular or demyelinating thalamic lesions causing taste loss, usually

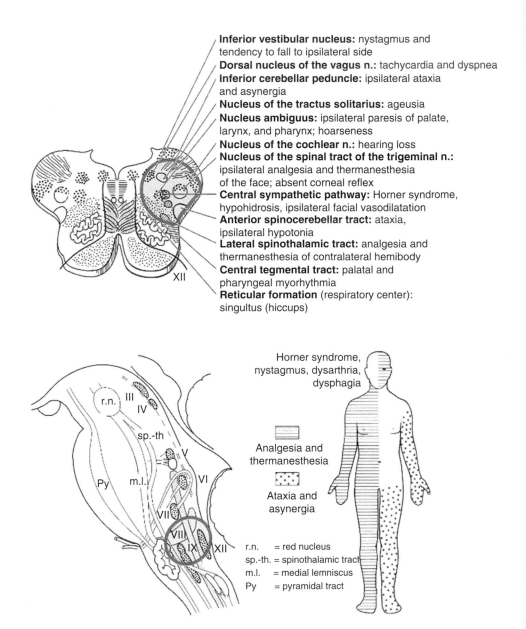

Inferior vestibular nucleus: nystagmus and tendency to fall to ipsilateral side
Dorsal nucleus of the vagus n.: tachycardia and dyspnea
Inferior cerebellar peduncle: ipsilateral ataxia and asynergia
Nucleus of the tractus solitarius: ageusia
Nucleus ambiguus: ipsilateral paresis of palate, larynx, and pharynx; hoarseness
Nucleus of the cochlear n.: hearing loss
Nucleus of the spinal tract of the trigeminal n.: ipsilateral analgesia and thermanesthesia of the face; absent corneal reflex
Central sympathetic pathway: Horner syndrome, hypohidrosis, ipsilateral facial vasodilatation
Anterior spinocerebellar tract: ataxia, ipsilateral hypotonia
Lateral spinothalamic tract: analgesia and thermanesthesia of contralateral hemibody
Central tegmental tract: palatal and pharyngeal myorhythmia
Reticular formation (respiratory center): singultus (hiccups)

XII

Horner syndrome, nystagmus, dysarthria, dysphagia

Analgesia and thermanesthesia

Ataxia and asynergia

r.n.   = red nucleus
sp.-th. = spinothalamic tract
m.l.   = medial lemniscus
Py   = pyramidal tract

Figure 6.4 Wallenberg Syndrome. Typically, this results from occlusion/dissection of a vertebral artery with damage to the dorsolateral medulla. It is rare to find all the features listed in the figure. Reproduced with permission from Baehr & Frotscher (2012), p. 149.

when the nucleus ventralis posteromedialis parvicellularis (VPMpc) is injured (Ito & Suzuki, 1993). A lesion of VPMpc would produce ageusia and given the proximity of this area to the termination of the main trigemino-thalamic tract, it is associated with contralateral sensory loss that includes the face. This was confirmed in a study of 11 patients with thalamic infarction by Fujikane et al. (1999), four of whom had taste impairment resulting from a VPMpc lesion. Two had the cheiro-oral syndrome, i.e., numb hand and face. In their four dysgeusic patients, the taste impairment was contralateral to the infarct, a finding that contradicts neurophysiological studies (see Chapter 2). Anecdotally, bilateral thalamotomy for Parkinson's disease has been noted to produce taste dysfunction.

There is one case report of bilateral thalamic deep brain stimulation of the ventral intermediate nucleus, undertaken for essential tremor, that produced ageusia during stimulation. When the stimulation was turned off, normal taste perception returned (Sajonz et al., 2011). Gustatory impairment is recognized with cortical lesions, particularly the orbitofrontal cortex (OFC) or anterior insular zone, and head injury is the most common cause. In the Fujikane study (1999), 3 of 13 patients had contralateral taste impairment following an infarct in the corona radiata. The final pathway for smell and taste travels from the insula to OFC, particularly its lateral part. In theory, a small lesion in this or its interconnecting fibers could affect taste while sparing smell, but this awaits description. Hemisensory neglect, which results typically from lesions of the right parietal lobe, thalamus, or basal ganglia, has been described for taste (Andre et al., 2000). In this condition, neglect of food products in the left side of the mouth impairs initiation of chewing and swallowing, leading to choking or a tendency to drool and regurgitate undetected food.

Traumatic Brain Injury

Trauma to the brain can result in taste impairment in addition to smell loss. The overall prevalence of trauma-related taste dysfunction has been estimated at 0.5% (Sumner, 1967), although studies in which modern psychophysical testing was performed suggest the prevalence may be around 5% (Deems et al., 1991). In one study, it was estimated that about 6% of those with post-traumatic anosmia also have ageusia (Sumner, 1967). Although few would doubt that taste can be impaired after head injury, no study to date has taken into account the prevalence of gustatory impairment in a non-injured population. Lesions that result in cortical ageusia are typically bilateral and involve the orbitofrontal cortex, thalamus, or insula. Many head injuries cause antero-posterior oscillation of the brain, resulting in the classic frontal and temporal polar damage (see Chapter 5, Figure 5.3). Such lesions impair smell and taste regularly and carry a poor prognosis. The chances for regaining taste is said to be better than for smell, perhaps because most lesions causing taste loss are peripheral and there are (for each side) three nerves (CN VII, IX, X) that subserve taste compared to just one for olfaction. It is suspected that sweet taste recovers more rapidly than bitter (Reiter et al., 2004). Based on Sumner's literature review of 18 head-injured patients and eight of his own cases with bilateral ageusia, there was a crude relationship between duration of post traumatic amnesia (PTA) and recovery of taste: If there was no PTA or it did not exceed 24 hours, then recovery of taste generally occurred within 3 months. If PTA lasted more than 24 hours, then recovery was found to take up to 5 years. Despite this, 4 subjects with no PTA had ageusia for an unspecified time.

Epilepsy

In general, a gustatory aura is less common than an olfactory aura. The seizure focus is usually located in the opercular region or amygdaloid nucleus and it is claimed to be more frequent in right hemisphere lesions (West and Doty, 1995). Among the reported symptoms are "peculiar," "rotten," "sweet," "bitter," "like a cigarette," "like rotten apples," and "like vomitus" (West & Doty, 1995). Many of these experiences are likely smell sensations misidentified as tastes by both the patients and their physicians. An aura of taste produced by partial seizures usually abates following treatment with anticonvulsants. Temporal lobe resection for drug-resistant seizures commonly eliminates most gustatory auras (Acharya et al., 1998). There are few empirical investigations that consider the influence of epilepsy, per se, on taste. In one study, Pal et al. (2004) measured phenylthiocarbamide (PTC) thresholds of 400 epileptic patients and in 100 normal controls. The number of non-tasters was higher in the epileptic patients (34%) than in the controls (20%).

Migraine

It is not clear whether the prodrome or acute headache phase associated with migraine involves definable gustatory phenomena, as seen with olfaction. Anecdotally, some patients report a metallic or mustard-like taste occurring hours or days prior to a migraine attack. Their descriptions are more suggestive of taste phenomena than olfactory, but no one has made proper measurements of taste threshold or identification in the prodromal stage. In one questionnaire-based study of 727 migraineurs, subjective taste abnormality was reported in about one quarter of patients during the headache phase (Kelman, 2004b). Patients sometimes report that certain tastes will provoke a migraine attack but to our knowledge there are no published studies supporting this concept.

Immune-Related Diseases

Diseases of the immune system that are associated with taste dysfunction include multiple sclerosis, myasthenia gravis, and Sjögren's syndrome, as described in detail below.

Multiple Sclerosis (MS)

It is surprising there that are not more reports of taste dysfunction in MS given its widespread nature that damages the cerebral hemispheres, brain stem, and cranial nerves. One uncontrolled prevalence study that used taste identification strips found impairment in 4 of 16 patients (25%) (Fleiner et al., 2010). In another small study, 7/30 MS patients (23%) scored abnormally on the same taste strip test compared to 2/30 of controls (Schmidt, Goktas et al., 2011), a figure very similar to that of a more recent study applying the same test procedure (5/23; 21.7%) (Dahlslett et al., 2012). Using standard liquid tastants, Combarros et al. (2000) described a 46-year-old lady with hemiageusia associated with sensory loss in the tongue and face – all on the left side. The MRI scan showed a plaque of demyelination involving the left central tegmental tract at mid-pontine tegmentum level, in keeping with the known ipsilateral projection of taste afferents in the brain stem. Another case report described a demyelinating lesion in the right midbrain accompanied by left-sided trigeminal sensory symptoms and dysgeusia, thus implying that taste afferents cross in the midbrain before entering their thalamic relay station – the VPMpc (Hisahara et al., 1994). During relapse, individuals with MS may develop subjective impairment of taste (Benatru et al., 2003; Combarros, Miro et al., 1994) and rarely as a presenting feature (Benatru et al., 2003; Bartosik-Psujek et al., 2004).

In the most definitive study to date, a 96-trial test of sweet (sucrose), sour (citric acid), bitter (caffeine), and salty (NaCl) taste perception was administered to the left and right anterior and posterior tongue regions of 73 MS patients and 73 matched controls (Doty et al., 2016). The number and volume of lesions were assessed using quantitative MRI in 52 brain regions of 63 of the MS patients. Taste identification scores were significantly lower in the MS patients for sucrose (p = .0002), citric acid (p = .0001), caffeine (p = .0372), and NaCl (p = .0004) and were present in both the anterior and posterior tongue regions. The percentage of MS patients with identification scores falling below the 5th percentile of controls was 15.07% for caffeine, 21.9% for citric acid, 24.66% for sucrose, and 31.50% for NaCl. Such scores were inversely correlated with lesion *volumes* in the temporal, medial frontal, and superior frontal lobes, and with the *number* of lesions in the left and right superior frontal lobes, right anterior cingulate gyrus, and left parietal operculum. This work clearly demonstrates that a significant proportion of people with MS exhibit taste dysfunction.

Myasthenia Gravis

Classically, MG is viewed as a primary peripheral immune disorder reflecting damage to the postsynaptic nicotinic receptor zone (i.e., muscle end plate). Although it was widely assumed at one time that muscarinic receptors were the sole cholinergic receptors in the brain, this concept is outdated. In the case of the taste system, for example, both muscarinic and nicotinic cholinergic receptors are found within the nucleus of the solitary tract, with muscarinic receptors largely mediating inhibition and nicotinic receptors excitation (Uteshev & Smith, 2006). All studies of taste in MG have been from Japan, of which the largest was a questionnaire and interview-based study of 371 patients who were simply asked about taste disorder. The prevalence was 2.4 percent when relevant confounders were excluded (Kabasawa et al., 2013). All had thymoma and raised acetylcholine receptor antibodies. Five reported onset of taste disorder particularly sweet loss, two–three months prior to their muscle symptoms. Prodromal dysgeusia to sweet was noted in an earlier single case report, again from Japan (Nakazato, 2008). Likewise, the patient had elevated acetylcholine receptor antibodies and a thymoma. It was suggested that the thymoma had produced antibodies to leptin, the hormone concerned with energy intake for which there are receptors in type 3 cells of the taste bud (see Figure 6.5). Other isolated reports mention taste impairment that improved after thymectomy (Iseki et al., 2007). All these studies appear to have relied on patient reports and none have performed any basic taste testing. Given that taste is often confused with smell, and that smell loss is profound in MG (Leon-Sarmiento et al., 2012), quantitative testing of taste, per se, is sorely needed.

Sjögren's Syndrome (SS)

This autoimmune disorder of exocrine glands results in dryness of the mouth and eyes and affects an estimated 1 million Americans. The situation is compounded if there is an associated trigeminal neuropathy as this will affect common sensory *and* taste afferents in the lingual nerve. This can depress taste function and the tactile pleasure of food and drink in addition to the untoward effects of a dry mouth. SS may occur in isolation – the "primary" form. The secondary variety follows other autoimmune conditions such as rheumatoid arthritis, systemic lupus, scleroderma, or primary biliary cirrhosis.

In pioneering study on this topic, Henkin et al. (1972) recorded taste complaints and evaluated taste function in 29 female SS patients, of whom more than half reported decreased taste acuity. The patients' performance on taste tests was markedly impaired. In particular, their taste detection and recognition sensitivity was reduced, and their perception of taste intensity was diminished. Compared to controls, patients judged each

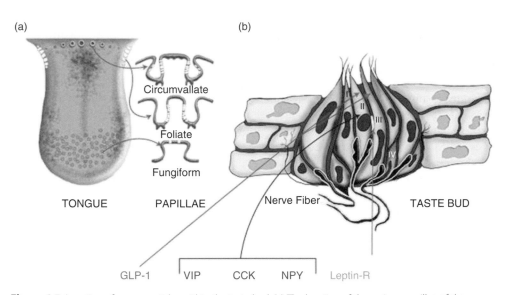

(a) (b)

Circumvallate

Foliate

Fungiform

TONGUE   PAPILLAE   Nerve Fiber   TASTE BUD

GLP-1   VIP   CCK   NPY   Leptin-R

Figure 6.5 Location of neuropeptides within the taste bud. (a) The location of the various papillae of the tongue are shown. (b) The type of taste cell within the taste buds of the tongue and the corresponding hormones. The arrows demarcate the location of each hormone within taste cell types 2, 2, 3, and 4. Abbreviations: GLP-1, glucagon-like peptide 1; VIP, vasoactive intestinal peptide; CCK, cholecystokinin; NPY, neuropeptide Y; leptin-R, leptin receptor. Modified with permission from Martin, Maudsley et al. (2009). (A black and white version of this figure will appear in some formats. For the color version, please refer to the plate section.)

concentration of all four qualities to be less intense. These findings suggest that the taste complaints of SS patients reflect sensory impairment. The SS patients' taste complaints, taste threshold deficits, and reductions in taste intensity were attributed to their lack of saliva, given that they were not reversed by moisturizing the mouth.

A more thorough subsequent investigation of gustation in SS patients measured taste intensity by direct scaling and detection thresholds using a two-alternative forced-choice procedure to sucrose, citric acid, sodium chloride, and quinine sulfate (Weiffenbach et al., 1995). There were 31 women with SS and 101 healthy female controls. Taste complaints were common and affected 55% of the cases and 28% of the controls. These investigators documented a clear alteration in threshold sensitivity between the two groups, but differences in taste intensity judgments were less striking. Although salivary flow was markedly impaired in the SS group, those with negligible flow were no more likely to have more complaints or taste impairment on testing. It was suggested that the taste problem in SS is not simply that of impaired saliva production.

A decade later, Gomez et al. (2004) tested 21 women with primary SS and 20 healthy controls. Detection and recognition thresholds to the standard four tastants in solution were determined by the method of least noticeable differences. Saliva production was determined by Saxon's test on two separate occasions. Although saliva production was severely reduced in SS patients compared to controls, all subjects recognized the 4 basic tastes when these were tested at suprathreshold concentrations. As in the two previous studies, detection thresholds for sweet, sour, and bitter tastes were higher in SS patients than in the controls. Elevations in recognition thresholds for salty, sour, and bitter tastes were also noted.

A different perspective on the taste disorder of SS was cast by a group from Japan (Negoro et al., 2004). Their study included patients with primary and secondary SS (group

A) and a non-SS group (Group B) that suffered from dry eyes and mouth. Eighteen percent of group A and 11% of group B complained of taste disorder. Quantitative testing with electrogustometry (EGM) gave higher figures, with 27% and 38% in groups A and B, respectively. Implementing a filter paper disk method gave comparable figures of 30% and 40%. In group A, unstimulated and stimulated salivary flows correlated with the ability to discriminate taste by the filter paper disk method, but not with the EGM threshold. Their data give a lower prevalence of taste disorder in SS than the investigation by Weiffenbach et al. (1995). These authors suggest that the dysgeusia may relate primarily to a deficiency in salivary flow that prevents tastants reaching the taste buds, again in contrast to the other studies cited above.

Taste threshold was evaluated in SS by filter strips impregnated with representatives of sweet, sour, bitter, and salty tastants (Kamel et al., 2009). There were 28 participants with well-validated primary SS matched to 37 controls. None was taking medication known to alter taste appreciation. Taste threshold was significantly reduced in the SS group and there was significant elevation of taste threshold irrespective of age that affected 70% of their SS sample. Interestingly, sweet thresholds were reduced the least, a finding they attributed to the independence of saliva production from sweet appreciation. It is not known whether this hypogeusia was secondary to simple dryness of the mouth or a coexistent trigeminal neuropathy.

In summary, there is no doubt that patients with SS have a high prevalence of taste complaints and impairment of taste on objective testing. The defects probably do not relate simply to hyposalivation. Not all investigators appear to have studied primary SS; some may have included the secondary form, which may have a different chemosensory profile. The contribution of trigeminal neuropathy, which is common in SS, has not been evaluated in any study and this important aspect clearly warrants further assessment.

Metabolic and Endocrine Diseases

Taste is affected by a range of metabolic and endocrine diseases. We describe disorders associated with dysfunction of the pancreas, thyroid, kidneys, and liver, as well as major metabolic diseases that impact taste perception.

Diabetes

One of the first clinical studies compared *Type 1 (insulin-dependent) diabetics* with controls using detection and recognition thresholds to representatives of the four classic taste qualities (Hardy et al., 1981). These investigators found that taste was affected by both diabetes and age. Subsequently, Le Floch et al. (1989) assessed gustation electrically (EGM) and chemically in 57 type 1 diabetics and 38 controls and found deficits on both types of tests. These investigators further examined 50 type 1 diabetics by EGM and screened for major complications of this condition; namely, retinopathy, renal disease, peripheral neuropathy, and autonomic neuropathy (Le Floch et al., 1990). Raised taste thresholds were found in 54% of the diabetics and the threshold change was associated most strongly with assessment of peripheral neuropathy, microalbuminuria, age, and duration of diabetes, but was not related to glycosylated hemoglobin level (HbA1$_c$), retinopathy, or autonomic neuropathy. In their 5-year follow-up study, hypogeusia at baseline had a predictive value of 88% for subsequent peripheral neuropathy, which led them to suggest that EGM might be a helpful screening tool for early identification of complications (Le Floch et al., 1992).

Influences on taste function similar to those observed in type 1 diabetes have been documented for type 2 (non-insulin dependent) diabetes. Stolbova et al. (1999) reported elevated EGM thresholds indicative of either hypogeusia or ageusia in 32/73 (45%) patients with type 2 disease and of 4/11 (35%) with the type 1 variety. Interestingly, raised taste threshold was discovered in 5 of their 12 non-diabetic obese subjects. Another survey that implemented whole-mouth threshold testing to the four primary tastants found abnormality in 50/80 (62.5%) type 2 diabetics, regardless of whether they were controlled well or not (Gondivkar et al., 2009). Impairment was most marked to sucrose, followed by sour and salt, suggesting that this difference might create a preference for sweet tasting compounds and aggravate hyperglycemia. A similar preferential effect on sweet taste threshold in type 2 disease was shown by others, again using the whole-mouth method (Bustos-Saldana et al., 2009). Once more, the quality of blood glucose control appeared to have no influence on the taste findings.

Insight concerning one possible mechanism for the adverse influence of diabetes on taste function stems from a study of α-gustducin expression in the circumvallate papillae of streptozotocin-induced diabetes in rats (Zhou et al., 2009). Gustducin is a transducin-like G protein that is expressed selectively in about one-third of taste receptor cells and it is probably concerned with mediation of bitter, sweet, and umami tastes. There was higher expression of α-gustducin in taste buds compared to controls, a finding that might explain the impairment to these three tastants (bitter, sweet, and umami). Interestingly, knockout mice lacking α-gustducin are unable to taste bitter, sweet, and umami compounds, whereas sour and salty tastes are unaffected (Wong et al., 1996). Genetic variation in the sweet receptor subunit, TAS1R3, and the second messenger, gustducin (GNAT3), affects the ability of people to sort ascending concentrations of sucrose correctly (Fushan et al., 2009). This raises the possibility of genetic susceptibility in the development of type 2 diabetes and obesity.

Another protein potentially linked with taste dysfunction in diabetics is the neuropeptide, cholecystokinin (CCK). The cholecystokinin receptor (CCK-1) mediates satiety in the central *and* peripheral nervous systems and it is thought to be concerned with bitter appreciation. CCK-1 is expressed in type 2 taste receptor cells (Figure 6.5) and may be concerned with peripheral regulation of sweet intake. OLETF rats are born without the CCK-1 receptor and have increased avidity for concentrated sweet solutions, leading to its overconsumption, obesity, and type 2 diabetes (Herness & Zhao, 2009). One group explored taste responsiveness of the rat chorda tympani (Tsunoda et al., 1998) and found that the relative response magnitude to concentrations of sucrose >1 M was greater in OLETF rats compared with their lean mouse model (LETO), thus supporting the concept of peripheral modulation of sweet appreciation.

Other gut neuropeptides expressed in taste buds are *glucagon-like peptide 1* (GLP-1), *neuropeptide Y* (NPY), and *vasoactive intestinal peptide* (VIP; see Figure 6.5). GLP-1 is expressed in type 2 and 3 taste cells (Figure 6.5). In the gut it is concerned with regulation of insulin secretion and its agonist Exenatide is used in treatment of type 2 diabetes. Conversely, Exendin, a GLP-1 receptor antagonist, elevates blood glucose levels. Mice that lack the GLP-1 receptor have reduced taste sensitivity to sucrose and hypersensitivity to umami and citric acid (Martin et al., 2009). NPY is expressed in type 2 taste cells and inhibits the effect of CCK, but its potential role in taste and diabetes is not clear at present. Both GLP-1 and NPY may be concerned with appetite regulation, obesity and subsequent diabetes. VIP is expressed in type 2 taste cells (Figure 6.5*)*. VIP knock-out mice show increased preference for sweet solutions and have elevated blood glucose levels (Martin et al., 2010). Furthermore, their taste cells showed a decrease in leptin receptor expression and elevated expression of GLP-1, factors which may explain sweet taste preference.

In summary there is convincing evidence regarding the influence of several taste cell neuropeptides on sensitivity to sweet compounds and this finding may have a bearing on predispositions to diabetes and obesity. This susceptibility may be connected to recently defined polymorphisms in the sweet receptor subunit, TAS1R3. Both type 1 and type 2 diabetes are associated with hypogeusia, particularly for sweet, and this impairment correlates with some of the recognized diabetic complications, notably peripheral neuropathy and renal disease. A raised taste threshold on EGM might be a useful guide for future complications, in particular peripheral neuropathy.

Thyroid Disease

A potential role of hypothyroidism in altering taste function was noted in two studies of congenital hypothyroidism (formerly termed cretinism) published in the early 1960s. This congenital disorder is associated with the absence of the thyroid gland and markedly stunted physical and mental growth that begins within 4 to 12 weeks after birth. In one study that used the Harris-Kalmus taste threshold procedure (see Chapter 2), only a third of congenital hypothyroid (CH) patients who could be tested were classified as PTC tasters (i.e., 9 of 27), as compared to 78.2% of controls of similar age (104 of 133) (Shepard & Gartler, 1960). In another study, only 2 PTC tasters were found in 17 CH youngsters (11.8%), in contrast to 70.6% of normal controls (Fraser, 1961).

The influences of hypothyroidism on taste function in adults is less clear. In one study, McConnell, Menendez et al. (1975) reported that 18 patients with hypothyroidism had decreased sensitivity to the tastes of NaCl, sucrose, urea, and HCl, as measured by both detection and recognition thresholds. Repletion of thyroid hormone was said to return the thresholds to normal levels. Indeed, chemosensory abnormalities of one patient were said to be completely corrected after 16 days of thyroid hormone replacement therapy. Unfortunately, this work lacked a control group and confounded test order with the treatment condition. Thus, the improvement attributed to hormone repletion could simply reflect improved performance due to repeated testing.

More recently, Bhatia et al. (1990) reported that hypothyroid patients were much more likely to be PTC non-tasters than tasters (60% vs. 40%). Furthermore, the non-tasters rated sweet (glucose) and bitter (quinine sulfate) sensations as weaker in intensity than tasters. Both hypothyroid PTC tasters and non-tasters rated NaCl solutions as more pleasant than did the controls and patients with hyperthyroidism, although no statistical analyses were performed. In a subsequent study, 30 hypothyroid patients, 20 hyperthyroid patients, and 100 normal controls were asked to rate the perceived intensity and pleasantness of various concentrations of glucose, NaCl, quinine sulfate, and citric acid on a 6-point category scale (Bhatia et al., 1991). No information regarding the ages of the groups was indicated and many of the controls were apparently college students. Although the authors claimed that differences existed in the ratings of the hypothyroid and hyperthyroid subjects and indicated significant p values, analysis of their tabulated data based on the reported means and standard deviations (or SEMs) do not support this concept.

In contrast to the claims of adverse effects, a study performed 10 years before the study by McConnell et al. (1975) that used the same testing procedure reported on 10 hypothyroid and 10 hyperthyroid subjects. They all had normal thresholds for NaCl, potassium chloride (KCl), sodium bicarbonate, sucrose, urea, and HCl (Pittman & Beschi, 1967). These authors noted that a few hypothyroid patients actually performed *better* than normal on the tests. Subsequently, Mattes et al. (1986), using a staircase forced-choice threshold procedure, measured recognition thresholds to NaCl and urea in 11 hypothyroid patients and 11 controls. No differences in threshold values were observed. Likewise, Lewitt et al. (1989) found no evidence that 16 hypothyroid subjects differed from 17 controls in their ability to recognize low concentrations of NaCl, sucrose, citric acid, and caffeine.

In a more recent investigation of 750 patients presenting to the University of Pennsylvania Smell and Taste Center for chemosensory disturbances, those who were taking thyroid medication such as levothyroxine complained of taste loss significantly more often than those who were not taking such medications (Deems et al., 1991). Unexpectedly, these subjects performed somewhat *better* on a taste identification test and rated low concentrations of caffeine as *more intense* than did the comparison subjects. Their taste thresholds for citric acid, NaCl, and sucrose were within normal limits.

Animal studies have also failed to show significant influences of hypothyroidism on taste sensitivity. Signal detection analysis is a sophisticated test procedure that assesses sensitivity and response biases independently. An investigation that applied this method to an operant task in rats with propylthiouracil-induced hypothyroidism found no change in their ability to detect NaCl, HCl, sucrose, or quinine sulfate (Brosvic et al., 1992). Moreover, no effects on the response bias measure were observed. However, during the period of propylthiouracil treatment and briefly thereafter, preferences for NaCl, HCl, and quinine sulfate were increased relative to controls, but returned to normal by two weeks after treatment had stopped. The latter observations are in accord with earlier studies that also found rats made hypothyroid by propylthiouracil increased their consumption and apparent preference for NaCl (Fregly, 1962; Fregly et al., 1965; Fregly & Waters, 1965, 1966). Desoxycorticosterone reversed these effects (Fregly & Waters, 1966). Preferential ingestion of other tastants, such as saccharine, by hypothyroid rats has also been noted by others (Gordon et al., 1992).

In summary, the effect of hypothyroidism on taste function is not clear. Test paradigms that differentiate between preferences and sensitivity need to be instituted and they should include procedures that separate response biases from measures of sensory sensitivity, incorporating, for example, signal detection analyses. Until such studies are performed, the effects of thyroid disease on human taste perception will remain speculative.

Renal Disease

Patients with diseases of the kidney, especially end-stage renal disease, commonly report dysgeusia, such as a metallic sensation (Dirschnabel et al., 2011). They often exhibit a range of oral conditions directly or indirectly associated with taste dysfunction, including dry mouth, gingival bleeding, pallor, halitosis, increased incidence of caries and calculi, and overexpression of opportunistic pathogens, e.g., fungal or herpetic (types 1 and 2) (Kho et al., 1999; de la Rosa et al., 2006; Thorman et al., 2009; Otero et al., 2011; Patil et al., 2012; Kaushik et al., 2013). Interestingly, sufferers of the late-onset kidney disease Balkan Endemic Nephropathy are frequent carriers of the TAS2R43 gene, which in theory should produce aversions to bitter-tasting nephrotoxins such as aristolochic acid (Wooding et al., 2012). The significance of this association is not clear.

Taste recognition thresholds are elevated in many patients with renal disease, particularly for sweet and sour stimuli (Burge et al., 1978). The mechanisms responsible are not known. Although dialysis improves the deficit, thresholds for some tastants remain elevated relative to those of healthy controls (Burge et al., 1979). In one study, patients described increased sensitivity and decreased preferences for NaCl in soup after dialysis (Shepherd et al., 1987). Another group reported that taste thresholds of younger uremic patients were more conspicuously elevated than those of older uremic patients relative to age-matched controls (Ciechanover et al., 1980). Importantly, lowered taste thresholds have been noted in patients after renal transplantation (Mahajan et al., 1984) and at least one double-blind study found improved taste threshold when zinc salts were added to the dialysis fluid (Sprenger et al., 1983).

Liver Disease

Liver disease is associated with altered taste, as well as smell, function. In one study, about 40% of over a hundred patients with various liver diseases reported recent changes in taste perception, compared to 6% of age- and gender-matched healthy controls (Deems et al., 1993). Elevated thresholds for all four classic taste qualities have been reported in liver disease (Burge et al., 1978), particularly thresholds for salty- and bitter-tasting stimuli (Smith et al., 1976). Such effects have not been observed in some studies that employed whole-mouth test procedures, presumably a reflection of redundancy in sensory innervation and greater sensitivity of those regional taste procedures. A recent exploration of 40 patients with chronic hepatitis documented elevated recognition thresholds for umami and, paradoxically, higher ratings for the intensity of sucrose (Van Daele et al., 2011). Improvement in detection of NaCl is reported after liver transplantation (Bloomfeld al., 1999).

Addison's Disease (Adrenal Insufficiency)

Complementing olfaction, one study reported that patients with Addison's disease are *hypersensitive* to the taste of salt (Henkin & Solomon, 1962). In this investigation, NaCl detection thresholds of 6 untreated or inadequately treated patients with adrenal insufficiency fell below the average thresholds of 75 hospitalized non-endocrine patients and 16 normal controls. These findings differ from observations in rats, where adrenalectomy has no effect on NaCl taste sensitivity but does alter NaCl preference thresholds (Richter, 1936, 1939; Carr, 1952; Harriman & Macleod, 1953; Brosvic et al., 1989).

Hypertension

Raised blood pressure independent of diabetes has been linked to taste dysfunction, although the nature of the testing and conclusions are variable. Since the early work of Richter (Richter, 1936, 1939), the association with salt intake and hypertension has been a major area of research. In a pioneering experiment, Fallis et al. (1962) obtained NaCl thresholds from 20 non-medicated hypertensive and 20 age-, sex-, and race-matched non-hypertensive subjects. An ascending series threshold procedure was used in which one of four cups at each concentration contained the stimulus and the other three cups held distilled water. Rinsing occurred after each trial. Half the subjects were instructed to check for the salty taste, whereas the rest were asked to identify only the different sample. The procedure was completed twice for each subject. Recognition thresholds for dextrose (sweet) were obtained for half of the subjects. In the hypertensive group, NaCl thresholds (but not dextrose thresholds) were significantly lower than the normotensive subjects, implying that hypertensive patients consume more salt because they are less sensitive to it. Similar elevations of NaCl thresholds have been observed in subsequent studies employing whole-mouth testing (Bisht et al., 1967; Wotman et al., 1967). Investigations that employ the three-drop protocol of Henkin have not found such changes (Schechter et al., 1973; Henkin, 1974; Schechter et al., 1974), emphasizing the importance of test procedure. Most suprathreshold assessments of NaCl perception indicate that hypertensive subjects, compared to those with normal blood pressures, rate NaCl concentrations less intense (e.g., Contreras, 1978; Barylko-Pikielna et al., 1985).

Turner's Syndrome (TS)

Turner's syndrome (TS) is a condition where a female has just one X chromosome, i.e., a 45,X0 genotype. Patients are short, dysmorphic, and do not menstruate. Diabetes and hypothyroidism are more frequent than expected. It is not clear whether TS is associated with gustatory deficits. In 1967, Henkin evaluated detection and recognition thresholds for sucrose (sweet), sodium chloride (NaCl; salty), hydrochloric acid (HCL; sour), and urea (bitter) of nine TS patients (Henkin, 1967). The median detection and recognition thresholds for HCl and urea were abnormally elevated, whereas thresholds for NaCl and sucrose were reported to be within normal limits. Treatment with gonadal steroids had no influence on the test measures. In an addendum to the paper, it was noted that an additional 12 TS patients were tested and identical thresholds were found. No specific control group was assessed.

More recently, Ros et al. (2012) claimed that 30 patients with TS had normal taste when "four (unnamed) powdered tastes" representing sweet, sour, bitter, and salt were spread over the tongue. Two questions were asked: "Did you taste any substance?" and "How did the powder taste: sweet, salty, sour, or bitter?" All patients detected a taste. However, 23% of the patients wrongly identified sour compared to only 5% of 43 healthy controls who were taking contraceptive medication (p = 0.082). The patients scored the same as controls in identifying the sweet, bitter, and salty stimuli.

Clearly more research is needed on this topic with exclusion of those who may have diabetes or thyroid disorder. As it stands, there is no convincing evidence in support of a taste disorder in TS. If there is a defect, the available data suggest it is likely to be mild.

Vitamin and Mineral Deficiencies

Surprisingly, little is known about the relationship between vitamin or mineral deficiencies and taste perception. The few empirical studies on this topic have employed animal models. Gradual loss of preferences for sucrose and NaCl, as well as aversions to quinine, has been reported in vitamin A-deficient rats (Bernard & Halpern, 1968; Reifan et al., 1998). Such deficits are reversed by vitamin A repletion. The taste disturbances are likely related to increased keratinization of the lingual papillae, including the region of the taste bud pores, adjacent epithelial, and glandular tissues (Bernard et al., 1961).

Frank zinc deficiency is linked to taste dysfunction, a defect that reverses readily with repletion of zinc stores (Takaoka et al., 2010). Double blind studies indicate that most patients with taste or smell deficits do not benefit from zinc supplements (Henkin et al., 1976; Greger & Geissler, 1978; Gibson et al., 1989). No differences in smell or taste test scores are evident in patients with chemosensory disorders whether or not they are receiving zinc supplements (Deems et al., 1991). Furthermore, significant adverse effects may be observed at the zinc dose levels that are often recommended, e.g., gastric problems, copper deficiency, iron-deficiency anemia, and neutropenia (Fosmire, 1990; Takaoka et al., 2010).

Medication-related Taste Disturbances

A wide range of medications may affect chemosensation, although taste is involved more frequently than smell (See Table 6.2). Most drug-related taste disorders disappear after removal of treatment, but polypharmacy can complicate matters and, in many cases, taste symptoms persist months after drug withdrawal. The physiologic basis of taste disorders associated with medications has, for the most part, received little scientific attention. A number of the main causes of dysgeusia related to pharmacologic agents are discussed below.

Antimicrobials

Several antimicrobials are associated with distorted taste sensations, including antibiotic and antiviral agents. The major classes of such agents are described below.

1. **Antibiotics.** It has been known for many years that antibiotics produce unpleasant taste sensations, although systematic studies of this phenomenon are relatively recent. An early report, for example, suggested that Griseofulvin produced "tastelessness" to all foods and flavors, but no formal tests were performed (Fogan, 2007). It should be noted that the taste of antibiotics is influenced by the medium in which they are ingested. Thus, some antibiotics, when taken with acidic foods or suspended in acidic sports drinks, taste more bitter than when consumed with water, reflecting their more rapid dissolution in acidic conditions and the failure of sweeteners to block their bitterness (Ishizaka et al., 2004).

Even though it is now common practice to prescribe antibiotics, such as amoxicillin and clarithromycin, with a proton pump inhibitor (PPI) such as omeprazole, rabeprazole, and pantoprazole, to eliminate *Helicobacter pylori* infections, dysgeusia remains a common side effect, although prevalence estimates vary considerably. For example, a large-scale study of triple therapy, with amoxicillin, clarithromycin, and rabeprazole (Fujioka et al., 2012) found that dysgeusia and diarrhea were the main adverse drug reactions that affected only 4.4% of the sample. Baena Diez et al. (1998) attempted to eliminate helicobacter pylori infection in 121 patients with a one-week course of similar therapy (omeprazole, amoxycillin, and clarithromycin). The incidence of self-reported dysgeusia was 67%, much higher than that reported by Fujioka et al. A further study implemented clarithromycin and amoxycillin without a PPI and noted an intermediate incidence of 28% (al-Assi et al., 1994). Despite high prevalence estimates, the associated dysgeusia reportedly recovers within a few weeks or months. It is also possible that PPIs may contribute to taste impairment rather than the antibiotics themselves.

Table 6.2. Medication and toxins that may cause taste disorder. For simplicity, only examples are given.

Drug group	Example	Type of taste disorder
Antimicrobials	Ampicillin	Bitter or metallic
Proton pump inhibitors	Omeprazole	Dysgeusia
Antiviral	HAART (protease inhibitors)	Oily aftertaste
Antifungal	Terbenafine	"Taste loss"
Antimicrobial mouth washes	Chlorhexidine	Increased intensity of quinine and salts.
Cancer chemotherapy	Cisplatin. Taxanes	Metallic
ACE inhibitors	Captopril	Distortion or metallic taste
Angiotensin II antagonists	Losartan	Metallic or burning. Raised threshold
Lipid lowering	Statins	Dysgeusia and ageusia
Calcium channel blockers	Amlodipine	Dysgeusia
Diuretics	Amiloride	Dysgeusia
Tricyclic antidepressants	amitriptyline	Reduced intensity
Selective serotonin reuptake inhibitors	Citalopram	Taste loss and perverted taste quality
Antianxiety agents	Benzodiazepines	Dysgeusia
Anti-manics / mood stabilizers	Lithium carbonate	Dysgeusia
Anti-epileptic	Phenytoin, carbamazepine & lamotrigine	Dysgeusia
CNS stimulants	Caffeine	Lowered threshold
Hypnotics	Zolpidem tartrate	Taste perversion. Metallic/ bitter dysgeusia
Botulinum toxin	Botulinum Toxin A	Improvement of dysgeusia
Snake, fish, and insect venoms	Ciguetera	Metallic taste
Heavy metals	Arsenic	Bitter or metallic taste
Intranasal sprays	Sumatriptan	Bitter

Most antibiotics, with the notable exception of pyrimidines (i.e., pyrimethamine and trimethoprim), alter the taste of sodium, potassium, and/or calcium salts when applied locally to the tongue. For example, ampicillin and the anti-fungal agent, pentamidine, decrease the perception of sodium chloride; tetracycline, pentamidine, and ethambutol decrease potassium chloride perception; and ampicillin, pentamidine, ethambutol, and sulfamethoxazole reduce $CaCl_2$ perception (Schiffman et al., 2000). The typical antibiotic-induced dysgeusias experienced by non-medicated subjects of all ages are bitter or metallic. Interestingly, older individuals use a broader range of adjectives than younger people to describe the abnormal taste sensations. Schiffman et al. (2000) found that thresholds for most antimicrobials were elevated in the elderly, in keeping with age-related changes in taste sensitivity. Importantly, antibiotics applied directly to the tongue were found to modify the experience of other taste qualities, such as salty and sour. The half-life of some antibiotics is quite long (up to three days for azithromycin), and since many antibiotics are excreted in saliva, it is not surprising that they can induce unpleasant tastes.

Several antimicrobial agents gain access to the nasal and salivary secretions from the blood. For example, Enoxacin, a fluoroquininone broad spectrum antibiotic used for urinary tract infection, is known to produce changes in taste and smell. The concentration of this drug in nasal secretions is nearly twice as high as plasma (Schiffman et al., 2000). Pentamidine, another antimicrobial used typically for pneumocystis pneumonia infection, induces a rapid bitter or metallic sensation when injected intravenously, presumably through stimulation of taste receptors via blood- or saliva-borne routes.

2. **Antivirals.** Bitter and metallic tastes are reported from ingestion of these compounds. In addition to provoking such dysgeusias, protease inhibitors used in the treatment of AIDS can alter the flavor of a number of tastants. Highly active antiretroviral therapies (HAARTs) cause taste perversions in HIV-positive adults such as an oily aftertaste (Eiznhamer et al., 2002; Johnson et al., 2003). Amantadine (Symmetrel®) and oseltamivir (Tamiflu®) used in treatment of influenza, taste bitter in oral suspension, particularly amantadine. The bitterness is stronger when they are presented in a more acidic milieu in common with antibiotics (Ishizaka et al., 2004). Acyclovir (Zovirax®), a drug employed as prophylaxis or treatment of herpes virus infections, often produces a bitter taste. The bitterness is more prominent in children, who may need to crush the large tablets before ingestion, resulting in poor compliance (Eksborg et al., 2002). Marivavir, a member of a new class of benzimidazole riboside antivirals, produces dysgeusia in most patients. In a double-blind Phase I study, 13 normal and 17 HIV type 1-infected subjects received increasing doses of the Marivavir (Wang et al., 2003). Taste disturbance occurred in 83%, notably bitter, metallic, or chemical dysgeusia.

Unpleasant tastes have been reported for some anti-rhinovirus intranasal spray preparations (Hayden et al., 1992; Hsyu et al., 2002). For example, pirodavir (R77975), a capsid-binding anti-picornaviral agent, induced an unpleasant taste in 59% of 66 subjects compared to 27% of 65 subjects who received the carrier medium alone (Hayden et al., 1992). Such sensations are usually mild, begin within 4–15 minutes after administration and last less than an hour. This effect may relate to movement of secretions from the nasopharynx to the taste buds.

Unpleasant tastes are recognized for over-the-counter oral zinc preparations that are alleged to have antiviral properties and decrease the duration of common cold symptoms. In one randomized, double-blind, placebo-controlled study, bad tastes were mentioned by 80% of the treated group compared to 30% on placebo (Mossad et al., 1996). Forty-one percent of zinc recipients and 6% of placebo recipients described the aftertaste as moderate to severe.

3. **Antifungals.** Terbinafine (Lamisil) is an oral antimycotic used for fungal infections of the finger and toe nails. It is estimated that 0.6% to 2.8% of those who have received the drug for at least 4 weeks mention taste impairment (Doty et al., 2008). According to case reports, recovery occurs about 4 months after drug withdrawal (Beutler et al., 1993; Stricker et al.,

1996), although long-lasting effects have been noted (Beutler et al., 1993; Bong et al., 1998; Doty et al., 2008).

Shortly after the introduction of Terbinafine there were several reports of subjective taste disorder. An early study, using a relatively insensitive whole-mouth threshold test, found no taste dysfunction in someone who complained of taste loss secondary to terbinafine (Lemont & Sabo, 2001). A more recent analysis of six patients who were prescribed terbinafine in standard dosage (250 mg daily), found significant deficits, relative to controls, for all four major tastants (Doty & Haxel, 2005) (Figure 6.6). The 96-trial taste test comprised 15μL of single concentrations of sucrose (0.49 M), sodium chloride (0.31 M), citric acid (0.015 M), and caffeine (0.04 M), equated for perceived intensity and physical viscosity (1.53mm^2/s^2). These were presented six times each to specified left and right anterior and posterior tongue regions. On a given trial, the subject indicated whether a sweet, sour, bitter, or salty taste was perceived by pointing to answers located on a chart before retracting the tongue and rinsing the mouth with purified water. The percentage of trials on which the tastants were correctly identified

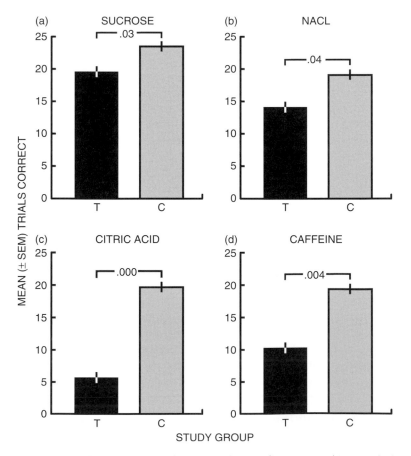

Figure 6.6 Mean (SEM) number of trials correct for the identification of sweet-, sour-, bitter-, and salty-tasting substances in six patients complaining of taste deficits following terbinafine usage (T) and in six matched controls (C). The P values reflect the main effects of group in separate analyses of variance performed for each tastant.

served as the test measure. Identification of all four tastants was impaired significantly, especially for citric acid and caffeine (Figure 6.6).

4. **Antimicrobial Mouthwashes.** The broad-spectrum antimicrobial, chlorhexidine, which is used in mouthwashes to control the build-up of plaque, can impair taste perception. In addition to its bitter taste, chlorhexidine decreases the intensity of quinine (bitter), the saltiness of sodium chloride, potassium chloride, and ammonium chloride, but not the sweetness of sucrose, the savory (umami) taste of monosodium glutamate, or the sourness of citric acid (Breslin & Tharp, 2001; Frank et al., 2001). Some of these influences are region specific. For example, chlorhexidine reduces sodium chloride intensity more in anterior (CN VII) than in posterior tongue regions (CN IX) (Grover & Frank, 2008). While the perceived intensity of a sodium chloride solution increases after rinsing the mouth with chlorhexidine, it is proposed that the subject's ability to identify the stimulus as salty decreases (Lang et al., 1988). Such effects, which can occur at chlorhexidine concentrations found in commercially available mouthwashes (e.g., 0.12% in Peridex®; 0.2% in Cordosyl®), have led to the suggestion that chlorhexidine-containing mouthwashes may be useful in mitigating salty or bitter dysgeusias (Helms et al., 1995).

Chemotherapeutic Agents

Self-reported chemosensory disturbances are associated with chemotherapy, particularly those administered for breast and gynecological cancers. Much depends on the type of therapy prescribed. In a study of 518 such patients, 75% reported changes in smell and taste (Bernhardson et al., 2008). Strikingly similar numbers of taste-centered complaints have been noted in other chemotherapy studies, e.g., 76.1% in a study of 74 breast cancer and 35 gynecological cancer subjects (Gamper et al., 2012) and 84% in an investigation of 45 with breast carcinoma (Jensen et al., 2008). In the latter investigation, over a third developed oral mucosal lesions and 11% had oral candidiasis, problems which may impair taste function. In a study of cisplatin, the anti-proliferative agent, 77% of the infused patients developed a metallic taste that lasted from a few hours to 3 weeks (Wickham et al., 1999).

Given the multiple oral problems in many patients receiving chemotherapy, some "taste" complaints likely reflect alterations in olfaction. A case report of severe chemotherapy-induced parosmia discovered that blocking the nose with a nose clip eliminated the parosmia and restored normal eating behavior (Muller et al., 2006). In an extensive study, a battery of psychophysical taste and smell tests was administered to 87 patients undergoing chemotherapy for breast cancer or a gynecologic malignancy at the beginning, midway (9 weeks), and immediately after (18 weeks) chemotherapy, and 12 weeks after cessation of therapy (Steinbach et al., 2009). Impairment of sweet, sour, bitter, and salty perception was noted at the 18-week test, with particular impact on the ability to detect salt. Tests of odor detection, identification, and discrimination were similarly altered, chiefly detection. Both taste and smell function generally returned to normal 12 weeks after cessation of therapy. In this study, Taxane-based agents caused most dysfunction. Taxanes, such as paclitaxel (Taxol) and docetaxel (Taxotere), are diterpenes produced from Yew plants and work by radiosensitizing and disrupting microtubule function, thus inhibiting cell division. These observations underpin previous subjectively based observations that poor appetite and weight loss are connected more to the chemosensory disturbance than the effect of the underlying cancer itself (Wismer, 2008).

Chemotherapy may affect taste more directly by inducing oral inflammation, mouth infection, and salivary gland dysfunction. Furthermore, chemotherapy permits overgrowth of oral commensals such as candida or there may be ulcer formation presumably related to diminished immunity. Salivary production can be reduced by these mechanisms but if there has been neck irradiation salivation is impaired significantly.

In summary, it is likely that cancer chemotherapy, particularly that based on Taxane, may cause impairment of smell and taste by a direct neurotoxic action. There are undoubted secondary effects on taste as a result of impaired salivation, microbial overgrowth, and reduced oral hygiene.

Cardiovascular Medications

Over a third of the 92 blood pressure modifying agents named in the Physicians' Desk Reference (PDR) are reported to have taste-related adverse side effects (Doty et al., 2003). Among those implicated are antilipemic agents, adrenergic stimulants, α-and β-adrenergic blockers, angiotensin-converting enzyme (ACE) inhibitors, angiotensin II agonists and antagonists, calcium channel blockers, group I-IV anti-arrhythmics, combination diuretics, and coronary vasodilators. Most such drugs reduce submandibular/sublingual salivary gland secretions under both stimulated and unstimulated conditions (Wolff et al., 2008). In this section we describe those cardiovascular medications for which the most data are available.

1. **Angiotensin-Converting Enzyme (ACE) Inhibitors.** ACE inhibitors are the antihypertensive drugs most frequently associated with gustatory disturbances. Approximately 70% of ACE inhibitors listed in the PDR are reported to alter perception, described as "loss of taste," "metallic taste," "taste disturbance," and "taste distortion," albeit in a relatively small percentage of individuals (Doty et al., 2003). Sixty-five percent of ACE inhibitors that are combined with calcium channel blocking or diuretic drugs have been associated with such disturbances (Doty et al., 2003). Captopril is notorious for such side effects, producing more frequent taste complaints than any other orally active ACE inhibitor (Boyd, 1993). This agent can make food that is normally sweet taste salty; it can reduce the perceived intensity of sucrose and potassium chloride, and may produce chronic bitter or salty taste sensations (Zervakis et al., 2000). The effects are dose related, with a prevalence increasing from 1.6% at less than 150 mg per day to 7.3% at doses above 150 mg per day (Griffin, 1992).

Although it has been suggested that the sulfhydryl group of Captopril may cause its adverse effects, other ACE inhibitors that lack this functional group also produce such actions, although at lower frequencies (DiBianco, 1990). Cessation of therapy usually eliminates the unwanted tastes within a few weeks (McNeill et al., 1979; Grosskopf et al., 1984).

2. **Angiotensin II Antagonists.** Angiotensin antagonists inhibit the renin-angiotensin-aldosterone (RAAS) system by blocking angiotensin receptors, rather than inhibiting the enzyme that converts angiotensin I to angiotensin II. The most widely used of these drugs, Losartan, can produce ageusia and dysgeusia (Schlienger et al., 1996; Heeringa & van Puijenbroek, 1998). The disturbance is often metallic or burning but usually reverses on drug withdrawal. The related product, Candesartan, may also produce minor change in taste sensitivity. This was shown in a trial of Candesartan given to eight healthy subjects who were evaluated by threshold testing to the four classic tastants and by electrogustometry (EGM) (Tsuruoka et al., 2004). There was a subclinical reduction of

threshold sensitivity to all four tastants, particularly bitter and sour. Likewise, an elevated EGM threshold was found, but the taste changes reversed after two weeks. This and other reports of gustatory disorder with the related compound, Valsartan, suggest that mild reversible hypogeusia is probably a class effect of angiotensin-II receptor blockers.

3. **Lipid Lowering.** Seven of the 10 main lipid lowering drugs listed in the PDR (2005) have been associated with subjective reports of taste disturbance. All six of the hydroxymethyl-glutaryl-coenzyme A (HMG-CoA) reductase inhibitors (statins) were listed as having "altered taste." Dysgeusia, ageusia, and parosmia were noted to be additional side effects for some of these drugs (Doty et al., 2003). Altered taste, parosmia, and ageusia were observed with Atorvastatin (Lipitor®) in one placebo-controlled study described in the PDR. Similar alterations were reported in clinical trials for Cerivastatin (Baycol®), Fluvastatin (Lescol®), Pravastatin (Provachol®), Lovastatin (Mevacor®), and Simvastatin (Zocor®).

4. **Calcium Channel Blockers.** Over half of the calcium channel blockers (CCB) found in the PDR have been implicated in taste or smell disturbances, although most via single case reports. Such agents as Amlodipine (Norvasc®, Lortel®), Bepridil (Vascor®), Diltiazem (Cardizem®, Dilaclor®), Nifedipine (Adalat®, Procardia®), and Nisoldipine (Sular®) have all been associated with dysgeusia (Levenson & Kennedy, 1985). CCB have been linked to gingival hyperplasia with a prevalence ranging from 20–83 percent, especially in those receiving Diltiazem. This implies that the effect on taste may result at least in part from gum disease itself.

5. **Diuretics.** The influences of diuretics on human taste function are not clear. Although amiloride itself can have a bitter taste, its association with "bad taste" in a study of 607 subjects noted in the PDR was less than 1 percent. In most subjects, 100 μM of amiloride placed on the tongue for 5 minutes reduces the perceived intensity of solutions of NaCl and LiCl, but not KCl (Anand & Zuniga, 1997). Paradoxically, whole-mouth NaCl threshold values of subjects who have been taking amiloride for long periods suggest increased, rather than reduced, sensitivity (Mattes et al., 1988). Subjects who had received amiloride displayed decreased salivary Na^+ levels, conceivably reflecting a perceptual imbalance between the stimulated and adapted states.

Psychoactive Drugs

Several psychoactive drugs are associated with taste disorders. These compounds are classified by type in this section.

1. **Antidepressants.** According to the PDR, numerous tricyclic antidepressants are listed as having a "peculiar taste." Drugs of this class include amitriptyline (Elavil), clomipramine (Anafranil), desipramine (Norpramin), doxepin (Sinequan), imipramine (Tofranil), nortriptyline (Pamelor), and trifluoperazine (Stelazine). Some not only have a taste of their own, but they can alter the perceived intensity of taste qualities such as sweet and salty (Schiffman et al., 1998). Amitriptyline, a widely used tricyclic antidepressant, decreased sensitivity to all four tastants when continuously applied to the tongue, although only salty taste was significantly altered when the drug was applied intermittently (Schiffman et al., 1999). In common with some other medications, amitriptyline likely affects taste receptors by excretion into saliva or through entry into the lingual

blood supply, where it may block sodium, potassium, and calcium membrane channels, as well as influence the metabolism of second messenger systems. Members of the tricyclic class have anticholinergic properties that result in a dry mouth which in turn could impair taste perception.

Serotonin reuptake inhibitors (SSRIs), such as citalopram (Celexa) and fluoxetine (Prozac), which are widely prescribed for depression, post-traumatic stress disorder, and phobias, are associated with taste loss and perversions of taste quality. Paroxetine (Paxil) decreases sucrose and quinine recognition thresholds (i.e., increased sensitivity) in humans by 27 percent and 53 percent, respectively (Heath et al., 2006). In the same study, reboxetine (4 mg), a norepinephrine reuptake inhibitor with little serotonin reuptake action, increased sensitivity to quinine and HCl, but not to sucrose or NaCl. Associations of taste thresholds to measures of anxiety were also noted.

2. **Antianxiety Agents.** This class of drug is used in the treatment of anxiety states, phobias, post-traumatic stress syndrome, and sleep disorders. Benzodiazepines, the most frequently prescribed antianxiety drugs, act on $GABA_A$ receptors and enhance GABAergic transmission in the brain. Along with other antianxiety agents such as flurazepam (Dalmane) and alprazolam (Xanax), they are reported in the PDR to cause dysgeusia in a very small number of cases. In rodents, benzodiazepines appear to enhance the palatability of fluids and foods in a receptor-specific manner. This is likely mediated at the level of the brainstem, given that the effects are present in decerebrate animals (Berridge & Pecina, 1995). However, no human studies have demonstrated a significant influence of benzodiazepines on taste, although trends have been noted. In one study, for example, intensity ratings for bitter obtained from 20 individuals receiving anxiolytics were nominally lower than those of controls, although the effects were not significant (respective means (SDs) = 9.6 (0.5) & 9.0 (1.6), p = 0.11) (de Matos et al., 2010). It is not clear whether these and other seemingly negative findings reflect the use of inappropriate study paradigms, the low dosages employed in humans, or species differences, including variable responsiveness of an apparent brainstem palatability system (Berridge & Pecina, 1995).

3. **Antipsychotics.** Traditional (typical) antipsychotics, such as the phenothiazines, butyrophenones, and thioxanthenes, block D-2 dopamine receptors and alter the balance between central cholinergic and dopaminergic systems. Haloperidol, the prototypical antipsychotic, and trifluoperazine (Stelazine) are both associated with taste disturbances according to the PDR. Atypical antipsychotics have largely replaced typical antipsychotics for psychotic disorder with marked positive symptoms. They are antagonists of most receptors for 5-hydroxytryptamine, dopamine, muscarine, and histamine. Olanzapine (Zyprexa), the prototype for this class, and risperidone (Risperdal), may both induce bitter dysgeusia (Thyssen et al., 2007).

4. **Antimanics/Mood Stabilizers.** Some anti-manic/mood stabilizers are accompanied by dysgeusia. Lithium, the widely used medication for bipolar disorders, is one such example (Bressler, 1980; Vestergaard et al., 1988; Terao et al., 2011). In an early case report, Duffield (1973) described a 50-year-old physicist who experienced "a strange and unpleasant taste" from food soon after taking lithium carbonate (250 mg t.i.d.). According to his account, butter and celery were the first tastes to be affected, both having a novel flavor superimposed on the original taste. While many vegetables smelled and tasted normal, cooked celery had a strong and unpleasant smell. In another report, dysgeusia was noted in ~5% of 450 patients treated with lithium. The dysgeusia reversed a few days after drug withdrawal. (Himmelhoch &

Hanin, 1974). In these reports, alterations in olfaction, rather than taste per se, may have been involved.

5. **Anti-Epileptic Drugs.** It is likely that many anti-epileptic drugs influence taste appreciation, including phenytoin (Dilantin), carbamazepine (Tegretol), and lamotrigine (Lamictal). Most descriptions are based on subjective complaints from just a few patients, and have not been followed up by empirical studies. In one case study, phenytoin (Dilantin) was associated with hypogeusia (Baumann et al., 2004). In another single report, 750 mg phenytoin was given intravenously over 3 hours to a 52-year-old man with a right parietal glioma who was affected by simple focal and secondary generalized seizures. Soon thereafter he was unable to detect saccharin, sodium chloride, citric acid, or quinine hydrochloride. Two weeks later the problem remained (Zeller et al., 1998). Subseqently, phenytoin was discontinued because of hepato-toxicity and replaced with phenobarbitone, following which taste function returned to normal. There are isolated reports of taste loss with carbamazepine (Tegretol) (Iniguez et al., 1994; Barajas Garcia-Talavera, 1988). In another report of three epileptic patients receiving several anti-convulsants, it was suspected that lamotrigine (Lamictal) was the likely cause of bitter or salt dysgeusia (Avoni et al., 2001). A uniting factor with all three drugs (phenytoin, carbamazepine, and lamotrigine) is the ability to block sodium channels and possibly impair transduction in taste buds or within the major afferent taste nerves.

6. **Central Nervous System Stimulants.** A number of stimulants, particularly caffeine, influence taste function. In one study of normal subjects that employed the Harris-Kalmus technique (see Chapter 4), caffeine lowered thresholds to quinine by 59% over baseline (DeMet et al., 1989). In another investigation (Schiffman et al., 1986), caffeine increased the suprathreshold intensity of various sweeteners, including sodium saccharin, stevioside, thaumatin, D-tryptophan, and neohesperidin dihydrochalcone, but sensitivities to aspartame, sucrose, fructose, or calcium cyclamate were unaltered. Adenosine reversed this effect, leading the authors to suggest that the inhibitory A_1 adenosine receptor may modulate the intensity of such sweeteners. Dextro-amphetamine the stimulant sometimes used in attention deficit hyperactivity disorder may decrease taste thresholds to quinine hydrochloride (Mata, 1963).

7. **Hypnotics.** Several sleep-inducing drugs are associated with taste distortions. According to the PDR, Zolpidem tartrate (Ambien), one of the most widely employed sleeping aids, can produce "taste perversion" and "parosmia." Eszopiclone (Lunesta®), a short-acting, non-benzodiazepine sedative hypnotic, is associated with dysgeusia. For example, in a 24-week randomized double-blind study of 164 elderly and 161 non-elderly people, the adverse event most often observed was dose-related dysgeusia (Uchimura et al., 2012). This problem was reported in 18.5% of the elderly group at the 1 mg dose, and 27.7% at the 2 mg dose. In the non-elderly, 42.9% reported dysgeusia at the 2 mg dose and 57.1% at the 2 mg dose. In a double-blind placebo-controlled study of eszopiclone, 66% of 24 women and 53% of 15 men reported metallic/bitter dysgeusia during the two-week period of drug administration, in contrast to 17% and 7%, respectively, who reported dysgeusia when on placebo (Doty et al., 2009). The intensity of dysgeusia was positively correlated with saliva and blood levels of Eszopiclone, implying that the dysgeusia was probably induced by taste bud stimulation. The altered taste was stronger in the morning than in the evening prior to taking the drug, and independent of age and PTC taster status. Taste function, per se, was not influenced by the drug.

Miscellaneous Agents (See Table 6.2)

1. **Botulinum Toxin A (BTX-A).** In a case report, a 44-year-old woman who had received Botulinum Toxin A for glabellar frown and crow's feet lines experienced a self-limiting metallic taste (Murray & Solish, 2003). This drug is frequently used intramuscularly to treat dystonia, hyperhidrosis, refractory migraine, and wrinkles. The toxin prevents release of acetylcholine at the presynaptic neuromuscular junction of striated muscles and eccrine glands but the relevance of this to dysgeusia is not clear. There is one report of dysgeusia in a patient with resection of an acoustic neuroma that was followed by hemifacial spasm (Heman-Ackah and Pensak, 2005). Paradoxically, after three courses of BTX-A there was relief of both the dysgeusia and facial spasm with relapse of dysgeusia between injections

2. **Snake, Fish, and Insect Venoms.** Ciguatera, the most common food poisoning from eating fish, as well as toxic reactions to a variety of insect and snake bites, have all been associated with temporary or prolonged taste disorders. In the case of ciguatera poisoning, one survey found that a metallic taste was noted by 55 percent of the affected individuals (Azziz-Baumgartner et al., 2012). Ciguatera has cholinergic effects; in particular, it influences sodium channels (Lehane & Lewis, 2000) chiefly through locking open this channel and permitting spontaneous firing of sensory neurons.

Metallic tastes are reported after bites from several poisonous snakes, although other chemosensory sensations are recognized. One case report refers to an 18-year-old man who was bitten on the hand by a Southern Pacific rattlesnake, *Crotalus viridis helleri* (Bush & Siedenburg, 1999). Within minutes, generalized weakness, difficulty breathing, diplopia, dysphagia, and dysphonia developed. Partial improvement took place after anti-venom therapy, but the weakness and walking difficulties continued. Subsequently a metallic taste developed that lasted several days, apparently coincident with the onset of intense muscle fasciculations involving the face, tongue, and upper extremities, implying over-stimulation of both nicotinic and muscarinic receptors. A similar case concerned a professional herpetologist who was bitten by a juvenile Red-bellied Black Snake, *Pseudechis porphyriacus* (Pearn et al., 2000). Within a minute he experienced nausea and severe stinging in the bitten finger. There was retching within five minutes which continued for several hours. Over the following weeks, abdominal pains continued and he experienced a persistent "horrible taste in his mouth." No taste or smell testing was performed, but permanent anosmia was said to be present. A bite from the cobra snake is alleged to abolish taste and according to Indian folklore a test for cobra envenomation is to place chili powder on the tongue. If the patient reports no sensation then the bite is likely from a cobra!

3. **Other Toxins and Pollutants.** Chronic arsenic poisoning has been associated with a metallic taste (Hall, 2002). Some employees having repeated contact with pesticides (e.g., agricultural workers) report a persistent bitter or metallic taste in the mouth. A garlic-like taste or odor is characteristic of organophosphorus exposure and may be accompanied by other complaints such as hypersalivation, small pupils, muscle twitching, or psychiatric problems. Sweet metallic taste is reported by workers cutting brass pipes ("metal fume fever") and in silver jewelry workers because of lead poisoning (Armstrong et al., 1983). In a study of 351 welders, over half (51.3%) experienced taste symptoms at some point in the welding process, and 3.7% specifically complained of a metallic taste at the beginning of the working week, typically 3–10 hours after exposure to welding fumes (El-Zein et al., 2003). Symptoms of manganese poisoning in welders include iron deficiency anemia with glossitis, loss of filiform papillae, and swollen fungiform

papillae. These changes would clearly affect the ability to taste. Similar changes on the tongue have been noted in the mouse model of manganese poisoning (Fortoul et al., 2010).

Industrial solvents vaporize readily and are more likely affect smell than taste (Doty, 2015). To our knowledge, there are no empirical studies of acute or chronic influences of solvent exposure on the taste function of industrial workers. Taste is rarely measured but on theoretical grounds such exposure would influence taste, just like other sensory systems and cognition. Research is sorely needed on this topic.

4. **Intranasal Sprays.** Acute migraine is treated effectively by Triptans, which are specific serotonin 1D and 1B agonists. About 5–20 percent of patients receiving the triptan-based nasal sprays Sumatriptan (Imigran) or zolmitriptan (Zomig) are troubled by an unpleasant bitter taste (Dahlof, 2003; Tepper et al., 2013). One explanation might relate to medication that enters the retronasal space and pharynx. Triptan-related paresthesias are common and, by implication, a direct effect on nerve fibers is also possible.

Antihistamine nasal sprays such as azelastine and olopatadine hydrochloride given for seasonal allergic rhinitis are both liable to produce a bitter taste in a small percentage of patients. Likewise a variety of intranasal steroids such as fluticasone furoate or triamcinolone also prescribed for seasonal allergic rhinitis are connected with an unpleasant immediate or after-taste in some individuals. The frequency of dysgeusia after such varied medication would favor a non-specific effect from inadvertent entry of medication into the nasopharynx.

Summary

In this chapter we reviewed a wide range of factors that can influence taste function. Insults to, or influences on, peripheral (e.g., taste buds, taste receptors, taste nerves, lingual epithelium, salivary glands) or central (e.g., brainstem, thalamus, cortex) taste-related neural structures are common. A wide range of non-neurodegenerative disorders, medications, and iatrogenic interventions can significantly impact taste function. Common diseases associated with taste dysfunction are diabetes, hypothyroidism, liver disease, hypertension, and immune system-related disorders such as multiple sclerosis, myasthenia gravis, and Sjögren's syndrome. Iatrogenic interventions include third-molar extraction and tonsillectomy. Medications that most commonly involve the perception of tastes are antimicrobials, antihypertensives, antilipid agents, and numerous psychoactive agents. It is clear that relatively few well-controlled studies are presently available, particularly in relation to the influences of medication on gustation. Much more research is needed to assess the validity of many claims based predominantly on anecdotal reports.

References

Acharya, V., Acharya, J., Luders, H., 1998. Olfactory epileptic auras. *Neurology* 51, 56–61.

Adour, K.K., Bell, D.N., Hilsinger, R.L. Jr., 1975. Herpes simplex virus in idiopathic facial paralysis (Bell palsy). *JAMA* 233, 527–530.

Akal, U.K., Kucukyavuz, Z., Nalcaci, R., Yilmaz, T., 2004. Evaluation of gustatory function after third molar removal. *International Journal of Oral & Maxillofacial Surgery* 33, 564–568.

al-Assi, M.T., Genta, R.M., Karttunen, T.J., Graham, D.Y., 1994. Clarithromycin-amoxicillin therapy for Helicobacter pylori infection. *Alimentary Pharmacology & Therapeutics* 8, 453–456.

Anand, K.K., Zuniga, J.R., 1997. Effect of amiloride on suprathreshold NaCl, LiCl, and KCl salt taste in humans. *Physiology & Behavior* 62, 925–929.

Andre, J.M., Beis, J.M., Morin, N., Paysant, J., 2000. Buccal hemineglect. *Archives of Neurology* 57, 1734–1741.

Armstrong, C.W., Moore, L.W. Jr., Hackler, R.L., Miller, G.B. Jr., Stroube, R.B., 1983. An outbreak of metal fume fever. Diagnostic use of urinary copper and zinc determinations. *Journal of Occupational Medicine* 25(12), 886–888.

Avoni, P., Contin, M., Riva, R., et al. 2001. Dysgeusia in epileptic patients treated with lamotrigine: report of three cases. *Neurology* 57, 1521.

Azziz-Baumgartner, E., Luber, G., Conklin, L., et al. 2012. Assessing the incidence of ciguatera fish poisoning with two surveys conducted in Culebra, Puerto Rico, during 2005 and 2006. *Environmental Health Perspectives* 120, 526–529.

Baehr, M., Frotscher, M., 2012. *Duus' Topical Diagnosis in Neurology* 5th edition. New York: Thieme, p. 149.

Baena Diez, J.M., Sancho, P.A., Lopez, M.C., et al. 1998. [Treatment with omeprazole, clarithromycin and amoxicillin for one week. Their efficacy and tolerance in eradicating Helicobacter pylori in primary care]. *Atención Primaria* 22, 547–551.

Barajas García-Talavera, F., 1988. [Ageusia in a patient treated with carbamazepine]. *Neurologia* 3(3), 126–127 (in Spanish).

Bartel, D.L., 2012. Glial responses after chorda tympani nerve injury. *Journal of Comparative Neurology* 520, 2712–2729.

Bartoshuk, LM., Miller, IJ., Jr., 1991. Taste perception, taste bud distribution, and spatial relationships. In: TV Getchell, RL Doty, LM Bartoshuk, JB Snow, Jr. (Eds.), *Smell and Taste in Health and Disease* New York: Raven Press, pp. 205–233.

Bartosik-Psujek, H., Psujek, M., Stelmasiak, Z., 2004. Rare first symptoms of multiple sclerosis. *Annales Universitatis Mariae Curie-Sklodowska. Sectio D: Medicina* 59, 242–244.

Barylko-Pikielna, N., Zawadzka, L., Niegowska, J., Cybulska, I., Sznajderman, M., 1985. Taste perception of sodium chloride in suprathreshold concentration related to essential hypertension. *Journal of Hypertension, Suppl* 3, S449–S452.

Baumann, C.R., Ott, P.M., Siegel, A.M., 2004. Hypogeusia as an adverse reaction to phenytoin. *British Journal of Clinical Pharmacology* 58, 678–679.

Benatru, I., Terraux, P., Cherasse, A., et al. 2003. [Gustatory disorders during multiple sclerosis relapse]. *Revue Neurologique* 159, 287–292.

Bernard, R.A., Halpern, B.P., 1968. Taste changes in vitamin A deficiency. *Journal of General Physiology* 52(3), 444–464.

Bernard, R.A., Halpern, B.P., Kare, M.R., 1961. Effect of vitamin A deficiency on taste. *Proceedings of the Society for Experimental Biology* 108, 784–786.

Bernhardson, B.M., Tishelman, C., Rutqvist, L.E., 2008. Self-reported taste and smell changes during cancer chemotherapy. *Supportive Care in Cancer* 16, 275–283.

Bernstein, I.L., 1985. Learned food aversions in the progression of cancer and its treatment. *Annals of the New York Academy of Sciences* 443, 365–380.

Berridge, K.C., Pecina, S., 1995. Benzodiazepines, appetite, and taste palatability. *Neuroscience & Biobehavioral Reviews* 19, 121–131.

Berteretche, M.V., Dalix, A.M., d'Ornano, A.M., et al. 2004. Decreased taste sensitivity in cancer patients under chemotherapy. *Supportive Care in Cancer* 12, 571–576.

Berteretche, M.V., Eloit, C., Dumas, H., et al. 2008. Taste deficits after middle ear surgery for otosclerosis: taste somatosensory interactions. *European Journal of Oral Sciences* 116, 394–404.

Beutler, M., Hartmann, K., Kuhn, M., Gartmann, J., 1993. Taste disorders and terbinafine. *British Medical Journal* 307, 26.

Bhatia, S., Sircar, S.S., Ghorai, B.K., 1990. Gustatory differences in hypothyroid and hyperthyroid tasters and non-tasters. *Indian Journal of Physiology & Pharmacology* 34, 201–205.

Bhatia, S., Sircar, S.S., Ghorai, B.K., 1991. Taste disorder in hypo and hyperthyroidism. *Indian Journal of Physiology & Pharmacology* 35, 152–158.

Bisht, D.B., Krishnamurthy, M., Rasgaswamy, R., 1967. Studies on threshold of taste for salt with special reference to hypertension. *Indian Heart Journal* 23, 137–140.

Bloomfeld, R.S., Graham, B.G., Schiffman, S.S., Killenberg, P.G., 1999. Alterations of chemosensory function in end-stage liver disease. *Physiology & Behavior* 66, 203–207.

Bolze, M.S., Fosmire, G.J., Stryker, J.A., Chung, C.K., Flipse, B.G., 1982. Taste acuity, plasma zinc levels, and weight loss during radiotherapy: a study of relationships. *Radiology* 144, 163–169.

Bong, J.L., Lucke, T.W., Evans, C.D., 1998. Persistent impairment of taste resulting from terbinafine. *British Journal of Dermatology* **139**, 747–748.

Boyd, I., 1993. Captopril-induced taste disturbance. *The Lancet* **342**, 304.

Breslin, P.A., Tharp, C.D., 2001. Reduction of saltiness and bitterness after a chlorhexidine rinse. *Chemical Senses* **26**, 105–116.

Bressler, B., 1980. An unusual side-effect of lithium. *Psychosomatics* **21**, 688–689.

Brewin, T.B., 1982. Appetite perversions and taste changes triggered or abolished by radiotherapy. *Clinical Radiology* **33**, 471–475.

Brosvic, G.M., Doty, R.L., Rowe, M.M., Harron, A., Kolodiy, N., 1992. Influences of hypothyroidism on the taste detection performance of rats: A signal detection analysis. *Behavioral Neuroscience* **106**, 992–998.

Brosvic, G.M., Risser, J.M., Doty, R.L., 1989. No influence of adrenalectomy on measures of taste sensitivity in the rat. *Physiology & Behavior* **46**, 699–705.

Burge, J.C., Park, H.S., Whitlock, C.P., Schemmel, R.A., 1979. Taste acuity in patients undergoing long-term hemodialysis. *Kidney International* **15**, 49–53.

Burge, J.C., Schemmel, R.A., Park, H.S., Green, J.A., 1978. Taste acuity and zinc status in chronic renal disease. *Archives of Internal Medicine* **138**, 743–746.

Bush, S.P., Siedenburg, E., 1999. Neurotoxicity associated with suspected southern Pacific rattlesnake (Crotalus viridis helleri) envenomation. *Wilderness & Environmental Medicine* **10**, 247–249.

Bustos-Saldana, R., Alfaro-Rodriguez, M., Solis-Ruiz, M.L., et al. 2009. [Taste sensitivity diminution in hyperglycemic type 2 diabetics patients]. *Revista Médica del Instituto Mexicano del Seguro Social* **47**, 483–488.

Caputo, J.B., Campos, S.S., Pereira, S.M., et al. 2012. Masticatory performance and taste perception in patients submitted to cancer treatment. *Journal of Oral Rehabilitation* **39**, 905–913.

Carr, W.J., 1952. The effect of adrenalectomy upon the Nacl taste threshold in rats. *Journal of Comparative and Physiological Psychology* **45**, 377–380.

Carrai, M., Steinke, V., Vodicka, P., et al. 2011. Association between TAS2R38 gene polymorphisms and colorectal cancer risk: a case-control study in two independent populations of Caucasian origin. *PLoS One* **6**(6), e20464.

Carrell, L.E., Cannon, D.S., Best, M.R., Stone, M.J., 1986. Nausea and radiation-induced taste aversions in cancer patients. *Appetite* **7**, 203–208.

Chencharick, J.D., Mossman, K.L., 1983. Nutritional consequences of the radiotherapy of head and neck cancer. *Cancer* **51**, 811–815.

Ciechanover, M., Peresecenschi, G., Aviram, A., Steiner, J.E., 1980. Malrecognition of taste in uremia. *Nephron* **26**, 20–22.

Combarros, O., Miro, J., Berciano, J., 1994. Ageusia associated with thalamic plaque in multiple sclerosis. *European Neurology* **34**, 344–346.

Combarros, O., Sanchez-Juan, P., Berciano, J., De, P.C., 2000. Hemiageusia from an ipsilateral multiple sclerosis plaque at the midpontine tegmentum. *Journal of Neurology, Neurosurgery, & Psychiatry* **68**, 796.

Conger, A.D., 1973. Loss and recovery of taste acuity in patients irradiated to the oral cavity. *Radiation Research* **53**, 338–347.

Contreras, R.J., 1978. Salt taste and disease. *American Journal of Clinical Nutrition* **31**, 1088–1097.

Dahlof, C., 2003. Clinical applications of new therapeutic deliveries in migraine. *Neurology* **61**, S31–S34.

Dahlslett, S.B., Goektas, O., Schmidt, F., et al. 2012. Psychophysiological and electrophysiological testing of olfactory and gustatory function in patients with multiple sclerosis. *European Archives of Oto-Rhino-Laryngology* **269**, 1163–1169.

Danielides, V., Milionis, H.J., Karavasilis, V., Briasoulis, E., Elisaf, M.S., 2005. Syndrome of inappropriate antidiuretic hormone secretion due to recurrent oral cancer. *B-ENT* **1**, 151–153.

de la Rosa, G.E., Mondragon, P.A., Aranda, R.S., Bustamante Ramirez, M.A., 2006. Oral mucosa symptoms, signs and lesions, in end stage renal disease and non-end stage renal disease diabetic patients. *Medicina Oral Patologia Oral y Cirugia Bucal* **11**, E467–E473.

de Matos, L.F., Pereira, S.M., Kaminagakura, E., et al. 2010. Relationships of beta-blockers and anxiolytics intake and salivary secretion, masticatory performance and taste perception. *Archives of Oral Biology* 55, 164–169.

Deems, D.A., Doty, R.L., Settle, R.G., et al. 1991. Smell and taste disorders, a study of 750 patients from the University of Pennsylvania Smell and Taste Center. *Archives of Otolaryngology - Head and Neck Surgery* 117, 519–528.

Deems, R.O., Friedman, M.I., Friedman, L.S., Maddrey, W.C., 1991. Clinical manifestations of olfactory and gustatory disorders associated with hepatic and renal disease. In: T.V Getchell, R.L Doty, L.M Bartoshuk, J.B Snow, Jr. (Eds.), *Smell and Taste in Health and Disease* Raven Press, pp. 805–827.

Deems, R.O., Friedman, M.I., Friedman, L.S., Munoz, S.J., Maddrey, W.C., 1993. Chemosensory Function, Food Preferences and Appetite in Human Liver-Disease. *Appetite* 20, 209–216.

DeMet, E., Stein, M.K., Tran, C., et al. 1989. Caffeine taste test for panic disorder: adenosine receptor supersensitivity. *Psychiatry Research* 30, 231–242.

DiBianco, R., 1990. ACE inhibitors in the treatment of heart failure. *Clinical Cardiology* 13, VII32–VII38.

Dirschnabel, A.J., Martins, A.S., Dantas, S.A., et al. 2011. Clinical oral findings in dialysis and kidney-transplant patients. *Quintessence International* 42, 127–133.

Doty, R.L., 2015. Neurotoxic exposure and impairment of the chemical senses of taste and smell. *Handbook of Clinical Neurology* 131, 299–324.

Doty, R.L., Cummins, D.M., Shibanova, A., Sanders, I., Mu, L., 2009. Lingual distribution of the human glossopharyngeal nerve. *Acta Otolaryngologica* 129, 52–56.

Doty, R.L., Heidt, J.M., MacGillivray, M.R., et al. Influences of age, tongue region, and chorda tympani nerve sectioning on signal detection measures of lingual taste sensitivity. *Physiology & Behavior* 17, 202–207.

Doty, R.L., Philip, S., Reddy, K., Kerr, K.L., 2003. Influences of antihypertensive and antihyperlipidemic drugs on the senses of taste and smell: a review. *Journal of Hypertension* 21, 1805–1813.

Doty, R.L., Shah, M., Bromley, S.M., 2008. Drug-induced taste disorders. *Drug Safety* 31, 199–215.

Doty, R.L., Tourbier, I.A., Pham, D.L., et al. 2016. Taste dysfunction in multiple sclerosis. *Journal of Neurology*, 263, 677–688.

Doty, R.L., Treem, J., Tourbier, I., Mirza, N., 2009. A double-blind study of the influences of eszopiclone on dysgeusia and taste function. *Pharmacology, Biochemistry & Behavior* 94, 312–318.

Duhra, P., Foulds, I.S., 1988. Methotrexate-induced impairment of taste acuity. *Clinical and Experimental Dermatology* 13, 126–127.

Duffield, J.E., 1973. Side effects of lithium carbonate. *British Medical Journal* 1, 491.

Dzaman, K., Rapiejko, P., Szczygielski, K., Pleskacz, W., Jurkiewicz, D., 2009. [Taste perception in patients with chronic rhinosinusitis with nasal polyps treated with oral glucocorticosteroid therapy]. *Otolaryngologia Polska* 63, 236–241.

Eiznhamer, D.A., Creagh, T., Ruckle, J.L., et al. 2002. Safety and pharmacokinetic profile of multiple escalating doses of (+)-calanolide A, a naturally occurring nonnucleoside reverse transcriptase inhibitor, in healthy HIV-negative volunteers. *HIV Clinical Trials* 3, 435–450.

Eksborg, S., Pal, N., Kalin, M., Palm, C., Soderhall, S., 2002. Pharmacokinetics of acyclovir in immunocompromised children with leukopenia and mucositis after chemotherapy: Can intravenous acyclovir be substituted by oral valacyclovir? *Medical & Pediatric Oncology* 38, 240–246.

El-Zein, M., Malo, J.L., Infante-Rivard, C., Gautrin, D., 2003. Prevalence and association of welding related systemic and respiratory symptoms in welders. *Occupational and Environmental Medicine* 60, 655–661.

Fallis, N., Lasagna, L., Tetreault, L., 1962. Gustatory thresholds in patients with hypertension. *Nature* 196, 74–75.

Fleiner, F., Dahlslett, S.B., Schmidt, F., Harms, L., Goektas, O., 2010. Olfactory and gustatory function in patients with multiple sclerosis. *American Journal of Rhinology & Allergy* 24, e93–e97.

Flesch, F., Rigaux-Barry, F., Saviuc, P., et al. 2011. Dysgeusia following consumption of pine nuts: More than 3000 cases in France. *Clinical Toxicology* 49, 668–670.

Fogan, L., 2007. Griseofulvin and dysgeusia: implications? *Annals of Internal Medicine* **74**, 795–796.

Fortoul, T.I., Velez-Cruz, M., Antuna-Bizarro, S., et al. 2010. Morphological changes in the tongue as a consequence of manganese inhalation in a murine experimental model: Light and scanning electron microscopic analysis. *Journal of Electron Microscopy* **59**, 71–77.

Fosmire, G.J., 1990. Zinc toxicity. *American Journal of Clinical Nutrition* **51**(2), 225–227.

Frank, M.E., Gent, J.F., Hettinger, T.P., 2001. Effects of chlorhexidine on human taste perception. *Physiology & Behavior* **74**, 85–99.

Fraser, G.R., 1961. Cretinism and taste sensitivity to phenylthiocarbamide. *Lancet* **1**, 964–965.

Fregly, M.J., 1962. Effect of hypothyroidism on sodium chloride aversion of renal hypertensive rats. *Endocrinology* **71**, 683–692.

Fregly, M.J., Cade, J.R., Waters, I.W., Straw, J.A., Taylor, R.E., Jr., 1965. Secretion of aldosterone by adrenal glands of propylthiouracil-treated rats. *Endocrinology* **77**, 777–784.

Fregly, M.J., Waters, I.W., 1965. Effect of propylthiouracil on preference threshold of rats for NaCl solutions. *Proceedings of the Society for Experimental Biology and Medicine* **120**, 637–640.

Fregly, M.J., Waters, I.W., 1966. Effect of desoxycorticosterone acetate on NaCl appetite of propylthiouracil-treated rats. *Physiology & Behavior* **1**, 133–138.

Fujikane, M., Itoh, M., Nakazawa, M. et al. 1999. [Cerebral infarction accompanied by dysgeusia– a clinical study on the gustatory pathway in the CNS]. *Rinsho Shinkeigaku* **39**(7): 771–4.

Fujioka, T., Aoyama, N., Sakai, K., et al. 2012. A large-scale nationwide multicenter prospective observational study of triple therapy using rabeprazole, amoxicillin, and clarithromycin for Helicobacter pylori eradication in Japan. *Journal of Gastroenterology* **47**, 276–283.

Fushan, A.A., Simons, C.T., Slack, J.P., Manichaikul, A., Drayna, D., 2009. Allelic polymorphism within the TAS1R3 promoter is associated with human taste sensitivity to sucrose. *Current Biology* **19**, 1288–1293.

Gamper, E.M., Giesinger, J.M., Oberguggenberger, A., et al. 2012. Taste alterations in breast and gynaecological cancer patients receiving chemotherapy: Prevalence, course of severity, and quality of life correlates. *Acta Oncologica* **51**, 490–496.

Gomez, F.E., Cassis-Nosthas, L., Morales-de-Leon, J.C., Bourges, H., 2004. Detection and recognition thresholds to the 4 basic tastes in Mexican patients with primary Sjogren's syndrome. *European Journal of Clinical Nutrition* **58**, 629–636.

Gondivkar, S.M., Indurkar, A., Degwekar, S., Bhowate, R., 2009. Evaluation of gustatory function in patients with diabetes mellitus type 2. *Oral Surgery, Oral Medicine, Oral Pathology, Oral Radiology, and Endodontology* **108**, 876–880.

Gordon, B.H., Wong, G.Y., Liu, J., Rivlin, R.S., 1992. Abnormal taste preference for saccharin in hypothyroid rats. *Physiology & Behavior* **52**, 385–388.

Graham, C.S., Graham, B.G., Bartlett, J.A., Heald, A.E., Schiffman, S.S., 1995. Taste and smell losses in HIV infected patients. *Physiology & Behavior* **58**, 287–293.

Greger, J.L., Geissler, A.H., 1978. Effect of zinc supplementation on taste acuity of the aged. *American Journal of Clinical Nutrition* **31**(4), 633–637.

Griffin, J.P., 1992. Drug-induced disorders of taste. *Adverse Drug Reactions & Toxicological Reviews* **11**, 229–239.

Grosskopf, I., Rabinovitz, M., Garty, M., Rosenfeld, J.B., 1984. Persistent captopril-associated taste alteration. *Clinical Pharmacy* **3**, 235.

Grover, R., Frank, M.E., 2008. Regional specificity of chlorhexidine effects on taste perception. *Chemical Senses* **33**, 311–318.

Guder, E., Bottcher, A., Pau, H.W., Just, T., 2012. Taste function after stapes surgery. *Auris Nasus Larynx* **39**, 562–566.

Hall, A.H., 2002. Chronic arsenic poisoning. *Toxicology Letters* **128**, 69–72.

Hardy, S.L., Brennand, C.P., Wyse, B.W., 1981. Taste thresholds of individuals with diabetes mellitus and of control subjects. *Journal of the American Dietetic Association* **79**, 286–289.

Harriman, A.E., Macleod, R.B., 1953. Discriminative thresholds of salt for normal and adrenalectomized rats. *American Journal of Psychiatry* **66**, 465–471.

Hayden, F.G., Andries, K., Janssen, P.A., 1992. Safety and efficacy of intranasal pirodavir (R77975) in experimental rhinovirus infection. *Antimicrobial Agents and Chemotherapy* 36, 727–732.

Heath, T.P., Melichar, J.K., Nutt, D.J., Donaldson, L.F., 2006. Human taste thresholds are modulated by serotonin and noradrenaline. *Journal of Neuroscience* 26, 12664–12671.

Heeringa, M., van Puijenbroek, P.E., 1998. Reversible dysgeusia attributed to losartan [letter]. *Annals of Internal Medicine* 129, 72.

Heiser, C., Landis, B.N., Giger, R., et al. 2010. Taste disturbance following tonsillectomy–a prospective study. *Laryngoscope* 120, 2119–2124.

Helms, J.A., Della-Fera, M.A., Mott, A.E., Frank, M.E., 1995. Effects of chlorhexidine on human taste perception. *Archives of Oral Biology* 40, 913–920.

Heman-Ackah, S., Pensak, M.A., 2005. Incidental finding of dysgeusia relieved by injections of botulinum toxin A. *Laryngoscope* 115, 844–845.

Henkin, R.I., 1967. Abnormalities of taste and olfaction in patients with chromatin negative gonadal dysgenesis. *The Journal of Clinical Endocrinology and Metabolism* 27, 1436–1440.

Henkin, R.I., 1974. Salt taste in patients with essential hypertension and with hypertension due to primary hyperaldosteronism. *Journal of Chronic Diseases* 27, 235–244.

Henkin, R.I., Larson, A.L., Powell, R.D., 1975. Hypogeusia, dysgeusia, hyposmia, and dysosmia following influenza-like infection. *Annals of Otology, Rhinology, and Laryngology* 84, 672–682.

Henkin, R.I., Schecter, P.J., Friedewald, W.T., Demets, D.L., Raff, M., 1976. A double blind study of the effects of zinc sulfate on taste and smell dysfunction. *Am J Med Sci* 272(3), 285–299.

Henkin, R.I., Solomon, D.H., 1962. Salt-taste threshold in adrenal insufficiency in man. *The Journal of Clinical Endocrinology and Metabolism* 22, 856–858.

Henkin, R.I., Talal, N., Larson, A.L., Mattern, C.F., 1972. Abnormalities of taste and smell in Sjogren's syndrome. *Annals of Internal Medicine* 76, 375–383.

Herness, S., Zhao, F.L., 2009. The neuropeptides CCK and NPY and the changing view of cell-to-cell communication in the taste bud. *Physiology & Behavior* 97, 581–591.

Heymans, F., Lacroix, J.S., Terzic, A., Landis, B.N., 2011. Gustatory dysfunction after mandibular zoster. *Neurological Sciences* 32, 461–464.

Himmelhoch, J.M., Hanin, I., 1974. Letter: Side effects of lithium carbonate. *British Medical Journal* 4, 233.

Hisahara, S., Makiyama, Y., Yoshizawa, T., Mizusawa, H., Shoji, S., 1994. [A case of unilateral gustatory disturbance produced by the contralateral midbrain lesion]. *Rinsho Shinkeigaku – Clinical Neurology* 34, 1055–1057.

Holmes, S., 1993. Food avoidance in patients undergoing cancer chemotherapy. *Supportive Care in Cancer* 1, 326–330.

Hsyu, P.H., Pithavala, Y.K., Gersten, M., Penning, C.A., Kerr, B.M., 2002. Pharmacokinetics and safety of an antirhinoviral agent, ruprintrivir, in healthy volunteers. *Antimicrobial Agents and Chemotherapy* 46, 392–397.

Iniguez, C., Perez-Trullen, J.M., Jimenez-Escrig, A., 1994. Loss of taste and carbamazepine. *European Journal of Neurology* 1, 177–178.

Iseki, K., Mezaki, T., Kawamoto, Y. et al. 2007. Concurrence of non-myasthenic symptoms with myasthenia gravis. *Neurological Sciences* 28:114–5.

Ishizaka, T. Miyanaga, Y., Mukai, J., et al. 2004. Bitterness evaluation of medicines for pediatric use by a taste sensor. *Chemical & Pharmaceutical Bulletin* 52, 943–948.

Ito, N., Suzuki, N., 1993. [Ipsilateral gustatory disturbance by thalamic hemorrhage]. *Rinsho Shinkeigaku* 33, 559–561.

Jensen, S.B., Mouridsen, H.T., Bergmann, O.J., et al. 2008. Oral mucosal lesions, microbial changes, and taste disturbances induced by adjuvant chemotherapy in breast cancer patients. *Oral Surgery, Oral Medicine, Oral Pathology, Oral Radiology, and Endodontology* 106, 217–226.

Johnson, M.O., Stallworth, T., Neilands, T.B., 2003. The drugs or the disease? Causal attributions of symptoms held by HIV-positive adults on HAART. *AIDS & Behavior* 7, 109–117.

Kabasawa, C., Shimizu, Y., Suzuki, S., et al. 2013. Taste disorders in myasthenia gravis: A multicenter cooperative study. *European Journal of Neurology* 20, 205–207.

Kamel, U.F., Maddison, P., Whitaker, R., 2009. Impact of primary Sjogren's syndrome on smell and taste: Effect on quality of life. *Rheumatology. (Oxford)* 48, 1512–1514.

Kaushik, A., Reddy, S.S., Umesh, L., et al. 2013. Oral and salivary changes among renal patients undergoing hemodialysis: A cross-sectional study. *Indian Journal of Nephrology* 23, 125–129.

Kelman, L., 2004. Osmophobia and taste abnormality in migraineurs: A tertiary care study. *Headache* 44(10), 1019–1023.

Kho, H.S., Lee, S.W., Chung, S.C., Kim, Y.K., 1999. Oral manifestations and salivary flow rate, pH, and buffer capacity in patients with end-stage renal disease undergoing hemodialysis. *Oral Surgery, Oral Medicine, Oral Pathology, Oral Radiology, and Endodontology* 88, 316–319.

Klasser, G.D., Grushka, M., Su, N., 2016. Burning Mouth Syndrome. *Oral and Maxillofacial Surgery Clinics of North America* 28(3), 381–396.

Kveton, J.F., Bartoshuk, L.M., 1994. The effect of unilateral chorda tympani damage on taste. *Laryngoscope* 104, 25–29.

Kwegyir-Afful, E.E., Dejager, L.S., Handy, S.M., et al. 2013. An investigational report into the causes of pine mouth events in US consumers. *Food and Chemical Toxicology* 60, 181–187.

Lang, N.P., Catalanotto, F.A., Knopfli, R.U., Antczak, AA.A., 1988. Quality-specific taste impairment following the application of chlorhexidine digluconate mouth rinses. *Journal of Clinical Periodontology* 15, 43–48.

Le Floch, J.P., Le, L.G., Labroue, M., Peynegre, R., Perlemuter, L., 1992. Early detection of diabetic patients at risk of developing degenerative complications using electric gustometry: A five-year follow-up study. *The European Journal of Medicine* 1, 208–214.

Le Floch, J.P., Le, L.G., Sadoun, J., et al. 1989. Taste impairment and related factors in type I diabetes mellitus. *Diabetic Medicine* 12, 173–178.

Le Floch, J.P., Le, L.G., Verroust, J., et al. 1990. Factors related to the electric taste threshold in type 1 diabetic patients. *Diabetic Medicine* 7, 526–531.

Lehane, L., Lewis, R.J., 2000. Ciguatera: Recent advances but the risk remains. *International Journal of Food Microbiology* 61, 91–125.

Lehman, C.D., Bartoshuk, L.M., Catalanotto, F.C., Kveton, J.F., Lowlicht, R.A., 1995. Effect of anesthesia of the chorda tympani nerve on taste perception in humans. *Physiology & Behavior* 57, 943–951.

Lemont, H., Sabo, M., 2001. Terbinafine-associated taste disturbance with normal taste threshold scores. *Journal of the American Podiatric Medical Association* 91, 540–541.

Leon-Sarmiento, F.E., Bayona, E.A., Bayona-Prieto, J., Osman, A., Doty, R.L., 2012. Profound olfactory dysfunction in myasthenia gravis. *PLoS One* 7, e45544.

Levenson, J.L., Kennedy, K., 1985. Dysosmia, dysgeusia, and nifedipine. *Annals of Internal Medicine* 102, 135–136.

Lewitt, M.S., Laing, D.G., Panhuber, H., Corbett, A., Carter, J.N., 1989. Sensory perception and hypothyroidism. *Chemical Senses* 14, 537–546.

Lloyd, S., Meerton, L., Di, C.R., Lavy, J., Graham, J., 2007. Taste change following cochlear implantation. *Cochlear Implants International* 8, 203–210.

Luker, J., Scully, C., 1990. The lateral medullary syndrome. *Oral Surgery, Oral Medicine and Oral Pathology* 69, 322–324.

Mahajan, S.K., Abraham, J., Migdal, S.D., Abu-Hamdan, D.K., McDonald, F.D., 1984. Effect of renal transplantation on zinc metabolism and taste acuity in uremia. *A Prospective Study. Transplantation* 38, 599–602.

Mareska, M., Gutmann, L., 2004. Lambert-Eaton myasthenic syndrome. *Seminars in Neurology* 24, 149–153.

Marinone, M.G., Marinone, M.G., Quaglini, S., Merlini, G., Cattaneo, V., 1994, [Taste changes in patients with AL amyloidosis. Preliminary studies]. *Minerva Stomatologica* 43), 473–477.

Martin, B., Maudsley, S., White, C.M., Egan, J.M., 2009. Hormones in the naso-oropharynx: Endocrine modulation of taste and smell. *Trends in Endocrinology and Metabolism* 20, 163–170.

Martin, B., Shin, Y.K., White, C.M., et al. 2010. Vasoactive intestinal peptide-null mice demonstrate enhanced sweet taste preference, dysglycemia, and reduced taste bud leptin receptor expression. *Diabetes* **59**(5), 1143–1152.

Mason, D.A., 1988. Lingual nerve damage following lower third molar surgery. *International Journal of Oral & Maxillofacial Surgery* **17**, 290–294.

Mata, F., 1963. Effect of dextro-amphetamine on bitter taste threshold. *Journal of Neuropsychiatry* **4**, 315–320.

Mattes, R.D., 1994. Prevention of food aversions in cancer patients during treatment. *Nutrition & Cancer* **21**, 13–24.

Mattes, R.D., Arnold, C., Boraas, M., 1987. Learned food aversions among cancer chemotherapy patients. Incidence, nature, and clinical implications. *Cancer* **60**, 2576–2580.

Mattes, R.D., Christensen, C.M., Engelman, K., 1988. Effects of therapeutic doses of amiloride and hydrochlorothiazide on taste, saliva, and salt intake in normotensive adults. *Chemical Senses* **13**, 33–44.

Mattes, R.D., Curran, W.J.J., Alavi, J., Powlis, W., Whittington, R., 1992. Clinical implications of learned food aversions in patients with cancer treated with chemotherapy or radiation therapy. *Cancer* **70**, 192–200.

Mattes, R.D., Heller, A.D., Rivlin, R.S., 1986. Abnormalities in suprathreshold taste function in early hypothyroidism in humans. In: HL Meiselman, R.S Rivlin (Eds.), *Clinical Measurement of Taste and Smell* New York: Macmillan Publishing Company, pp. 467–486.

McConnell, R.J., Menendez, C.E., Smith, F.R., Henkin, R.I., Rivlin, R.S., 1975. Defects of taste and smell in patients with hypothyroidism. *American Journal of Medicine* **59**, 354–364.

McManus, L.J., Stringer, M.D., Dawes, P.J.D., 2012. Iatrogenic injury of the chorda tympani: A systematic review. *The Journal of Laryngology & Otology* **126**, 8–14.

McNeill, J.J., Anderson, A., Christophidis, N., Jarrott, B., Louis, W.J., 1979. Taste loss associated with oral captopril treatment. *British Medical Journal* **2**, 1555–1556.

Michael, P., Raut, V., 2007. Chorda tympani injury: Operative findings and postoperative symptoms. *Otolaryngology-Head and Neck Surgery* **136**, 978–981.

Mirza, N., Machtay, M., Devine, P.A., et al. 2008. Gustatory impairment in patients undergoing head and neck irradiation. *Laryngoscope* **118**, 24–31.

Mossad, S.B., Macknin, M.L., Medendorp, S.V., Mason, P., 1996. Zinc gluconate lozenges for treating the common cold. A randomized, double-blind, placebo-controlled study. *Annals of Internal Medicine* **125**, 81–88.

Mossman, K.L., Chencharick, J.D., Scheer, A.C., et al. 1979. Radiation-induced changes in gustatory function: Comparison of effects of neutron and photon irradiation. *International Journal of Radiation Oncology, Biology, Physics* **5**, 521–528.

Mossman, K.L., Shatzman, A.R., Chencharick, J.D., 1981. Effects of radiotherapy on human parotid saliva. *Radiation Research* **88**, 403–412.

Muller, A., Landis, B.N., Platzbecker, U., et al. 2006. Severe chemotherapy-induced parosmia. *American Journal of Rhinology* **20**, 485–486.

Murakami, S., Mizobuchi, M., Nakashiro, Y., et al. 1996. Bell palsy and herpes simplex virus: Identification of viral DNA in endoneurial fluid and muscle. *Annals of Internal Medicine* **124**(1 Pt 1), 27–30.

Murray, C., Solish, N., 2003. Metallic taste: An unusual reaction to botulinum toxin A. *Dermatologic Surgery* **29**, 562–563.

Musialik, J., Suchecka, W., Klimacka-Nawrot, E., et al. 2012. Taste and appetite disorders of chronic hepatitis C patients. *European Journal of Gastroenterology – Hepatology* **24**, 1400–1405.

Nakazato, Y., Imai, K., Abe, T., Tamura, N., Shimazu, K., 2006. Unpleasant sweet taste: A symptom of SIADH caused by lung cancer. *Journal of Neurology, Neurosurgery, & Psychiatry* **77**, 405–406.

Nakazato, Y., Ito, Y., Naito, S., Tamura, N., Shimazu, K., 2008. Dysgeusia limited to sweet taste in myasthenia gravis. *Internal Medicine* **47**(9), 877–878.

Najafizade, N., Hemati, S., Gookizade, A., et al. 2013. Preventive effects of zinc sulfate on taste alterations in patients under irradiation for head and neck cancers: A randomized placebo-controlled trial. *Journal of Research in Medical Sciences* **18**, 123–126.

Negoro, A., Umemoto, M., Fujii, M., et al. 2004. Taste function in Sjogren's syndrome patients with special reference to clinical tests. *Auris Nasus Larynx* **31**, 141–147.

Nickel, A.A., 1993. Trigeminal nerve injury. *Journal of the American Dental Association* **124** (6), 17–18, 20.

Onoda, K., Ikeda, M., 1999. Gustatory disturbance due to cerebrovascular disorder. *Laryngoscope* **109**, 123–28.

Otero, R., Martins, C., Ferreira, D., et al. 2011. Identification of herpesvirus types 1–8 in oral cavity of children/adolescents with chronic renal failure. *Journal of Oral Pathology Medicine* **40**, 610–615.

Pal, S.K., Sharma, K., Pathak, A., Sawhney, I.M., Prabhakar, S., 2004. Possible relationship between phenylthiocarbamide taste sensitivity and epilepsy. *Neurology India* **52**, 206–209.

Patil, S., Khaandelwal, S., Doni, B., Rahuman, F., Kaswan, S., 2012. Oral manifestations in chronic renal failure patients attending two hospitals in North Karnataka, India. *Journal of Oral Health and Dental Management* **11**, 100–106.

Patten, J., 1995. *Neurological Differential Diagnosis* 2nd edition. London: Springer-Verlag.

Pearn, J., McGuire, B., McGuire, L., Richardson, P., 2000. The envenomation syndrome caused by the Australian Red-bellied Black Snake Pseudechis porphyriacus. *Toxicon* **38**, 1715–1729.

Pittman, J.A., Beschi, R.J., 1967. Taste thresholds in hyper- and hypothyroidism. *The Journal of Clinical Endocrinology and Metabolism* **27**, 895–896.

Medical Economics Company, Inc. 2005. *Physicians' Desk Reference* Montvale, NJ.

Pruszewicz, A., 1981. Zaburzenia powonienia i czucia w nosie. In: A. Zakrzewski (Ed.), *Otolaryngolgia Kliniczna* Warsqawa: PZWL, pp. 66–68.

Raja, J.V., Rai, P., Khan, M., Banu, A., Bhuthaiah, S., 2013. Evaluation of gustatory function in HIV-infected subjects with and without HAART. *Journal of Oral Pathology & Medicine* **42**, 216–221.

Rathi, S.S., Chaturvedi, V.N., Raizada, R.M., Jain, S.K., 1986. Electrogustometry in Hansen's disease (study of 225 cases). *International Journal of Leprosy and Other Mycobacterial Diseases* **54**, 252–255.

Reddaway, R.B., Davidow, A.W., Deal, S.L., Hill, D.L., 2012. Impact of chorda tympani nerve injury on cell survival, axon maintenance, and morphology of the chorda tympani nerve terminal field in the nucleus of the solitary tract. *Journal of Comparative Neurology* **520**, 2395–2413.

Reifen, R., Agami, O., Weiser, H., Biesalski, H., Naim M., 1998. Impaired responses to sweet taste in vitamin A-deficient rats. *Metabolism* **47**(1), 1–2.

Reiter, E.R., DiNardo, L.J., Costanzo, R.M., 2004. Effects of head injury on olfaction and taste. *Otolaryngologic Clinics of North America* **37**, 1167–1184.

Richter, C.P., 1936. Increased salt appetite in adrenalectomized rats. *American Journal of Physiology* **115**, 155–161.

Richter, C.P., 1939. Salt taste thresholds of normal and adrenalectomized rats. *Endocrinology* **24**, 367–371.

Ros, C., Alobid, I., Centellas, S., Balasch, J., Mullol, J., Castelo-Branco, C., 2012. Loss of smell but not taste in adult women with Turner's syndrome and other congenital hypogonadisms. *Maturitas* **73**(3), 244–250.

Rud, J., 1984. Reevaluation of the lingual split-bone technique for removal of impacted mandibular third molars. *Journal of Oral & Maxillofacial Surgery*. **42**, 114–117.

Rydzewski, B., Pruszewicz, A., Sulkowski, W.J., 2000. Assessment of smell and taste in patients with allergic rhinitis. *Acta Otolaryngologica* **120**, 323–326.

Saito, T., Ito, T., Narita, N., Yamada, T., Manabe, Y., 2011. Light and electron microscopic observation of regenerated fungiform taste buds in patients with recovered taste function after severing chorda tympani nerve. *Annals Otology Rhinology Laryngology* **120**, 713–721.

Saito, T., Narita, N., Yamada, T., Manabe, Y., Ito, T., 2011. Morphology of human fungiform papillae after severing chorda tympani nerve. *Annals Otology Rhinology Laryngology* **120**, 300–306.

Sajonz, B., Mädler, B., Herberhold, S., Paus, S., Coenen, V.A., 2011. A case of tremor reduction and almost complete ageusia under bilateral thalamic (VIM) deep brain stimulation in essential tremor–a therapeutic dilemma. *Acta Neurochirurgica* **153**, 2361–2363.

Sakagami, M., 2009. Taste disorder after middle ear surgery. *Journal of International Advanced Otology* **5**, 382–390.

Sakaguchi, A., Katsura, H., Nin, T., et al. 2012. Preoperative Assessment of taste function in patients with middle ear disease. *Otology & Neurotology* **33**, 761–764.

Sakashita, S., Takayama, K., Nishioka, K., Katoh, T., 2004. Taste disorders in healthy "carriers" and "non-carriers" of Candida albicans and in patients with candidosis of the tongue. *The Journal of Dermatology* **31**, 890–897.

Salisbury, P.L., III, 1997. Diagnosis and patient management of oral cancer. *Dental Clinics of North America* **41**, 891–914.

Schechter, P.J., Horwitz, D., Henkin, R.I., 1973. Sodium chloride preference in essential hypertension. *JAMA* **225**, 1311–1315.

Schechter, P.J., Horwitz, D., Henkin, R.I., 1974. Salt preference in patients with untreated and treated essential hypertension. *American Journal of the Medical Sciences* **267**, 320–326.

Schiffman, S.S., Diaz, C., Beeker, T.G., 1986. Caffeine intensifies taste of certain sweeteners: Role of adenosine receptor. *Pharmacology, Biochemistry & Behavior* **24**, 429–432.

Schiffman, S.S., Graham, B.G., Suggs, M.S., Sattely-Miller, E.A., 1998. Effect of psychotropic drugs on taste responses in young and elderly persons. *Annals of the New York Academy of Sciences* **855**, 732–737.

Schiffman, S.S., Zervakis, J., Suggs, M.S., Shaio, E., Sattely-Miller, E.A., 1999. Effect of medications on taste: example of amitriptyline HCl. *Physiology & Behavior* **66**, 183–191.

Schiffman, S.S., Zervakis, J., Westall, H.L., et al. 2000. Effect of antimicrobial and anti-inflammatory medications on the sense of taste. *Physiology & Behavior* **69**, 413–424.

Schlienger, R.G., Saxer, M., Haefeli, W.E., 1996. Reversible ageusia associated with losartan [letter]. *Lancet* **347**, 471–472.

Schmidt, F.A., Goktas, O., Harms, L., et al. 2011. Structural correlates of taste and smell loss in encephalitis disseminata. *PLoS One* **6**, e19702.

Shafer, D.M., Frank, M.E., Gent, J.F., Fischer, M.E., 1999. Gustatory function after third molar extraction. *Oral Surgery, Oral Medicine, Oral Pathology, Oral Radiology, & Endodontics* **87**, 419–428.

Shepard, T.H., Gartler, S.M., 1960. Increased incidence of non-tasters of phenylthiocarbamide among congenital athyreotic cretins. *Science* **131**, 929.

Shepherd, R., Farleigh, C.A., Atkinson, C., Pryor, J.S., 1987. Effects of haemodialysis on taste and thirst. *Appetite* **9**, 79–88.

Shih, C.T., Hao, S.P., Ng, S.H., Yen, K.C., 1999. Necrosis of the tongue after arterial chemotherapy. *Otolaryngology - Head and Neck Surgery* **121**, 655–657.

Shikama, Y., Kato, T., Nagaoka, U., et al. 1996. Localization of the gustatory pathway in the human midbrain. *Neuroscience Letters* **218**, 198–200.

Shimura, T., Norgren, R., Grigson, P.S., 1997. Brainstem lesions and gustatory function: I. The role of the nucleus of the solitary tract during a brief intake test in rats. *Behavioral Neuroscience* **111**, 155–168.

Sinnatamby, C.S. *Last's Anatomy* 2006. 11th edition. New York: Churchill Livingstone Elsevier.

Smith, F.R., Henkin, R.I., Dell, R.B., 1976. Disordered gustatory acuity in liver disease. *Gastroenterology* **70**, 568–571.

Smith, J.C., Blumsack, J.T., 1981. Learned taste aversion as a factor in cancer therapy. *Cancer Treatment Reports* **65** Suppl 5, 37–42.

Smith, J.C., Hollander, G.R., Spector, A.C., 1981. Taste aversions conditioned with partial body radiation exposures. *Physiology & Behavior* **27**, 903–913.

Solemdal, K., Sandvik, L., Willumsen, T., Mowe, M., Hummel, T., 2012. The impact of oral health on taste ability in acutely hospitalized elderly. *PLoS One* **7**, e36557.

Sprenger, K.B., Bundschu, D., Lewis, K., et al. 1983. Improvement of uremic neuropathy and hypogeusia by dialysate zinc supplementation: A double-blind study. *Kidney International* **16**, S315–S318.

Stathas, T., Mallis, A., Naxakis, S., et al. 2010. Taste function evaluation after tonsillectomy: A prospective study of 60 patients. *European*

Archives of Oto-Rhino-Laryngology **267**, 1403–1407.

Steinbach, S., Hummel, T., Bohner, C., et al. 2009. Qualitative and quantitative assessment of taste and smell changes in patients undergoing chemotherapy for breast cancer or gynecologic malignancies. *Journal of Clinical Oncology* **27**, 1899–1905.

Stolbova, K. Hahn, A., Benes, B., Andel, M., Treslova, L., 1999. Gustometry of diabetes mellitus patients and obese patients. *The International Tinnitus Journal* **5**, 135–140.

Stricker, B.H., Van, R.M., Sturkenboom, M.C., Ottervanger, J.P., 1996. Taste loss to terbinafine: A case-control study of potential risk factors. *British Journal of Clinical Pharmacology* **42**, 313–318.

Sumner, D., 1967. Post-traumatic ageusia. *Brain* **90**, 187–202.

Takahashi, H., Hitsumoto, Y., Honda, N., et al. 2001. Mouse model of Bell's palsy induced by reactivation of herpes simplex virus type 1. *Journal of Neuropathology and Experimental Neurology* **60**, 621–627.

Takaoka, T., Sarukura, N., Ueda, C., et al. 2010. Effects of zinc supplementation on serum zinc concentration and ratio of apo/holo-activities of angiotensin converting enzyme in patients with taste impairment. *Auris Nasus Larynx* **37**(2), 190–194.

Teker, A.M., Gedikli, O., Altun, H., Korkut, A.Y., Ahishali, B., 2010. Chorda tympani nerve analysis with electron microscopy in chronic suppurative otitis media. *Acta Oto-Laryngologica* **130**, 859–864.

Tepper, S.J., Chen, S., Reidenbach, F., Rapoport, A.M., 2013. Intranasal zolmitriptan for the treatment of acute migraine. *Headache* **53** Suppl 2, 62–71.

Terao, T., Watanabe, S., Hoaki, N., Hoaki, T., 2011. Strange taste and mild lithium intoxication. *BMJ Case Repotrs*. doi: 10.1136/bcr.05.2011.4267

Thorman, R., Neovius, M., Hylander, B., 2009. Prevalence and early detection of oral fungal infection: A cross-sectional controlled study in a group of Swedish end-stage renal disease patients. *Scandinavian Journal of Urology and Nephrology* **43**, 325–330.

Thyssen, A., Remmerie, B., D'Hoore, P., Kushner, S., Mannaert, E., 2007. Rapidly disintegrating risperidone in subjects with schizophrenia or schizoaffective disorder: A summary of ten phase I clinical trials assessing taste, tablet disintegration time, bioequivalence, and tolerability. *Clinical Therapeutics* **29**, 290–304.

Tomita, H., Ohtuka, K., 2002. Taste disturbance after tonsillectomy. *Acta Otolaryngologica* 164–172.

Tomofuji, S., Sakagami, M., Kushida, K., et al. 2005. Taste disturbance after tonsillectomy and laryngomicrosurgery. *Auris Nasus Larynx* **32**, 381–386.

Tsunoda, K., Osada, K., Komai, M., et al. 1998. Effects of dietary biotin on enhanced sucrose intake and enhanced gustatory nerve responses to sucrose seen in diabetic OLETF rat. *Journal of Nutritional Science & Vitaminology* **44**, 207–216.

Tsuruoka, S., Wakaumi, M., Nishiki, K., et al. 2004. Subclinical alteration of taste sensitivity induced by candesartan in healthy subjects. *British Journal of Clinical Pharmacology* **57**, 807–812.

Uchimura, N., Kamijo, A., Takase, T., 2012. Effects of eszopiclone on safety, subjective measures of efficacy, and quality of life in elderly and nonelderly Japanese patients with chronic insomnia, both with and without comorbid psychiatric disorders: A 24-week, randomized, double-blind study. *Annals of General Psychiatry* Ann Gen Psychiatry. 2012 Jun 25;**11**(1):15.

Uteshev, V.V., Smith, D.V., 2006. Cholinergic modulation of neurons in the gustatory region of the nucleus of the solitary tract. *Brain Research* **1084**, 38–53.

Valmaseda-Castellon, E., Berini-Aytes, L., Gay-Escoda, C., 2000. Lingual nerve damage after third lower molar surgical extraction. *Oral Surgery, Oral Medicine, Oral Pathology, Oral Radiology, and Endodontology* **90**, 567–573.

Van Daele, D.J., Fazan, VP.S., Agassandian, K., Cassell, M.D., 2011. Amygdala connections with jaw, tongue and laryngo-pharyngeal premotor neurons. *Neuroscience* **177**, 93–113.

Vestergaard, P., Poulstrup, I., Schou, M., 1988. Prospective studies on a lithium cohort. 3.

Tremor, weight gain, diarrhea, psychological complaints. *Acta Psychiatrica Scandinavica* **78**, 434–441.

Wang, L.H., Peck, R.W., Yin, Y., et al. 2003. Phase I safety and pharmacokinetic trials of 1263W94: A novel oral anti-human cytomegalovirus agent, in healthy and human immunodeficiency virus-infected subjects. *Antimicrobial Agents & Chemotherapy* **47**, 1334–1342.

Weiffenbach, J.M., Schwartz, L.K., Atkinson, J.C., Fox P.C., 1995. Taste performance in Sjogren's syndrome. *Physiology & Behavior* **57**, 89–96.

West, S.E., Doty, R.L., 1995. Influence of epilepsy and temporal lobe resection on olfactory function. *Epilepsia* **36**, 531–542.

Wickham, R.S., Rehwaldt, M., Kefer, C., et al. 1999. Taste changes experienced by patients receiving chemotherapy. *Oncology Nursing Forum* **26**, 697–706.

Wilken, M.K., Satiroff, B.A., 2012. Pilot study of "miracle fruit" to improve food palatability for patients receiving chemotherapy. *Clinical Journal of Oncology Nursing* **16**, E173–E177.

Wismer, W.V., 2008. Assessing alterations in taste and their impact on cancer care. *Current Opinion in Supportive and Palliative Care* **2**, 282–287.

Wolff, A., Zuk-Paz, L., Kaplan, I., 2008. Major salivary gland output differs between users and non-users of specific medication categories. *Gerodontology* **25**, 210–216.

Wong, G.T., Gannon, K.S., Margolskee, R.F., 1996. Transduction of bitter and sweet taste by gustducin. *Nature* **381**, 796–800.

Wooding, S.P., Atanasova, S., Gunn, H.C., et al. 2012. Association of a bitter taste receptor mutation with Balkan Endemic Nephropathy (BEN). *BMC Medical Genetics* **13**, 96.

Wotman, S., Mandel, I.D., Thompson, R.H Jr., Laragh, J.H., 1967. Salivary electrolytes and salt taste thresholds in hypertension. *Journal of Chronic Diseases* **20**, 833–840.

Xiao, C., Hanlon, A., Zhang, Q., et al. 2013. Symptom clusters in patients with head and neck cancer receiving concurrent chemoradiotherapy. *Oral Oncology* **49**, 360–366.

Yanagisawa, K., Bartoshuk, L.M., Catalanotto, F.A., Karrer, T.A., Kveton, J.F., 1998. Anesthesia of the chorda tympani nerve and taste phantoms. *Physiology & Behavior* **63**, 329–335.

Yu, Z., Kryzer, T.J., Griesmann, G.E., et al. 2001. CRMP-5 neuronal autoantibody: Marker of lung cancer and thymoma-related autoimmunity. *Annals of Neurology* **49**, 146–154.

Yung, M., Smith, P., Hausler, R., et al. 2008. International Common Otology Database: Taste disturbance after stapes surgery. *Otology & Neurotology* **29**, 661–665.

Zeller, J.A., Machetanz, J., Kessler, C., 1998. Ageusia as an adverse effect of phenytoin treatment [letter]. *Lancet* **351**, 1101.

Zervakis, J., Graham, B.G., Schiffman, S.S., 2000. Taste effects of lingual application of cardiovascular medications. *Physiology & Behavior* **68**, 405–413.

Zhou, L.H., Liu, X.M., Feng, X.H., Han, L.O., Liu, G.D., 2009. Expression of alpha-gustducin in the circumvallate papillae of taste buds of diabetic rats. *Acta Histochemica* **111**, 145–149.

Neurodegenerative Chemosensory Disorders

Olfactory Disorders

Of great interest to the neuroscientist is the fact that several conditions associated with progressive neuronal cell loss are accompanied in their earliest stages by olfactory disturbances. These diseases, loosely termed "neurodegenerative," include Alzheimer's disease (AD) and "parkinsonism," which is a broad term that includes the classic variety of Parkinson's Disease (PD) (see Tables 7.1 and 7.2). Such disorders are common. AD, for example, affects more than 25 million people worldwide (Ziegler-Graham et al., 2008). Somewhat less frequent neurodegenerative diseases, such as progressive supranuclear palsy (PSP) and corticobasal syndrome (CBS), are not associated with major smell dysfunction, making olfactory testing useful in differential diagnosis (e.g., PD and PSP are often confused and misclassified).

It is noteworthy that most neurodegenerative diseases that influence olfaction appear in later life and that age is the most important variable affecting olfactory function in the general population. Thus, after 80 years of age, over 70 percent of apparently healthy people have marked impairment of olfaction and, between 65 and 80 years, 50 percent have a demonstrable deficit (Doty et al., 1984; Murphy et al., 2002), with men exhibiting a greater overall average decline than women. In one study of 211 healthy control subjects in the UK, identification ability was found to decline significantly as early as 36 years of age and thereafter more steeply, with women scoring, on average, 1–2 points higher than men at all ages on the UPSIT (Hawkes et al., 2005; Figure 7.1). Whether, and to what degree, AD, PD, and similar diseases represent an acceleration of the aging process within the olfactory pathways is unknown. It is very relevant that a wide variety of xenobiotics, such as viruses, pesticides, and heavy metals, cumulatively damage the olfactory epithelium across the age span and, in some instances, enter the brain via the olfactory route. Such observations, along with patterns of developmental brain pathology, have led to the hypothesis that some neurodegenerative diseases may be caused or catalyzed by xenobiotics that damage the olfactory system and enter the brain via the nose, possibly by acting upon genetically determined substrates. The strengths and weakness of this hypothesis – termed the "olfactory vector hypothesis" (OVH) – are discussed in detail later in this chapter.

Alzheimer's Disease (AD)

Pathology. The key pathologic changes in AD are the presence of amyloid plaques and neurofibrillary tangles throughout the cerebral cortex that lead to neuronal death. According to the seminal studies of Braak and colleagues based on the examination of 2,332 brains with sporadic AD (Braak, et al., 2011), this disorder most

Table 7.1. Relative degree of olfactory dysfunction in various "neurodegenerative" conditions on an arbitrary scale. Olfactory changes in those with PARK mutations are given in Table 7.2.

Disease	Relative severity of smell defect
Classic PD; Alzheimer's disease; Dementia with Lewy Bodies; Pure autonomic failure. Guam complex; Down syndrome; Adult onset Gaucher disease	++++
Pallido-ponto-nigral degeneration; drug induced PD (some); semantic dementia; Huntington disease; frontotemporal dementia; prion diseases?; Wilson's disease	+++
Schizophrenia; SCA2; Multiple System Atrophy (type-P); Corticobasal syndrome; X-linked dystonia-parkinsonism ("Lubag"); Progressive supranuclear palsy.	++
Motor neuron disease (ALS); Essential tremor; SCA3 (Marchado-Joseph disease); Friedreich's ataxia; Segawa syndrome?; DYT25 (adult onset focal dystonia)	+
Vascular parkinsonism; MPTP parkinsonism; idiopathic dystonia (SWEDD)	0

Key: ++++ severe impairment; + mild; 0 normal. ALS=amyotrophic lateral sclerosis. SCA = spinocerebellar atrophy. SWEDD = scans without evidence of dopamine deficiency. MPTP= methyl-phenyl-tetrahydro-pyridine. NB. Most of these scores, except for classic PD, are based on relatively small patient numbers and should be interpreted conservatively.

likely begins in the brain stem decades before clinical presentation, predominantly affecting initially the locus coeruleus. Although not widely appreciated, it is likely that this early involvement of the coeruleus complex will affect alertness and sustained concentration and result in cognitive changes particularly affecting executive function, an often overlooked point of major relevance for psychometric testing. According to Braak et al., the first *cortical* area to be involved is the transentorhinal cortex (Figure 7.2), a region concerned with transmission of sensory input from the parietal cortex to the posterior temporal lobe. From the transentorhinal cortex the pathology spreads to the hippocampus (particularly entorhinal cortex) and subsequently to the rest of the temporal lobe, finally affecting high order association areas of the frontal, parietal, and occipital neocortex. The major pathological and clinical findings connected with AD-related changes in the olfactory system are described in the following sections.

Pathology of the Olfactory System. There was considerable interest when it was suggested that AD could be diagnosed from postmortem samples of nasal olfactory neuroepithelium (Talamo et al., 1989) and the clear implication that an accurate diagnosis could be made via biopsy of the olfactory epithelium (Lovell et al., 1982). Although changes in morphology, distribution, and immunoreactivity of neuronal structures typical of AD were noted, subsequent studies have cast doubt on this finding, partly because the control subjects were significantly younger than the cases and because the changes were not specific for AD; there was similarity to those found in other neurodegenerative diseases and even in some healthy elderly control subjects (Trojanowski et al., 1991; Kishikawa et al., 1994). Nevertheless, one cannot discount the possibility that the apparently healthy elderly control

Table 7.2. Currently proposed monogenic forms of parkinsonism with some associated pathological features and olfactory deficit where known.

PARK number	Gene & common mutations	Inheritance pattern & locus	Age onset	Function or effect of mutation	LB	OLF	Comment
1/4	Alpha synuclein (SNCA). G209A. Missense mutations: A53T, A30P & E46 K. Also duplications and triplications.	AD 4q21.3-q22	30–40	Dopamine transmission	++	++	Early onset. Good response to levodopa. Impaired olfaction in 1 case (Markopoulou, Larsen et al, 1997) Abnormal in 2/7 Greek cases (Bostantjopoulou, Katsarou et al, 2001) and in 6 Japanese (Nishioka, Ross et al, 2009). Severe olfactory defect in two cases from Germany (Kertelge, Bruggemann et al, 2010). Duplications resemble classic PD. Dementia prominent in duplications & triplications
2	Parkin Over 200 mutations	AR 6q26	<40	Mitochondral disorder. UPS, E3-ubiquitin ligase	+?	+	Early onset, slow progression. Good response to levodopa. No dementia. Normal/mild impairment of olfaction in manifesting and non-manifesting carriers, heterozygotes but not compound heterozygotes. Susceptibility to glioma, lung cancer, possibly leprosy & TB
3 & 5					Not confirmed		
6	PINK1 Over 60 mutations	AR 1p36.12	20–50	Mitochondrial kinase	+	++	Early onset and slow progression. Good response to levodopa.

Table 7.2. (cont.)

PARK number	Gene & common mutations	Inheritance pattern & locus	Age onset	Function or effect of mutation	LB	OLF	Comment
				Defective mitophagy			Dementia. Moderate impairment of olfaction in all cases & some asymptomatic heterozygotes. One autopsy showed LB but sparing of locus coeruleus and amygdala. OB not examined (Samaranch, Lorenzo-Betancor et al., 2010)
7	DJ-1 10 mutations	AR 1p36	20–40	Oxidative stress; Defective mitophagy	?	0?	Good response to levodopa. Normal olfaction based on one patient. (Verbaan, Boesveldt et al., 2008)
8	LRRK2 / Dardarin G2019S; N1437H	AD 12q12	40–60y	Membrane trafficking, Kinase	++	+++	Moderate – severe olfactory impairment in manifesting patients from London, New York, Lisbon, Brazil, and Germany. Variable or no impairment in non-manifesting carriers. Dementia and tremor common. Good response to levodopa. Susceptibility to leprosy & TB
9	ATP13A2 10 mutations	AR 1p36	11–16	Lysosome ATPase	?	++	Kufor-Rakeb disease. Based on 4 subjects (Kertelge, Bruggemann et al., 2010). Similar to Hallervorden-Spatz disease. Levodopa responsive PD with pyramidal signs, supranuclear gaze palsy and dementia (Klein, 2009)
10–13							Not confirmed

	Gene/Syndrome	Inheritance/Locus	Onset (y)	Function			Clinical features
14	PLA2G6 Karak syndrome	AR 22q13.1	20–25	Phospholipase enzyme	+++	?	Karak syndrome. Adult onset dystonia-parkinsonism. Temporary response to levodopa. Dementia. Cortical LB in 4 autopsies. No OB data but hippocampus involved in some (Paisan-Ruiz, Li et al, 2010)
15	FBOX7 AR	AR 22q11.2-qter	10–19	Ubiquitin protein ligase	?	?	Early onset levodopa-responsive parkinsonism with dystonia and spasticity
16					Not confirmed		
17	Heterozygous mutation (D620 N) in VPS35 gene	AD 16q12	40–60y	Membrane trafficking.	0 (One limited autopsy)	?	Indistinguishable from tremor dominant PD. Dementia uncommon. Good response to levodopa

GBA = glucocerebrosidase mutation. POLG1 = mitochondrial DNA polymerase subunit gamma one. LB=Lewy bodies. OLF = olfactory defect. AD= autosomal dominant. AR=autosomal recessive.

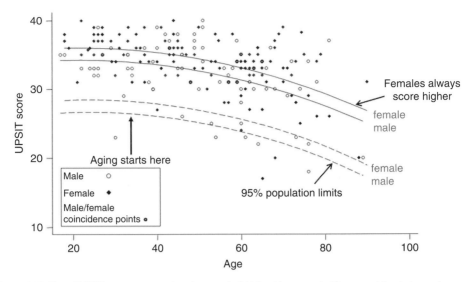

Figure 7.1 Plot of UPSIT score regressed against age in 211 healthy controls. Men are white circles and women black circles. Note that olfactory scores decline with age but at all ages females score 1–2 points higher than males. The vertical arrow indicates the age (36 years) at which UPSIT scores deviate significantly from horizontal. From Hawkes et al. (2005).

subjects were in the preclinical phase of AD and that olfactory or cognitive measurement before death may have detected early changes of this disorder.

Further light has been shed on this problem by Kovacs (2013). In the olfactory neuroepithelium, amyloid beta (Aβ, a hallmark of AD) was found in epithelial cells in 71% of neuropathologically confirmed AD cases compared to 22% of controls. Also present was another AD hallmark, namely, hyperphosphorylated tau (HPτ) in 55%, mainly as neuropil threads compared to 34% of controls. Neuropil threads and neurofibrillary tangles are already present in the OB in cases with only low neuritic Braak stages, implying that HPτ pathology in the OB develops in early stage AD, whereas Aβ plaques occur mostly in cases with severe cortical Aβ pathology.

Other attempts have been made to diagnose AD by nasal biopsy, but tissues from this region have limitations, particularly sampling problems. Apart from lack of specific changes, it can be difficult to identify olfactory neurons even with the specific immunofluorescent olfactory marker protein. With advancing years, the olfactory neuroepithelium is replaced progressively by respiratory epithelium (Yamagishi et al., 1994). Furthermore, it is not known whether the progressive deterioration of the neuroepithelium occurs more rapidly in patients with AD than in normal people of similar age.

Despite the arguments surrounding olfactory nasal mucosal involvement, olfactory bulb (OB) changes in AD are well recognized and probably universal (Kovacs et al., 2001). Neurofibrillary tangles (NFTs) and amyloid plaques are found in all cell layers of the bulb, as well as the anterior olfactory nucleus (AON), a structure whose most peripheral segments are dispersed in patches within the main part of the bulb and its tract. A subsequent study by Mundiano et al. (2011) confirmed and extended these observations by demonstrating tau pathology and beta-amyloid in the OB of nearly all of their 41 AD

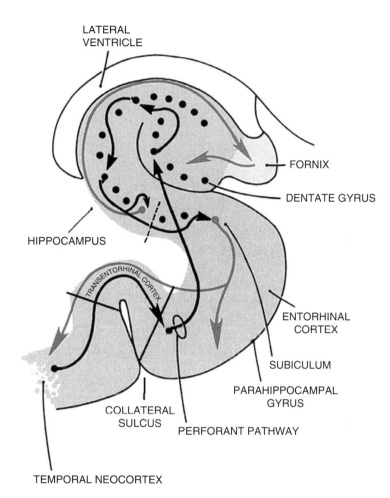

LATERAL
VENTRICLE

FORNIX

DENTATE GYRUS

HIPPOCAMPUS

TRANSENTORHINAL CORTEX

ENTORHINAL
CORTEX

SUBICULUM

PARAHIPPOCAMPAL
GYRUS

COLLATERAL
SULCUS

PERFORANT PATHWAY

TEMPORAL NEOCORTEX

Figure 7.2 Coronal section of the hippocampus to show the position of the transentorhinal cortex. This lies in the depths of the collateral sulcus between the two straight lines as shown. It is one of the first areas to be affected in Alzheimer's disease. From Braak & Braak (1998).

patients. They also demonstrated an increased number of dopaminergic periglomerular neurons compared to age-matched controls, and suggested this might be a compensatory mechanism. Several MRI studies report decrements in the volume of the AD olfactory bulb (Thomann et al., 2009a, 2009b), mirroring the known atrophy of these structures seen at autopsy (Esiri, 1991). Importantly, a significant reduction in cholinergic innervation into the olfactory bulbs of AD patients has been noted – a reduction essentially equivalent to that observed in PD (Mundinano et al., 2013).

It is not certain whether the earliest olfactory pathological changes occur in the nasal neuroepithelium, bulb, or more centrally in the temporal cortex. As noted above, Braak & Braak (1998) suggested that the earliest area of cortical damage is within the transentorhinal cortex, a bottleneck zone for cortical sensory afferents to the hippocampus (Figure 7.2). However, Kovacs et al. (2001) found NFTs in the AON of some AD cases before any change was seen in the entorhinal cortex. The primary olfactory cortex was less severely affected than the medial orbitofrontal cortex (an olfactory association area) and there was a correlation between the pathology of the olfactory bulb and some non-olfactory areas. This led to the suggestion that NFTs developed independently of synaptic connections, i.e., it was not a process that advanced along established fiber pathways, in contrast to Braak's observations. In a study of 93 olfactory bulbs by Tsuboi et al., (2003), tau pathology was found in *all* definite cases of AD. Likewise, Attems et al., (2005) confirmed the universal presence of tau and neuritic plaque pathology in the AD olfactory bulb and showed a strong correlation between tau deposits in the olfactory and limbic systems, both of which showed a similar increase of severity, implying that the peripheral and central olfactory structures were affected simultaneously. Perhaps the most definitive information on the central/peripheral origin debate comes from a unique study based on autopsy of 42 people all below the age of 29 years (Braak & Del Tredici, 2011). Tau pathology was found in the temporal lobes (transentorhinal region) as in classic disease, but the olfactory bulbs were spared, suggesting that AD begins centrally and that OB involvement is a later feature. The balance of human evidence would favor a central to peripheral spread for olfactory impairment, but this view is not supported uniformly by transgenic mouse models, as explained below.

Transgenic Mouse Models. Several researchers have explored the olfactory deficit in a variety of AD transgenic mice. In the first study, Macknin et al. (2004) used an odor habituation paradigm and found olfactory deficits in Tα1–3RT transgenic mice that overexpress tau, a key pathogenic protein in AD. Histology showed that these mice variably developed tau-related pathology within the anterior olfactory nucleus and external plexiform layer of the olfactory bulb, mostly in neurons, but not glia. Although olfactory cortical areas were affected (e.g., the amygdala), it was not stated whether this preceded or followed the OB pathology. Another group assayed olfactory perception and Aβ deposition throughout the olfactory system in Tg2576 transgenic mice that overexpress a mutated form of the human Aβ precursor protein (AβPP) (Wesson et al., 2010). At around age three months, the mice displayed progressive olfactory deficits with nonfibrillar Aβ deposits in the olfactory bulb that occurred earlier than deposition within any other brain region. Subsequently, Wu et al. (2013) assessed behavior and olfactory system pathology in the similar AβPP/PS1 transgenic mouse using a variety of olfactory tests. In keeping with Wesson's findings, they observed a spatial-temporal deposition of Aβ that appeared first in the olfactory epithelium at one–two months, olfactory bulb at three–four months, anterior olfactory nucleus, piriform cortex, entorhinal cortex, and hippocampus at six–seven months and at nine–ten months in more central cortices. Potentially opposing results come from a study by Martel et al. (2015), who employed another strain of transgenic mice (THY-Tau22) and found that age, but not the expression of tau pathology throughout olfactory cortical structures, was associated with decrements in olfactory function. Unlike previous studies, these authors employed a wide range of sophisticated behavioral olfactory tests, including habituation tests and operant discrimination and memory conditioning tasks.

The overall picture is confusing. Two longitudinal studies from transgenic mice favor a centripetal pattern of spread, whereas two other "snap-shot" investigations employing different mouse strains are less conclusive. The best human information would favor centrifugal spread.

Clinico-Pathological Studies. Among the most definitive autopsy-based studies are those by Wilson and colleagues (2007a; 2009). These investigators conducted a large prospective assessment of 471 elderly community-dwelling subjects free of olfactory deficit, as measured by the Brief Smell Identification Test (B-SIT), and cognitive disorder at baseline. Lower B-SIT scores were associated with a more rapid decline in episodic memory and increased risk of developing mild cognitive impairment (MCI), even after controlling for the baseline level of episodic memory and the presence of an apolipoprotein E ε4 allele. In 34 people who died without evidence of cognitive impairment, lower B-SIT scores were associated with higher levels of AD pathology (principally NFT in the entorhinal cortex and CA1/subiculum area), again after controlling for ε4 and episodic memory function when olfaction was assessed. They concluded that among older people without clinical manifestations of AD or MCI, olfactory dysfunction is related to the level of AD pathology in the brain and the risk of subsequent prodromal symptoms of the disease, an effect that is independent of ε4 status. As the authors note, their study conflicts with two prospective post-mortem-based studies: McShane et al. (2001), where the perception of lavender water odor was assessed, and Olichney et al. (2005), who used butanol. Neither of these two studies found an association between smell measurement and AD pathology, but there was a good correlation between smell impairment and the presence of Lewy bodies (dementia with Lewy bodies or Lewy body variant). The studies by Wilson and colleagues (2007b; 2009) are likely to be more accurate as validated olfactory testing was used, but it is probably true that the olfactory defect in dementia with Lewy bodies is more severe than the deficit of AD (Williams et al., 2009).

Clinical Studies of Olfaction in Alzheimer's Disease

Predictive Studies. In one of the first prospective population-based studies, 1,836 healthy people were tested at baseline using the B-SIT and a cognitive screening procedure (Graves et al., 1999). Reduced smell identification ability, in particular anosmia, was significantly associated with increased risk of cognitive dysfunction several years later. Persons who were anosmic and who had at least one ApoE ε4 allele, a risk factor for AD, had 4.9 times the risk of developing future cognitive decline, compared to a 1.23 risk of normosmic persons who carried this allele and a 1.92 risk of anosmic persons not carrying the allele. Other associations of decreased olfactory function with the ApoE ε4 allele also have been reported (e.g., Bacon et al., 1998; Hozumi et al., 2003; Gilbert & Murphy, 2004; Salerno-Kennedy et al., 2005; Handley et al., 2006; Doty et al., 2015) and some first-degree relatives of AD patients exhibit lower olfactory test scores than those of healthy non-relative controls, emphasizing the genetic component (Serby et al., 1996; Schiffman et al., 2002). Another group examined prospectively UPSIT scores in 90 older patients with mild cognitive impairment (MCI; Devanand et al., 2000). Those scoring 34 or less who were unaware of their defect were more at risk of developing AD within two years. In a subsequent prospective study (Devanand et al., 2008), 33 of 126 MCI patients converted to AD after 3 years follow up. Five items were found to have high predictive value for conversion from MCI to AD, namely UPSIT score less than 32/40; informant report of functioning; verbal memory; MRI hippocampal and entorhinal cortex volume. Several longitudinal studies have demonstrated similarly that olfactory dysfunction is predictive of future cognitive decline in older subjects with minimal or no cognitive defect on initial assessment (Bacon et al., 1998; Royall et al., 2002; Swan & Carmelli, 2002; Schubert et al., 2008; Roberts et al., 2016). Schiffman et al. (2002) found that at-risk relatives of AD patients had higher phenylethyl alcohol detection thresholds than control subjects, as well as decreased ability to remember smells, tastes, and narrative information. Oddly enough, ApoE-4 status was not associated with at-risk status. This could mean that ApoE-4 status is not a "proximity" marker but mainly indicates long-term risk.

A further study sought to find which subset of the 40 UPSIT items predicted best the conversion to dementia in people with minimal cognitive impairment (Tabert et al., 2005). The authors identified 10 items (leather, clove, menthol, strawberry, pineapple, natural gas, lemon, lilac, soap, and smoke) that had high predictive power after a mean follow-up of 42 months, but as they point out, the odors may not be able to predict AD specifically and could indicate other dementias or PD. Importantly, the focus on odor qualities, per se, may be misleading, since most UPSIT items are complex mixtures of odorant chemicals. The difficulties associated with this approach, which also has been applied to PD, are discussed in more detail later in this chapter.

One study potentially at variance with the aforementioned studies examined the predictive value of the UPSIT in AD patients with the autosomal dominant presenilin-1 mutation (Nee & Lippa, 2001). The test was administered to 18 at-risk family members 10 years previously and although four individuals subsequently developed dementia, the UPSIT was not predictive. This variant of AD is, of course, genetically distinct but it does raise the possibility that olfaction may decline simultaneously with cognitive function as proposed for Huntington's disease (see Figure 7.13 and Paulsen et al., 2008), as discussed later in this chapter.

Studies During Established Phase of AD. Numerous studies employing quantitative psychophysical tests have found olfactory abnormalities in patients with AD, often at an early stage of disease (for review, see Doty et al., 2015). Most have used clinical criteria for diagnosis, as autopsy data has been available only rarely. Severe abnormalities were documented in many instances for identification, recognition, and threshold detection. An early and detailed study undertaken without autopsy and before readily available CT/MRI brain scans compared 19 healthy controls with 18 clinically diagnosed probable AD and 18 with vascular dementia (VD) (Knupfer & Spiegel, 1986). Mini-Mental State Examination (MMSE) scores were in the severely abnormal range, with means ranging from 12.3 to 13.7/30. The AD group fared worse with the greatest difference seen in smell identification and recognition tests. Olfactory threshold and naming tasks also differentiated the three groups, but there was more overlap. There was a strong negative correlation between threshold and MMSE, which lead the authors to recommend adjustment of odorant concentrations individually in smell recognition and identification experiments, and argued against the isolated use in dementia of fixed threshold identification methods. In one meta-analysis, Mesholam et al. (1998) found that the AD- and PD-related defects in olfaction were relatively uniform, although there was a non-significant trend toward better performance on threshold tests than recognition and identification tests. Unfortunately, no measure distinguished AD from PD. A study of 90 patients with AD by (Westervelt et al., 2007) found that some had normal, or near normal, scores on the B-SIT. It was suggested that there might be a subgroup of patients with apparently typical AD who were male, without a family history of dementia, and performed less well on visuospatial tests. The B-SIT utilizes 12 odors compared to the 40 employed by the UPSIT, so some reduction in sensitivity in a relatively small series is inevitable. The deficit in AD reportedly progresses with time (Nordin et al., 1997), although the validity of psychophysical test results from more demented individuals would seem questionable. The majority (over 90 percent) of AD patients seem unaware of their defective smell sense until they are formally tested (Doty et al., 1987), probably reflecting the fact that complete anosmia is rare. Only patients who did well on the Picture Identification Test (PIT) were included, thus the results are unlikely to be the effect of dementia itself.

An interesting study by Stamps et al. (2013) compared the ability to detect the odor of peanut butter at varying distances from either nostril; in essence a crude single-odor threshold procedure. This approach stemmed from the observations that in some patients with early AD the left hippocampus is more atrophic than the right (Shi et al., 2009) and that the projections from the olfactory bulbs are mainly ipsilateral. Surprisingly, it was found that their 18 patients with AD had greater difficulty at detecting the presence of an odor with the left compared to the right nostril and that this was significantly different from patients with other types of dementia and controls. It was suggested that this simple test might be useful as a rapid screening procedure. A more recent study failed to replicate these observations (Doty et al., 2014). It was pointed out that if the unaffected nostril was in fact normal (as indicated by Stamps et al., 2013), then bilateral measurements should also be normal, which is clearly inconsistent with the available literature on AD, but may not be so relevant to early AD. Other studies on asymmetry have found either no asymmetry or asymmetry with no consistent laterality, both in normal subjects and in subjects with AD or mild cognitive impairment (Murphy et al., 1990; Bahar Fuchs et al., 2010; Huart et al., 2015; Oleson & Murphy 2015). That being said, Stamps and colleagues have recently extended their work and have, in essence, confirmed their original findings, suggesting that the effects are present mainly in the least demented subjects (Stamps et al., 2016).

Olfactory Event-Related Potentials. Controversy surrounds the influence of AD on olfactory event-related potentials. In a study of eight non-depressed patients with AD, all of whom had mild or moderately severe forms of the disease, age-matched UPSIT scores were all abnormal (Hawkes & Shephard, 1998). However, the H_2S olfactory event-related potential (OERP) was normal in the four subjects who could be tested. Morgan & Murphy (2002) found significant delay in the OERP to amyl acetate in all of 12 AD cases. The same group found that healthy individuals, positive for the ApoE4 allele, exhibited more delayed OERP than healthy ApoE4 negative persons (Wetter & Murphy, 2001). The basis for the differing OERP findings is not clear, but may relate to the fact that odor identification tests are more sensitive and specific than OERPs in distinguishing AD from control subjects (Hawkes & Shephard, 1998). If AD pathology starts centrally then preservation of OERP would be expected in the early disease phase and, by definition, only subjects with mild dementia will be amenable to testing, given the technical difficulties of a relatively complex test and the required level of patient co-operation. As mentioned in Case report 7.1, it is possible that the OERP is reaching central olfactory areas but that cognitive impairment prevents interpretation of identification tests.

These physiological observations in AD are complemented by measurements of regional cerebral blood flow that show decreased activation of central olfactory struc-tures such as the piriform cortex (Kareken et al., 2001; Imamura et al., 2009), as well as hippocampal atrophy (see Figure 7.3). Changes were more pronounced on the right side, a finding that is at odds with the unconfirmed laterality findings of Stamps et al. (2013). In the context of the central/peripheral debate is the common factor that reductions in central activation can be due to lack of peripheral input and do not necessarily imply central dysfunction, per se.

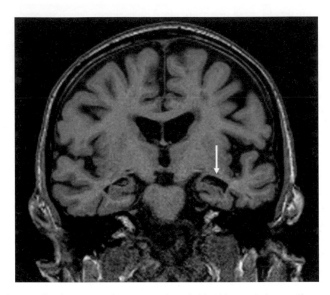

Figure 7.3 Coronal T1-weighted MRI scan of a patient with probable Alzheimer's disease. The temporal horns are markedly enlarged (down-pointing arrows) and the temporal lobes (T) are atrophic. The parahippocampal fissures are atrophic also (horizontal white arrow). Modified and reproduced from Yousem et al. (2001), with permission from Elsevier.

No form of treatment has demonstrated improvement of olfaction in AD but one preliminary non-blinded study suggested that the UPSIT predicted response to the anticholinesterase, Donepezil (Velayudhan & Lovestone, 2009; Bak & Chandran, 2011).

A rare variant of AD is posterior cortical atrophy (PCA). Olfactory processing was assessed in 15 subjects with PCA and in 10 with AD using a modified UPSIT (Witoonpanich et al., 2013). For each trial, the subject was asked to categorize the source of the odor as edible or inedible before identifying it. To maximize available response cues, the target-foil choices were name-picture combinations rather than odor names alone. Most had volumetric MRI studies. In both AD and PCA categories, about 30% showed significant impairment of olfactory identification, but there was no difference between these two groups. Performance on the odor identification task was positively associated with atrophy in the right entorhinal cortex and parahippocampal gyrus, leading to the suggestion that olfactory impairment in PCA reflected its pathologic similarity to AD.

Other Varieties of Dementia

Relatively little is known about olfaction in other varieties of dementia, such as semantic dementia, frontotemporal dementia, and vascular dementia. Normal pressure hydrocephalus is described in Chapter 6.

1. **Semantic Dementia (SD)** is a multimodal disorder of meaning in which patients have difficulty recognizing the significance of words, objects, faces, nonverbal sounds, and tastes, despite their normal perception of such stimuli. SD is potentially a very important test case for understanding the cognitive organization of chemosensory processing as it is the paradigmatic disorder of human semantic memory. One would expect a parallel loss of meaning for odors but no impairment in their detection and discrimination. Pathologically SD is associated with severe atrophy of the amygdala, middle, and inferior temporal gyri

with relative sparing of the posterior hippocampal formation. This spatial gradient distinguishes SD from AD where the major pathology is in the posterior hippocampus.

One study examined olfaction in mild AD (14 cases) compared to SD (8 cases), FTD (11 cases), and corticobasal syndrome (CBS; 7 cases, described later in this chapter) – all defined by clinical, rather than pathologic, criteria (Luzzi et al., 2007). In this study, patients of Italian and British origin were evaluated by a specially designed test battery. As expected, the AD group performed weakly on odor discrimination, naming, and odor picture-matching tasks. The SD group had particularly low scores on odor naming in the presence of normal discrimination, in keeping with the concept of olfactory agnosia. In another study, flavor processing was examined in three patients with probable SD and someone with the logopenic variant of primary progressive aphasia (Piwnica-Worms et al., 2010). They employed a modified UPSIT in which words and pictures were presented simultaneously. A novel battery incorporated tests of flavor perception, flavor identification, and congruency of flavor combinations. Those with SD equaled healthy controls on the perceptual subtest, while their ability to identify flavors or to determine congruence of flavor combinations was impaired. Classification of flavors according to affective valence was similar to controls. In contrast, the patient with logopenic variant of primary progressive aphasia exhibited a perceptual deficit with relatively preserved identification of flavors, but impaired ability to determine flavor congruence, which did not benefit from affective valence. It was proposed that SD produces a true deficit of flavor knowledge (associative agnosia).

2. **Frontotemporal dementia (FTD)** is a disorder of behavior, characterized by striking personality change, breakdown in social conduct and executive impairment. Some are parkinsonian, others have motor neuron disease (amyotrophic lateral sclerosis). Atrophy is most prominent in the frontal lobes, with involvement of the anterior temporal cortex, in contrast to AD where the posterior temporal cortex is more severely affected, but resembling the anterior temporal predominance of SD. Some of the olfactory deficits of SD would be expected, although to lesser degree, in view of the effortful search involved in odor identity that might also be compromised by patients' executive impairment. Furthermore, orbitofrontal atrophy might compromise smell perception. In the study by Luzzi et al. (2007), those with FTD and CBS exhibited mild impairment of olfactory naming and discrimination. It was concluded that the marked impairment of naming in the presence of normal discrimination in semantic dementia (i.e., olfactory agnosia) might permit differentiation from other dementias. Defects in odor identification with preservation of discrimination were also observed in three male patients with FTD (Rami et al., 2007) and the deficiency was more pronounced in those with greater involvement of the temporal lobes on MRI. McLaughlin and Westervelt (2008) studied 17 patients with a clinical diagnosis of FTD. B-SIT scores were low and of similar severity to their patients with AD. Pardini et al. (2009) tested 22 subjects with the frontal variant of FTD and 25 with CBS both defined clinically rather than pathologically. There was severe reduction of UPSIT score in FTD with only one person scoring in the normal range. Those with CBS were affected to lesser degree with 8/25 scoring in the normal range. A further study of 22 cases of FTD (Magerova et al., 2014) implemented an in-house multiple-choice 18-odor identification test and observed that those with primary non-fluent dysphasia, semantic dementia, and the behavioral variant all displayed significant impairment of identification and that there was no difference between these groups. A weakness of all these studies on SD and FTD is the absence of pathological confirmation and sometimes lack of agreed clinical diagnostic criteria. Until this is available these findings will remain provisional.

In a unique investigation (Omar et al., 2013), flavor identification was examined prospectively in 25 patients with FTD, 12 with behavioral variant frontotemporal dementia (bvFTD), 8 with semantic variant primary progressive aphasia (svPPA), 5 with non-fluent variant primary progressive aphasia (nfvPPA), and 17 healthy control subjects using a new test based on cross-modal matching of flavors to words and pictures. Odor identification was assessed using a modified UPSIT. Relative to the healthy control group, the bvFTD and svPPA subgroups showed significant impairment of flavor identification and all three FTD subgroups exhibited deficits of odor identification. Flavor identification performance did not differ significantly between the FTD syndromic subgroups. Such performance was associated with atrophy in the anteromedial temporal lobe network in the combined FTD cohort.

3. **Vascular Dementia (VD).** This is a doubtful entity and it is suggested that in many instances the correct diagnosis is AD with co-incidental infarcts. The classic clinical profile is that of an elderly hypertensive ateriopath who experiences step-wise decline in motor function. In other patients there is gradual cognitive decline, pseudobulbar palsy with relatively late onset of memory impairment. Little is known about olfaction in VD. The study by Knupfer and Spiegel (1986), described above, examined 18 patients with presumed VD and found moderate impairment of olfactory threshold, recognition, identification, and naming tasks, but not to the same degree as AD. In the investigation by Duff et al. (2002), also detailed above, there were 20 patients with VD and their scores on the basic 3-odor Pocket Smell Test (PST) were superior to those with AD or depression. Conversely the study by Gray et al. (2001) using the UPSIT found no significant difference between 13 patients with AD and 13 with vascular dementia. This important area is in dire need of further clarification supported by autopsy. On basic principles and by comparison with vascular PD, one would not expect marked olfactory impairment in VD unless there were very extensive ischemic lesions in both temporal lobes.

An important issue is the need to differentiate between operational aspects of nominally disparate olfactory tests such as identification, discrimination, memory, and detection, which are not necessarily specific to olfaction and the actual olfactory percept. Hence, errors on an odor discrimination test, for example, may not reflect difficulties in discriminating odors, per se, but in performing the discrimination task itself. In the case of odor identification, particularly if dementia is involved, it is important to ascertain whether the patient is familiar with the odorant source or name. Thus, in some studies employing the UPSIT, the picture test equivalent to the UPSIT (PIT) has been administered to ensure that the olfactory data comes from individuals who are cognizant of the inherent odor concepts (e.g., a picture of an apple which is identified as an apple) (Doty et al., 1987). If a subject performs poorly on the PIT, then their UPSIT test scores are of questionable validity.

4. **Depression.** A recurrent clinical problem is to decide whether difficulty with short-term memory represents an organic dementia, anxiety-depressive disorder, or both. Olfactory testing may be helpful as shown in case Report 7.1 This dilemma is discussed in detail in Chapter 5 but in brief, depression, per se, appears to have relatively little or no influence on most measures of olfactory function.

Case Report 7.1: Early Probable AD. A 62-year-old taxi driver presented with a two-year history of progressive failure of short-term memory and bouts of confusion. He had been driving until one year previously but gave up after a minor road traffic accident that was probably caused by poor concentration or lack of visuospatial awareness (one aspect of Balint syndrome). There was no family history of dementia and according to his wife his general health was good apart from difficulties with smelling since the age of 50 years. Examination revealed weakly positive grasp and pout reflexes. Blood pressure was 155/95 mmHg. The Mini-Mental State Examination (MMSE) score was 27/30 (normal/ borderline). The UPSIT score was in the anosmic range (13/40). OERP showed an H_2S, P2 latency of 700ms which was within the unit's 95 percent population limits. Psychometric evaluation revealed a mild degree of general intellectual decline. A magnetic resonance imaging (MRI) brain scan was normal, including views of the hippocampus and sinuses. A brain single photon emission computed tomography (SPECT) scan with Ceretec showed reduced perfusion in both temporal lobes. There was slight improvement in cognitive function with Rivastigmine (Exelon), the centrally acting anticholinesterase drug. *Comment:* The most likely diagnosis is early AD, in which there is often a long prior history of microsmia. It is interesting that the OERP was within normal limits, despite anosmia on identification testing. This could mean that signals arrive at the central processing areas (temporal lobes), thus eliciting an evoked response, but cognitive difficulty impairs the ability to identify smells on the UPSIT. Olfactory tests are useful in this situation as many who present with memory problems have pseudo-dementia secondary to depression.

In summary, there is strong evidence that impairment of olfaction in otherwise healthy elderly people may predict the development of MCI or AD and that the smell defect in established AD is severe, whether measured by psychophysical, neurophysiological, or regional blood flow studies. It still has to be determined whether olfactory neuropathology appears first in the nasal receptor zone, bulb, or temporal cortex, but at present the balance of evidence favors origin in the hippocampus prior to more peripheral olfactory structures. The characteristics of the AD olfactory defect in terms of selective odor loss or general severity are insufficiently reliable to distinguish it from other types of dementia. A patient with short-term memory impairment associated with normal olfactory identification is unlikely to have AD. If olfactory tests are abnormal, then AD or other dementias need consideration. Olfactory dysfunction may predict future cognitive decline, but prior smell loss is not specific for AD and could reflect the early development of other dementias or parkinsonian syndromes, especially those associated with Lewy bodies. Clinico-pathological correlation is badly needed for all dementia varieties, except for AD.

Down Syndrome

Down syndrome (DS) is a disorder caused by trisomy of chromosome 21. It is characterized by several dysmorphic features, including slanting eyes, broad hands, short fingers, a broad skull, and mild to severe mental impairment. DS carries a high risk of subsequent AD and is more likely to occur in those with a family history of Alzheimer's disease (Katzman, 1986). Alzheimer type pathology is observed inevitably in patients who live to the fourth decade and worsens with advancing years (Berger & Vogel, 1973; Ball & Nuttall, 1980; Wisniewski et al., 1985; Mann, 1988). Neurons in layer 2 of the entorhinal cortex and the CA1/subiculum field of the hippocampus are first to be affected by tangle formation, suggesting early involvement of structures critical to olfactory processing (Oliver & Holland, 1986).

Initial clinical observations suggested that DS is accompanied by smell dysfunction (Brousseau & Brainerd, 1928). Subsequent empirical studies have confirmed this, showing deficits on tests of identification, detection, and memory, as well as OERP (Warner et al., 1988; Hemdal et al., 1993; Zucco & Negrin, 1994; McKeown et al., 1996; Murphy & Jinich, 1996; Wetter & Murphy, 1999). It has been proposed that the olfactory defect is progressive (Nijjar & Murphy, 2002). In general, the average degree of smell loss observed in DS is close to that observed in AD, i.e., mean UPSIT scores around 20 (Warner et al., 1988; McKeown et al., 1996). Scores on the San Diego Odor Identification Test were noted to be worse in those carrying the ApoE 4 allele (Sliger et al., 2004). It is relevant that patients with DS may have increased tendency to upper-respiratory infections and sleep-disordered breathing (Chen et al., 2006). These features could influence smell test results if not addressed at the time of evaluation.

It is not clear *when* individuals with DS exhibit olfactory loss. In the sole study designed to shed light on this question, McKeown et al. (1996) administered the UPSIT and a 16-item odor discrimination test to 20 adolescents with DS and to 20 non-DS mentally impaired children matched on the basis of mental age using the Peabody Picture Vocabulary Test-Revised (Dunn et al., 1981). Twenty non-mentally impaired children similarly matched on mental age were also tested. Although no meaningful differences in olfactory function were found among the three study groups, the test scores of both the DS and non-DS mentally impaired subjects were lower than non-mentally impaired age-matched children and of similar magnitude to those of adult DS subjects. The DS subjects were at an early age where AD pathology is unlikely to be present, suggesting that the olfactory deficit might occur prior to the development of typical AD-related pathology.

Fragile X Syndrome

This is a common cause of intellectual disability in males and the most common single gene cause of autism. It is caused by a CGG trinucleotide repeat of the fragile X mental retardation gene (FMR1). There are two main varieties of the syndrome. In the early onset form there is a full mutation expressed in children who display intellectual disability, elongated face, prominent ears, and large testes. In the late-onset type there are fewer trinucleotide repeats (premutation) and patients suffer tremor and ataxia abbreviated to FXTAS. Clinical features of FXTAS consist of ataxia and cerebellar tremor, but it is sometimes confused with Parkinson's disease and essential tremor. Knock-out mice lacking the FMR1 gene were found to have impairment of olfactory discrimination learning (Larson et al., 2008), but no change in threshold, implying that there may be a human correlate. Another group who used the same knock-out mouse model found lowering of olfactory sensitivity but no change in habituation or discrimination (Schilit et al., 2015). In a human study of 41 subjects with FXTAS (Juncos, Lazarus et al., 2012), UPSIT scores were depressed but not to the same degree as PD or AD. Cognitive impairment affected the scores adversely. It is therefore unlikely that olfactory testing alone will help distinguish FXTAS from PD.

Parkinson's Disease

Parkinson's disease is one the most prevalent movement disorders affecting more than 1 percent of people over the age of 65. The main features are muscle rigidity, akinesia (hesitancy or slowness of movement), and rest tremor. Sensory abnormalities are not prominent in PD and until recently many textbooks stated that sensory systems were spared. Although the major senses (vision, hearing, touch, taste) are all damaged mildly, an important exception is the sense of smell which is affected severely. This fact was overlooked by James Parkinson in his treatise (1817) and not reported until 1970

(Constantinidis & De Ajuriaguerra, 1970). This important defect is now reviewed from the pathological and clinical aspects with particular attention to the familial varieties of PD

Pathological Studies of the Olfactory System

Olfactory Neuroepithelium. Dystrophic neurites without Lewy bodies have been found in the olfactory epithelium in autopsies from individuals with PD. Several patients also display accumulation of amyloid precursor protein fragments apparently equivalent to those observed in Alzheimer's disease (Crino et al., 1995). All varieties of synuclein (α, β, γ) are expressed in olfactory receptor neurons, particularly α-synuclein which, when phosphorylated and misfolded, becomes highly insoluble and forms the hallmark pathology of PD. The expression of abnormal α-synuclein within the olfactory mucosa was found to be no different from that of Lewy body disease, AD, multiple system atrophy (MSA), and seemingly healthy older controls (Duda et al., 1999). More recently, nasal biopsy specimens from seven patients with symptomatic PD (Witt et al., 2009) were compared to nasal biopsies from nine microsmic controls and seven with normal olfaction using antibodies against olfactory marker protein (OMP), protein gene product 9.5 (PGP 9.5), beta-tubulin (BT), proliferation-associated antigen (Ki 67), the stem cell marker nestin, cytokeratin, p75NGFr, and alpha-synuclein. Irregular areas of olfactory epithelium were positive for PGP 9.5 and neurotubulin, but mostly negative for OMP even though mRNA for OMP was found in the olfactory cleft and respiratory mucosa. There was no clear difference between the PD patients and the controls. The investigators concluded that the olfactory loss in PD is more likely to be explained by more central pathology (e.g., olfactory bulb or primary olfactory cortex) than changes in the nasal epithelium. This complex problem was addressed further in a study of the olfactory pathways in 105 autopsied Japanese individuals (Funabe et al., 2013). There were 39 with Lewy-related alpha-synucleinopathy (LBAS, Lewy neurites) in the central or peripheral nervous system, of whom seven showed Lewy neurites in the olfactory mucosa and bulb. There were six of eight cases with LBAS in olfactory neurons of the lamina propria (the layer just deep to the olfactory epithelium) in those with clinically or pathologically confirmed PD (four cases) and one instance of LBAS with incidental Lewy body disease. No one has found Lewy bodies, only dystrophic neurites, in the olfactory epithelium, but this may have been bad luck, as the Lewy body is composed of clumps of phosphorylated alpha-synuclein. It remains possible that healthy subjects coincidentally found to have α-synuclein containing dystrophic neurites in the nasal receptor zone by Duda et al. (1999) were in the preclinical stage of PD and that the changes actually represent a disease-related, if not disease-specific, finding. A major difficulty is that with age the olfactory neuroepithelium is replaced progressively by respiratory epithelium and, for safety reasons, many have sampled from the more accessible anterior part of the middle turbinate where ORN are less numerous. At present the presence of specific PD related Lewy pathology in the nasal olfactory epithelium is possible but not proven.

Olfactory Bulb and Anterior Olfactory Nucleus (AON)

Unlike the nasal olfactory epithelium, considerable disease-related changes are readily demonstrable in the olfactory bulbs and tracts of patients with PD. In an early study of eight PD patients and eight controls, all PD cases contained Lewy bodies that were most numerous in the AON but also present in mitral cells – structures that receive direct input from the bipolar olfactory cells (Daniel & Hawkes, 1992). The Lewy body morphology at this site resembled that observed in the cortex, although inclusions showing a classic tri-laminar structure were rarely present. Within the AON, the loss of neurons correlated with the number of Lewy bodies, as well as with disease duration (Pearce et al., 1995).

It is likely that olfactory bulb α-synucleinopathy is associated with Lewy Body disorders. Thus, Beach and co-workers (2009) found that 55 of 58 olfactory bulbs from patients with PD contained Lewy bodies, thereby achieving a sensitivity of 95% and specificity of 91% versus elderly controls, an observation echoed in a smaller study by Jellinger (2009). They showed that the α-synucleinopathy density score in the bulb correlated well with such scores in other brain regions, together with measures on the MMSE and Unified Parkinson's Disease Rating Scale (UPDRS), and suggested boldly that olfactory bulb biopsy might be used to confirm a diagnosis of PD prior to surgical therapy for this disease. The latter statement is probably unwarranted at present given the number of conditions other than classic PD (e.g., MSA, PSP, Dementia with Lewy bodies) that are associated with Lewy pathology in the bulb.

It should be noted that the human olfactory bulb (OB) contains at least 20 different neurotransmitters in addition to dopamine (see Chapter 1). Oddly enough, dopamine deficiency within the bulb has not been observed in PD at autopsy. Indeed, a significant *increase* in the number of periglomerular dopaminergic neurons was reported in an initial study of the human OB (Huisman et al., 2004), as well as up-regulation of tyrosine hydroxylase (TH) expression. As TH is the precursor of dopamine synthesis, such upregulation was a proposed mechanism for the microsmia in PD. Their subsequent study, which adjusted for gender, failed to confirm the initial findings although a trend was still apparent (Huisman et al., 2008). An elevation of TH expression relative to three controls was reported in the olfactory bulbs of three Macaca monkeys who had been injected with methyl-phenyl-tetrahydropyridine (MPTP) (Belzunegui et al., 2007) and in transgenic rats and mice bearing the common PD alpha-synuclein mutations, A30P and A53T (Ubeda-Banon et al., 2010b; Lelan et al., 2011). In the MPTP mouse model of PD, a 4-fold increase of dopamine expression in the olfactory bulb has also been reported (Yamada et al., 2004). Such dopamine increase may reflect attempts to compensate for loss of a dopamine-responsive substrate, conceivably via increased migration of dopamine secreting cells from the sub-ventricular zone/rostral migratory stream into the olfactory bulb (Bedard & Parent, 2004).

The importance of alpha-synuclein (ASN) pathology in explaining the anosmia of PD was highlighted in experiments involving Thy1-aSyn transgenic mice that over-expressed ASN under the Thy1 promoter (Fleming et al., 2008). These mice have high levels of ASN expression throughout the brain but no loss of nigrostriatal dopamine neurons up to eight months. Compared with wildtype littermates, Thy1-aSyn mice could still detect and habituate to odors but showed olfactory impairments in aspects of all three testing paradigms they employed, i.e., latency to find an exposed or hidden odorant, a block test centered on exposure to self- and non-self-odors, and a habituation/dishabituation test based on exposure to non-social odors.

The picture has become more complex following a study by Ubeda-Bañon et al. (2010a) who evaluated the distribution of abnormal α-synuclein in the olfactory bulbs of 11 cases of Parkinson's Disease. Immuno-histochemical distribution of α-synuclein was measured in the olfactory bulb, AON, and more central olfactory regions. Also determined was its co-localization with (1) TH, the dopamine precursor, situated in periglomerular and tufted cells, (2) somatostatin and substance P, peptides present in most layers of the OB, (3) calbindin, a calcium binding protein, present in granule cells, short axon neurons and interneurons of the external plexiform layer (EPL), (4) calretinin, a calcium binding protein localized to granule, periglomerular cell and interneurons of the EPL, and (5) parvalbumin, a calcium binding albumin, which is a marker for short axon and periglomerular cells. Lewy pathology was localized in mitral cells, the inner plexiform layer, and all divisions of the AON, but less conspicuous in the olfactory tubercle and olfactory cortices. In the olfactory bulb, AON, and olfactory cortices, those cells affected by α-synucleinopathy seldom co-localized TH or somatostatin, but they frequently co-localized calbindin, calretinin, parvalbumin, and substance P. Dopamine and somatostatin-positive cells *were rarely affected*, whereas the cell types most vulnerable to neurodegeneration were glutamate (mitral cells), and calcium-binding protein- and substance P-positive cells. This detailed study and others mentioned above suggest that it is naïve to attribute the anosmia of PD to dopamine deficiency in the OB. Immunohistochemistry suggests that multiple cell types are affected, particularly those concerned with calcium protein binding. The study from Japan cited above (Funabe et al., 2013) analyzed the olfactory bulb as well as the olfactory epithelium. The main Lewy pathology in their seven cases was found in the glomerular apparatus, granular cells, and tufted cells, but less frequently in the mitral cells.

Even further complexity has been shown with respect to the distribution of abnormal ASN in more central olfactory structures, i.e., AON, olfactory tubercle, piriform cortex, posterolateral cortical amygdala, and lateral entorhinal cortex (Ubeda-Banon et al., 2012). They examined homozygous transgenic mice, aged two–eight months, that overexpressed the human A53T variant of alpha-synuclein, which is the equivalent of PARK1/4 (see Table 7.2). A significant increase of ASN expression in the transgenic strain was found in the piriform cortex at eight months compared to other brain structures. Double-labeling experiments using neural tracers showed axonal collaterals of mitral cells entering layer 2 of the piriform cortex in close proximity to alpha-synuclein-positive cells. No changes were observed in the substantia nigra (up to age 8 m), but the OB and piriform cortex were both affected at two months' age. This is in keeping with the concept of olfactory damage preceding motor changes. At present there are few published studies of olfaction in PARK1/4 patients bearing the A53T mutation but one would expect impaired smell to precede the motor phenomena of classic PD.

The corticomedial nucleus of the amygdala and primary olfactory cortices, i.e., the piriform and entorhinal cortices, receive direct projections from the olfactory bulb and have high concentrations of dopamine receptors and dopaminergic fibers. The main innervation of the piriform cortex is the olfactory tubercle, which has markedly decreased dopamine levels in PD (Bogerts et al., 1983). In a study of PD central olfactory structures, there were deposits of abnormal alpha-synuclein predominantly in the temporal division of the piriform cortex, olfactory tubercle, or anterior portions of the entorhinal cortex (Silveira-Moriyama et al., 2009), in keeping with Braak staging (Braak et al., 2003b).

Dopamine repletion has no influence on the olfactory deficit of PD, implying that if the dopamine system is involved, the olfactory receptors in the nose nose or elsewhere in the olfactory pathways are dysfunctional or so severely depleted that they cannot respond.

Conclusions. It is still unclear whether the nasal neuroepithelium is specifically damaged in PD beyond age-related effects, but there is no doubt about the olfactory bulb and AON – they

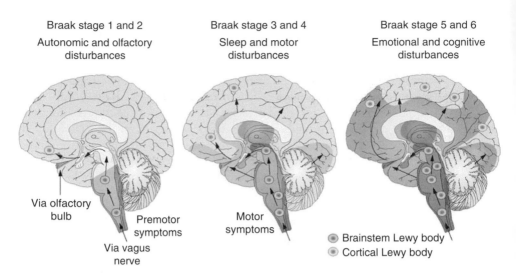

Braak stage 1 and 2
Autonomic and olfactory disturbances

Braak stage 3 and 4
Sleep and motor disturbances

Braak stage 5 and 6
Emotional and cognitive disturbances

Via olfactory bulb

Premotor symptoms

Via vagus nerve

Motor symptoms

⦿ Brainstem Lewy body
⦿ Cortical Lewy body

Figure 7.4 The Braak staging system of Parkinson's disease, showing the initiation sites in the olfactory bulb and the dorsal motor nucleus of the vagus, through to the later Lewy pathology into cortical regions (see text). Figure reproduced with permission from Halliday et al. (2011).

are injured early in the disease process and probably beyond repair. Simple dopamine deficiency is not sufficient to explain the microsmia of PD. Immunohistochemical studies in PD suggest that several cell types are affected, particularly those concerned with glutamate release (mitral cells), calcium-binding protein, and substance P, but the main dopaminergic neurons – the periglomerular cells – are spared. This information tallies with the lack of olfactory improvement in response to levodopa, assuming there are sufficient neurons remaining to generate a signal. Despite this, significant correlations have been found between UPSIT scores and dopamine transporter activity in the basal ganglia (Siderowf et al., 2005; Bohnen et al., 2007, 2008, 2010; Deeb et al., 2010; Berendse et al., 2011). Whether this reflects the close association between dopamine and acetylcholine is not clear, but certainly plausible (Doty, 2017). Overall, the picture is confusing and awaits further elaboration. Speculatively, these findings support the use of cholinergic, noradrenergic, or glutamatergic medication in an attempt to improve the sense of smell.

Braak Staging and Central olfactory changes

In 2003, Braak and colleagues performed a landmark detailed neuropathological analysis of PD by α-synuclein immunostaining (Braak et al., 2003a). In brief, their data suggested that the pathological process advances in a caudo-rostral sequence, with the earliest changes (which develop before any motor symptoms) occurring within the olfactory bulb, particularly the AON, and the dorsal motor nuclear complex (DMC) of the glossopharyngeal and vagus nerves (Figure 7.4).

Where Lewy bodies could be found in the substantia nigra, invariably there were similar and more severe changes in the olfactory bulb and the dorsal medulla. Interestingly, the involvement of DMC and demonstration of Lewy pathology in the gastric submucosal plexus led to the proposal that PD starts in the enteric plexus (Braak et al., 2006 and Figure

Central nervous system

dorsal motor
nucleus

Enteric nervous system

muscularis   muscularis
propria   mucosa

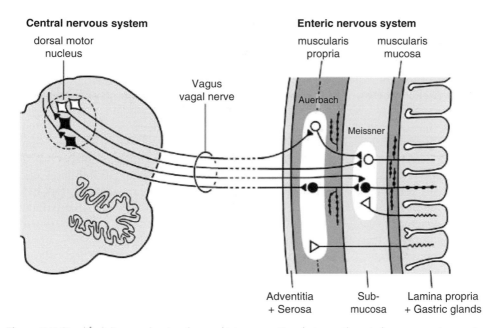

Vagus
vagal nerve

Auerbach

Meissner

Adventitia   Sub-   Lamina propria
+ Serosa   mucosa   + Gastric glands

Figure 7.5 Simplified diagram showing the vagal interconnections between the enteric nervous system and medulla oblongata. A neurotropic agent capable of passing through the mucosal epithelial barrier of the stomach could enter terminal axons of postganglionic VIPergic neurones (black, rounded cell somata) in the submucosal Meissner plexus and, via retrograde axonal and transneuronal transport (black, rounded cell somata in the Auerbach plexus), reach the preganglionic cholinergic neurones (black, diamond-shaped cell somata) of the dorsal motor nucleus of the vagus in the lower brainstem. Reproduced with permission from Braak et al. (2006).

7.5) and that a pathogen, possibly viral or chemical, ascends the motor vagal fibers in retrograde fashion to the dorsal medulla (Braak et al., 2006).

Limited support for a vagal pathogenic pathway has come from a retrospective study of subjects who underwent vagotomy from 1977 to1995 (Svensson et al., 2015). In comparison to the general population, those who underwent complete (truncal) vagotomy appeared less likely to develop PD if follow-up exceeded 20 years (adjusted HR = 0.53; 95% CI: 0.28–0.99). Conversely those who received selective vagotomy had a subsequent PD risk similar to the general population. However, their observations had limited statistical precision and their findings were not confirmed in a separate analysis using the same database (Tysnes et al., 2015).

The enteric origin theory, while appealing because it explains the presence of abnormal α-synuclein deposits in the enteric plexus, does not explain the olfactory bulb changes or the probable early deposits in the autonomic nervous system, i.e., hypothalamus, sympathetic ganglia, cardiac and pelvic plexus, spinal cord, and adrenal medulla (Wakabayashi & Takahashi, 1997). An alternative explanation is that a "dual hit" occurs where a pathogen simultaneously enters the olfactory bulb and enteric plexus (Hawkes et al., 2007), but even this concept does not explain easily the sympathetic involvement. It is of interest that there is a higher prevalence of ulcers in patients with PD, with the presence of ulcers often preceding the diagnosis of PD by 10 to 20 years (Strang, 1965; Altschuler, 1996). Conceivably, uptake of viruses or other xenobiotics is facilitated by the ulcerated exposure of nerve endings within the gut. It has been shown in the rhesus monkey that it is difficult to induce poliomyelitis by introducing polio virus into the gastrointestinal tract. However, when the tract is disturbed by operative procedures, induction occurs readily (Toomey, 1935, 1936). Such observations led Toomey to propose that a combination of virus and other toxic process or material is required for induction in the monkey. Could the same be the case with PD? These issues are elaborated later in this chapter under the olfactory vector hypothesis.

Given that at least 50 percent of substantia nigra cells have to die before clinical symptoms emerge (Fearnley & Lees, 1991; Ross et al., 2004), it is possible that the clinical motor manifestations of PD represent the late stage of a pathological process that probably started many years previously. This point is borne out by anecdotal clinical observations from patients with PD who report regularly that smell impairment occurred years before their first motor symptoms. According to the study by Braak et al. (2003a), Lewy pathology in central olfactory areas such as the entorhinal cortex develops much later – in the fourth of six phases, implying that olfactory dysfunction in PD starts peripherally.

The proposed sequential development of PD, as formulated by Braak and colleagues (2003a), has been challenged (Parkkinen et al., 2005; Kalaitzakis et al., 2008). Many exceptions have been identified to the proposed caudo-rostral spread in the brain stem with demonstration of substantia nigra or cerebral cortex pathology without any DMC change. However, such differences may relate to variation in the pattern and accuracy of case selection. For example, in Lewy body dementia, which is sometimes confused clinically with PD, the pathology is more severe in the cerebral cortex than in the brain stem. Inadvertent inclusion of such cases will run counter to the Braak staging. As mentioned above, the picture is complicated further by the presence of Lewy pathology in the sympathetic and enteric nervous systems probably at a very early stage. The consensus view is that Braak staging of PD is broadly correct and concurs well with "premotor" symptoms (Duda et al., 2007; Hawkes et al., 2010).

Clinical Evidence for Olfactory Dysfunction in Parkinson's Disease

Constantinidis and De Ajuriaguerra (1970) noted anosmia in two subjects with familial and slightly atypical parkinsonism. Subsequently, olfactory loss in 10 of 22 patients with typical PD was documented by Ansari & Johnson (1975). There were elevated thresholds to the banana-smelling substance amyl acetate. They noted an association between higher threshold scores (i.e., greater olfactory dysfunction) and more rapid disease progression. There appeared to be no influence from medication (levodopa, anticholinergic drugs) or smoking behavior. In a subsequent study of 78 PD patients and 40 controls, Quinn et al. (1987) similarly found elevated amyl acetate thresholds but there was no influence on the threshold measures from age, sex, on–off state, disease duration, or use of levodopa.

Further studies suggested that olfactory dysfunction, as measured by the UPSIT and detection threshold for phenylethyl alcohol, is independent of disease duration or disability, and not meaningfully correlated with measures of motor function, tremor, or cognition (Doty et al., 1988, 1989, 1992a). It was also demonstrated that the olfactory deficit was typically bilateral and uninfluenced by anti-Parkinsonian medication. Evaluation of clinically defined PD subtypes showed that females with mild disability and tremor dominant disease had slightly better UPSIT scores than males with moderate to severe disability and little or no tremor; age at disease onset was not a factor (Stern et al., 1994). A comparable

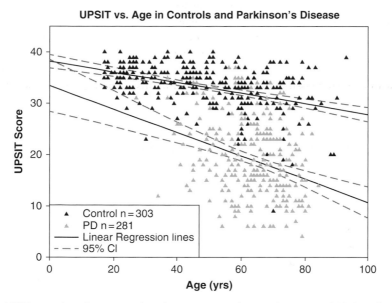

Figure 7.6 UPSIT score plotted against age based on 281 cognitively normal patients with PD (grey diamonds) and 303 controls (black diamonds). Linear regression lines and 95% confidence limits are shown for each group.

survey was subsequently undertaken by Hawkes et al. (1997) in 155 cognitively normal, depression-free PD patients and 156 age-matched controls. UPSIT scores for the PD patients were dramatically lower than the UPSIT scores of the age-matched controls (see Figure 7.6 from a later study). Only 19% (30/155) of the PD patients had a score within the normal range defined by 95% population limits. Sixty-five (42 percent) were classified as anosmic, i.e., scoring less than 17/40. There was no correlation between disease duration and UPSIT score (r = 0.074). A somewhat lower prevalence of abnormality (65 percent) was obtained for odor identification in 404 Dutch PD patients assessed by the extended version of Sniffin' Sticks test (Boesveldt et al., 2008). Sobel and colleagues (2001) found sniffing to be impaired in PD, resulting in a slight reduction in their performance on identification and detection threshold tests. In the case of the UPSIT, this reduction was not-significant and less than 2 UPSIT points (see below). Increasing sniff vigor improved olfactory scores. It may be argued that investigations into PD that have not allowed for this effect may tend to exaggerate slightly the severity of any defect, especially where the disease has affected bulbar function.

Altered olfactory event related potentials (OERP) are found in PD (Kobal & Plattig, 1978; Hawkes & Shephard, 1992, see Figure 7.7). In a detailed study, Hawkes et al. (1997) evaluated OERP in 73 non-depressed, cognitively normal patients with PD and in 47 control subjects of similar age and sex. In 36 of 73 patients (49 percent), responses were either absent or unsatisfactory for technical reasons. Regression analysis on the 37 individuals with a measurable trace showed a highly significant latency difference between PD patients and control subjects for the odorant hydrogen sulfide (H_2S).

Similar results were reported in 31 PD patients using vanillin and H_2S (Barz et al., 1997). Prolonged latencies were observed whether or not medication was being taken for the condition. However, more marked change was evident for those receiving treatment,

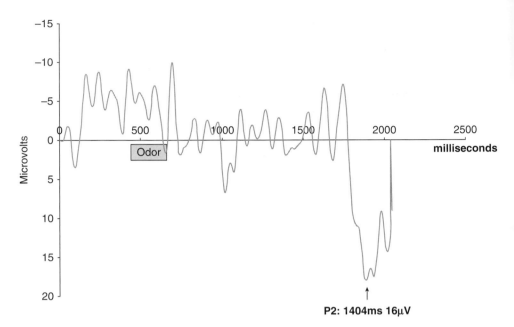

Figure 7.7 Olfactory event-related potential obtained from PZ in a patient with classic PD. The 200 ms stimulus (hydrogen sulfide, 20 ppm) is shown as a rectangle at 500 ms from recording onset. Latency to P2 is significantly delayed at 1404 ms (upper limit ~937mS) but the amplitude is normal. Note the poor signal-noise ratio which is typical but adds to the difficulty of recording such potentials.

conceivably reflecting greater PD-related disability. A correlation between disability, as measured by Webster score, and latency to the H_2S derived OERP was noted. Finally, a multimodal study in 73 patients with early PD (Deeb et al., 2010) confirmed increased OERP latency (but not amplitude) in 49 patients, but this did not correlate with dopamine transporter uptake. Typically, increased latency indicates demyelination, but in PD there is no evidence of this and a satisfactory explanation for such prolongation has yet to be found.

There is debate about the temporal characteristics of the olfactory defect in PD, i.e., whether it is stable or progressive and whether it correlates with indicators of disease severity. An age-related decline in smell function particularly after 60 years is unavoidable, even in apparently healthy people, but the critical issue is whether there is additional progressive impairment from PD, superimposed on aging effects. Several studies of smell identification or detection threshold sensitivity found no correlation with disease duration (Quinn et al., 1987; Doty et al., 1988; Hawkes et al., 1997). This contrasts with the early observations of Ansari & Johnson (1975), who reported an association between olfactory thresholds and rapid progression. Others describe an association between disability and olfactory event-related potentials (Barz et al., 1997).

Support for the concept of pathological progression within the olfactory system derives from studies that show neuronal loss in the AON, along with progressive accumulation of Lewy bodies and neurites which advance with disease duration (Pearce et al., 1995) and increasing Braak stage (Braak et al., 2003a). The concept of functional progression receives tangential support from the finding of a significant correlation ($r = 0.66$) between dopamine transporter uptake, as measured by dopamine transporter SPECT, and UPSIT scores (Siderowf et al.,

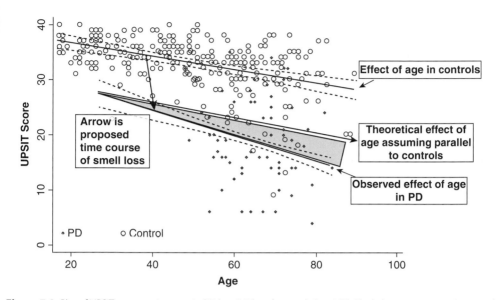

Figure 7.8 Plot of UPSIT score against age in PD (n = 263) and controls (n = 266). Black dots represent patients and open circles are controls. The lines show age-related decline of UPSIT scores in controls (upper black line) and patients (lower black line), assuming linear regression. If the PD olfactory defect is stable with age, then its regression line (center line) should remain parallel to the controls, but in fact the control and PD lines diverge, suggesting an additional variable. The large downsloping arrow indicates a proposed acute event causing a decline in olfaction from the healthy control level. If there is accelerated deterioration of smell function with age in PD, this additional component would be represented by the gray shaded area between the center and bottom lines. Modified from Hawkes (2008a).

2005), but not with symptom duration or disability, as measured by the Unified Parkinson's Disease Rating Scale (UPDRS). Using "Sniffin' Sticks" in 40 non-demented Parkinson's disease subjects, Tissingh & colleagues (2001) found a negative correlation between olfactory discrimination and both the UPDRS motor score and Hoehn and Yahr stage. Hawkes (2008a) compared the UPSIT scores of 266 patients with Parkinson's disease with those of 263 healthy control subjects. The linear regression lines on age, apart from showing a lower mean UPSIT score at all ages, *diverged* with age (Figure 7.8). Although this is a cross-sectional rather than a longitudinal study, it implies that the olfactory disorder reflects the combined effect of aging and Parkinson's disease itself. Deeb et al. (2010) reported a significant correlation between UPSIT and motor scores in early cases of Parkinson's disease. Another group analyzed 19 patients with PD over five-year intervals using Sniffin' Sticks and OERP (Meusel et al., 2010). At follow up five years later, some initially hyposmic subjects had become anosmic and 3/19 with initially detectable OERP were no longer recordable. Strangely, OERPs were detectable in another three subjects whose OERPs were absent at baseline. These observations reopen the question of an association between olfactory function, the passage of time, and the motor deficit of Parkinson's disease. Given the compelling evidence from neuropathology and dopamine transporter data, it is likely that there is progression of the olfactory defect with time.

Selective Anosmia in Sporadic PD? If a small number of odors could be found which distinguish reliably between PD patients and healthy control subjects, then a brief test based on these would have clinical utility. In the first formal study to address this issue, two UPSIT odors, pizza and wintergreen, were found to best discriminate between British PD patients and control subjects, with a sensitivity of 90 percent and specificity of 86 percent (Hawkes & Shephard, 1993). Other investigators using UPSIT, B-SIT, or Sniffin' Sticks have found different sets of odors to be useful discriminators (Daum et al., 2000; Double et al., 2003; Silveira-Moriyama et al., 2005; Bohnen et al., 2007; Boesveldt et al., 2008). Although it is conceivable that genetically based specific anosmias are present in PD, the use of complex odorants such as those indicated above, which are not equally intense, would be unlikely to identify them. Even oregano, a major component of pizza, is composed of multiple volatile components (Diaz-Maroto et al., 2002). Moreover, different response alternatives are present for a variety of odor items in the currently employed tests, making the stimulus–response complexes even more multifaceted. Cultural or socioeconomic factors may play a role, bringing forth issues related to familiarity or frequency of interactions with specific odors. If progress is to be made in this area, a dedicated test battery will be needed to include odors that are less complex and of equal intensity.

Olfactory Hallucinations in PD. Olfactory hallucinations (OH) that are usually unpleasant and short-lived are found moderately frequently in PD if one troubles to ask. Prevalence estimates range from 10 percent (Bannier et al., 2012) to 36 percent (Goetz et al., 2011). The latter study was based on a 10-year follow up of hallucination-naïve patients with PD and found, not surprisingly, that the prevalence of OH increased with time and that OH were regularly associated with auditory or tactile hallucinations. OH may represent the olfactory equivalent of the Charles Bonnet syndrome – where blind people experience visual hallucinations. Interestingly, OH may predate the onset of classic motor symptoms, a phenomenon probably first identified by Sandyk (1981). In this brief letter, there were three patients in which OH preceded motor manifestations by several months and a further instance where the hallucinations developed at the time of motor presentation. A later publication described pleasant OHs that disappeared with the onset of Parkinson's disease (Landis & Burkhard, 2008). Mitral cell denervation hypersensitivity or excess dopaminergic activity in the olfactory bulb were proposed mechanisms. Another report described unpleasant OH in 4/188 patients with PD, giving a prevalence of 2.1% (McAuley & Gregory, 2012). These patients had a long duration of disease treated with dopaminergic medication. None were demented but they all failed to report the OH spontaneously. The only authors who actually measured olfactory function (using the extended Sniffin' Stick Test) found microsmia in one patient and normal smell function in the other (Landis & Burkhard, 2008). It has been proposed that development of hallucinations (including olfactory) in those with established PD may indicate a co-morbid psychotic illness or parkinsonism (Goetz et al., 1998).

Case Report 7.2: PD with Longstanding Prior Anosmia. A 63-year-old retired male electrical engineer presented with a three- year history of slight impairment of walking and tendency to stumble. Relatives remarked that he had become more stooped and did not swing the arms on walking. His handwriting had become smaller and there was increased fatigue when playing a round of golf. Twenty years previously he developed what was thought to be Bornholm's disease (intercostal myalgia) and shortly after that it was noticed that he could not detect the smell of gas. Examination, including cognitive tests, was unremarkable apart from reduced arm swing and minimal increase of arm tone on reinforcement. The provisional diagnosis was early classic PD corresponding to Hoehn and Yahr stage I. MRI brain scan showed no abnormality and there were no significant inflammatory changes in the paranasal sinuses, implying that local nasal disease did not contribute to the smell deficit. The olfactory bulbs and tracts appeared normal. The UPSIT score was 16/40 (anosmic range) and there was delay on OERP at 1120 ms (normal less than 937 ms). Electrogustometry showed a markedly raised threshold over the fungiform and circumvallate papillae. The DATScan showed significant loss of dopamine transporter uptake in the putamen of both sides. One year later there was slight progression of disability and he was placed on levodopa (Sinemet CR), to which he made an excellent response. *Comment:* This patient had signs of early PD, which was confirmed by the DATScan and his excellent response to levodopa. The prior history of anosmia in the absence of local nasal disease is in keeping with the proposal that smell impairment is an early warning sign of PD – here by as much as 20 years. The taste involvement is an intriguing aspect. Initial reports suggested that taste is unaffected in PD (Sienkiewicz-Jarosz et al., 2005), but this has now been challenged, as explained later in this chapter.

Case Report 7.3: Anosmia and Ageusia with Unclear Diagnosis. A 61-year-old man presented initially with a two-year history of difficulty in appreciating the smell or taste of food. The problem appeared to have evolved over a few days in the absence of local nasal infection. The smell symptoms showed no tendency to fluctuate, as might be expected if there was an element of obstructive anosmia. Strong perfume made him sneeze but he could not smell the fragrance. He thought that his appreciation of food flavor was impaired – for example, salted potato crisps tasted completely bland. Physical examination, including nasal endoscopy, was normal. The UPSIT score was 19/40 (severe microsmic range) and he was unable to detect bitter, sweet, sour, or salt using supra-threshold filter strips to the four main tastants. MRI brain scan showed minor vascular changes in keeping with his age and blood pressure (167/89 mm Hg). Three years later he was referred because of involuntary kicking movements in bed, suggestive of restless legs syndrome – an occasional precursor of PD. A dopamine transporter scan (DATScan) showed reduced uptake in the left putamen, confirming the possibility of preclinical PD. Routine clinical examination showed no obvious sign of PD, but he was advised that he might develop this disorder over the next 5–10 years. *Comment:* The patient's history suggests that the olfactory impairment might be a precursor of Parkinsonism, but the coexistence of taste impairment early on is not typical of classic PD (Shah et al., 2009). The abnormal DATScan gives objective confirmation of a Parkinsonian syndrome, but time will tell whether this patient will turn out to have classic PD.

Smoking and Classic Parkinson's Disease. Numerous epidemiologic studies find that the majority of people with classic PD are either never smokers or not current smokers. Indeed, it is very unusual to find a patient with typical PD who continues to smoke, and if so, the question is always raised of parkinsonism such as vascular PD or progressive supranuclear palsy (Type-P). Furthermore, most studies do not have autopsy verification, thus there is always the risk of misclassification that affects at least 10% (Hughes et al., 2001). The most popular explanation for the under-representation of smokers with PD is that smoking is protective. This concept has been challenged with the suggestion that it may be a false association due to reversed causation (Ritz et al., 2014). It is proposed that smoking and PD are related through a reduction in nicotinic reward, such that ease of quitting might represent an early prodromal marker. Conversely, studies of olfactory identification in PD suggest that smoking is protective. In one preliminary case-control study of 68 patients with PD (Moccia et al., 2014), there was no significant difference in UPSIT scores between PD current smokers compared to PD current non-smokers. However, 10 currently smoking controls underperformed 51 never-smoking controls, implying that smoking may have protected against olfactory dysfunction in their PD cohort. A slightly larger case-control study

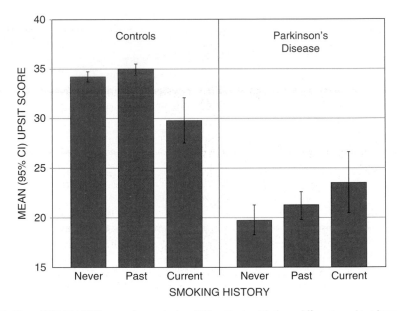

Figure 7.9 Mean (95% CI) UPSIT scores for control and PD patients with three different smoking histories. Reproduced with permission from Sharer, et al. (2015).

comprising 76 PD subjects (Lucassen et al., 2014) showed a fractionally higher but significant UPSIT mean score for PD ever-smokers compared to PD never-smokers. Only one PD patient was a current smoker. In a substantive study by Sharer et al. (2015), UPSIT scores were measured in 323 PD patients and 323 controls closely matched individually on age, sex, and smoking history (never, past, current). PD current smokers scored significantly higher than past and never-smoker PD subjects. The difference in PD mean UPSIT score between current and never-smokers was around four points higher (10%) whereas for current smoking controls, the mean score was four–five UPSIT points *lower* (~10%) than never- or past smokers (Figure 7.9). There was no association between test scores and pack years. Sceptics might argue that the apparent protective effect from smoking was due partly to over-representation of those with vascular PD who would be more likely to smoke, have normal olfaction (see above) or may relate to the recognized 10% diagnostic error rate. Nonetheless, at face value, these findings provide further support to the concept of protection against PD by cigarette smoking and concur with epidemiologic studies reporting that smokers exposed to workplace solvents and acrylates score higher on the UPSIT than their non-smoking counterparts (Schwartz et al., 1989; Schwartz et al., 1990). The question of reversed causality has yet to be resolved.

Evidence of olfactory bulb involvement *in vivo* is now emerging with the advent of high resolution MRI techniques. Visualization of the olfactory bulb and its tract is hampered by so-called susceptibility artifacts where it is difficult to obtain a clear image of structures close to the bones of the skull. Scherfler & colleagues (2006) reported increased diffusivity of the olfactory tract in PD using diffusion-weighted MRI and showed it was possible to differentiate PD subjects from controls by this procedure. Reliable imaging of the olfactory bulb has been achieved to some extent using 3.0-Tesla MRI "constructive interference in the steady state sequence" (CISS). This technique has produced acceptable images of the olfactory bulbs, as

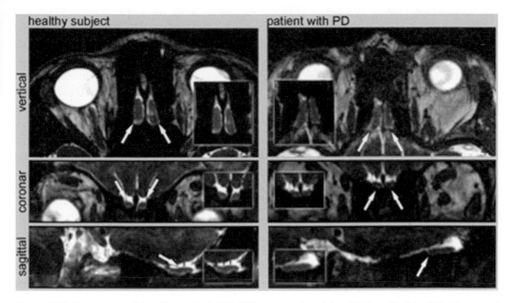

Figure 7.10 Visualization of the olfactory bulb (OB). CISS sequence (voxel size: 0.064 mm3) of the OB (white arrows) of a healthy control subject (left) and a PD patient. Manually traced OB after segmentation are highlighted in red. Although comparable slices are selected, the OB volumes of the 2 individuals do not exhibit a major visible discrepancy, although the OB height in the coronal slice is moderately decreased in the PD patient. Reproduced with permission from Brodoehl, Klingner et al. (2012). (A black and white version of this figure will appear in some formats. For the color version, please refer to colour plate section, Figure 3.28)

shown in Figure 7. 10. Olfactory bulb volume was measured more recently in another study of 41 PD subjects (Altinayar et al., 2014). It was found that olfactory bulb volume (OBV) was similar to controls in those with tremor-dominant disease but there was a reduction of OBV in those without tremor. A more recent MRI evaluation of OBV sampled 52 patients with idiopathic PD and found no significant volume reduction (Paschen et al., 2015). These conflicting findings probably reflect difficulties in examining such a small structure (approximately 42 mm^3). More sophisticated imaging sequences in the future should clarify this issue and determine whether OBV changes have potential diagnostic value.

Summary. Data from pathological, psychophysical, and neurophysiological investigations suggest that smell impairment is a frequent (at least 80 percent) early sign of PD that is independent of cognitive function. Thus, olfactory test information may be used to identify apparently healthy people who are at risk of future disease. Moreover, such investigations may permit early neuroprotective therapy if this becomes available.

Familial and Prodromal Parkinson's Disease

Olfaction and Familial Parkinson's Disease

Preliminary data about smell dysfunction in families with known monogenetic disorder are available, but most observations are based on small numbers and must be regarded as provisional (see Table 7.2). On top of this, the nomenclature has become unwieldy. Some have a "PARK" number and at present range from 1–17. PARK 1 and 4 are thought to be the same condition and although PARK 3, 5, and 16 have been allocated numbers, the original claims for a mutation have not been confirmed. Other familial disorders such as Lubag and the Gaucher-associated mutation are known as such and do not have a PARK number – but that may change. The whole nomenclature of these conditions is in dire need of revamping, but given the wide variety of clinical presentations and numerous mutations a simple classification will be challenging.

In the pioneering Michigan study of familial Parkinsonism (Markopoulou et al., 1997), the UPSIT was administered to six kindreds with various types of parkinsonism. The typical PD families were subsequently found to have the PARK 1, 3, and 8 mutations (Hentschel et al., 2005), although the claim for PARK 3 association has not been confirmed. A single case of PARK 1 was anosmic. There were seven cases of genetically confirmed pallidopon-tonigral degeneration in the atypical group and their UPSIT score indicated anosmia. Four cases with the PARK 8 mutation scored an average of 29.7 on the UPSIT, which appeared lower than those at risk, whose mean score was in the normal range at 34. There was no obvious relationship between olfaction and parkinsonian phenotype.

Genome-wide association studies have since shed further light on the genetic basis for many varieties of familial parkinsonism. The major varieties are detailed below and summarized in Table 7.2 and 7.3. Pathologic studies are few but they are important as those with Lewy body pathology are likely to be more similar to the classic form of PD.

PARK 1 and PARK 4. These two autosomal dominant conditions are now known to be identical and due to either various point mutations in the gene coding for alpha-synuclein (SNCA), of which the commonest is A53T with either duplication or triplication of the normal SNCA gene. The disorder, described initially in Italian families, presents typically in the fourth and fifth decades, although a late onset form is recognized (Krüger et al., 2000). Clinically the disorder may be hard to distinguish from sporadic PD but many have dementia at an early stage, particularly those with SNCA triplication. In a study of Greek kindreds bearing the G209A mutation, two of seven patients from separate families were found to be anosmic using the UPSIT (Bostantjopoulou et al., 2001). This was confirmed by a study of Japanese families with SNCA gene duplication (Nishioka et al., 2009). Using Sniffin' Sticks, it was noted that all six symptomatic patients were abnormal but non-manifesting carriers had normal olfaction. A single case report from Spain (Tijero et al., 2010) concerned an asymptomatic carrier of the rarer E46 K substitution in the α-synuclein gene and found no evidence of smell loss. Finally, there are two cases from Germany with the SNCA mutation (no further details available) whose mean scores on UPSIT were 17, which is in the anosmic range (Kertelge et al., 2010). In summary, the limited data available suggest that the olfactory defect is severe in subjects with the SNCA mutation.

PARK 2 (Parkin Disease). This is the most common autosomal recessive form of juvenile-onset parkinsonism. It was described first in Japanese families, but it is now well recognized in young onset European and North American populations. It is caused by a mutation of the Parkin gene located on the long arm of chromosome 6. Parkin is involved in proteasome-dependent breakdown of proteins and degradation of damaged mitochondria ("mito-phagy"). Most subjects are under the age of 40 years and progression is slower than classic disease. Dystonia is common but the response to levodopa is good. The sense of smell was

Table 7.3. Further familial disorders with features of parkinsonism that do not have a PARK number.

Disorder	Gene & common mutations.	Inheritance & locus	Age onset	Function or effect of mutation	LB	Olfactory deficit	Comment
X-linked recessive dystonia-parkinsonism	TATA-binding protein-associated factor-1 (TAF1)	XLR Xq13	~40y	Impaired expression of TAF1 in striatum	0	++	"Lubag." Also known as DYT3. Mainly males from Panay, Philippines. Patients have dystonia and levodopa responsive parkinsonism.
Gaucher Disease	Gluco cerebro sidase (GBA). N370S, L444P, & c.84dupG	AR 1q21	42–77y	Accumulation of glucocere brosidase in Lewy bodies	+++	++++	Classic PD. Mild-severe olfactory loss in manifesting carriers. McNeil (2012). Equivocal results for non-manifesting carriers.
POLG1	DNA polymerase gamma. POLG 1	AR? 15q25	Early adult	Mitochondrial disorder	?	++	Mitochondrial disorder. Have progressive external ophthalmoplegia. One unpublished case was microsmic.

Table 7.3. (cont.)

Disorder	Gene & common mutations.	Inheritance & locus	Age onset	Function or effect of mutation	LB	Olfactory deficit	Comment
Spinocerebellar ataxia type 2 (SCA2)	CAG expansion in ATXN2 gene	AD	30–40y	Unclear.	+	++	Smell identification tests show mild to moderate abnormalities
Spinocerebellar ataxia type 3 (SCA3). Machado Joseph disease	CAG expansion in ATXN3 gene	AD	30–40y	Codes for Ataxin-3. Involved in ubiquitin-proteasome system	-?	+?	Olfactory tests are normal or mildly affected. One autopsy report.
Waisman syndrome	RAB39B	XLR Xq28	Early adult	Vesicular trafficking	++	?	Early onset parkinsonism with intellectual disability. Affects Wisconsin and Australian families. Alpha synuclein pathology and Lewy bodies present

Key: AD = autosomal dominant. AR = autosomal recessive. XLR = X-linked recessive. SCA= spinocerebellar ataxia relatively preserved (mean UPSIT score 27.3) on a culturally modified UPSIT in 17 subjects (Khan et al., 2004), an observation that concurs with the scarcity of Lewy bodies in this condition. A similar normal finding for smell identification was documented in a Dutch study of five patients with PARK 2 (Verbaan et al., 2008). In keeping with these observations in humans, Parkin knockout mice displayed no defect in tests of olfactory discrimination, cookie-finding, or electro-olfactogram recordings (Kurtenbach et al., 2013; Rial et al., 2014). Conversely, olfaction was significantly reduced in Parkin heterozygotes with parkinsonism but, oddly enough, not in compound heterozygotes (Alcalay et al., 2011). Slight reduction of UPSIT score was seen in a study of 14 manifesting and non-manifesting carriers (Kertelge et al., 2010). These partially contradictory findings may relate to the type of mutation and ethnic variables, but emphasize the need for larger, more definitive studies. Interestingly, subjects with Parkin disease have susceptibility to glioblastoma, lung cancer, and possibly leprosy (Veeriah et al., 2010; Bakija-Konsuo et al., 2011).

PARK 3 and PARK 5. The proposed loci have not been confirmed to have an association with parkinsonism.

PARK 6. This is an autosomal recessive form of parkinsonism caused by mutations in the mitochondrial phosphatase and tensin homolog (PTEN)-induced kinase 1 (PINK1) located on the short arm of chromosome 1. PINK1 is concerned with limiting oxidative stress, i.e., neuroprotection and regulation of mitochondrial turnover. Typically, the condition is early-onset, slowly progressive, and levodopa responsive. It is rare and the only post-mortem study showed Lewy bodies in the brain stem, but sparing the locus coeruleus (Samaranch et al., 2010) – the nucleus that is invariably damaged in sporadic PD. In PINK1 mutant drosophila there was evidence of olfactory impairment according to electro-antennogram recordings (Poddighe et al., 2013). PINK1 knockout mice were found to have abnormalities of gait and olfaction (Glasl et al., 2012). This change was supported by abnormalities in the glomerular layer of the olfactory bulb with reduction of serotonergic neuronal density. In humans, an Italian group investigated olfaction by Sniffin' Sticks in PARK 6 (Ferraris et al., 2009). They found quite significant impairment of identification and discrimination in their 19 cases and mild defects in some asymptomatic heterozygotes, suggesting they could be in a prodromal phase of disease. Similar findings were documented in 17 subjects who were manifesting or non-manifesting carriers of the PINK1 mutation (Kertelge et al., 2010). In a German family, Eggers and colleagues found mild to moderate hyposmia using the UPSIT in 7/10 heterozygotes and mild to severe hyposmia in all four homozygotes (Eggers et al., 2010). Once more findings vary between centers, but it can be concluded that there is a significant defect of olfaction in carriers of the PINK1 mutation.

PARK 7. This autosomal recessive form was described first in Dutch families and related to one of several mutations in DJ-1, a gene located on the short arm of chromosome 1. The properties of DJ1 are not yet clear, but it is probably concerned with mitochondrial function and resistance to oxidative stress as in PARK 6. The parkinsonism is characterized by young onset and slow progression similar to the first descriptions of PARK 2 in Japan. In a study that included one DJ-1 mutation carrier, olfaction was normal (Verbaan et al., 2008). There are no reported pathologic studies as yet.

PARK 8. This is an autosomal dominant condition caused by a heterozygous mutation on the long arm of chromosome 12 in Leucine-Rich Repeat Kinase 2 (LRRK2), a gene that codes for the protein dardarin, which is a Basque word for "tremor." Dardarin is concerned with manufacture of leucine but the role of the mutation in PARK 8 is not understood fully. PARK 8 is one of the most prevalent causes of familial PD, accounting for 2 to 5 percent of all PD in Europe with a higher level in Spain, Portugal, North Africa, and Ashkenazi Jews (Ferreira et al., 2007). Penetrance of the commonest LRRK2 mutation (G2019S) is incomplete and age dependent (Lesage et al., 2007). Clinically the disorder gives rise to late onset benign tremor and may be indistinguishable from sporadic PD; dementia is not an early feature. Limited pathologic studies show Lewy and tau pathology in olfactory pathways at all levels (Silveira-Moriyama et al., 2009). Olfaction in PARK 8 families with the G2019S mutation was assessed by UPSIT in 5 patients from London and 16 from Lisbon (Ferreira et al., 2007; Silveira-Moriyama et al., 2008). There was severe impairment in the London and Lisbon populations; both sets of UPSIT scores and clinical phenotypes were indistinguishable from their classic PD subjects. Unaffected relatives at 50 percent risk of PARK 8 could not be identified reliably by smell testing. In a preliminary study from three centers in Brazil, Silveira-Moriyama and co-workers found impaired olfaction on Sniffin' Sticks in 22 LRRK2 patients carrying the G2019S mutation but it was less severe than patients with classic PD (Silveira-Moriyama et al., 2010). Moderate impairment of UPSIT score in 7 subjects was found in four manifesting carriers in a study from Germany and some non-manifesting carriers (Kertelge et al., 2010). Less clear-cut results were documented in a large French pedigree that carried the G2019S mutation (Lohmann et al., 2009). Three of 5 affected carriers of this mutation, 10/12 non-affected carriers, and 8/8 non-carriers had varying degrees of olfactory impairment on the UPSIT. These changes did not allow clear distinction of gene-carriers from those without the mutation, but this apparent anomaly, as the authors point out, may be explained by the presence of depression or cognitive change in affected and unaffected family members. In a study from New York, the UPSIT scores of 31 LRRK2 manifesting and non-manifesting carriers were slightly better than those of sporadic PD patients, but worse than controls and a sub-set of non-manifesting LRRK2 carriers (Saunders-Pullman et al., 2011).

These findings were confirmed in their larger study of 126 G2019S mutation carriers (Saunders-Pullman et al., 2014). Non-manifesting carriers did not show significant olfactory deficit, a finding that led the authors to suggest that microsmia is not predictive of LRRK2-related parkinsonism. In their latest, largest sample (134 LRRK2 mutation carriers and 119 noncarriers), Mirelman et al. (2015) found that non-motor symptoms such as constipation, urinary urgency, and sleep disorders were more frequently reported in carriers, but olfaction, as measured by UPSIT, did not significantly differ between carriers and non-carriers.

Another investigation from Spain examined olfaction by the UPSIT in (1) 29 subjects with parkinsonism due to the G2019S mutation, (2) 49 asymptomatic mutation carriers, (3) 47 non-carrier relatives, (4) 50 with idiopathic PD, and (5) 50 community-based controls (Sierra et al., 2013). Their findings are summarized in Figure 7.11. In the G2019S manifesting carrier group, 50% were hyposmic compared to 82% in the IPD group and there was no significant difference between these two. Hyposmia was less frequent in the asymptomatic carrier group (26%) and asymptomatic non-carriers (28%). Although the groups were matched on age and gender, the cut off point for UPSIT was derived from published American norms. Also, the Mini-Mental State Examination Score cut-off point was rather low at >25/30. If these limitations are ignored, their study implies that olfactory disorder is

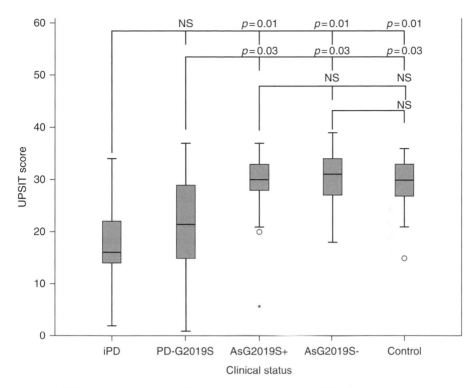

Figure 7.11 UPSIT score according to the clinical and mutational status. AsG2019S– = asymptomatic non-carriers; AsG2019S+ = asymptomatic G2019S mutation carriers; Control = unrelated healthy controls; iPD = idiopathic Parkinson disease. NS = statistically non-significant (p > 0.05); PD-G2019S = patients with Parkinson disease with the G2019S mutation; p values adjusted by age. Reproduced with permission from Sierra, Sanchez-Juan et al. (2013).

not found in asymptomatic carriers of the G2019S mutation. It seems odd that so many relatives (28%) had microsmia.

A different pattern was noted in a Norwegian study where the B-SIT was administered to 47 *non-symptomatic* family members of LRRK2 PD patients, of whom 32 were positive and 15 negative for either the G2019S or the N1437H mutation (Johansen et al., 2011) Unlike measures of urinary and sleep dysfunction, B-SIT scores were normal in both groups and did not differ significantly from one another. This unexpected finding may relate to the reduced sensitivity of B-SIT, which employs only 12 odors.

In summary, patients with parkinsonism due to LRRK2 mutations have an impaired sense of smell, but the severity is less than that seen in idiopathic PD (IPD). Non-manifesting carriers appear to have no olfactory impairment, but before it is concluded that hyposmia is not a premotor feature, much larger populations should be examined.

PARK 9 (Kufor-Rakeb syndrome). This is a rare autosomal recessive degenerative disorder due to a mutation in the short arm of chromosome 1 for the ATP13A2 gene that encodes a lysosomal type 5 ATPase described first in Jordan (Najim Al-Din, 1994). The condition affects the substantia nigra, striatum, pallidum, and pyramidal tracts, and is sometimes associated with iron deposits in these zones, thus creating an overlap with iron overload syndromes such as NBIA (Neurodegeneration with Brain Iron Accumulation). Onset is in teenage years with clinical features of levodopa responsive parkinsonism, spasticity, supranuclear upgaze paresis, and dementia. One study from Germany assessed olfaction in PARK 9 and found marked impairment in four subjects who were manifesting carriers (Kertelge et al., 2010). There are isolated reports of olfactory impairment from China and Pakistan (Park et al., 2015). Of indirect relevance is an exploratory study that examined 25 patients with NBIA resulting from aceruloplasminemia, PKAN, and ferritinopathy (Dziewulska et al., 2013). The pooled median UPSIT score (30/40) was slightly but significantly depressed compared to controls and there was iron deposition in the olfactory bulb and tract in two cases that came to autopsy. Those with PKAN had the most severe olfactory deficit.

PARK 10–13. The status of these four newly claimed mutations has not been confirmed.

PARK 14. This autosomal recessive disorder, sometimes known as Karak syndrome, is due to a homozygous mutation in the PLA2G6 gene located on the long arm of chromosome 22. This is usually an adult onset form of dystonia-parkinsonism. Cortical Lewy bodies and tau pathology have been noted in four autopsies (Paisan-Ruiz et al., 2010), but there were no specific studies of the olfactory bulb. Involvement of the hippocampus and entorhinal cortex was noted in some instances, an observation suggesting that olfaction should be affected clinically.

PARK 15. This autosomal recessive disorder is due to a mutation in the gene coding for FBOX7 located on the long arm of chromosome 22. It is another ubiquitin protein ligase that affects children who develop spastic weakness and later on, parkinsonism. Autopsy and olfactory data are awaited.

PARK 17. This is an autosomal dominant adult onset form of mainly tremulous parkinsonism that may be indistinguishable from classic disease. It relates to a mutation in the VPS35 gene located on chromosome 16q. There is a single report of severe olfactory impairment (10th percentile on UPSIT) in a German male with tremor-dominant levodopa responsive PARK17 that commenced at the age of 45 (Kumar et al., 2012). A limited autopsy from another family showed no abnormal alpha-synuclein immunostaining and no Lewy bodies which would make it a pathologically distinct form of parkinsonism, if this study is representative (Wider et al., 2008).

Apart from the above list of PARK-numbered conditions, there are several inherited parkinsonian syndromes that do not have a number for unclear reasons. These include Gaucher-variant Parkinsonism and POLG1, to be described below. X-linked recessive dystonia-parkinsonism (Lubag) has prominent dystonia and is described below under the Dystonia section.

Gaucher-Variant Parkinsonism. Mutations in the gene encoding the lysosomal enzyme glucocerebrosidase (GBA) result in Gaucher's disease (GD), a disorder predominantly of childhood that affects the skeletal, hematologic, and nervous systems with varying severity. Several years ago Neudorfer et al. (1996) found that a late presenting form of Gaucher's disease was associated with parkinsonism. However, the significance of this relationship was not fully appreciated until some 15 years later when several families were identified with parkinsonism, mostly of Ashkenazi Jewish origin. Presentation is similar to sporadic PD with asymmetric rest tremor, bradykinesia, and gait disturbance, but age of onset is younger (around 50 years), there are frequent hallucinations, and cognitive decline is evident. A large prevalence study of mainly French inhabitants (Lesage et al., 2011) estimated that 6.7 percent of apparently sporadic PD cases carried GBA mutations, a frequency that slightly exceeds the European rate for PARK 8. In one detailed pathological study (Neumann et al., 2009), examination of 17 genetically proven cases revealed widespread and abundant alpha-synuclein pathology graded at Braak stage 5–6. There was also limbic or diffuse neocortical Lewy body-type pathology. Non-motor aspects of classic PD are documented including microsmia (Goker-Alpan et al., 2008). The latter authors tested six patients, of whom three were anosmic, two severely microsmic, and one moderately microsmic with an UPSIT mean score similar to sporadic PD. Observations in 10 further cases revealed severe olfactory impairment on the UPSIT (Saunders-Pullman et al., 2010; Alcalay et al., 2011). A preliminary study, currently available only in abstract form, examined 42 first-degree relatives of GBA "severe" mutation carriers who had no extrapyramidal signs and documented mildly impaired olfaction again using the UPSIT (Rosenberg et al., 2011).

McNeill and colleagues studied 30 patients with Gaucher parkinsonism, their heterozygous GBA mutation carriers, and 30 mutation negative controls matched for age, gender, and race (McNeill et al., 2012). It was found that olfactory scores on the UPSIT were significantly lower in the Gaucher patients and heterozygous carriers. In a subsequent paper it was shown that odor identification scores declined slightly from baseline over a two-year period with respective UPSIT means = 31.85 vs. 30.71 (Beavan et al., 2015). It is not clear from either paper whether any carriers free of clinical evidence of parkinsonism, as measured by the Unified Parkinson's Disease Rating Scale (UPDRS), had abnormal UPSIT or whether any carrier with normal olfaction had an abnormal UPDRS score.

In the PREDICT-PD cohort study, healthy UK adults were screened online by questionnaire, a keyboard tapping test, and the UPSIT to identify the presence of early phenotypic features and risk factors (Noyce et al., 2014). Higher-risk and lower-risk subjects were compared by using various markers for PD and eventual clinical outcome. In their high-risk group (n = 195), there were six people with GBA mutations which was a significant result compared to their low-risk group (Noyce et al., 2015). This is a preliminary study but it suggests that impaired olfaction (among other factors) is relevant to the identification of adult onset Gaucher's disease, i.e., a prodromal feature.

POLG 1. This rare disorder is due to a mutation in the mitochondrial gene, DNA polymerase gamma 1 (POLG1). Onset is earlier than sporadic PD, and comprises typical parkinsonian features overlain with those of mitochondrial disorder such as ptosis, myopathy, and peripheral neuropathy. The authors are aware of just one hitherto unpublished case where olfaction was moderately impaired.

Clearly these observations in genetic disorders might pave the way for predictive testing in at-risk family members. Although patients with PARK 6 and PARK 8, for example, have severe smell dysfunction comparable to that of classic PD, the smell status of their relatives, whether they are symptomatic, asymptomatic, homozygous, heterozygous, or compound heterozygous, is not clear, partly because of small subject numbers, variable stringency of olfactory measurement, and ethnic, cultural, and environmental variables. The initial hope that microsmia would be a robust predictive biomarker in relatives has yet to be realized. It is possible that the prodrome may be a matter of just a few years or that it develops in synchrony with the motor defects, as suggested in Huntington's disease (Paulsen et al., 2008). It might be questioned why so much effort has gone into prodromal biomarkers such as olfaction when there are readily available, highly specific genetic tests, albeit costly. The answer is that for classic PD there is no specific genetic marker and the onset time of olfactory impairment (or other biomarkers) may be the stage of disease expression and the point at which protective therapy, once available, should be initiated. This desirable goal is crucially related to the time that smell impairment really begins.

Another approach to assessing familial PD has been to administer tests of motor function, olfaction, and mood to first-degree relatives of PD patients (Montgomery et al., 1999, 2000). Using this procedure, significant differences were found in sons and daughters, in particular where the affected parent was the father. Ponsen et al. (2004) evaluated olfactory function and dopamine striatal transporter activity (DATScan) in a prospective study of 78 asymptomatic first-degree relatives of non-familial PD patients. Forty relatives were hyposmic at baseline. When evaluated two years later, four had abnormal DATScans and displayed clinical evidence of PD. In the remaining 36 individuals with hyposmia who displayed no sign of PD, the rate of decline of dopamine transporter binding was higher than in normosmic relatives. Sommer & colleagues (2004) tested 30 patients with unexplained smell impairment to determine whether any might be in the premotor phase of PD. Apart from detailed olfactory testing, subjects were evaluated by DATScan and transcranial sonography (TCS) of the substantia nigra. Eleven displayed increased (pathologic) echogenicity on TCS, five were abnormal on DATScan, and two were borderline, suggesting they might be in a presymptomatic phase of Parkinsonism. At follow-up four years later two had developed PD (Haehner et al., 2007). In one large study of olfaction and sleep, nearly all of 30 patients with rapid eye movement (REM) sleep behavioral disorder (RBD) had significantly increased olfactory thresholds and there was evidence of Parkinsonism in eight, implying that olfaction and RBD are early features of PD (Stiasny-Kolster et al., 2005). Similar findings were documented by Iranzo et al. (2006). In keeping with many sleep studies, no pathological confirmation was available, and where such confirmation was done (e.g., Boeve et al., 2003), the changes in RBD were more in keeping with parkinsonism than classic PD. Interestingly, acute sleep deprivation per se has a specific but mild adverse influence on the ability to identify odors – an influence that cannot be explained on the basis of task difficulty (Killgore & McBride, 2006). As yet, it is not clear whether this phenomenon compromises the RBD findings described above.

Olfaction and Presymptomatic Parkinson's Disease

In the first long-term prospective community-based olfactory study of the development of PD, smell function was tested with the 12-item B-SIT in 2,263 healthy Japanese-American males aged 71–95 years who participated in the Honolulu Asia Aging Study (Ross et al., 2004; Ross et al., 2006; Ross et al., 2008; Ross et al., 2012). After 7 years' follow-up, 19 individuals developed PD at an average latency of 2.7 years from baseline assessment. Adjustment for multiple confounders gave relative odds for PD in the lowest B-SIT score tertile of 4.3 (95 percent confidence interval 1.1–16.1; $p = 0.02$) compared with those in the highest tertile, thus indicating the moderately strong predictive power of olfactory testing. In the same cohort, those who later died underwent autopsy of the brainstem exploring for Lewy bodies in the substantia nigra and locus coeruleus (Ross et al., 2006). Of 163 autopsied men *without* clinical PD or dementia, there were 17 with incidental Lewy bodies. Those who scored in the lowest tertile of the B-SIT were significantly more likely to have Lewy body changes at autopsy. Impaired olfaction, constipation, slow reaction time, excessive daytime sleepiness, and impaired executive function were all associated with future development of PD and/or with increased likelihood of incidental Lewy bodies or neuronal loss in the substantia nigra or locus coeruleus. Compared to persons without any proposed risk factors, those with combinations of two or more pre-motor features had up to a 10-fold increase in risk for development of PD (Ross et al., 2012).

At present there are several prospective studies that are examining the predictive value of microsmia, RBD, MIBG, transcranial ultrasound of the substantia nigra, dopamine transporter scans, etc. The largest is PARS (Parkinson At-Risk Syndrome Study) (Siderowf et al., 2012) which has a longitudinal database of 4,999 subjects with no neurologic disease at baseline. Of these, 669 were at or below the 15th percentile based on age and gender, indicating marked impairment of olfactory identification. Hyposmics were significantly more likely to report other features such as anxiety and depression, constipation, RBD, or change in motor function, implying that they were in the early stages of PD. In the PREDICT-PD cohort (see above) 1,323 healthy UK adults were screened online by questionnaire (notably for family history, non-motor symptoms, and lifestyle factors), a keyboard tapping test, and the UPSIT to identify early risk factors (Noyce et al., 2014). PD was diagnosed in seven individuals during follow-up and this was significantly associated with baseline risk score (Noyce et., al 2017).

Findings that potentially diverge from the above studies were reported by Marras et al. (2005) in a study of 62 male twin pairs discordant for PD. At baseline, these authors found impaired UPSIT scores in the affected twins, but not in their brothers who were rated normal by clinical examination. After a mean of 7.3 years, 28 brothers were still alive and, of these, 19 were retested using the B-SIT. Two of the 28 brothers had developed PD. Neither of the two had impaired UPSIT scores at baseline, but the average decline in their UPSIT scores was greater than that of the remaining 17 brothers who had not developed the disease. Although it was suggested that smell testing may not be a reliable predictor of PD, the dropout rate was unusually high and smell function was reassessed by two different methods: initially the UPSIT, which is a 40-odor sensitive research tool, followed by the B-SIT, which uses 12 odors and is more appropriate for rapid screening.

Pre-Symptomatic Period. If we assume that the staging of PD by Braak et al. (2003a) is correct, and that there is a prodromal phase, then the duration of this pre-symptomatic period can be estimated. Approximations based on patients' reports of olfactory loss are not reliable, as most individuals will report such abnormality only if they are anosmic – as in just 40 percent of patients (see above). The remaining microsmic patients may be unaware of any deficit. Therefore, more reliance must be placed on prospective measurement derived from outwardly healthy people.

Applying cross-sectional modeling of UPSIT scores in 266 patients with PD (Hawkes, 2008b), two models were proposed that addressed the problem of pre-symptomatic disease. In the first, back-projection of the UPSIT regression lines on age implied disease onset around the time of birth, and likely genetically determined. In the second version, an abrupt event was proposed, which inferred an acute environmental exposure (Figure 7.8).

The latent period for development of PD from the onset of a smell problem according to the study by Ponsen et al. (2004) was about two years; in the clinically and pathologically based study by Ross et al. (2008), the mean latency was 4.0 years, although the range was wide (1.9–8 years). The latter study was based on 35 cases of PD in 2,267 subjects and the onset of smell impairment in those who subsequently developed PD clearly would be *prior to the date of baseline testing*, so this estimate would represent a minimum prodromal period. In a follow-up study of 30 subjects with idiopathic anosmia, two developed PD after a four-year interval (Haehner et al., 2007). Personal observations (CHH) from patients who have been aware of their smell loss suggest that many have a much longer latent period – in some cases over 30 years. A major question is whether the olfactory deficit represents an epiphenomenon that is just easy to measure, or whether it reflects some underlying predilection of the basic pathological process for olfactory neurons. Is there, for example, some underlying shared neurotransmitter or metabolic process in olfactory and vagal neurons? Both structures utilize dopamine, but this transmitter is widely distributed throughout the nervous system. According to Braak et al. (2003b), the selective pathological change may be explained by preferential damage to fibers with long, thin, incompletely myelinated axons. Nevertheless, it has yet to be shown beyond reasonable doubt whether olfactory dysfunction *precedes* or *develops synchronously* with changes in the nigra-striatal system – the "multicentric" theory vs. the "sequential spread" theory.

Issues yet to be resolved are why some patients with apparently typical PD have normal olfaction. According to one review of PD (Ondo & Lai, 2005), olfaction was more likely to be better if there was a family history of tremor. Another group who reported on 208 drug-naïve PD patients found that normosmic subjects were younger, had fewer motor deficits, and required less levodopa medication (Lee et al., 2015).

Also to be resolved is why patients at risk of PD who display smell impairment do not develop the disease. These problems are discussed in more detail in the Olfactory Vector Hypothesis section later in this chapter.

Case Report 7.4. Akinetic-Rigid Classic PD with Prominent Pre-motor Features. A 63-year-old retired gentleman presented on account of slowed limb movements but no tremor. His wife mentioned that on their honeymoon 35 years ago he punched her in the face during his sleep when he appeared to be acting out a dream. Ten years before presentation he had noted impaired sense of smell and nocturia. For around five years he had become constipated, was drowsy in the afternoons, and became intermittently depressed. One year before attending hospital his mobility had declined slightly, balance was less secure, and he was unable to swim. Examination showed he was mentally alert with a normal Mini-Mental State Examination score. The UPSIT score was 19/40, which is in the severe microsmic range for a male age 63 years. There was moderate impairment of arm swing on walking and asymmetric cogwheeling in both arms more on the right side. Balance tests were normal and he was placed in Hoehn and Yahr stage 2/5. *Comment.* The diagnosis was asymmetric akinetic-rigid classic PD with multiple prodromal (pre-motor) features. Acting out a dream suggests REM sleep behavior disorder (RBD), a frequent non-motor precursor of parkinsonism, although not necessarily of the classic variety. Many other symptoms above (excess daytime somnolence, depression, constipation) are suspected precursor features of PD. He became aware of olfactory problems 10 years before visiting his primary care physician but it is likely the defect was there several years before then, to a milder degree.

Non-motor Correlations

Olfactory test scores are associated with other deficits in the established phase of PD, including REM sleep behavior disorder (RBD), reduced color vision in sporadic and monogenic forms (Kertelge et al., 2010), constipation, and altered UPDRS scores

(Stiasny-Kolster et al., 2005; Postuma & Montplaisir, 2010; Postuma et al., 2011). Associations are also present between hyposmia and measures of transcranial ultrasound of the substantia nigra, MIBG heart scans, olfactory bulb size, and dopamine transporter imaging (Lee et al., 2007; Deeb et al., 2010; Iijima et al., 2010; Postuma et al., 2010; Postuma & Montplaisir, 2010). In the prodromal period, RBD, abnormal dopamine transporter imaging, and incidental brain stem Lewy bodies (Ross et al., 2004) all appear in conjunction with olfactory dysfunction (Ross et al., 2006; Hawkes, 2008b; Jennings et al., 2014).

Parkinsonism

Parkinsonism ("Parkinson plus" syndromes) refers to those diseases that resemble typical Parkinson's disease but differ on pathological, clinical, or genetic grounds. Among such disorders are Lewy body disease, multiple system atrophy, progressive supranuclear palsy, corticobasal syndrome, drug-induced PD, the PD–dementia complex of Guam, X-linked dystonia–parkinsonism ("Lubag"), vascular parkinsonism, and pure autonomic failure. Olfactory data in this group have been obtained by psychophysical measurement. Since pathological verification has rarely been made, and the number of patients studied has been small, most observations should be regarded as provisional. These diseases are described separately below.

Lewy Body Disease (LBD)

Incidental Lewy bodies (ILB). Many who die from non-neurologic diseases are found to have ILB, the suspected pathologic precursor of classic PD (Ross et al., 2006; Markesbery et al., 2009). It is proposed that the presence of ILB may be inferred from olfactory testing. Thus, in a prospective study from Chicago (Wilson et al., 2011), 201 people were tested by the B-SIT at baseline and their scores compared to the distribution of Lewy pathology at autopsy. There were 26 subjects with Lewy bodies that were either neocortical, limbic, or nigral. Impaired olfaction was associated with ILB in neocortical and limbic areas after adjustment for age, gender, education, and time to death. It was proposed that ILB may be responsible for the late life decline in olfactory function in outwardly healthy individuals. Similar findings were obtained in a smaller pathologically verified study from Arizona (Driver-Dunckley et al., 2014).

Dementia Associated with Parkinson Disease. Classic Parkinson disease is associated with widespread deposition of Lewy bodies; thus, PD may be considered the major form of Lewy body disease. It is well recognized that many patients with typical PD develop dementia after 10 or more years – a process that may reflect spread of pathology into the cerebral hemispheres, as defined by Braak stages 4–6. There are several subtypes of Lewy body disease that show variable degrees of dementia which develop before, synchronously with parkinsonism, or at varying intervals thereafter. If dementia comes on before, at the same time, or at the latest within one year of the motor symptom onset then it is called dementia with Lewy bodies (DLB; McKeith, 2006). If dementia develops more than a year after well-established PD, it is called Parkinson disease dementia (PDD). Pathologically, many consider that dementia with Lewy bodies, Parkinson disease dementia, and classic PD are indistinguishable (Ballard et al., 2006; Galvin et al., 2006). In the clinical setting it may also be difficult to distinguish PDD from DLB; hence the generic term "Lewy body disease" is often used. Many alternative names have been adopted, leading to further confusion. Thus, dementia with

Lewy bodies has been termed "diffuse Lewy body disease," "Lewy body dementia," "Lewy body variant of AD," "senile dementia of Lewy body type," and "dementia associated with cortical Lewy bodies" (Geser et al., 2005). The sole histological study of olfactory bulbs from patients with DLB (Tsuboi et al., 2003) found 9 of 10 cases with tau pathology, Lewy bodies, and a-synuclein deposits, suggesting it would be difficult to distinguish from PD on pathological grounds alone. In a study of clinically defined DLB, but without pathological verification, severe impairment of olfactory identification and detection was observed, and test scores were independent of disease stage and duration (Liberini et al., 2000). In another investigation, McShane et al. (2001) examined simple smell perception to one uncalibrated odor (lavender water) in 92 patients with autopsy-confirmed dementia, of whom 22 had DLB and 43 had only AD pathology. They were compared with 94 age-matched controls. The main finding was impaired smell perception in the DLB group, but little or no defect in patients with AD. In their subsequent investigation of mild forms of DLB and AD using Sniffin' Sticks, more pronounced olfactory impairment was found in the DLB group compared to the AD and mild cognitive impairment groups (Williams et al., 2009). Their studies afford pathological confirmation for the clinically based conclusion of Liberini et al. (2000) that impairment of smell is significant in DLB, given that we are dealing with a disorder separate from PD. In a study of what was termed "Lewy body variant" (equivalent to DLB) with autopsy confirmation, smell dysfunction was common and its presence was thought useful to improve the sensitivity for detecting Lewy body variant, but it did not improve discrimination between AD and Lewy body variant because of false positives (Olichney et al., 2005). The overall picture awaits considerable clarification, but a "best-guess" is given earlier in Table 7.1.

Case Report 7.5: Dementia with Lewy Bodies? An 82-year-old woman complained of loss of taste and smell function for the previous five years. She recalled no upper respiratory infection or other specific incident associated at the outset of the symptoms. About two years after the onset of the smell loss, she was diagnosed with PD. Olfactory testing revealed anosmia with an UPSIT score of 9/40 and markedly elevated phenylethyl alcohol odor detection threshold values both bilaterally and unilaterally. Performance on the 12-item Odor Memory Test was at chance level. Nasal cross-sectional area, as measured by acoustic rhinometry, and nasal airway resistance, assessed by anterior rhinometry, were normal. Whole-mouth and regional taste test results were unremarkable, likewise scores on the Beck Depression Inventory (4), the Picture Identification Test (40/40), and the Mini-Mental State Examination (30/30). On follow-up approximately two years later, the patient was admitted to a nursing home with a revised diagnosis of AD. *Comment:* This lady's complaint of taste dysfunction was most likely secondary to loss of smell. The subjective olfactory impairment that occurred approximately two years previously was probably a precursor of the parkinsonian syndrome. In the absence of further details on examination and brain imaging, it is difficult to be certain of the disease label. Assuming the initial diagnosis of "PD" was correct and that this was revised to AD of sufficient severity to warrant nursing home care, a clinical diagnosis of dementia with Lewy bodies would seem likely. As described, these patients present with characteristic features of PD but within one year show cognitive decline typical of AD. In this context, smell testing is of value in separating other parkinsonian syndromes associated with dementia, such as corticobasal syndrome and progressive supranuclear palsy, where in general, the sense of smell is preserved.

Case Report 7.6: Parkinson Disease Dementia. A 66-year-old male former insurance worker had noted that for three years his golf handicap was worsening progressively. Six months previously he became aware of mild symmetrical hand tremor. He reckoned his sense of smell had been poor for 40 years at least, i.e., during his twenties. More recently there was some clumsiness on eating, slowing of walking speed, and reduction of speech volume. Examination showed an expressionless face and quiet monotonous speech. Upgaze was slightly impaired and ocular saccades were jerky. There was marked axial rigidity, failure of arm swing on walking, and mild hand tremor at rest. An MRI brain scan showed multiple small ischemic lesions mostly in the sub-cortical white matter but not in the deep white matter or basal ganglia regions. His UPSIT score was 18 (severe microsmia) and there was significant asymmetric reduction of tracer uptake on DATScan in keeping with a parkinsonian syndrome. This patient responded moderately well to levodopa and his golf handicap improved. However, four years later (which would be after seven years of symptoms), he developed visual hallucinations, further cognitive decline, and levodopa-related involuntary movements. *Comment:* The initial presentation was compatible with classic PD except for the possibility of cognitive decline during the second or third years of illness. The abnormalities on olfactory tests and DATScan would be in keeping with typical PD. Development of hallucinations and cognitive decline within the first year of presentation is characteristic of dementia with Lewy bodies, but in this instance the symptoms occurred later. According to many, dementia with Lewy bodies is pathologically indistinguishable from classic PD (Ballard et al., 2006), suggesting that there is a continuous spectrum from typical PD to dementia with Lewy bodies. Olfactory testing cannot distinguish these varieties since olfaction is probably affected severely in both (see Table 7.1). The most likely clinical diagnosis here is Parkinson disease – dementia which is an Alzheimer-like disorder that develops during the course of PD, typically 10 or more years after its onset.

Multiple System Atrophy (MSA)

There are two major varieties of multiple system atrophy (MSA). A common, predominantly parkinsonian variety (MSA-P, Shy–Drager syndrome), in which akinesia and rigidity predominate. This form comprises 80 percent of the total cases. In the remaining 20 percent, cerebellar ataxia prevails (MSA-C). Both varieties display comparatively rapidly evolving parkinsonism with dysautonomia that affects principally bladder and orthostatic blood pressure control. In just one publication, pathological changes in the MSA olfactory bulb (OB) have been documented and characterized by cytoplasmic inclusions in oligodendrocytes, sometimes called Papp–Lantos filaments (Kovacs et al., 2003). Despite this, there was no impairment on olfactory preference tests in a transgenic mouse model of MSA (Krismer, Wenning et al., 2013). Furthermore, there was no reduction of OB volume in MSA patients on MRI images of the OB or central olfactory areas, such as the piriform cortex, amygdala, and entorhinal cortex (Chen et al., 2014). As expected, there was significant OB volume reduction in the PD group.

Psychophysical tests paint a less confused picture. Nee et al. (1993) and Muller et al. (2002) each found reduced smell function in seven of eight patients (in both publications), although neither distinguished between the parkinsonian and cerebellar varieties. Odor identification in 29 patients with a clinical diagnosis of MSA-P revealed mild impairment of odor identification ability, with a mean UPSIT score of 26.7 compared with the control mean of 33.5 (Wenning et al., 1995). There were no UPSIT differences between the parkinsonian and cerebellar types. Abele et al. (2003) focused particularly on MSA-C in comparison to other ataxias of unknown etiology and found no useful difference in olfactory test scores between the two categories. As shown in Figure 7.12, Goldstein et al. (2008) examined multiple

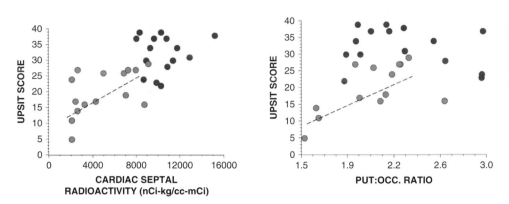

Figure 7.12 University of Pennsylvania Smell Identification Test (UPSIT) results in patients with Parkinson disease (red) or Multiple System Atrophy (blue). Left graph: this shows individual UPSIT scores, expressed as a function of septal myocardial fluorodopamine derived radioactivity. Right graph. This shows individual UPSIT scores, expressed as a function of the putamen: occipital cortex ratio of fluorodopa-derived radioactivity. Dashed lines indicate line of best fit among PD patients. Reproduced with permission from Goldstein, Holmes et al. (2008). (A black and white version of this figure will appear in some formats. For the color version, please refer to the plate section.)

potential biomarkers in an attempt to differentiate clinically-defined PD (77 subjects) from MSA (57 subjects). The PD group had a lower mean UPSIT score (20 ± 2) than did the MSA group (32 ± 2; p = 0.0002) and around half the MSA patients had normal olfaction, something that was not observed in any PD patient. About 50 percent of PD patients had anosmia (defined as a score of 17/40 or less), a finding that was not observed in any MSA patient. Among PD patients, UPSIT scores correlated positively with cardiac fluorodopamine-derived radioactivity and the putamen: occipital ratio of fluorodopa-derived radioactivity. Most PD patients had both an UPSIT score below 30 and diminished cardiac fluorodopamine-derived radioactivity less than 7,500 nCi-kg/cc-mCi, a combination not seen in any MSA patient, and most MSA patients had both an UPSIT score of at least 30 and cardiac 6-fluorodopamine-derived radioactivity more than 7500 nCi-kg/cc-mCi, a combination not seen in any PD patient. Separate olfactory data on the two varieties of MSA (parkinsonian and cerebellar) were not given. There is just one small autopsy-based study that examined the correlation with olfaction in life (Glass et al., 2011). Age- and gender-adjusted UPSIT scores of their four cases lay between the 43rd and 79th percentiles of their healthy UK control population and thought to be within normal limits. The unreliability of the clinical diagnosis of MSA was emphasized, but it is likely some MSA patients have olfactory impairment given the known pathology in the olfactory bulb as mentioned above.

In summary, studies to date suggest that mild to moderate olfactory impairment is present in MSA, but its overall severity is far less than that of PD.

Corticobasal Syndrome (CBS)

The original term, "corticobasal degeneration," has been renamed "corticobasal syndrome" because of the very high rate of diagnostic errors prior to autopsy. In the classic disorder, parkinsonian features are compounded by limb dystonia, ideomotor apraxia, myoclonus, and ultimately, cognitive decline. The condition is classed as a tauopathy because there is accumulation of tau protein typically in the fronto-parietal cortex and basal ganglia. In a large pathological survey of 93 olfactory bulbs there were three cases of CBS (Tsuboi et al.,

2003), but none displayed tau pathology, an observation that was thought to explain the relative preservation of olfaction in some with CBS. In the first survey of seven patients with clinically suspected CBS (Wenning et al., 1995), UPSIT scores were in the low normal range with a mean of 27, a value not significantly different from their age-matched controls. A more recent study comprising seven patients with clinically defined CBS (described in the Dementia section above) showed mild impairment of odor-naming and odor picture-matching in the presence of normal discrimination (Luzzi et al., 2007). However, a more recent and larger study of olfaction in CBS showed significant olfactory involvement (Pardini et al., 2009). They studied 25 patients with CBS and found that only 8 were normal on UPSIT, with a mean percentile score of 31.6 percent. Two patients with autopsy confirmation of CBS were both anosmic.

In conclusion, it cannot be assumed that a normal olfactory assessment is necessarily supportive of CBS. Complete loss of smell would be unexpected, but it now appears that the microsmia of CBS occupies a position intermediate between PD and healthy controls.

Progressive Supranuclear Palsy (PSP)

In progressive supranuclear palsy (PSP), also known as the Steele–Richardson syndrome, there is failure of voluntary vertical gaze, progression of motor dysfunction at a rate more rapid than that seen in PD, marked imbalance, and advancing cognitive decline. The characteristic pathology in PSP is a tauopathy with widespread deposits of tau protein in degenerating neurons, but (like CBS) tau and α-synuclein pathology was absent in the olfactory bulbs of 27 patients studied by Tsuboi et al. (2003). On the basis of a large clinic-pathological study of 103 cases, Williams et al. (2005) proposed a new classification to distinguish two major varieties. The first, which these authors termed the "Richardson syndrome," accounted for 54 percent of their patients and was characterized by early onset of postural instability and falls, supranuclear vertical gaze palsy, and cognitive dysfunction. The second, entitled PSP-P, applied to 32 percent of patients who exhibited asymmetric onset tremor with moderate initial therapeutic response to levodopa. Patients were frequently misdiagnosed as classic PD. The remaining 14 percent of the patients were difficult to classify.

In the first substantial olfactory study on PSP that involved 21 patients and matched control subjects (Doty et al., 1993), no significant difference was observed, either in UPSIT scores or phenylethyl alcohol threshold values, although there was a trend toward higher threshold values. Subjects were included only if they performed well on the Picture Identification Test (PIT). This procedure ensures that subjects are not too demented to understand the sources of odorants to be identified. Similar results were found in 15 cases of PSP that were also tested with the UPSIT (Wenning et al., 1995). In all instances, the diagnosis was clinically, not autopsy, based. A different perspective has been raised by a further study of 36 patients with PSP, six of whom were pathologically confirmed (Silveira-Moriyama et al., 2010). Although some had low UPSIT scores that may have related, in part, to co-existing dementia, others who had normal values on the Mini-Mental State Examination had impairment of UPSIT, but of less severity than classic PD. The relative absence of tau or α-synuclein pathology in the olfactory bulb of these patients gives some support to the clinically based observation of relatively preserved olfactory function. A more complex picture was found in relatives of patients with PSP (Baker & Montgomery, 2001). These workers used the same test battery as in their PD study, i.e., measures of motor function, odor identification, and mood. In 23 first-degree relatives, nine (39 percent) scored in the abnormal range, which is a remarkably high value, raising the possibility that this study may be confounded by self-selection of at-risk relatives, as the familial risk of PSP is nowhere near this magnitude. While there is clearly a need for further pathologically confirmed studies, evidence at present suggests that olfaction is normal or mildly impaired in the commoner, Richardson variant, which is the easier of the two syndromes to diagnose. The existence of the PSP-P variety, which may simulate PD, might explain why some patients with apparent classic PD have normal olfactory function.

A form of PSP accounting for 29 percent of all cases of parkinsonism is found in the Caribbean island of Guadeloupe and its pathology has similarity to the sporadic form of PSP observed elsewhere. At present there are no studies of olfaction in this PSP variant.

Vascular Parkinsonism (VP)

Some patients with cerebrovascular disease involving the basal ganglia, in particular the putamen and striatum, may develop a syndrome that mimics PD, but the response to levodopa is variable. If someone has significant cerebrovascular disease and unilateral parkinsonism develops acutely, then the diagnosis is relatively straightforward. The diagnosis is more difficult when the onset is insidious or stepwise. Although brain MRI may show extensive vascular lesions, it can be tricky to know whether this is coincidental, especially if cerebrovascular disease co-exists. In one study, those with acute onset vascular parkinsonism (VP) had lesions located in the subcortical gray nuclei (striatum, globus pallidus, and thalamus), whereas those with insidious-onset displayed lesions distributed diffusely in borderzone (watershed) areas (Zijlmans et al., 1995). Dopamine transporter imaging in the striatal region is usually normal in VP (Tzen et al., 2001), although it may show a "punched out" appearance reflecting local ischemia. One study of odor identification in 14 patients fulfilling strictly defined clinical criteria for VP showed no significant difference compared with age-matched controls (mean UPSIT score of 25.5 in VP and 27.5 in control subjects), suggesting that identification tests may aid differentiation from idiopathic PD (Katzenschlager et al., 2004). Conversely, a recent study of 15 cases of clinically diagnosed VP (Navarro-Otano et al., 2014) found quite severe impairment of odor identification with a mean score on UPSIT of 18.3 compared to their PD group of 15.3. In fact, the cardiac MIBG scan yielded better differentiation of VP from PD. The value of olfactory testing in VP is not clear chiefly because autopsy data are lacking, but the severity of loss is probably less than classic PD.

Case Report 7.7: Probable Parkinson Disease with a Vascular Component. A 62-year-old housewife found that for one year previously her automatic watch kept stopping. This was an old-fashioned analog watch that was worn on the left wrist. It had been checked over by her jeweler several times, but no fault was discovered. Over the same period it was found that, on swimming, the left lower limb felt peculiar – like a balloon and she had a tendency to swim in circles. The leg was starting to drag when walking. She reported that for 20 years her sense of smell had been poor for no obvious reason. She had mild untreated hypertension with systolic pressures around 180 mm Hg. Examination showed a staring facial expression with a brisk, non-fatiguing glabella tap reflex. There was moderate rigidity of the trunk and neck muscles and limbs, more pronounced on the left side, and no arm swing on walking. The blood pressure was 190/110 mm Hg. Her UPSIT score was 27/40, which was just below the local 95 percent population limit (28/40) for a female of her age. Olfactory event-related potential latency to P2 was 1120ms, which is above the 2 standard deviation (SD) limit for control subjects (937 ms). DATScan imaging was not performed. An MRI brain scan showed multiple small white matter high signal changes in the right supraventricular and subcortical white matter, in keeping with small-vessel disease. The basal ganglia were normal and so were the sinuses. There was a good response to levodopa, confirming the diagnosis of classic PD of the akinetic rigid type. *Comment:* The presentation with recurrent stopping of an automatic watch is well recognized among neurologists and sometimes known as the "Marsden sign" after the late Queen Square neurologist, David Marsden, who contributed so much to the field of movement disorders. This sign reflects the relative immobility of the arm on which the watch is worn. Other limb features are in keeping with this condition, with rigidity in the limbs more marked on the left side. The longstanding hypertension would explain the MRI changes but their distribution is not suggestive of vascular PD. Furthermore, smell function is often normal in vascular PD. A DATScan would have clinched the diagnosis but this is still an expensive investigation, not undertaken routinely. Smell testing showed minor abnormalities in keeping with microsmia. The likely onset of smell impairment 20 years prior to the initial signs of PD is consistent with the concept that smell dysfunction along with vagal motor disorder are among the earliest features of PD.

Drug-Induced PD (DIPD)

This disorder can be clinically indistinguishable from PD and it was common when broad-spectrum dopamine antagonists were used widely for psychotic disorders – e.g., Haloperidol (Serenace), Trifluoperazine (Stelazine), etc. With the advent of selective D2 blockers such as Clozapine (Clozaril), Olanzepine (Zyprexa), Quetiapine (Seroquel), and Risperidone (Risperdal), the prevalence has subsided dramatically. A small initial study of drug-induced PD (DIPD) was undertaken in 10 patients (Hensiek et al., 2000), all of whom scored normally (27/30 or more) on the Mini-Mental State Examination. Parkinsonism had developed in response to a variety of phenothiazine preparations that were administered for at least two weeks. Of the 10 patients, five had an abnormal age-matched UPSIT score and none made a complete recovery from DIPD even when the offending medication was changed or stopped. Of the remaining five who did regain motor function after their treatment was adjusted, all but one had normal smell function. Unfortunately, a number of these patients had a psychotic disorder which may have contributed or even caused their smell problem. Nonetheless, it is possible that some individuals with DIPD are predisposed to develop PD and that exposure to a dopamine-depleting drug unmasks underlying disease and its associated olfactory dysfunction. Thus their clinician, without realizing it, may have been treating a patient with prodromal features of PD. A further study of DIPD using Sniffin' Sticks was undertaken by Krüger et al. (2008). In 15 patients that had received selective or non-selective dopamine-blocking medication for depression (Haloperidol, Flupenthixol, and Risperidone), they found significant impairment of identification and threshold but not discrimination. Depressed patients that received similar medication or those who had not received any neuroleptic and did not develop DIPD had normal olfactory scores confirming that the observed effect on olfaction did not relate to depression itself. Follow-up study of these subjects to determine whether the DIPD was reversible has not been published. Bovi et al. (2010) administered odor identification and detection tests to 16 DIPD patients who had received a variety of non-selective dopamine blocking agents. Seven received Haloperidol, five Amisulpride, two Perphenazine, one Fluphenazine, and one Clomipramine. There were 13 PD patients, and 19 age- and sex-matched normal controls.

The DIPD patients were classified according to their dopamine transporter SPECT imaging as normal (n = 9) or abnormal (n = 7). Only those DIPD patients with a pathologic putamen uptake had abnormal olfactory test scores – values which like those for PD, correlated with putamen uptake values. DIPD patients with *normal* putamen uptake showed odor function similar to controls. These findings suggested that the olfactory loss in DIPD is more closely associated with central dopamine (DA) damage than with drug-induced DA receptor blockade. In contrast are the observations of Lee et al. (2007), who administered the B-SIT to 15 DIPD and 15 matched normal controls. DIPD had been provoked by Levosulpiride, Haloperidol, Flunarizine, Perphenazine, Metoclopramide, or Risperidone. The B-SIT scores of the DIPD patients did not differ from those of their 15 controls and were significantly higher than 24 patients with sporadic PD (6.9 vs. 4.4; p < 0.001). The most recent study examined retrospectively a variety of motor and non-motor features associated with PD that had the potential to predict persistent drug-induced PD (Morley, Pawlowski et al., 2014). Only 13/97 DIPD had undergone smell identification tests by three different methods (pocket smell test, B-SIT, and UPSIT). They found that those with persistent DIP (6/7) were more likely to have severe hyposmia than those with reversible DIPD (1/6). In conclusion, there is no doubt that DA-blocking medication, especially the non-selective variety, may cause parkinsonism. Whether this is explained by an unmasking process or whether the drug causes parkinsonism *de novo* is not clear, but the presence of abnormal olfactory tests in DIPD would favor the onset or unmasking of permanent PD.

In a unique study of parkinsonism induced by methyl-phenyl-tetrahydro-pyridine (MPTP), all six drug addicts exhibited normal values on both the UPSIT and on a phenylethyl alcohol detection threshold test (Doty et al., 1992b). However, there was a trend toward higher threshold values in the exposed group relative to age-matched controls and there is some evidence that MPTP may produce damage to the olfactory system in monkeys. Thus, three common marmosets injected with MPTP had difficulty locating bananas by smell and were not averse to eating bananas odorized with skatole (putrid, fecal) or isovaleric acid (dirty socks, rancid cheese). This was not the case in two controls or prior to MPTP treatment (Miwa et al., 2004). The reason for dissimilarity between humans and monkeys is not clear, but could reflect differences in age, species, or drug concentrations. Rotenone, the pesticide and complex I inhibitor, reproduces features of PD in animals, including selective nigrostriatal dopaminergic degeneration and alpha-synuclein-positive cytoplasmic inclusions (Betarbet et al., 2000; Sherer et al., 2003). Brains from rotenone-treated animals demonstrate oxidative damage, notably in the same midbrain and olfactory bulb dopaminergic regions that are affected by PD (Sherer et al., 2003). There are no reported human cases of rotenone-induced PD, but it is freely available and certainly has the potential to cause a form of parkinsonism.

Guam PD–Dementia Complex (PDC)

The Guam PD–dementia complex (PDC) is largely confined to the Chamorro population that inhabits the Pacific Island of Guam and is typified by coexistence of Alzheimer-type dementia, parkinsonism, and motor neuron disease (amyotrophic lateral sclerosis; ALS), either alone or in combination. The cause of the disorder is still debated, i.e., whether it is mainly environmental or genetic, but the marked decline in prevalence since 1970 favors an environmental toxin such as the plant excitotoxins derived from Cycad nuts, high aluminium, or low calcium and magnesium level in drinking water (Oyanagi, 2005). Pathologically, it is classed as a tauopathy with neurofibrillary tangles and no Lewy bodies, quite distinct from idiopathic PD. Like PD, the number of cells within the AON are significantly decreased (Doty et al., 1991b). Administration of a culturally adjusted UPSIT to 24 patients with PDC revealed severe olfactory dysfunction of magnitude similar to that seen in idiopathic PD, although a few had additional cognitive impairment which could have lowered the scores slightly (Doty et al., 1991a). The latter observations were confirmed subsequently by Ahlskog & colleagues (1998) in Chamorros who suffered any one of the four varieties of Gaumanian degenerative disease, namely ALS, pure parkinsonism, pure dementia, or PDC.

Dystonia

Dystonia is a broad term that encompasses sustained or intermittent muscle contractions resulting in abnormal, often repetitive, movements and postures. Where a mutation is known, the dystonia is given the prefix "DYT" followed by a number that relates to the time of discovery. At the time of writing, DYT27 is the most recent variety. Primary (inherited) dystonias are rare, consequently there is very limited information about olfaction. Some of the primary dystonic conditions have features of parkinsonism and levodopa responsiveness, notably DYT5 (Dopa responsive dystonia; DRD; Segawa syndrome), which is associated with mutations in tyrosine hydroxylase (TH) or the GTP cyclohydrolase 1 gene. Parkinsonian features occur late on. In one autopsy there was no evidence of Lewy pathology although TH levels were reduced (Rajput et al., 1994), and there was no examination of the olfactory pathways. A 66-year-old man with a 20-year history of hemiparkinsonism, dystonia, and loss of smell was presented at the International Movement Disorders meeting, San Diego, 2015. There was a mutation in GTP cyclohydrolase 1, response to levodopa associated with significant fluctuations, and dyskinesia. In DYT12, a rapid onset dystonia-parkinsonism syndrome that does not respond to levodopa. A single limited autopsy, showed no Lewy pathology or cell loss in the substantia nigra (Pittock et al., 2000).

X-Linked Recessive Dystonia–Parkinsonism (see Table 7.3). This X-linked disorder, also termed "Lubag," or DYT3, predominantly affects Filipino male adults with maternal roots from the Philippine Island of Panay. There are infrequent cases affecting females who have a milder form of disease and the condition is now recognized in people born outside the Philippines. Lubag is caused by a mutation in a gene at Xq13.1 that codes for TATA-binding protein- associated factor-1 (TAF1), which is expressed in the striatum. There are few pathological studies, but Lewy bodies have not been found (Lee et al., 2001; Waters et al., 1993). The average age of onset is approximately 40 years and the disorder commences with progressive dystonia, mainly affecting the jaw, neck, and trunk, followed after a few years by parkinsonism. A single study of 20 affected males, using a culturally modified UPSIT, showed that olfaction was mildly impaired in Lubag (mean score of 18 of 25 items compared to a control score of 20), even in the early stages. The smell loss was independent of the degree of dystonia, rigidity, severity, and disease duration (Evidente et al., 2004)

DYT25. One group from Tennessee studied Afro-American families with cervical, laryngeal, or upper limb dystonia not explained by known dystonia genes (Vemula et al., 2013). Whole-exome sequencing revealed a missense mutation (V228F) in GNAL (guanine nucleotide-binding protein) G(olf), that, in turn, plays a role in olfaction, coupling G-protein receptors to adenylyl cyclase. G(olf) is expressed in the olfactory neuroepithelium and striatum, thus providing a plausible association between dystonia and olfactory disorder. Subjects harboring the p.V228F mutation exhibited mild reduction of UPSIT score with a mean value of 30.8 compared to non-carrier healthy family members who scored a mean of 35.1. The differences were not significant probably because of small case numbers. The authors suggest that mutant Gα(olf) and Gα(olf) deficiency may precipitate dystonia by limiting activation of adenylate cyclase in dopamine D1 receptors in striatal medium spiny neurons of the direct pathway. It is also commented that two Iranian families with isolated congenital anosmia showed linkage to 18p11.23-q12.2 (Ghadami, Majidzadeh et al., 2004), an area that is close to the GNAL coding region and that mice deficient in Gα(olf) are anosmic (Belluscio et al., 1998).

Little information is available for other forms of dystonia. These include dystonic tremor, tremor associated dystonia, focal dystonia (e.g., cervical dystonia (spasmodic torticollis)), facial dystonias, drug-induced dystonia, and the primary dystonias affecting children and young adults such as torsion dystonia, myoclonus dystonia, and "degenerative" conditions such as Pantothenate Kinase-Associated Neurodegeneration (PKAN) (Hallervorden-Spatz disease). In one study all 16 patients with idiopathic adult onset dystonia (mostly cervical) scored well within the normal range on the UPSIT (Silveira-Moriyama et al., 2009).

Wilson's Disease (Hepatolenticular Degeneration)

This is an autosomal recessive disorder of copper metabolism described by the famous British neurologist Kinnear Wilson in 1912. It is due to a mutation in the ATP7B gene located on the long arm of chromosome 13. Copper accumulates in the liver and basal ganglia, leading to progressively severe dystonia and parkinsonism if untreated or diagnosed late. The largest investigation of olfaction in Wilson's disease related to 24 patients all on treatment (Mueller et al., 2006). Eleven patients had just liver disease and 13 displayed neurological symptoms as well. Compared to the hepatic group, those with neurological manifestations had mild–moderate impairment of olfaction as measured by the extended Sniffin' Sticks test. Olfactory function was unrelated to long-term treatment with penicillamine, which might impair taste and smell (Nores et al., 2000), but in theory its copper-clearing effect would improve olfactory function. There was no correlation between olfactory score and MRI or regional glucose metabolism as measured by fluoro-deoxy-glucose PET scans. The authors suggest that the microsmia related to "specific functions of the basal ganglia in the processing of odorous stimuli." There appear to be no pathological studies of the olfactory bulb in Wilson's disease, but involvement of the amygdala has been noted (Shimoji et al., 1987) and would provide a basis for olfactory loss.

There is one description of "olfactory paranoid syndrome" (presumably the same as the olfactory reference syndrome) in a Japanese patient with Wilson's disease associated with idiopathic thrombocytopenic purpura. With penicillamine treatment the patient recovered from the psychiatric and physical symptoms (Sagawa et al., 2003).

Pure Autonomic Failure (PAF)

This disorder is typified by neurogenic orthostatic hypotension probably due to reduction of noradrenalin (norepinephrine) secretion in sympathetic nerves, without other neurological features. Lewy bodies are present in the brain stem, pre- and postganglionic autonomic neurons, and the peripheral sympathetic and parasympathetic nerves

(Hague et al., 1997). Although parkinsonism is absent in PAF, it shares pathological features and some consider PAF belongs to the spectrum of Lewy Body disorders and that PAF may be a precursor of PD. An early example concerns a patient who underwent lumbar sympathectomy for peripheral vascular disease. Biopsy showed Lewy bodies in the sympathetic ganglia and three years thereafter the patient developed typical PD (Stadlan et al., 1965). Kaufmann et al. (2004) described one patient with PAF who appeared to progress to PD after 20 years, and another subject with marked dysautonomia who developed DLB after 18 months.

Goldstein et al. (2009) studied olfaction by the UPSIT in 8 patients with PAF, 23 with PD and 20 with MSA. The PAF group had a low UPSIT score (mean 22/40) similar to PD and significantly worse than MSA (mean 31/40). Individual UPSIT scores correlated positively with cardiac fluorodopamine radioactivity in the septum but not with fluorodopamine brain PET scans, implying that the olfactory dysfunction was independent of striatal dopamine deficiency. A similar approach was taken by Silveira-Moriyama et al. (2009) in a group of 16 subjects with PAF, 14 with MSA, and 191 with PD. After adjustment for age, gender, and smoking habit, they found the lowest UPSIT score in PD and equal impairment in MSA and PAF, suggesting that the olfactory defect in PAF occupied a position intermediate between classic PD and healthy controls. Another survey used the UPSIT to evaluate 12 patients with PAF, 10 with MSA, and 4 with dopamine beta hydroxylase deficiency (Garland et al., 2011). Severe olfactory impairment was noted for the PAF group with little or no change in the other two groups.

In conclusion, it appears well established that patients with PAF are likely to have severe olfactory loss and that some may progress to parkinsonism.

Essential Tremor

Classic essential tremor (ET) is characterized by a relatively rapid postural and action tremor that disappears on rest. It is sometimes known as "tea-cup tremor" given the tendency for the spoon to rattle on the saucer! There is often a family history in keeping with autosomal dominant inheritance but onset is bimodal with peaks in young and late adult life. It is usually diagnosed without difficulty but occasionally there are problems when the tremor appears to be dystonic or there is coexisting rigidity. Also, there may be confusion between ET and benign tremulous PD where cogwheeling is absent or equivocal. There have been no detailed pathological studies of the olfactory pathways in ET, and only a few on the rest of the brain (Louis et al., 2006). The major pathology is in the cerebellum, where Purkinje cell axonal swelling ("torpedoes") are found more frequently than in control brains (Louis et al., 2011). The first appraisal of identification ability, which was completed in 15 subjects with benign ET, found all to be normal on the UPSIT (Busenbark et al., 1992). This study was subsequently challenged by Louis & colleagues (2002), who reported that a significant proportion of ET patients had mild impairment, prompting the suggestion that this defect may relate to the postulated olfactory function of the cerebellum. In a subsequent study of ET patients with isolated rest tremor (Louis & Jurewicz, 2003), the UPSIT score was no different from typical ET patients, suggesting that involvement of the basal ganglia is part of the ET syndrome. Recent olfactory findings using the UPSIT in ET (Adler et al., 2005; Shah et al., 2005; Quagliato et al., 2009; Silveira-Moriyama et al., 2009) are normal overall, but errors may creep in if a patient with apparent ET is confused with benign tremulous PD, a condition where olfactory function is impaired. Ondo & Lai (2005) found that PD patients

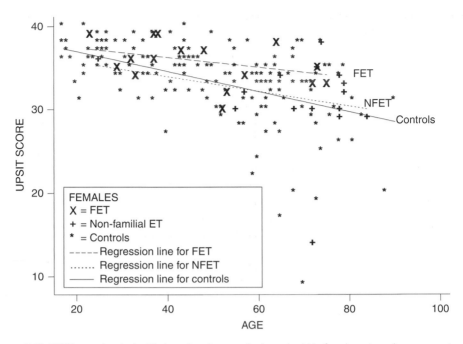

Figure 7.13 UPSIT score (vertical axis) plotted against age (horizontal axis) in females using a linear regression on age. Individual subject data points are shown by the symbols referenced in the key box. Fitted lines to show a slower rate of age-related decline in familial ET.

with a family history of tremor had better olfactory function than other Parkinson's patients, including those with tremor-predominant disease. Djaldetti et al. (2008) did not find a relation with the extent of dopaminergic innervation measured by DATScan, and ET patients with and without rest tremor did not have abnormal smell tests. Finally, a study by Louis et al. (2008) suggested a correlation between the cerebellar neurotoxin Harmane (methylpyridoindole) and UPSIT score, although the mean UPSIT score of ET patients and controls were similar.

Clearly it would help diagnostically if ET subjects had normal olfactory function, as this would allow better distinction of ET from PD subjects with tremor. One study has addressed this problem by comparing ET in 59 healthy control subjects with 64 subjects suffering from tremor-dominant PD (Shah et al., 2007). There was almost complete separation of the two groups on the basis of UPSIT scores and to lesser degree on the olfactory-event-related potential (OERP). If there was a family history of essential tremor in a first-degree relative (FET), this group scored significantly better than age- and gender-matched control subjects (Figure 7.13). There was a suggestion of resistance to the effects of olfactory aging in the FET category as well. These unexpected findings need to be verified but it is likely that patients with ET have no important disorder of olfaction.

In practical terms, the expectation of normal olfactory function in ET (whether familial or not) could be used diagnostically: if a patient with suspected ET has abnormal olfactory test scores, when allowing for age and gender, then the diagnosis would merit review. If the patient is thought to have tremor-dominant PD then olfaction should be abnormal. At present it would be unwise to use a smell test in isolation, but olfactory testing may provide a useful initial guide to the diagnosis.

Case Report 7.8: Benign Tremulous PD with Positive Family History. A 64-year-old former engineer presented on account of left-sided tremor for the preceding two years. It started in the foot and spread to the hand, and was diminished slightly by alcohol. He was unaware of any problem with the sense of smell. Both parents developed tremor late in life, neither of whom were significantly disabled. Examination showed a moderately severe rest tremor on the left with slight cogwheel rigidity on that side. There was mild postural tremor and increased fatigue on repeated hand movement. The provisional diagnosis was either benign tremulous PD with a positive family history of the same condition or familial ET. The UPSIT score was in the severe microsmic range (23/40) and OERP was delayed at 1116 ms (normal less than 937 ms). The MRI brain scan was normal but there was mild mucosal prominence in the sphenoid air sinus. DATScan showed bilateral reduction of transporter uptake in the putamen. Response to levodopa was good and the final clinical diagnosis was benign tremulous PD. *Comment:* The clinical assessment here pointed to tremulous PD with a family history of tremor, which is unusual, although it is increasingly recognized. The fact that neither parent was disabled suggests that they had essential tremor or benign tremulous PD, neither of which is characterized by severe disability. In some families with typical PD in one generation, there may be others with typical ET (Yahr et al., 2003). The diagnosis of PD in our case is confirmed by clinical examination, abnormality of smell identification, good response to levodopa, delayed OERP, and by an abnormal DATScan. If this patient had essential tremor all smell tests should be normal (Shah et al., 2007).

Inherited Cerebellar ataxias

If the cerebellum is concerned with olfaction, either through control of sniffing or actual identification, then abnormalities might be present in the inherited ataxias. Some varieties may simulate classic Parkinson disease with rigidity or dystonia as seen in Machado-Joseph syndrome (autosomal dominant spino-cerebellar ataxia type 3; SCA3). Indeed, in SCA3 there is neuronal loss in the substantia nigra and sometimes levodopa responsiveness. Given the possibility of confusion between cerebellar tremor and parkinsonism, olfactory tests might aid the differential diagnosis.

Friedreich's Ataxia (FRDA). This is a recessively inherited ataxia associated with progressive corticospinal tract damage, peripheral neuropathy, diabetes, and cardiac abnormalities. Given earlier suggestions that the cerebellum might play a role in olfaction it was logical to examine the sense of smell in ataxic disorders. In the first such study, recognition thresholds were measured in seven FRDA patients and found to be elevated compared to controls (Satya-Murti & Crisostomo, 1988). Subsequently mild but significant abnormalities in UPSIT scores were found in 23 patients with FRDA (Connelly et al., 2003) but there was no correlation between UPSIT score and GAA trinucleotide repeat length, disease duration, or walking disability. A study from Brazil, currently available only in abstract, examined 17 genetically verified Friedreich's ataxia patients compared to 34 healthy controls (Branco Germiniani et al., 2014). They used the screening version of the Sniffin' Sticks test and found significant hyposmia in eight patients compared to controls. There was no correlation with age of onset, duration of disease, ataxia severity, or number of GAA repeats. Based on these studies it may be concluded that olfaction is likely to be impaired in patients with

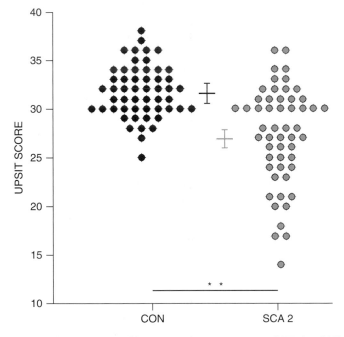

Figure 7.14 Distribution and mean number of correct UPSIT responses in control (CON) and SCA2 groups. Bars are SEM. Mann-Whitney test, ** = p < 0.01. Reproduced with permission from Velázquez-Pérez et al., 2006.

Friedreich's ataxia but the defect is not severe and confounding from diabetes that may co-exist has not been addressed.

Spinocerebellar Ataxia Type 2 (SCA2) and Machado-Joseph Syndrome (SCA3). In a preliminary study of various ataxic disorders, 12 patients with the SCA2 mutation were examined by the UPSIT (Fernandez-Ruiz et al., 2003). They found significant impairment of UPSIT score in the SCA2 group (but not SCA3). In a small study, Hentschel et al. (2005) observed normal UPSIT scores in seven individuals with the SCA2 mutation and one at risk patient. In a more definitive study, Velázquez-Pérez et al. (2006) evaluated UPSIT, olfactory threshold, and discrimination test scores in 53 genetically verified cases of SCA2. Mild to moderate olfactory impairment was found in about half of the subjects tested (Figure 7.14).

Conversely, in the Machado-Joseph Syndrome (SCA3) olfaction is probably normal or only slightly compromised. Thus, Fernandez-Ruiz et al. (2003) found normal UPSIT results in their five patients. Braga-Neto et al. (2011) found very mildly lowered Sniffin' Stick scores in 41 patients with the SCA3 mutation (11.5 ± 2.4 vs. 12.8 ± 1.5, p = 0.003) but this effect persisted after controlling for gender and Mini-Mental State Examination. A further study in 17 patients with the SCA3 mutation also using Sniffin' Sticks tests found no difference in olfactory scores compared to controls (11.5 ± 2.0 vs. 11.9 ± 2.3) after adjustment for age and cognitive function (Moscovich et al., 2012). Thus, a patient with Machado-Joseph Syndrome would be expected to display normal or very mild impairment of olfaction, a point that might assist distinction from classic PD and SCA2.

As mentioned, patients with SCA2 or SCA3 mutations may have parkinsonian tremor or dystonia, either of which might cause diagnostic difficulty; hence, the finding of normal or mildly impaired olfaction in suspected PD with imbalance could indicate an inherited cerebellar syndrome. In the newly identified SCA 8 and SCA 17 disorders there may be parkinsonian features but no olfactory data are available as yet. All these observations have been based on relatively small numbers of patients and should be interpreted conservatively. At present no form of spinocerebellar ataxia is associated with severe anosmia. Finally, it would be premature to suggest that the cerebellum is responsible for the smell defect in ataxic disorder until there has been pathological examination of the classic olfactory pathways.

Motor Neuron Disease (Amyotrophic Lateral Sclerosis)

Nomenclature varies worldwide, but here "motor neuron disease" (MND) will be used as a generic term for all varieties affecting motor neurons of which amyotrophic lateral sclerosis (ALS) is the most common, followed by bulbar forms and then the mildest form – progressive muscular atrophy (PMA). In the North American literature, ALS approximates to MND in the United Kingdom. The disorder is characterized by rapidly progressive weakness and wasting of limb muscles associated with muscle twitching (fasciculation) cramp and brisk deep tendon reflexes. The conditional invariably spreads to the bulbar muscles (i.e., those concerned with chewing, swallowing, and breathing) leading to death within three years. Pathologically there has been just one olfactory study and that examined the olfactory bulb. In eight autopsy cases of MND which were compared to age-matched controls, Hawkes et al. (1998) found marked accumulation of lipofuscin in both the neurons of the AON and other principal neuronal types of the olfactory bulb, suggesting increased lipid peroxidation. The first clinically based pilot study examined 15 patients with MND, of whom eight had moderate or severe bulbar involvement and eight were chair bound (Elian, 1991). No test for dementia was administered but a significant lowering of the UPSIT score was documented. In another study of 37 patients with ALS (Sajjadian et al., 1994), 28 (75.7%) had significantly lower scores on UPSIT compared with age-matched controls. Four of these 28 (i.e., 11%) had near or total anosmia. Hawkes et al. (1998) examined UPSIT scores in 58 cognitively normal patients with an established diagnosis of MND. Seven had PMA, 34 typical ALS, and 17 had bulbar disease. Overall, 9 of 58 patients (16%) displayed UPSIT scores that were significantly below those of age-matched controls. The effect of group status overall (i.e., MND versus control) was statistically significant (p = 0.02). However, analysis among the patient groups found that only bulbar patients differed meaningfully from control subjects. OERPs were performed in 15 patients: in nine the responses were normal for latency and amplitude measurements; one was delayed; in two the response was absent; and in three the recording could not be obtained. In this study, the reason for a proportionately larger number of patients with normal olfactory function is not clear, but it could reflect case selection effects or diagnostic bias. Also there is a possibility of falsely lowered identification scores from reduced sniffing, as seen in PD (Sobel et al., 2001), since many bulbar MND patients are likely to have respiratory weakness. The OERP findings, which circumvent the need to inhale actively, suggest that olfaction is affected in MND, although to a mild degree. There is one instance of ALS and smell loss in a 44-year-old worker in an Israeli battery factory (Bar-Sela et al., 2001). He developed symptoms of ALS, confirmed by electromyography, two years after exposure to high concentration of cadmium, the main component of nickel-cadmium batteries. It was suggested this may be connected with the ability of cadmium to reduce levels of brain copper-zinc superoxide dismutase and enhance the excitoxicity of glutamate. Just one study found normal smell (and taste) function in motor neuron disease (Lang et al., 2011). Here, olfaction was assessed with Sniffin' Sticks in 26 patients and 26 matched controls and group analysis showed no difference between the ALS and control subjects. Given that microsmia has a low prevalence in ALS, a minor difference could be overlooked in this small sample, i.e., only two–three abnormal cases would be expected (Type 2 error).

There are no olfactory studies as yet in the newly described variant of familial ALS caused by mutations in the C9ORF72 gene. This is associated with frontotemporal dementia (FTD) where olfactory impairment is recognized (see above). Thus, olfactory measurement might help identify FTD patients who have the C9ORF72 mutation. Other patients with a familial ALS type presentation have mutations in TDP-43 that result in neuronal inclusions. One study from Japan showed significant olfactory impairment in their ALS patients and at autopsy (in other ALS patients) they noted TDP-43 inclusions with maximum expression in central olfactory regions, especially the hippocampus, rather than the olfactory bulb (Takeda et al., 2015). It was suggested that olfactory impairment in someone with ALS should alert the clinician to this mutation.

Nine patients with the Guam form of ALS were tested with a culturally modified form of the UPSIT (Ahlskog et al., 1998). Marked impairment of smell identification was found in the Guam ALS variant as well as those with other categories, namely pure parkinsonism, pure dementia and the PD-dementia complex.

Huntington's Disease (HD)

This is a late-presenting autosomal dominant disorder of basal ganglia function typified by choreic movement, dementia, and, in rare cases, muscular rigidity similar to that of PD (Westphal variant). It is caused by an expansion of a CAG trinucleotide repeat in the HTT gene encoding huntingtin. HTT CAG heterozygous knock-in mice demonstrate several behavioral abnormalities consistent with the human disease, including hypoactivity, decreased anxiety, motor learning/coordination deficits, and impaired olfactory discrimination (Holter et al., 2013). We are not aware of any specific pathologic study of the human olfactory bulb (OB), but in the R6/2 knock-in HD rat model cell proliferation was reduced in the subventricular zone and OB of transgenic rats compared to wild type rats (Kandasamy, Rosskopf et al., 2015). Although OB cell survival was reduced, the frequency of neuronal differentiation was not altered in the granule cell layer, compared to normal rats despite increased dopaminergic neuronal differentiation in the glomerular layer. In humans there are widespread pathologic changes, particularly in the cerebral cortex (deep layers), globus pallidus, thalamus, subthalamic nucleus, substantia nigra, and cerebellum. These pathological abnormalities have been confirmed on voxel-based morphometric analysis (Barrios et al., 2007). Structures associated with the greatest impact on the HD olfactory defect, as measured by UPSIT, were the entorhinal cortex, thalamus, parahippocampal gyrus, and caudate nucleus.

An initial study of 38 Huntington's disease (HD) subjects reported early defective odor memory, in some cases prior to the expression of cognitive or marked involuntary movement (Moberg et al., 1987). Subsequent analysis, using tests of odor identification and detection, confirm the presence of moderate olfactory impairment in HD with established disease, but of less severity than PD (Nordin et al., 1995b; Bylsma et al., 1997; Moberg & Doty, 1997; Hamilton et al., 1999). According to one study (Hamilton et al., 1999), n-butanol threshold measurement in early-stage HD provided good classification of sensitivity and specificity between the patients (seven) and matched control subjects (seven), suggesting that olfactory testing may provide a sensitive measure of disease onset. Two studies explored smell function in relatives at risk of HD. In one (Moberg & Doty, 1997), UPSIT scores and phenylethyl alcohol thresholds were normal in 12 offspring at 50% risk but abnormal in 25 probands. In the other study (Bylsma et al., 1997), 20 healthy subjects known to have the HD mutation exhibited normal UPSIT scores, whereas those of the HD group (20) were mildly abnormal. In this study, a significant (r = −0.77) correlation was found between UPSIT scores and results on the Quantified Neurological Exam (QNE; total score), indicating that the more neurologically impaired subjects fared worse on the UPSIT. Patients with HD may show deficits in recognizing disgust in the facial expressions and vocal intonations of others (Gray et al., 1997), a feature that may relate to dysfunction in the amygdala. These difficulties with facial expression recognition were also seen in otherwise healthy HD gene carriers. Extending this principle, it has been suggested that disgust-related deficits may apply to foul-smelling olfactory stimuli and inappropriate combinations of taste stimuli (Mitchell et al., 2005). Subjects at 50 percent risk of future disease were not tested, but this would be an obvious extension of such work. Others have explored the use of "source memory" for olfactory and visual stimuli in HD (Pirogovsky et al., 2007), i.e., which person delivered a particular test. In the HD group (n = 10), as expected, there was impairment of olfactory item memory, and olfactory (and visual) source memory compared to controls (n = 20). Interestingly, they also demonstrated impaired olfactory (but not visual) source memory in asymptomatic gene carriers (n = 10) of magnitude similar to patients with HD. They conclude that olfactory source memory may be particularly sensitive to neuropathological changes in preclinical stages of HD. Just one study explored the value of OERP in eight subjects with established HD (Wetter et al., 2005), where it was shown that the major positive component (P3) was significantly delayed.

Until recently, most observations suggested that olfactory impairment in HD expresses itself near or at the time of clinical disease onset. Such a concept is supported indirectly by the negative correlation between UPSIT scores and QNE (see above), an index of neurological impairment (Bylsma et al., 1997). However, data from the long-term prospective PREDICT-HD study (Paulsen et al., 2008) suggest that the onset of dysfunction may occur much earlier. In this analysis of 438 non-manifesting carriers of the HD mutation, olfaction began to decline insidiously along with subtle motor and cognitive changes 10–20 years prior to the predicted time of clinical diagnosis (Figure 7.15). Despite this, olfactory testing may still have value (along with motor tests, for example), as it may indicate the onset of disease in apparent non-manifesting mutation carriers.

Several other conditions are now recognized that can simulate the HD phenotype: spinocerebellar atrophy type 17 (SCA-17), neuroacanthocytosis, benign hereditary chorea, and Huntington disease-like disorder (HDL1 and HDL2). In all of these, a molecular diagnosis can be made, but so far there are no published studies on olfactory function. This would clearly be an interesting line of research.

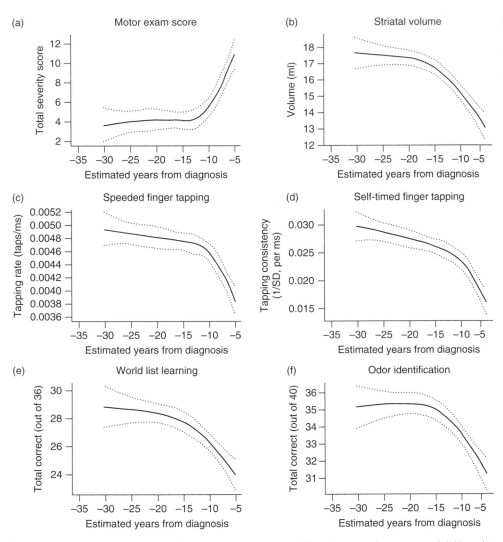

Figure 7.15 Relationship between estimated years to diagnosis of HD and various other measures. Solid line plots the predicted response; broken lines are 95% confidence limits for the estimated mean response. Reproduced with permission from Paulsen et al. (2008).

Prion-Related Disease

Prion diseases, also known as transmissible spongiform encephalopathies, are a family of rare neurodegenerative diseases of which Creutzfeldt-Jakob disease (CJD) is an example. In prion protein knock-out mice, olfactory behavior and oscillatory activity in the deep layers of the main olfactory bulb was disrupted, suggesting that the non-pathogenic cellular prion protein (PrP^c) is involved in the normal processing of sensory information in the olfactory system (Le Pichon et al., 2009). It is likely on the basis of animal experiments that the olfactory mucosa acts as a reservoir for pathogenic prions (PrP^{Sc}) and that such prions are shed into nasal secretions, which in turn may be infectious to other animals (Hamir et al., 2008; Bessen et al., 2010; Bessen et al., 2011).

In the sporadic form of Creutzfeldt-Jakob Disease (CJD), PrP^{Sc} was found in the olfactory cilia and central olfactory pathway of all nine patients examined, but not in the respiratory mucosa or control tissue (Zanusso et al., 2003). The same group suggested that olfactory pathway involvement is an early feature in all varieties of CJD and that in the MV2 and VV2 variants, pathology in the olfactory system is accompanied by damage in the dorsal motor nucleus of the vagus, solitary tract, and perihypoglossal nuclei (Zanusso et al., 2009), thus resonating in part, with Braak staging of classic PD. Their observations are supported by a case report of CJD on a 59-year-old woman who had a nasal olfactory neuroepithelial biopsy 45 days after initial symptoms (Tabaton et al., 2004). Prion protein immunostaining was observed in the olfactory cilia and olfactory mucosa. It was suggested that the presence of PrPSc in the olfactory epithelium at an early stage supported the concept of centrifugal spread of pathogenic prion protein along olfactory pathways.

Another case report described progressive impairment of smell and taste sense due to variant CJD in a 54-year-old ceramic tiler (Reuber et al., 2001). Over the course of 12 months he became unable to distinguish the taste of tea from beer and developed an unusual craving for vanilla ice cream, irritability, excess drowsiness, imbalance, and tremor, leading to a pathologically confirmed diagnosis of variant CJD. Crude olfactory testing showed impaired odor detection and recognition and at autopsy there was widespread prion staining in the cerebral cortex and basal ganglia. There was particularly marked prion staining and vacuolation in the olfactory tracts. Apart from this single case, there are no reports of olfactory loss in other prion-related conditions such as Gerstmann-Straussler Syndrome and Fatal Familial Insomnia, but extrapyramidal features are often seen in these disorders and may be confused initially with a variety of Parkinson's disease (Kovacs et al., 2002). Thus, it is likely that some chemosensory dysfunction is present in other prion-related conditions but due to the rapidity of progression, routine testing may be challenging.

Diagnostic Implications of Smell Disorders for Neurodegenerative Disease

It is well established that the olfactory system is impaired to varying degree in clinically evident parkinsonism (see Tables 7.1–7.3). Most severe changes are seen in Classic PD, Gaucher, Guamanian, and Lewy body varieties. Least involvement is found in vascular parkinsonism and various dystonias, with intermediate damage in MSA, PSP, and CBS. However, there is considerable variability and overlap of smell dysfunction in these syndromes, limiting the diagnostic value of olfactory testing. Broadly speaking, where the pathologic features are those of tauopathy, olfaction is likely to be normal or mildly affected (e.g., PSP, CBS); if the pathology is α-synucleinopathy (Classic PD, Lewy body disease, dementia with Lewy bodies), abnormal olfaction is to be expected. Such pathological diagnoses must be interpreted conservatively, since tau and a-synuclein may be expressed in several brain regions and in some instances both tau and alpha-synuclein pathology may be present in the olfactory bulb, e.g., AD, DLB, and PARK 8. At present there are too few studies on familial parkinsonism to state whether smell testing could help predict whether non-manifesting carriers will later express the disease, but the limited information at present is not encouraging.

With these caveats, differences in smell function can aid diagnosis. For example, if a patient is suspected to have classic PD, especially of the akinetic rigid variety, the presence of normal olfaction *on testing* should prompt review of the diagnosis. Thus, normal olfaction in alleged PD would imply seven alternative diagnoses: vascular parkinsonism; the parkinsonian variant of PSP; spinocerebellar ataxia type 3; corticobasal syndrome; idiopathic dystonia, Fragile-X tremor ataxia syndrome and benign tremulous PD, especially in women. Dopamine transporter imaging is useful in confirming a suspected diagnosis of PD, but it is not specific and cannot distinguish PD from parkinsonian syndromes. Its diagnostic utility is comparable to olfactory testing (Deeb et al., 2010), although at much greater expense and it is not yet known which test – DATScan, olfactory, or transcranial sonography – is best able to detect presymptomatic PD (Sommer et al., 2004). The minor abnormalities found in ALS are probably not useful clinically. In HD, smell impairment is an early feature, and although genetic testing makes olfactory measurement partially redundant, it may help indicate the time of disease onset. It is apparent that olfaction is severely impaired in the majority of cases with AD, probably reflecting more central than peripheral pathology, at least in the early disease phase.

Although early-stage AD may be assessed validly using psychophysical procedures, the results of such testing in later stages is questionable because of likely confounding by cognitive issues. Hence, there is need for studies that apply procedures less dependent upon cognitive responses, such as OERPs or measures of sniff magnitude (Chapter 3). Some argue that smell threshold or discrimination tests make less cognitive demand and that they would be useful for examining those in the early to moderately advanced stages of dementia. Although many investigations suggest that olfactory dysfunction is a pre-cognitive abnormality in AD, it might be argued that olfaction is just easier to measure than mild cognitive decline. A parallel argument may be applied to PD, although the studies of Braak and those from the Honolulu Asia Aging Study make this unlikely. Olfactory testing in asymptomatic relatives of those with Parkinson's disease or AD could act as a useful biomarker for those at risk of subsequent disease. Further long-term prospective studies in families with AD and PD containing substantial members at 50 percent risk will help solve this problem.

As mentioned, olfactory abnormalities of varying degree are found in familial syndromes such as: PARK1/4; 2; 6, 8, 9, Lubag, and those with adult onset Gaucher disease. Data are awaited for PARK 14, 15, 17, and POLG1 mutations. Some non-manifesting carriers of the PARK 6 and PARK 8 mutations may have abnormal olfaction, a finding that might assist predictive testing. These observations are all preliminary, based on small numbers and it cannot be assumed at present that hyposmia is a reliable predictive marker in carriers of any form of monogenic PD.

The Olfactory Vector Hypothesis

One of the interesting and controversial theories proposed to explain the olfactory loss and the etiology of some neurodegenerative diseases is the "olfactory vector hypothesis" (OVH; for review, see Doty, 2008). This theory suggests that olfactory loss, or perhaps even the neuro-degenerative disease itself, is induced, directly or indirectly, by environmental agent(s) that enter the brain via the olfactory fila (Roberts, 1986; Ferreyra-Moyano & Barragan, 1989). The olfactory receptor cells (ORC), whose cilia and dendritic knobs in the human have an extensive combined surface area of ~23 cm^2 (Doty, 2001), are in relatively direct contact with the potentially hostile external environment and, along with trigeminal free nerve terminals and nerve endings from the nervus terminalis, can incorporate and serve as a conduit into the brain. Invasion may relate to airborne viruses, nanoparticles, and other xenobiotics, including ionized metals (e.g., cadmium, gold, manganese) from the nose into the central nervous system (CNS) (Roberts, 1986; Ferreyra-Moyano & Barragan, 1989; Charles et al., 1995; Doty, 2008; Genter et al., 2015). In some cases, the rate of entry is higher than 2 mm an hour (Gottofrey & Tjalve, 1991; Tjalve et al., 1996; Tjalve & Henriksson, 1999).

Although some xenobiotics are actively detoxified in the epithelium by nasal enzyme systems, including the P450 cytochrome family, others are metabolized (paradoxically) into more neurotoxic or carcinogenic compounds (Bond, 1986; Dahl, 1986). Interestingly, herbicides, such as the dioxins (Gillner et al., 1987) or chlorthiamid (Brittebo et al., 1991), are selectively taken up by, and are harmful to, the olfactory epithelium, even when administered systemically. Some xenobiotics can be transported beyond the olfactory system to multiple brain regions, that include sites in common with the neuropathology of AD and PD. For example, Herpes simplex virus type 1, placed intranasally in six-week-old mice, subsequently spreads as far as the temporal lobe, hippocampus, and cingulate cortex (Tomlinson & Esiri, 1983). Horseradish peroxidase (HRP), when applied intranasally in the rat, is transported to the bulb, AON, and transmitter-specific projection neurones of the diagonal band (cholinergic), raphe nucleus (serotonergic), and locus coeruleus (noradrenergic) (Shipley, 1985). This is of particular relevance as the locus coeruleus and raphe nuclei are involved in the premotor phase of PD – Braak stage 2 (Braak et al., 2003a). HRP, when injected into the olfactory tubercle of the rat, results in retrograde labeling of the ipsilateral olfactory bulb, AON, and other primary olfactory areas, as well as anterograde labeling of the ipsilateral ventral tegmental area, substantia nigra, (pars reticulata), and ventral pallidum (Newman & Winans, 1980), emphasizing the existence of direct connections between primary olfactory areas and the substantia nigra. A direct dopaminergic innervation from neurons in the rat substantia nigra to the olfactory bulb has been demonstrated recently by axonal tracing (Höglinger et al., 2015). Injection of two dopaminergic neurotoxins (1-methyl-4-phenylpyridinium and 6-hydroxydopamine) into the olfactory bulb decreased the number of dopaminergic neurons in the substantia nigra. In turn, ablation of the nigral projection led to impaired olfactory perception. Many viruses, such as the Epstein–Barr virus, encode proteins that exploit the ubiquitin–proteasome system to regulate latency and allow the persistence of infected cells in immunocompetent hosts (Masucci, 2004; Shackelford & Pagano, 2005). Importantly, some inhaled neurotoxins may activate latent viruses; for example, trichloroethylene may reactivate herpes simplex 1 infection within the trigeminal nerve (Buxton & Hayward, 1967).

It should be emphasized that species differences exist in terms of transmission of agents from the nose to the brain and that, with rare exception, evidence for such transmission comes solely from animal studies. In the early twentieth century, it was shown that poliomyelitis readily infects monkeys by nasal instillation of the virus (Flexner & Lewis, 1910; Flexner & Clark, 1912). Subsequently, it was demonstrated, in mouse and monkey studies, that intranasal instillation of agents such as alum, aluminum sulfate, tannic acid, tinitrocresol, thionin, mercurochrome, picric acid, trinitrocesol, and zinc sulfate prevented infection by the nasally induced virus (Armstrong & Harrison, 1935; Sabin et al., 1936; Schultz & Gebhardt, 1936, 1937). In the rhesus monkey, olfactory bulb pathology was noted primarily in subjects that received the poliomyelitis virus intranasally, but not in those exposed intracerebrally, subcutaneously, or via the sciatic nerve (Sabin et al., 1936). Such studies led to clinical trials in Alabama and Toronto in which thousands of school children were inoculated intranasally with either picric acid or zinc sulfate in a generally ineffective effort to ward off polio infection (Rutty, 1996). Lack of effectiveness may have occurred because poliomyelitis virus is rarely found in the human olfactory bulb (Sabin & Ward, 1941; Faber & Silverberg, 1946). According to Faber & Silberg (1946), airborne virus-bearing particles are probably not often in contact with the human olfactory epithelium, although sporadic reports suggest the human olfactory system is not totally refractory to poliomyelitis infection,

In this section we address major arguments for and against the OVH (see summary in Table 7.4). The areas of focus are: (1) the degree to which environmental and genetic factors are implicated in most forms of AD and PD; (2) the types of xenobiotic agents implicated as risk factors for AD and PD which may enter the brain via the olfactory pathways; and (3) the pattern of direction, i.e., peripheral to central versus central to peripheral, of neurodegenerative pathology within the CNS. Theoretically, evidence of damage to the olfactory epithelium may shed light on the etiology of a given disease by implicating an environmental agent. For example, some viruses may be transported from the olfactory epithelium to the olfactory bulb without replicating within, or imparting major damage to, the epithelium, despite using this pathway into the brain (Genter et al., 2015). Moreover, different CNS cell types may be preferentially infected by certain viruses, depending, for example, on the presence or absence of receptors to which a given virus binds (Schlitt et al., 1991).

Environmental Agents Known to Be Transported into the Brain through the Nose. A number of environmental agents suspected to be risk factors for AD and PD can, in theory, enter the brain via the olfactory route, including viruses, toxic metals, air pollutants, herbicides, and defoliants (Doty, 2008, 2015). Calderon-Garciduenas et al. (2004) measured the expression of the inflammatory mediator cyclo-oxygenase-2 (COX2) and the 42-amino acid form of beta-amyloid (Abeta42) in autopsy brain tissues of cognitively and neurologically intact lifelong residents of cities having low or high levels of air pollution. Occupants of Mexico City, a city with severe air pollution, had significantly higher COX2 expression in the olfactory bulb, frontal cortex, and hippocampus, and greater neuronal and astrocytic accumulation of Abeta42 compared with residents in a low air pollution city. Brain inflammation and Abeta42 accumulation are believed to precede the appearance of neuritic plaques and NFTs. Interestingly, UPSIT scores were lower in the high pollution Mexico City cohort than in the cohort from the low air pollution city (Calderón-Garcidueñas et al., 2010).

Several large epidemiologic studies have found occupational herbicide or defoliant use linked to AD and PD (Semchuk et al., 1992; Liou et al., 1997; Tyas et al., 2001; Li et al., 2005; Ascherio et al., 2006). Such agents may be inhaled and enter the brain via the lungs and bloodstream; alternatively, they might accumulate initially within the olfactory neuroepithelium and then migrate to the olfactory bulb. Indeed, there is evidence that this occurs for rotenone (Sherer et al., 2003), a widely available herbicide. This toxin, which acts by complex I inhibition, causes selective nigrostriatal dopaminergic degeneration, Lewy body formation, and damage to areas typically associated with PD,

Table 7.4. Arguments for and against the Olfactory Vector Hypothesis in AD and PD

Proposal	For	Against
Low rate of inheritance	Fewer than 10% of sporadic cases are inherited and most have less severe smell loss than classic PD. Genetic forms may represent different diseases. Mutations may still produce susceptibility to environmental agents rather than cause disease directly.	More genes are being discovered. Down syndrome progresses to AD. Transgenic mice can be induced to over-express PD and AD pathology. Families with α-synuclein triplication always suffer a form of Parkinson's disease.
Transport of agents into brain from nose	Known to occur for herbicides, pesticides, toxins, heavy metals, viruses, and other agents.	Epidemiological data inconclusive. One case of AD in someone with imperforate cribriform plate.
Cerebrospinal fluid drains along olfactory perineural lymphatics from subarachnoid space through the cribriform plate into nasal cavity, terminating in cervical lymph nodes	Provides a portal for retrograde transmission of neuropathogens from cervical lymph nodes or the nasal cavity.	Needs proof.
Clinical evidence of early olfactory involvement	Long-term prospective studies, family surveys. 80–90% of patients with PD are microsmic. Those who are not microsmic may be misclassified.	10 20% patients with PD appear to have normal smell sense. Not all surveys that show microsmia have pathological confirmation. Patients with presenilin-1 mutation did not have prior olfactory loss, nor do all cases of apparently typical AD.
Pathological findings	Lewy pathology in Braak PD stage 1 involves nasal mucosa, olfactory bulb, and medullary vagal nucleus only. Honolulu-Asia aging study showed pre-symptomatic microsmia was predictive of later Lewy pathology.	Not yet clear whether AD starts in the bulb or (probably) more centrally. In PD some find no Lewy pathology in medulla or pons when the substantia nigra is involved.
Herbicide use and PD	Epidemiology suggests link with farming. Rotenone causes typical changes of PD in animals.	Epidemiological data inconclusive and often retrospective.

Table 7.4. (cont.)

Proposal	For	Against
Olfactory epithelium is metabolically highly active	Possibly a defective cytochrome system permits entry of neurotoxin.	Not much direct evidence in humans apart from disordered Debrisoquine metabolism.
Allergic rhinitis	Prevalence raised in PD. Suggests there may be reduced nasal protection or chronic inflammation that might facilitate entry of pathogen.	Single retrospective case-note based study.

including the olfactory bulbs (Betarbet et al., 2000; Sherer et al., 2003). In light of such observations, as well as work by Calderon-Garciduenas et al. (2004, 2010), it may not be coincidental that a disproportionate number of PD patients have significantly increased prevalence of intermediate-type hypersensitivity disorder, in particular allergic rhinitis (Bower et al., 2006), a condition with compromised olfactory function (Klimek, 1998). Antunes et al. (2007) found that 88 percent of 43 confined-space workers exposed to airborne metals such as cadmium, iron, manganese, and lead for standard shift periods over the course of one to two years exhibited olfactory dysfunction and 28 percent developed signs of parkinsonism. Whether this reflects movement of such metals into the brain via the olfactory receptors is unknown but clearly a possibility. An argument leveled at the OVH for AD concerns a 65-year-old anosmic non-demented woman who displayed plaques and tangles in typical AD distribution. The cribriform plate was imperforate, the olfactory bulbs and tracts were rudimentary, and there were sulcal abnormalities of the orbitofrontal region (Arriagada et al., 1991). However, it is possible that in this single case a pathogen entered the olfactory system several years prior to occlusion of the cribriform plate foramina (Doty, 2008). Indeed, such occlusion occurs in many elderly people (Kalmey et al., 1998).

Environmental versus Genetic Determinants. Although an increasing number of abnormal genes have been identified in AD and PD, at present they account for a small percentage of apparently sporadic cases. This would imply that heritability is low and that environmental agents may be critically involved in their etiology. Given that smell impairment is an early sign of such disorders, it is possible that such loss signifies early pathology relating to an offending xenobiotic agent, as implied by the OVH. Conversely, and as discussed already in this chapter, patients with an early-onset familial form of AD who express the presenilin-1 mutation may not have pre-symptomatic smell impairment (Nee & Lippa, 2001) and some with apparent AD have normal smell function (McShane et al., 2001; Westervelt et al., 2007).

The fact that AD-like pathology occurs inevitably in older people with Down syndrome implies a genetic causation for AD (Rebeck & Hyman, 1993). Olfactory impairment is probably minimal in PARK 2 and PARK 3 (but not in PARK 1,6, 8, and 9; see Table 7.2) and while the phenotype may be similar to classic PD, the olfactory features suggest that at least some may represent a different disease. According to Hardy (2005), the majority of *Classic* PD cases are probably genetically based and the key factor is the degree of genetic loading.

For example, where there is triplication of normal α-synuclein the disease is always expressed and at an earlier age (Singleton et al., 2004). Although genetic predisposition is undoubtedly relevant in AD and PD, multiple etiologies are likely and the contribution from environmental protection or facilitation cannot be ignored. Not all cases of AD or PD need be explained by the OVH, including the Alzheimer-type pathology associated with Down syndrome. Importantly, the OVH does not necessarily exclude other determinants within the same individual.

Primacy of Olfactory Involvement. As detailed above, numerous behavioral and pathological studies indicate compromise of the olfactory system in AD and PD, and suggest that, in some cases, this may take place years before typical signs of disease are expressed. According to the Braak staging of PD (sequential theory), Lewy pathology is found first within the olfactory bulb and dorsal motor nuclear complex of cranial nerves IX and X (Braak et al., 2003a). From here it is proposed that simultaneously the disease ascends the brainstem to the substantia nigra and travels along the olfactory tracts to the temporal lobes. However, as described earlier in this chapter, not all pathologists concur with this progressive staging (Parkkinen et al., 2005; Halliday et al., 2006; Kalaitzakis et al., 2008). In AD, the evidence for a peripheral origin of olfactory damage is less robust than for PD. Thus, Vogt et al. (1990) pointed out that sectors of the amygdala which receive olfactory projections are not those most reliably laden with plaques and tangles, and Mann (1989) proposed that AD-related degeneration begins in cortical, not subcortical, brain regions. He pointed out that the major subcortical nuclei damaged in AD (i.e., nucleus basalis, locus coeruleus, and dorsal raphe) project to the same cortical areas, whereas subcortical nuclei that do not project to such areas are not similarly damaged. Elsewhere he argued that because the frequency of plaques and tangles is lower in the olfactory bulbs and tracts than in the amygdala and hippocampus, the direction of damage must be centrifugal (Mann, 1988). A similar argument was made by Okamoto et al. (1990) in a study of 100 AD patients who exhibited plaques in the olfactory bulbs only when greater numbers were present in the cerebral cortex. As mentioned above, the seminal studies of Braak and colleagues based on examination of 2,332 brains with sporadic AD (Braak et al., 2011) suggest that AD likely begins in the brain stem, predominantly affecting the locus coeruleus, decades before clinical presentation. The transentorhinal cortex is affected next, long before any olfactory region. Despite this, not all pathological studies support the notion of centrifugal spread. For example, Kovacs et al. (2001), who examined 15 brains from patients with AD, discovered early involvement of the olfactory bulbs, sometimes before other brain structures. Moreover, it is possible that formation of senile plaques (SP) and NFTs within the amygdala and hippocampus results from other processes (e.g., a defect in blood–brain barrier function) in which areas "triggered off" by a pathogenic agent spread via the olfactory pathways. If so, formation of AD pathology in olfactory nuclei would not necessarily occur during orthograde transport of such an agent, but could result from later retrograde spread. Consequently, less severe changes in the bulb and tracts would be expected. Thus the pattern of AD pathology need not necessarily reflect the direction of movement of a xenobiotic in the CNS. Viruses or other pathogens that enter the CNS via the olfactory fila could selectively damage more central regions of the limbic system, beginning with the most vulnerable areas and subsequently produce centrifugal propagation of damage (Mann, 1988). Indeed, neurotropic viral and toxin selectivity is well documented. For example, Barnett et al. (1993) employed in situ hybridization to compare the spread of two viruses, herpes simplex virus type I and a mouse hepatitis virus strain (JHM), through the olfactory pathways of the mouse. While both viruses entered the brain via the olfactory system, only herpes simplex-infected noradrenergic neurons in the locus coeruleus. Although both viruses infected dopaminergic neurons in the ventral tegmental area, mouse hepatitis virus produced much more widespread infection. Although these arguments are somewhat circular, and the site of initial damage in AD is not yet established, on balance we favor a centrifugal process.

Nasal Metabolism of Xenobiotics. As a first line of defense against xenobiotics, several studies imply that the nasal cytochrome system is probably as important as that of the liver. In some instances, microsomes in the olfactory epithelium have higher levels of cytochrome P450 and other detoxification enzymes than those in the liver (Hext & Lock, 1992; Ding & Xie, 2015). In the monkey, P450 levels are higher in the olfactory bulb than in other brain structures (Iscan et al., 1990). Compounds shown to be metabolized in vitro by the nasal P450 dependent mono-oxygenase system include nasal decongestants, essences, anesthetics, alcohols, nicotine, cocaine, and many nasal carcinogens (Dahl, 1988). Importantly, individuals with a mutation in the P450 cytochrome CYP2D6-debrisoquine hydroxylase gene appear to have increased risk for PD (Smith et al., 1992; Elbaz et al., 2004), raising the possibility that a compromised P450 enzyme system may facilitate the penetration of xenobiotics into brain tissue, leading to neural damage. The existence of familial forms of AD or PD does not exclude the possibility that a breakdown occurs in metabolic pathways at some stage (such as cytochrome P450 within the olfactory mucosa), thereby rendering such individuals more susceptible to neurotoxic environmental agents. In accord with this are studies suggesting that tobacco smokers have reduced risk of contracting PD but not AD (Tanner et al., 2002; Aggarwal et al., 2006), and that smoking may protect the olfactory system from damage by industrial exposure to methacrylates, acrylates, and acetone (Schwartz et al., 1989; Schwartz et al., 1990). Cigarette smoke contains high levels (100–250 ng/cigarette) of polyaromatic hydrocarbons which are known to induce cytochrome P-450 enzyme activity. Stimulation of such enzymes leads to increased metabolism of xenobiotics in the olfactory epithelium (as well as the liver), conceivably preventing environmental neurotoxins from reaching their target organs (Gresham et al., 1993). Of possible relevance, although speculative, is the fact that elderly dogs may spontaneously display Alzheimer-type pathology (Papaioannou et al., 2001), but they do not develop PD spontaneously nor do they show Lewy pathology in the substantia nigra (Uchida et al., 2003). This may relate to their highly developed nasal detoxification system, which protects their brain against PD. If this preliminary observation is confirmed, it lends support to the OVH for PD but not for AD.

Clearly, the aforementioned evidence for nasal entry of a pathogen that might cause AD is less persuasive than for PD. If such an AD-related pathogen does enter the brain via the olfactory fila, it probably influences central more than peripheral brain structures. In PD, the argument is more convincing, but the presence of early CN IX and CN X pathology in the medulla presents a potential barrier to acceptance. It could be argued that a pathogen such as a neurotropic virus enters the nose, damages the sense of smell, and then travels along sensory fibers of CN IX and CN X in the pharynx to reach the medulla. However, the medullary nuclei of these cranial nerves are spared in the early stages of PD (Braak et al., 2003b). Wakabayashi (1990) and Braak et al. (2006) showed Lewy pathology in Auerbach's and Meissner's plexus in the stomach wall (Figure 7.5), which led to the proposal that the pathogen ascends retrogradely in the motor fibers of the vagus to its medullary nucleus (Braak et al., 2006). Retrograde vagal entry into the CNS, of course, will not explain the early peripheral olfactory changes. To explain such initial pathology, a pathogen would concurrently need to enter and damage the olfactory pathway via the nose, be swallowed in nasal secretions, invade the enteric plexus of the stomach, and ascend in motor vagal fibers. This sequence of somewhat tortuous events has been termed the "dual hit" hypothesis because of the simultaneous entry of pathogen via the nose and stomach (Hawkes et al., 2007). Further studies, now underway, may clarify this interesting lead.

Summary

The olfactory vector hypothesis for AD and PD proposes that an initiating event may be entry of a pathogen through the nose prior to brain invasion. Although this hypothesis has been discounted by many critics, its viability is still unclear and the possibility exists that exogenous agents are responsible for the olfactory loss and initiation of central pathology in genetically susceptible individuals. Whether and how this occurs is largely unknown, although it clearly represents a challenging question for future research.

Gustatory Disorders

Taste Disorder in Dementia

The majority of studies relating to taste dysfunction in dementia concern Alzheimer's disease (AD). Given the widespread involvement in the cerebral hemispheres, particularly the parieto-temporal areas, some impairment of taste in the later stages would not be surprising. The first and second order neurons in the brain stem and VPMpc thalamic nuclei are not involved in early stages of AD, thus it is likely that any taste impairment in AD will relate to pathology in the anterior insula and orbitofrontal cortex, i.e., stage IV, which is a moderately advanced stage of disease.

Probably the first, but somewhat rudimentary, evaluation of taste in dementia was made by Waldton in 66 females, with a diagnosis of "senile dementia" all verified (probably macroscopically) at autopsy (Waldton, 1974). He observed marked impairment of olfaction and taste that occurred relatively early in the disease course and progressed over a three-year period of follow-up. A subsequent study of taste assessed 10 males with early AD using a threshold procedure to sucrose and citric acid (Koss et al., 1988). No abnormality was found in taste or smell threshold but there was significant impairment of smell identification. A further investigation examined taste threshold in various dementias (Schiffman et al., 1990) and found that taste thresholds were raised to glutamic acid in most varieties of dementias, but this was not specific for AD. Thresholds to the bitter-tasting chemical, quinine, were no different from age-matched controls. Eight years later, Bacon and colleagues examined taste thresholds to sucrose in a small group of subjects at risk of AD and found no abnormality compared to controls (Bacon et al., 1998).

A different approach was employed in a group of 20 patients with a clinical diagnosis of AD by Broggio et al. (2001). They aimed to determine which of the three stages in gustatory information processing might be involved in AD, classified according to severity. These stages were represented by (a) same: difference testing (discrimination stage), (b) match-to-sample testing (associative stage), and (c) verbal taste quality identification testing (verbal stage). They used various foodstuffs found in a normal diet and discovered

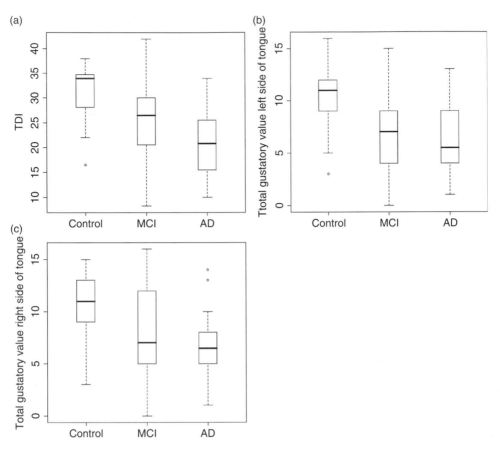

Figure 7.16 A. TDI (threshold-discrimination-identification olfactory score) in controls, MCI and AD groups. B. Total gustatory score on right side of tongue in controls, MCI and AD. C. Total gustatory score on left side of tongue in controls, MCI and AD. Adapted with permission from: Steinbach et al. (2010).

impairment in all three stages. It was suggested that patients with early AD had deficits in taste quality identification, suggesting to the authors that the origin of the problem affected central rather than peripheral areas of the CNS.

A detailed assessment of chemosensory function was undertaken in 33 subjects at risk for AD by Schiffman et al. (2002). Tests of taste threshold, memory recognition, and identification were performed. Of these three components, taste memory was impaired at baseline and at review 18 months later. Over time, taste memory worsened, likewise the threshold to glutamate but not to quinine (as shown earlier for AD by the same group). A further study employed taste strips and whole-mouth tastants in 24 subjects with AD and another group of non-Alzheimer type dementia but mostly the vascular form (Lang et al., 2006). Both the AD and non-AD groups had abnormal values and the severity of dementia correlated with the taste strip results. Steinbach et al. (2010) conducted a scholarly appraisal of taste in subjects with mild cognitive impairment and AD. Twenty-nine healthy controls were compared to 29 subjects with mild cognitive impairment (MCI) and 30 with AD. Taste was assessed with impregnated strips to the four basic tastants (sucrose, citric acid, sodium chloride, quinine) at varying concentration applied to either side of the tongue. There was a significant reduction of total taste scores and values for individual tastes on either side of the tongue between controls and the combined MCI/AD subjects, but no difference was found between the MCI and AD group (Figure 7.16). It was suggested that a taste test may be useful for differentiating healthy subjects from those with MCI or AD but separation of MCI from AD would require olfactory tests, cognitive screening, apo-E4 status, and imaging (MRI or PET).

In summary, and despite varying and sometimes conflicting opinions, in part relating to small numbers of patients and test procedures of varying reliability, the more robust studies (Schiffman et al., 2002; Steinbach et al., 2010) suggest that there is mild and slowly progressive impairment of taste in the early clinical stages of AD and probably in some family members at risk of future disease. Taste impairment in AD indicates moderately advanced disease (Braak stage IV) from the neuropathological aspect and should alert the clinician to this degree of severity – likewise for PD as described below. The magnitude of the taste defect is probably much less than that of olfaction both for existing cases and as a predictive marker.

Taste Disorder in Classic Parkinson Disease

Detailed studies of PD neuroanatomy show that the taste pathway is spared within the brain stem and thalamus, but there is Lewy pathology in the frontal insular region, an important relay station for taste fibers destined for the orbitofrontal cortex (Braak et al., 2003a; see Chapter 2). A recent study showed that Lewy bodies were present in submandibular glands of all nine PD patients examined (Del Tredici et al., 2010). This is relevant because disease in the salivary glands might affect the quantity and consistency of saliva and could have indirect effects on the ability to taste. Despite this there is uncertainly with regard to taste, in stark contrast to olfaction.

Questionnaire analyses, although fraught with recall problems and confusion with smell disorder (that usually co-exists), infer that impaired "taste" is moderately prevalent in PD. Thus, a study from London UK (Politis et al., 2010) assessed 265 consecutive PD patients and asked them to rank their three most troublesome complaints in the past six months. In their early PD group, disorder of smell and/or taste was listed in the five most prevalent complaints. Another study of 285 PD patients from Japan (Kashihara et al., 2011) found that 26 (9%) thought their taste appreciation was diminished.

In one of the earliest investigations of 25 PD patients and 16 normal controls, Travers et al. (1993) found that pleasantness ratings of their patients increased monotonically across six ascending suprathreshold concentrations of sucrose, whereas those of the controls reversed at one of the higher concentrations, resulting in an inverted U-shaped function. Conceivably the PD patients perceived the higher sucrose concentrations as weaker and therefore did not experience them as less pleasant; the latter is a well-established phenomenon in normal subjects.

In the first large study with detailed taste measurement (Sienkiewicz-Jarosz et al., 2005), 33 controls and 30 PD patients were assessed by (a) individual paper disks soaked in sucrose, quinine, citric acid, or sodium chloride, (b) 100 ml samples of chocolate and vanilla milk, and (c) taste threshold with the Rion TR-06 electrogustometer. No abnormalities were found in response to pleasant or unpleasant taste stimuli. Some PD patients rated, on average, a 0.025% concentration of quinine as *more intense* than did the controls (p < 0.04) and exhibited *lower* electrical taste thresholds on electrogustometry (p < 0.001). A subsequent study of 20 PD patients and 20 age-matched controls by this group did not replicate the electrogustometric finding; however, a 1% sucrose solution applied to the anterior tongue using a syringe was rated as *more intense* by the PD patients than by the controls in a fashion similar to that observed earlier for quinine (Sienkiewicz-Jarosz et al., 2013).

A further study (mentioned above in the Dementia section) examined taste in 52 patients with various forms of dementia (Lang et al., 2006), of whom 6 had non-Alzheimer type dementia with parkinsonism. Taste was assessed by whole-mouth and taste-strip tests and the patients' results compared to a control group consisting of 52 patients with minor strokes or vascular risk factors without stroke, some of whom had mild cognitive impairment as measured by the Mini-Mental State Examination (MMSE). In the six demented PD patients, taste was impaired in comparison to the dementia patients without parkinsonism. A year later, Moberg et al. (2007) found that only 24 % of 56 patients with PD were able to detect bitter-tasting phenylthiocarbamide (PTC), as compared to 75 % of 20 healthy controls, implying a bitter-taste deficit in PD.

This unclear position prompted further analysis of the possible association between non-demented PD subjects and taste appreciation by Shah et al. (2009). Taste was estimated using the Rion electrogustometer and olfaction by the UPSIT in 75 non-demented PD patients and 74 controls. There was significant impairment of taste threshold in 27 percent (20/75) of the patients and this involved both the chorda tympani (anterior) and the glossopharyngeal (posterior) innervated sectors of the tongue. Mean thresholds in the PD group were around three times higher than controls. The taste abnormality was uninfluenced by age, duration of symptoms, disability, and smoking. Although olfaction was profoundly disordered, there was no correlation between taste and smell dysfunction. Sensitivity analysis suggested that a provisional diagnosis of PD would be confirmed if smell or taste were abnormal; conversely the diagnosis would merit review if both modalities were normal. These findings were confirmed in a further study of taste in a separate group of 50 PD subjects (Deeb et al., 2010), but *lowered* thresholds were not observed. Given the sparing of the first- and second-order taste neurons in PD (Braak et al., 2003a), it was concluded that disorder of taste in PD most likely signifies involvement of the anterior insula or orbitofrontal cortex, in keeping with advanced disease, i.e., Braak stage 5, although confounding by drug effects and changes in salivary constitution cannot be excluded. Subsequently, Kim et al. (2011), in a study from Korea, that used taste strips, found that taste was slightly impaired overall in their 31 PD patients. However, they observed significant changes only in women, an effect suspected to be due to a lower MMSE score in males, echoing the findings in the German study described above (Lang et al., 2006).

More recently, Doty et al. (2015) evaluated taste in detail using whole-mouth and regional taste tests in multiple concentrations, as well as electrogustometry (limited to the anterior tongue). Twenty-nine early stage patients with PD and 29 matched controls were tested on and off dopamine-related medications. Whole-mouth taste identification scores for all stimuli were, on average, nominally lower for the PD patients than for the controls, but a trend in the *opposite* direction was noted for intensity ratings at the lower stimulus concentrations for all stimuli except caffeine. Regional testing demonstrated that PD subjects, relative to controls, generally rated sweet-, sour-, bitter-, and salty-tasting stimuli as more intense on the anterior tongue and less intense on the posterior tongue. Whole-mouth taste identification test scores for all stimuli were, on average, nominally lower for the PD patients than for the controls. No measurable effects were noted on EGM. There were no significant associations evident between taste and UPDRS scores, dopamine-related medications, or dopamine transporter uptake imaging. The authors suggested that PD-related damage to the posterior tongue (CN IX), which conceivably could occur from brainstem damage, might release central inhibition on the anterior tongue (CN VII), thereby enhancing taste on this segment of the tongue. Such a mechanism would be akin to the taste enhancement in the posterior tongue region after anesthetizing the lingual nerve, which supplies taste to the anterior tongue via the chorda tympani (Lehman et al., 1995). Thus, paradoxical increase of taste intensity would be compatible with damage to central taste pathways and is in accord with the earlier findings of Sienkiewicz-Jarosz et al. (2005, 2013).

Conclusion. Evidence for severe taste impairment is lacking for classic PD. Any changes in the early stage of disease are likely to be subtle and not noticed by patients. Overall. there is probably mild impairment of gustation affecting about one-quarter of patients. Interestingly, several studies find that PD patients report the intensity of various tastants as more intense on the anterior tongue than do normal controls. If taste loss in PD is secondary to Lewy pathology, then it has likely spread into the anterior insula, equating to at least Braak stage 5 and moderately severe disability.

Amyotrophic Lateral Sclerosis (Motor Neuron Disease)

Impairment of taste is described in ALS and it is sometimes mentioned informally by patients prior to disease onset. Two patients reported from Berlin experienced initial symptoms of persistent bitter or metallic taste, in one instance principally affecting the posterior tongue (Petzold et al., 2003). Whole-mouth testing to sodium chloride, sucrose, citric acid, and quinine was normal. Neither subject was taking Riluzole, which is standard ALS medication known to impair taste, and the dysgeusia antedated the diagnosis. Presumably these patients had true taste impairment rather than smell loss, given that the report of "bitter" or "metallic" would be unusual for an olfactory problem. There is no known ALS pathology in the taste pathways but it was speculated that their patients might have a mild sensory neuropathy affecting the chorda tympani or that there was a dysautonomia involving the solitary tract nucleus.

Facial Onset Sensori-Motor Neuropathy (FOSMN). This is a novel variant of motor neuron disease with superficial resemblance to syringomyelia (Vucic et al., 2006). Initial symptoms comprise facial sensory loss that spreads over the head, upper limbs, and trunk. Later, there is involvement of bulbar muscles and limb weakness. Three of the original four middle-aged male patients complained of taste loss (Vucic et al., 2006). In one case it accompanied trigeminal sensory loss five years before spread of the facial numbness. At autopsy there was neuronal loss in the solitary tract nucleus. In a subsequent article, "complete loss of taste and smell" was reported in another individual with FOSMN, but at post mortem involvement of the solitary tract nucleus was not commented on (Ziso et al., 2015). No chemosensory measurements appear to have been undertaken in any patient. In one personal case, symptomatic taste impairment preceded facial sensory symptoms by some 10 years, suggesting that ageusia might be a useful biomarker of future disease.

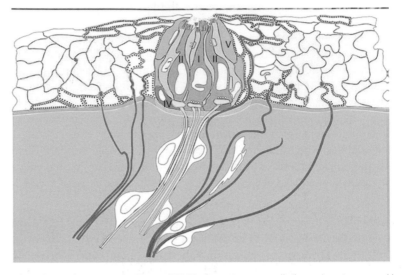

Figure 7.17 Brain-Derived Neurotrophic Factor (BDNF)-expressing taste cells (brown) are innervated by gustatory chorda tympani axons (yellow). Many of the cells surrounding the taste bud are innervated by somatosensory lingual nerve axons (light blue) and express neurotrophin-3 (NT3; light blue) and p75 Nerve Growth Factor Receptor (NGFR; dots). Types of taste bud cells (I-V) according to Reutter and Witt. Adapted with permission from Oakley & Witt (2004). (A black and white version of this figure will appear in some formats. For the colour version, please refer to the plate section.)

Other "Neurodegenerative" Conditions

We have been unable to locate any study of gustatory disorder in parkinson*ism* or familial PD and there appears to be no evidence that diminished taste is a prodromal feature of PD, although theoretically taste impairment is a potential late feature according to Braak staging of the classic pathology. In Huntington's disease (HD), there is indirect evidence of impaired taste perception. An abnormally dry mouth is reported in HD compared to controls (Wood et al., 2008), possibly resulting from elevated serum vasopressin levels and this may have a secondary effect on taste sensation. Two groups reported impaired feelings of disgust in response to unpleasant odors and tastes (Mitchell et al., 2005; Hayes et al., 2007), but there has been no detailed examination of taste in this disorder.

As mentioned in Chapter 1, support of developing neurons by neurotrophins is of major importance in the development of fungiform papillae and taste buds. There are four neurotrophins of potential relevance to human diseases: nerve growth factor (NGF), brain-derived neurotrophic factor (BDNF), neurotrophin-3 (NT3), and neurotrophin-4 (NT4) – see Figure 7.17. These are all responsible for axonal guidance to the appropriate target tissue and such support is required for the development of sensory receptors in the tongue. Thus, it was shown that BDNF double knockout mice (BDNF$^{-/-}$) had fewer fungiform papillae, malformed circumvallate papillae and a 35% reduction in the number of intragemmal fibers (i.e., within the taste bud) whereas NT3$^{-/-}$ mice had reduced somatosensory innervation to the tongue, under-developed filiform papillae, and some malformed or non-innervated circumvallate papillae (Nosrat, 1998).

According to a novel proposal (Gardiner et al., 2008), several neurological disorders may be grouped according to those with (a) reduced papillae such as Machado-Joseph disease,

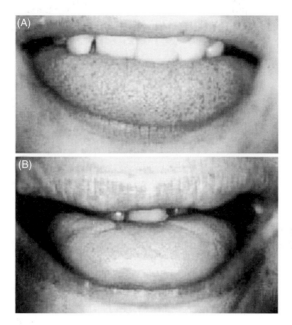

Figure 7.18 Images of normal (A) and familial dysautonomic (B) tongues. Red fungiform papillae are obvious on the normal tongue and missing on the familial dysautonomic tongue. Images courtesy of Professor Felicia Axelrod MD, New York University. (A black and white version of this figure will appear in some formats. For the color version, please refer to the plate section.)

Stüve-Wiedemann syndrome, familial dysautonomia, torsion dystonia, and Behçet's disease, and (b) those with taste defects only such as Alzheimer's disease, Huntington's disease, hereditary sensory and autonomic neuropathy type 4, and diabetes mellitus. Evidence for taste impairment in torsion dystonia and Behçet's disease is weak. Only the first three conditions in the reduced papillae group will now be reviewed.

Machado-Joseph Disease (MJD). This is autosomal dominant spino-cerebellar ataxia type 3 (SCA 3) which was described originally in people born in the Azores. It is now known to be due to a trinucleotide repeat disorder in the gene coding for Ataxin-3 located on 14q. Olfaction is either normal or mildly affected as reviewed above. In one Japanese family that comprised three people affected by MJD, fungiform papillae and taste buds were absent (Uchiyama et al., 2001) and one was ageusic to formal testing. This observation led to the proposal that the gustatory problem might relate to a neurotrophic defect in the pathway connecting the fungiform papillae and CN VII (Gardiner et al., 2008).

Stüve-Wiedemann Syndrome or Schwartz-Jampel Syndrome Type 2. This is an autosomal recessive condition due to a mutation in the leukemia inhibitory factor receptor gene (LIFR) located on chromosome 5p13. There are multiple skeletal abnormalities, contractures, dysautonomia, and a smooth tongue due to absent fungiform papillae. It is suggested that there may be a defect of neurotrophic support underlying this condition. There appear to be no published formal studies of taste in this disorder but impairment is likely to be found.

Familial Dysautonomia (FD; also called Riley-Day Syndrome, Hereditary Sensory and Autonomic Neuropathy Type 3). This is an autosomal recessive disorder mainly affecting Jewish people due to mutations in the IKBKAP gene located on chromosome 9q. Common features include defective lacrimation, absent fungiform papillae (Figure 7.18), impaired taste, vasomotor instability, and indifference to pain and temperature. The only examination of taste and smell ability in FD was somewhat crudely measured in nine patients by "psychophysical-cognitive and reflex-like facial-behavioral responses" to taste and smell (Gadoth et al., 1997). Five taste stimulants were presented to patients and 15 healthy controls. Those with FD showed a higher incidence of recognition failures for salty, bitter, sweet, and water stimuli than controls, but the rate of recognition of sour stimuli was similar in the two groups. There was relatively normal sensitivity for sour and to a lesser extent for bitter stimuli, findings which lead the authors to propose a specific rather than general dysgeusia. Smell responses were normal. Given the lack of taste buds these findings are not surprising.

Conclusion. It is likely that taste is slightly impaired early in Alzheimer's disease and that the defect gradually progresses. In Parkinson's disease the existence of dysgeusia is controversial but most likely taste is impaired mildly as a late feature in around one-quarter of subjects. Paradoxical increased taste sensitivity is sometimes found. It is unclear whether the deficiency progresses with time, but such a defect is ominous as it probably indicates spread of pathology to the frontal lobe (Braak stage 5). Of the miscellaneous conditions – Huntington's chorea, ALS, Machado-Joseph disease, Stüve-Wiedemann syndrome (Schwartz-Jampel syndrome), and familial dysautonomia – there is only indirect evidence of taste impairment either from psychophysical tests or assessment of fungiform papillae on the tongue surface. These disorders would all benefit from further appraisal.

References

Abele, M., Riet, A., Hummel, T., Klockgether, T., Wullner U. 2003.Olfactory dysfunction in cerebellar ataxia and multiple system atrophy. *Journal of Neurology* **250**, 1453–1455.

Adler, C.H., Caviness, J.N., Sabbagh, M.N., et al. 2005. Olfactory testing in Parkinson's disease and other movement disorders: Correlation with Parkinsonian severity. *Movement Disorders* **20**(Supplement 10), Abs: 231.

Aggarwal, N.T., Bienias, J.L., Bennett, D.A., et al. 2006. The relation of cigarette smoking to incident Alzheimer's disease in a biracial urban community population. *Neuroepidemiology* **26**(3), 140–146.

Ahlskog, J.E., Waring, S.C., Petersen, R.C., et al. 1998. Olfactory dysfunction in Guamanian ALS, parkinsonism, and dementia. *Neurology* **51**, 1672–1677.

Alcalay, R.N., Siderowf, A., Ottman, R., et al. 2011. Olfaction in Parkin heterozygotes and compound heterozygotes: The CORE-PD study. *Neurology* **76**, 319–326.

Altinayar, S., Oner, S., Can, S., Kizilay, A., Sarac, K., 2014. Olfactory disfunction and its relation olfactor bulbus volume in Parkinson's disease. *European Review for Medical and Pharmacological Sciences* **18**(23), 3659–3664.

Altschuler, E., 1996. Gastric Helicobacter pylori infection as a cause of idiopathic Parkinson disease and non-arteric anterior optic ischemic neuropathy. *Medical Hypotheses* **47**(5), 413–414.

Ansari, K.A., Johnson, A., 1975. Olfactory function in patients with Parkinson's disease. *Journal of Chronic Diseases* **28**, 493–497.

Antunes, M., Bowler, R.M., Doty, R.L., 2007. San Francisco/Oakland Bay Bridge Welder Study: Olfactory function. *Neurology* **69**, 1278–1284.

Armstrong, C., Harrison, W.T., 1935. Prevention of intranasally-inoculated poliomyelitis of monkeys by instillation of alum into the nostrils. *Public Health Reports* 50, 725–730.

Arriagada, P.V., Louis, D.N., Hedley-Whyte, E.T., Hyman, B.T., 1991. Neurofibrillary tangles and olfactory dysgenesis. *Lancet* 337, 559.

Ascherio, A., Chen, H., Weisskopf, M.G., et al. 2006. Pesticide exposure and risk for Parkinson's disease. *Annals of Neurology* 60, 197–203.

Attems, J., Lintner, F., Jellinger, K.A., 2005. Olfactory involvement in aging and Alzheimer's disease: an autopsy study. *Journal of Alzheimer's Disease* 7(2), 149–157.

Bacon, A.W., Bondi, M.W., Salmon, D.P., Murphy, C., 1998. Very early changes in olfactory functioning due to Alzheimer's disease and the role of apolipoprotein E in olfaction. *Annals of the New York Academy of Sciences* 855, 723–731.

Bahar-Fuchs, A., Moss, S., Rose, C., Savage, G., 2010. Olfactory performance in AD, aMCI, and healthy aging: A unirhinal approach. *Chemical Senses* 35, 855–862.

Bak, T.H., Chandran, S., 2011. What wires together dies together: Verbs, actions and neurodegeneration in motor neuron disease. *Cortex* 48, 936–944.

Baker, K.B., Montgomery, E.B. Jr., 2001. Performance on the PD test battery by relatives of patients with progressive supranuclear palsy. *Neurology* 56, 25–30.

Bakija-Konsuo, A., Mulic, R., Boraska, V., et al. 2011. Leprosy epidemics during history increased protective allele frequency of PARK2/PACRG genes in the population of the Mljet Island, Croatia. *European Journal of Medical Genetics* 54, e548–e552.

Ball, M.J., Nuttall, K., 1980. Neurofibrillary tangles granulovacuolar degeneration and neuron loss in Down's syndrome: Quantitative comparison with Alzheimer's dementia. *Annals of Neurology* 7, 462–465.

Ballard, C., Ziabreva, I., Perry, R., et al. 2006. Differences in neuropathologic characteristics across the Lewy body dementia spectrum. *Neurology* 67, 1931–1934.

Bannier, S., Berdague, J.L., Rieu, I., et al. 2012. Prevalence and phenomenology of olfactory hallucinations in Parkinson's disease. *Journal of Neurology, Neurosurgery, & Psychiatry* 83, 1019–1021.

Barnett, E.M., Cassell, M.D., Perlman, S., 1993. Two neurotropic viruses, herpes simplex virus type 1 and mouse hepatitis virus, spread along different neural pathways from the main olfactory bulb. *Neuroscience* 57, 1007–1025.

Barrios, F.A., Gonzalez, L., Favila, R., et al. 2007. Olfaction and neurodegeneration in HD. *Neuroreport* 18, 73–76.

Bar-Sela, S., Reingold, S., Richter, E.D., 2001. Amyotrophic lateral sclerosis in a battery-factory worker exposed to cadmium. *International Journal of Occupational and Environmental Health* 7, 109.

Barz, S., Hummel, T., Pauli, E., et al. 1997. Chemosensory event-related potentials in response to trigeminal and olfactory stimulation in idiopathic Parkinson's disease. *Neurology* 49, 1424–1431.

Beach, T.G., White, C.L. 3rd, Hladik, C.L., et al. 2009. Olfactory bulb alpha-synucleinopathy has high specificity and sensitivity for Lewy body disorders. *Acta Neuropathologica* 117(2), 169–174.

Beavan, M., McNeill, A., Proukakis, C., et al. 2015. Evolution of prodromal clinical markers of Parkinson disease in a GBA mutation-positive cohort. *JAMA Neurology* 72, 201–208.

Bedard, A., Parent, A., 2004. Evidence of newly generated neurons in the human olfactory bulb. *Developmental Brain Research* 151, 159–168.

Belluscio, L., Gold, G.H., Nemes, A., Axel, R., 1998. Mice deficient in G(olf) are anosmic. *Neuron* 20, 69–81.

Belzunegui, S., Sebastian, W.S., Garrido-Gil, P., 2007. The number of dopaminergic cells is increased in the olfactory bulb of monkeys chronically exposed to MPTP. *Synapse* 61, 1006–1012.

Berendse, H.W., Roos, D.S., Raijmakers, P., Doty, R.L., 2011. Motor and non-motor correlates of olfactory dysfunction in Parkinson's disease. *Journal of the Neurological Sciences* 310, 21–24.

Berger, P.C., Vogel, F.S., 1973. The development of the pathologic changes of Alzheimer's disease and senile dementia in patients with Down's syndrome. *American Journal of Pathology* 73, 457–476.

Bessen, R.A., Shearin, H., Martinka, S., et al. 2010. Prion shedding from olfactory neurons into nasal secretions. *PLoS Pathogens* **6**, e1000837.

Bessen, R.A., Wilham, J.M., Lowe, D., Watschke, C.P., Shearin, H., Martinka, S., Caughey, B., Wiley, J.A., 2011. Accelerated shedding of prions following damage to the olfactory epithelium. *Journal of Virology* **86**(3), 1777–1788.

Betarbet, R., Sherer, T.B., MacKenzie, G., et al. 2000. Chronic systemic pesticide exposure reproduces features of Parkinson's disease. *Nature Neuroscience* **3**, 1301–1306.

Boesveldt, S., Verbaan, D., Knol, D.L., et al. 2008. A comparative study of odor identification and odor discrimination deficits in Parkinson's disease. *Movement Disorders* **23**, 1984–1990.

Boeve, B.F., Silber, M.H., Parisi, J.E., et al. 2003. Synucleinopathy pathology and REM sleep behavior disorder plus dementia or parkinsonism. *Neurology* **61**, 40–45.

Bogerts, B., Hantsch, J., Herzer, M., 1983. A Morphometric Study of the Dopamine-Containing Cell Groups in the Mesencephalon of Normals, Parkinson Patients, and Schizophrenics. *Biological Psychiatry* **18**, 951–969.

Bohnen, N.I., Gedela, S., Herath, P., Constantine, G.M., Moore, R.Y., 2008. Selective hyposmia in Parkinson disease: association with hippocampal dopamine activity. *Neuroscience Letters* **447**, 12–16.

Bohnen, N.I., Gedela, S., Kuwabara, H., et al. 2007. Selective hyposmia and nigrostriatal dopaminergic denervation in Parkinson's disease. *Journal of Neurology* **254**, 84–90.

Bohnen, N.I., Muller, M.L., Kotagal, V., et al. 2010. Olfactory dysfunction, central cholinergic integrity and cognitive impairment in Parkinson's disease. *Brain* **133**, 1747–1754.

Bond, J.A., 1986. Bioactivation and biotransformation of xenobiotics in rat nasal tissue. In: *Toxicology of the Nasal Passages*. Ed. C.S. Barrow. Washington DC: Hemisphere Publishing Corporation pp. 249–261.

Bostantjopoulou, S., Katsarou, Z., Papadimitriou, A., et al. 2001. Clinical features of parkinsonian patients with the alpha-synuclein (G209A) mutation. *Movement Disorders* **16**, 1007–1013.

Bovi, T., Antonini, A., Ottaviani, S., et al. 2010. The status of olfactory function and the striatal dopaminergic system in drug-induced parkinsonism. *Journal of Neurology* **257**, 1882–1889.

Bower, J.H., Maraganore, D.M., Peterson, B.J., Ahlskog, J.E., Rocca, W.A., 2006. Immunologic diseases, anti-inflammatory drugs, and Parkinson disease: a case-control study. *Neurology* **67**, 494–496.

Braak, H., Braak, E., 1991. Neuropathological stageing of Alzheimer-related changes. *Acta Neuropathologica* **82**(4), 239–259.

Braak, H., Braak, E., 1998. Evolution of neuronal changes in the course of Alzheimer's disease. *Journal of Neural Transmission* **53**, 127–140.

Braak, H., de Vos, R.A., Bohl, J., Del Tredici, K., 2006. Gastric α-synuclein immunoreactive inclusions in Meissner's and Auerbach's plexuses in cases staged for Parkinson's disease-related brain pathology. *Neuroscience Letters* **396**(1), 67–72.

Braak, H., Del Tredici, K., 2011. The pathological process underlying Alzheimer's disease in individuals under thirty. *Acta Neuropathologica* **121**, 171–181.

Braak, H., Del Tredici, K., Rub, U., et al. 2003a. Staging of brain pathology related to sporadic Parkinson's disease. *Neurobiology of Aging* **24**, 197–211.

Braak, H., Rub, U., Gai, W.P., Del Tredici, K. 2003b. Idiopathic Parkinson's disease: Possible routes by which vulnerable neuronal types may be subject to neuroinvasion by an unknown pathogen. *Journal of Neural Transmission* **110**, 517–536.

Braak, H., Thal, D.R., Ghebremedhin, E., Del, T.K., 2011. Stages of the pathologic process in Alzheimer disease: Age categories from 1 to 100 years. *Journal of Neuropathology and Experimental Neurology* **70**, 960–969.

Braga-Neto, P., Felicio, A.C., Pedroso, J.L., et al. 2011. Clinical correlates of olfactory dysfunction in spinocerebellar ataxia type 3. *Parkinsonism & Related Disorders* **17**, 353–356.

Branco Germiniani, F., Cavalcante, T., Moro, A., et al. 2014. Evaluation of olfactory function in Friedreich's ataxia: A case-control study. *European Journal of Neurology* **21**, 175–175.

Brittebo, E.B., Eriksson, V.F., Bakke, J., Brandt, I., 1991. Toxicity of 2 6-dichlorothiobenzamide (Chlorthiamid) and 2 6-dichlorobenzamide in the olfactory nasal mucosa of mice. *Fundamental and Applied Toxicology* 17, 92–102.

Brodoehl, S., Klingner, C., Volk, G.F., et al. 2012. Decreased olfactory bulb volume in idiopathic Parkinson's disease detected by 3.0-Tesla magnetic resonance imaging. *Movement Disorders* 27, 1019–1025.

Broggio, E., Pluchon, C., Ingrand, P., Gil, R., 2001. Taste impairment in Alzheimer's disease. *Revue Neurologique* 157(4), 409–413.

Brousseau, K., Brainerd, H.G., *Mongolism: A Study of the Physical and Mental Characteristics of Mongolian Imbeciles.* Baltimore: Williams and Wilkins. 1928.

Busenbark, K.L., Huber, S.J., Greer, G., Pahwa, R., Koller, W.C., 1992. Olfactory function in essential tremor. *Neurology* 42, 1631–1632.

Buxton, P.H., Hayward, M., 1967. Polyneuritis cranialis associated with industrial trichloroethylene exposure. *Journal of Neurology, Neurosurgery, & Psychiatry* 30, 511–518.

Bylsma, F.W., Moberg, P.J., Doty, R.L., Brandt, J., 1997. Odour identification in Huntington's disease patients and their offspring with and without the genetic mutation for HD. *Journal of Neuropsychology and Clinical Neuroscience* 9, 598–600

Calderón-Garcidueñas, L., Reed, W., Maronpot, R.R., et al. 2004. Brain inflammation and Alzheimer's-like pathology in individuals exposed to severe air pollution. *Toxicologic Pathology* 32(6), 650–658.

Calderón-Garcidueñas, L., Franco-Lira, M., Henríquez-Roldán, C., et al. 2010. Urban air pollution: Influences on olfactory function and pathology in exposed children and young adults. *Experimental and Toxicologic Pathology* 62(1), 91–102.

Charles, P.C., Walters, E., Margolis, F., Johnston, R.E., 1995. Mechanism of neuroinvasion of Venezuelan equine encephalitis virus in the mouse. *Virology* 208, 662–671.

Chen, M.A., Lander, T.R., Murphy, C., 2006. Nasal health in Down syndrome: A cross-sectional study. *Otolaryngology – Head and Neck Surgery* 134, 741–745.

Chen, S., Tan, H.Y., Wu, Z.H., et al. 2014. Imaging of olfactory bulb and gray matter volumes in brain areas associated with olfactory function in patients with Parkinson's disease and multiple system atrophy. *European Journal of Radiology* 83, 564–570.

Connelly, T., Farmer, J., Lunch, D., Doty, R.L., 2003. Olfactory dysfunction in degenerative ataxias. *Journal of Neurology, Neurosurgery, & Psychiatry* 74(10), 1435–1437.

Constantinidis, J., de Ajuriaguerra, J., 1970. Syndrome familial avec tremblement parkinsonien et anosmie et sa thérapeutique par la L-dopa associée à un inhibiteur de la decarboxylase. *Thérapeutique (Semaine des Hôpitaux)*, 46, 263–269.

Crino, P.B., Martin, J.A., Hill, W.D., et al. 1995. Beta-amyloid peptide and amyloid precursor proteins in olfactory mucosa of patients with Alzheimer's disease Parkinson's disease and Down syndrome. *Annals of Otology, Rhinology, and Laryngology* 104, 655–661.

Dahl, A.R., 1986. Possible consequences of cytochrome P-450 dependent monooxygenases in nasal tissues. In: *Toxicology of the Nasal Passages*. Ed. Barrow, C.S. Hemisphere Publishing Corporation. Washington D.C.; 263–273.

Dahl, A.R., 1988. The effect of cytochrome P-450-dependent metabolism and other enzyme activities in olfaction. In: *Molecular Neurobiology of the Olfactory System*. Eds. Margolis, F.L., Getchell, T.V. Plenum press. New York; 51–70.

Daniel, S.E., Hawkes, C.H., 1992. Preliminary diagnosis of Parkinson's disease by olfactory bulb pathology [letter]. *Lancet* 340, 186.

Daum, R.F., Sekinger, B., Kobal, G., Lang, C.J., (2000) Riechprufung mit "sniffin' sticks" zur klinischen Diagnostik des Morbus Parkinson. *Nervenarzt* 71, 643–650.

Deeb, J., Shah, M., Muhammed, N., et al. 2010. A basic smeel test is as sensitive as a dopamine transporter scan: Comparison of olfaction, taste and DaTSCAN in the diagnosis of Parkinson's disease. *QJM* 103, 941–952.

Del Tredici, K., Hawkes, C.H., Ghebremedhin, E., Braak, H., 2010. Lewy pathology in the submandibular gland of individuals with incidental Lewy body disease and sporadic Parkinson's disease. *Acta Neuropathologica* **119**, 703–713.

Devanand, D.P., Liu, X., Tabert, M.H., et al. 2008. Combining early markers strongly predicts conversion from mild cognitive impairment to Alzheimer's disease. *Biological Psychiatry* **64**(10), 871–879.

Devanand, D.P., Michaels-Marston, K.S., Liu, X., et al. 2000. Olfactory deficits in patients with mild cognitive impairment predict Alzheimer's disease at follow-up. *American Journal of Psychiatry* **157**, 1399–1405.

Diaz-Maroto, M.C., Perez-Coello, M.S., Cabezudo, M.D., 2002. Headspace solid-phase microextraction analysis of volatile components of spices. *Chromatographia*, **55**, 723–728.

Ding Xie, F., 2015, Olfactory mucosa: Composition, enzymatic localization, and metabolism. In Doty R.L., (Ed.), *Handbook of Olfaction and Gustation*. Hoboken: John Wiley & Sons, pp. 63–91.

Djaldetti, R., Nageris, B.I., Lorberboym, M., et al. 2008 [(123)I]-FP-CIT SPECT and olfaction test in patients with combined postural and rest tremor. *Journal of Neural Transmission* **115**: 469–472.

Doty, R.L., 1991, Olfactory dysfunction in neurodegenerative disorders. In: Getchell, T.V., Doty, R.L., Bartoshuk, L.M., Snow, J.B., Jr. *Smell and Taste in Health and Disease*. New York: Raven Press, pp. 735–752.

Doty, R.L., 2001, Olfaction. *Annual Review of Psychology* **52**, 423–452.

Doty, R.L., 2008. The olfactory vector hypothesis of neurodegenerative disease: Is it viable? *Annals of Neurology* **63**, 7–15.

Doty, R.L., 2015a. Neurotoxic exposure and impairment of the chemical senses of taste and smell. *Handbook of Clinical Neurology* **131**, 299–324.

Doty, R.L., 2015b (Ed.), *Handbook of Olfaction and Gustation*. Hoboken: John Wiley & Sons.

Doty, R.L., 2017. Olfactory dysfunction in neurological diseases: Is there a common pathological substrate? *Lancet Neurology* **16**, 478–488.

Doty, R.L., Bayona, E.A., Leon-Ariza, D.S., et al. 2014. The lateralized smell test for detecting Alzheimer's disease: Failure to replicate. *Journal of the Neurological Sciences* **340**, 170–173.

Doty, R.L., Bromley, S.M., Moberg, P.J., Hummel, T., 1997. Laterality in human nasal chemoreception. Chapter 14. In: Christman S. (Ed.), *Cerebral Asymmetries in Sensory and Perceptual Processing*. Elsevier, pp. 497–542.

Doty, R.L., Deems, D.A., Stellar, S., 1988. Olfactory dysfunction in parkinsonism: A general deficit unrelated to neurologic signs, disease stage, or disease duration. *Neurology*, **38**, 1237–1244.

Doty, R.L., Golbe, L.I., McKeown, D.A., et al. 1993. Olfactory testing differentiates between progressive supranuclear palsy and idiopathic Parkinson's disease. *Neurology*, **43**, 962–965.

Doty, R.L., Hawkes, C.H., Good, K.P., Duda, J.E., 2015. Odor perception and neuropathology in neurodegenerative diseases and schizophrenia. In: Doty R.L. (Ed.), *Handbook of Olfaction and Gustation*. 3rd edition. Hoboken, NJ: John Wiley & Sons, pp. 403–451.

Doty, R.L., Nsoesie, M.T., Chung, I., et al. 2015. Taste function in early stage treated and untreated Parkinson's disease. *Journal of Neurology* **262**, 547–557.

Doty, R.L., Perl, D.P., Steele, J.C., et al. 1991a. Odor identification deficit of the parkinsonism-dementia complex of Guam: Equivalence to that of Alzheimer's and idiopathic Parkinson's disease. *Neurology* **41**, 77–80.

Doty, R.L., Reyes, P.F., Gregor, T., 1987, Presence of both odor identification and detection deficits in Alzheimer's disease. *Brain Research Bulletin* **18**, 597–600.

Doty, R.L., Riklan, M., Deems, D.A., Reynolds, C., Stellar, S., 1989. The olfactory and cognitive deficits of Parkinson's disease: Evidence for independence. *Annals of Neurology* **25**, 166–171.

Doty, R.L., Shaman, P., Applebaum, S.L., et al. 1984. Smell identification ability: Changes with age. *Science* **226**, 1441–1443.

Doty, R.L., Stern, M.B., Pfeiffer, C., Gollomp, S.M., Hurtig, H.I., 1992a. Bilateral olfactory dysfunction in early stage treated and untreated idiopathic Parkinson's disease. *Journal of Neurology, Neurosurgery, & Psychiatry* **55**, 138–142.

Doty, R.L., Singh, A., Tetrud, J., Langston, J.W., 1992b. Lack of major olfactory dysfunction in MPTP-induced parkinsonism. *Annals of Neurology* 32, 97–100.

Doty, R.L., Tourbier, I., Ng, V., et al. 2015. Influences of hormone replacement therapy on olfactory and cognitive function in postmenopausal women. *Neurobiology of Aging* 36(6), 2053–2059.

Double, K.L., Rowe, D.B., Hayes, M., et al. 2003. Identifying the pattern of olfactory deficits in Parkinson disease using the brief smell identification test. *Archives of Neurology* 60, 545–549.

Driver-Dunckley, E., Adler, C.H., Hentz, J.G., et al. 2014. Olfactory dysfunction in incidental Lewy body disease and Parkinson's disease. *Parkinsonism & Related Disorders* 20, 1260–1262.

Duda, J.E., Noorigian, J.V., Petrovitch, H., White, L.R., Ross, W.R., 2007. Pattern of Lewy body progression suggested Braak staging system is supported by analysis of a population based cohort of patients. *Movement Disorders* 22: Suppl 16, LB5 (late breaking abstract).

Duda, J.E., Shah, U., Arnold, S.E., Lee, V.M., Trojanowski, J.Q., 1999. The expression of alpha-beta- and gamma synucleins in olfactory mucosa from patients with and without neurodegenerative diseases. *Experimental Neurology* 160: 515–522.

Duff, K., McCaffrey, R.J., Solomon, G.S., 2002. The Pocket Smell Test: Successfully discriminating probable Alzheimer's dementia from vascular dementia and major depression. *Journal of Neuropsychiatry and Clinical Neurosciences*, 14(2), 197–201.

Dunn, L.M., 1981. *Peabody Picture Vocabulary Test-Revised Manual for Forms L and M.* American Guidance Service: Circle Pines, MN.

Dziewulska, D., Doi, H., Fasano, A., et al. 2013. Olfactory impairment and pathology in neurodegenerative disorders with brain iron accumulation. *Acta Neuropathologica* 126, 151–153.

Eggers, C., Schmidt, A., Hagenah, J., et al. 2010. Progression of subtle motor signs in PINK1 mutation carriers with mild dopaminergic deficit. *Neurology* 74, 1798–1805.

Elbaz, A., Levecque, C., Clavel, J., et al. 2004. CYP2D6 polymorphism pesticide exposure and Parkinson's disease. *Annals of Neurology* 55(3), 430–434.

Elian, M., 1991. Olfactory impairment in motor neuron disease: a pilot study. *Journal of Neurology, Neurosurgery, & Psychiatry* 54, 927–8

Esiri, M.M., 1991. Pathology of the olfactory and taste systems. In: Getchell, T.V., Doty, R.L., Bartoshuk, L.M., Snow, J.B., Jr. *Smell and Taste in Health and Disease.* N.Y.: Raven Press, pp. 683–701.

Evidente, V.G., Esteban, R.P., Hernandez, J.L., et al. 2004. Smell testing is abnormal in "lubag" or X-linked dystonia-parkinsonism: A pilot study. *Parkinsonism & Related Disorders* 10, 407–410.

Faber, H.K., Silverberg, R.J., 1946. A neuropathological study of acute human polio-myelitis with special reference to the inidtial lesio and various potential portals of entry. *Journal of Experimental Medicine* 83, 329–353.

Fearnley, J.M., Lees, A.J., 1991. Ageing and Parkinson's disease: substantia nigra regional selectivity. *Brain* 114, 2283–2301.

Fernandez-Ruiz, J., Diaz, R., Hall Haro, C., et al. 2003. Olfactory dysfunction in hereditary ataxia and basal ganglia disorders. *Neuroreport* 14(10), 1339–1341.

Ferraris, A., Ialongo, T., Passali, G.C., et al. 2009. Olfactory dysfunction in Parkinsonism caused by PINK1 mutations. *Movement Disorders* 24(16), 2350–2357.

Ferreira, J.J., Guedes, L.C., Rosa, M.M., et al. 2007. High prevalence of LRRK2 mutations in familial and sporadic Parkinson's disease in Portugal. *Movement Disorders*, 22, 1194–1201.

Ferreyra-Moyano, H., Barragan, E., 1989. The olfactory system and Alzheimer's disease. *International Journal of Neuroscience* 49, 157–197.

Fleming, S.M., Tetreault, N.A., Mulligan, C.K., et al. 2008. Olfactory deficits in mice overexpressing human wildtype alpha-synuclein. *European Journal of Neuroscience* 28, 247–256.

Flexner, S., Clark, P.F., 1912. A note on the mode of infection in epidemic poliomyelitis. *Proceedings of the Society for Experimental Biology & Medicine* 10, 1–2.

Flexner, S., Lewis, P.A., 1910. Experimental epidemic poliomyelitis in monkeys. *Journal of Experimental Medicine* 12, 227–255.

Funabe, S., Takao, M., Saito, Y., et al. 2013. Neuropathologic analysis of Lewy-related alpha-synucleinopathy in olfactory mucosa. *Neuropathology* 33, 47–58.

Gadoth, N., Mass, E., Gordon, C.R., Steiner, J.E., 1997. Taste and smell in familial dysautonomia. *Developmental Medicine and Child Neurology* 39, 393–397.

Galvin, J.E., Pollack, J., Morris, J.C., 2006. Clinical phenotype of Parkinson disease dementia. *Neurology* 67, 1605–1611.

Gardiner, J., Barton, D., Vanslambrouck, J.M., et al. 2008. Defects in tongue papillae and taste sensation indicate a problem with neurotrophic support in various neurological diseases. *Neuroscientist* 14, 240–250.

Garland, E.M., Raj, S.R., Peltier, A.C., Robertson, D., Biaggioni, I., 2011. A cross-sectional study contrasting olfactory function in autonomic disorders. *Neurology* 76, 456–460.

Genter, M.B., Krishan, M., Preditor, R.D., 2015. The olfactory system as a route of delivery for agents to the brain and circulation. In: Doty R.L. (Ed.), *Handbook of Olfaction and Gustation*. 3rd edition. Hoboken, NJ: John Wiley & Sons, pp. 453–484.

Geser, F., Wenning, G.K., Poewe, W., McKeith, I., 2005. How to diagnose dementia with Lewy bodies: state of the art. *Movement Disorders* 20 Suppl 12, S11–20.

Ghadami, M., Majidzadeh, A., Morovvati, S., et al. 2004. Isolated congenital anosmia with morphologically normal olfactory bulb in two Iranian families: A new clinical entity? *American Journal of Medical Genetics Part A* 127A, 307–309.

Gilbert, P.E., Murphy, C., 2004. The effect of the ApoE epsilon4 allele on recognition memory for olfactory and visual stimuli in patients with pathologically confirmed Alzheimer's disease, probable Alzheimer's disease, and healthy elderly controls. *Journal of Clinical Experimental Neuropsychology* 26, 779–794.

Gillner, M., Brittebo, E.B., Brandt, I., Soderkvist Appelgren, L-E., Gustafsson, J-A., 1987. Uptake and specific binding of 2 3 7 8-tetrachlorodibenzo-p-dioxin in the olfactory mucosa of mice and rats. *Cancer Research* 47, 4150–4159.

Glasl, L., Kloos, K., Giesert, F., et al. 2012. Pink1-deficiency in mice impairs gait, olfaction and serotonergic innervation of the olfactory bulb. *Experimental Neurology* 235, 214–227.

Glass, P.G., Lees, A.J., Mathias, C., Mason, L., Best, C., Williams, D.R., Katzenschlager, R., Silveira-Moriyama, L., et al. 2011. Olfaction in pathologically proven patients with multiple system atrophy. *Movement Disorders* 27(2), 327–328.

Goetz, C.G., Stebbins, G.T., Ouyang, B., 2011. Visual plus nonvisual hallucinations in Parkinson's disease: Development and evolution over 10 years. *Movement Disorders* 26, 2196–2200.

Goetz, C.G., Vogel, C., Tanner, C.M., Stebbins, G.T., 1998. Early dopaminergic drug-induced hallucinations in parkinsonian patients. *Neurology* 51, 811–814.

Goker-Alpan, O., Lopez, G., Vithayathil, J., et al. 2008. The spectrum of parkinsonian manifestations associated with glucocerebrosidase mutations. *Archives of Neurology* 65, 1353–1357.

Goldstein, D.S., Sewell, L., 2009. Olfactory dysfunction in pure autonomic failure: Implications for the pathogenesis of Lewy body diseases. *Parkinsonism & Related Disorders* 15(7), 516–520.

Goldstein, D.S., Holmes, C., Bentho, O., et al. 2008. Biomarkers to detect central dopamine deficiency and distinguish Parkinson disease from multiple system atrophy. *Parkinsonism & Related Disorders* 14, 600–607.

Gottofrey, J., Tjalve, H., 1991. Axonal transport of cadmium in the olfactory nerve of the pike. *Pharmacology & Toxicology* 69, 242–252.

Graves, A.B., Bowen, J.D., Rajaram, L., et al. 1999. Impaired olfaction as a marker for cognitive decline: Interaction with apolipoprotein E epsilon4 status. *Neurology* 53, 1480–1487.

Gray, A.J., Staples, V., Murren, K., Dhariwal, A., Bentham, P., 2001. Olfactory identification is impaired in clinic-based patients with vascular dementia and senile dementia of Alzheimer type. *International Journal of Geriatric Psychiatry* 16(5), 513–517.

Gray, J.M., Young, A.W., Barker, W.A., Curtis, A., Gibson, D., 1997. Impaired recognition of disgust in Huntington's disease gene carriers. *Brain* 120(Pt 11), 2029–2038.

Gresham, L.S., Molgaard, C.A., Smith, R.A., 1993. Induction of cytochrome P-450 enzymes via tobacco smoke: A potential mechanism for developing resistance to environmental toxins as related to parkinsonism and other neurologic diseases. *Neuroepidemiology* 12(2), 114–116.

Haehner, A., Hummel, T., Hummel, C., et al. 2007. Olfactory loss may be a first sign of idiopathic Parkinson's disease. *Movement Disorders* 22, 839–842.

Hague, K., Lento, P., Morgello, S., Caro, S., Kaufmann, H., 1997. The distribution of Lewy bodies in pure autonomic failure: autopsy findings and review of the literature. *Acta Neuropathol* 94, 192–196.

Halliday, G., Del Tredici, K., Braak, H., 2006. Critical appraisal of the Braak staging of brain pathology related to sporadic Parkinson's disease. *Journal of Neural Transmission Suppl* 70, 99–103.

Halliday, G.M., Barker, R.A., Rowe, D.B., 2011. *Non-dopamine Lesions in Parkinson's Disease.* Oxford: Oxford University Press.

Hamilton, J.M., Murphy, C., Paulsen, J.S., 1999. Odour detection learning and memory in Huntington's disease. *Journal of the International Neuropsychological Society* 5, 609–615.

Hamir, A.N., Kunkle, R.A., Richt, J.A., Miller, J.M., Greenlee, J.J., 2008. Experimental transmission of US scrapie agent by nasal, peritoneal, and conjunctival routes to genetically susceptible sheep. *Veterinary Pathology* 45, 7–11.

Handley, O.J., Morrison, C.M., Miles, C., Bayer, A.J., 2006. ApoE gene and familial risk of Alzheimer's disease as predictors of odour identification in older adults. *Neurobiology of Aging* 27, 1425–1430.

Hardy, J., 2005. Expression of normal sequence pathogenic proteins for neurodegenerative disease contributes to disease risk: "Permissive templating" as a general mechanism underlying neurodegeneration. *Biochemical Society Transactions* 33, 578–581.

Hawkes, C.H., Shephard, B.C., 1992. Olfactory impairment in Parkinson's disease: Evidence of dysfunction measured by olfactory event-related potentials and smell identification tests. *Annals of Neurology* 32, 248 (abstract).

Hawkes, C.H., Shephard, B.C., 1993, Selective anosmia in Parkinson's disease? *Lancet Neurology* 341, 435–436.

Hawkes, C.H., Shephard, B.C., 1998. Olfactory evoked responses and identification tests in neurological disease. *Annals of New York Academy of Science* 855, 608–615.

Hawkes, C., Shah, M., Fogo, A., 2005. Smell identification declines from age 36 years and mainly affects pleasant odours. *Movement Disorders* 20 (Suppl. 10) S48. P160 (abstract).

Hawkes, C.H., Del Tredici, K, Braak, H., 2007. Parkinson's disease: A dual-hit hypothesis. *Neuropathology and Applied Neurobiology* 33(6), 599–614.

Hawkes, C.H., 2008a. Parkinson's disease and aging: same or different process? *Movement Disorders* 23(1), 47–53.

Hawkes, C.H., 2008b. The prodromal phase of sporadic Parkinson's disease: Does it exist and if so how long is it? *Movement Disorders* 23, 1799–1807.

Hawkes, C.H., Del Tredici, K., Braak, H., 2010. A timeline for Parkinson's disease. *Parkinsonism & Related Disorders* 16, 79–84.

Hawkes, C.H., Shephard, B.C., Daniel, SE. (1997). Olfactory dysfunction in Parkinson's disease. *Journal of Neurology, Neurosurgery, & Psychiatry* 62, 436–436.

Hayes, C.J., Stevenson, R.J., Coltheart, M., 2007. Disgust and Huntington's disease. *Neuropsychologia* 45, 1135–1151.

Hemdal, P., Corwin, J., Oster, H., 1993. Olfactory identification deficits in Down's syndrome and idiopathic mental retardation. *Neuropsychologia* 31, 977–984.

Hensiek, A.E., Bhatia, K., Hawkes, C.H., 2000. Olfactory function in drug induced parkinsonism. *Journal of Neurology* 247(3), 303.

Hentschel, K., Baba, Y., Williams, L.N., et al. 2005. Olfaction in familial parkinsonism (FP). *Movement Disorders* 20, P175, S52–S52.

Hext, P.M., Lock, E.A., 1992. The accumulation and metabolism of 3-trifluoromethylpyridine by rat olfactory and hepatic tissues. *Toxicology* 72, 61–75.

Höglinger, G.U., Alvarez-Fischer, D., Arias-Carrión, O., et al. 2015. A new dopaminergic nigro-olfactory projection. *Acta neuropathologica* **130**(3), 333–348.

Holter, S.M., Stromberg, M., Kovalenko, M., et al. 2013. A broad phenotypic screen identifies novel phenotypes driven by a single mutant allele in Huntington's disease CAG knock-in mice. *PLoS One* **8**, e80923.

Hozumi, S., Nakagawasai, O., Tan-No, K., Niijima, F., Yamadera, F., Murata, A., Arai, Y., Yasuhara, H., Tadano, T., 2003. Characteristics of changes in cholinergic function and impairment of learning and memory-related behavior induced by olfactory bulbectomy. *Behavioural Brain Research* **138**(1), 9–15.

Huart, C., Rombaux, P., Gérard, T., Hanseeuw, B., Lhommel, R., Quenon, L., Ivanoiu, A., Mouraux, A., 2015. Unirhinal olfactory testing for the diagnostic workup of mild cognitive impairment. *Journal of Alzheimer's Disease* **47**(1), 253–270.

Hughes, A.J., Daniel, S.E., Lees, A.J. 2001. Improved accuracy of clinical diagnosis of Lewy body Parkinson's disease. *Neurology* **57**(8), 1497–1499.

Huisman, E., Uylings, H.B, Hoogland, P.V., 2004. A 100% increase of dopaminergic cells in the olfactory bulb may explain hyposmia in Parkinson's disease. *Movement Disorders* **19**, 687–692.

Huisman, E., Uylings, HB., Hoogland, PV., 2008. Gender-related changes in increase of dopaminergic neurons in the olfactory bulb of Parkinson's disease patients. *Movement Disorders* **23**, 1407–1413.

Iijima, M., Osawa, M., Momose, M., et al. 2010. Cardiac sympathetic degeneration correlates with olfactory function in Parkinson's disease. *Movement Disorders* **25**(9), 1143–1149.

Imamura, K., Matumoto, S., Mabuchi, N., et al. 2009. Relationship between the regional cerebral blood flow and the cognitive function and anosmia in patients with Parkinson disease and Alzheimer disease. *Brain Nerve* **61**(6), 683–690.

Iranzo, A., Molinuevo, J.L., Santamaria, J., et al. 2006. Rapid-eye-movement sleep behaviour disorder as an early marker for a neurodegenerative disorder: A descriptive study. *Lancet Neurology* **5**, 572–577.

Iscan, M., Reuhl, K., Weiss, B., Maines, M.D., 1990. Regional and subcellular distribution of cytochrome P-450-dependent drug metabolism in monkey brain: The olfactory bulb and the mitrochondrial fraction have high levels of activity. *Biochemical and Biophysical Research Communications* **169**, 858–863.

Jellinger, K.A. 2009. Olfactory bulb alpha-synucleinopathy has high specificity and sensitivity for Lewy body disorders. *Acta Neuropathologica* **117**(2), 215–6

Jennings, D., Siderowf, A., Stern, M., et al. 2014. Imaging prodromal Parkinson disease: the Parkinson Associated Risk Syndrome Study. *Neurology* **83**, 1739–1746.

Johansen, K.K., White, L.R., Farrer, M.J., Aasly, J.O., 2011. Subclinical signs in LRRK2 mutation carriers. *Parkinsonism & Related Disorders* **17**, 528–532.

Juncos, J.L., Lazarus, J.T., Rohr, J., et al. 2012. Olfactory dysfunction in fragile X tremor ataxia syndrome. *Movement Disorders* **27**, 1556–1559.

Kalaitzakis, M.E., Graeber, M.B., Gentleman, S.M., Pearce, R.K., 2008. The dorsal motor nucleus of the vagus is not an obligatory trigger site of Parkinson's disease: A critical analysis of alpha-synuclein staging. *Neuropathology and Applied Neurobiology* **34**, 284–295.

Kalmey, J.K., Thewissen, J.G., Dluzen, DE. 1998. Age-related size reduction of foramina in the cribriform plate. *Anatomical Record* **251**(3), 326–329.

Kandasamy, M., Rosskopf, M., Wagner, K., et al. 2015. Reduction in subventricular zone-derived olfactory bulb neurogenesis in a rat model of Huntington's disease is accompanied by striatal invasion of neuroblasts. *PLoS One* **10**, e0116069.

Kashihara, K., Hanaoka, A., Imamura, T., 2011. Frequency and characteristics of taste impairment in patients with Parkinson's disease: Results of a clinical interview. *Internal Medicine* **50**(20), 2311–2315.

Kareken, D.A., Doty, R.L., Moberg, P.J., et al. 2001. Olfactory-evoked regional cerebral blood flow in Alzheimer's disease. *Neuropsychology* **15**(1), 18–29.

Katzman, R., 1986. Alzheimer's disease. *New England Journal of Medicine* **314**, 964–973.

Katzman, R., 1986. Differential diagnosis of dementing illnesses. *Neurologic Clinics* **4**, 329–340.

Kaufmann, H., Nahm, K., Purohit, D., Wolfe, D., 2004. Autonomic failure as the initial presentation of Parkinson disease and dementia with Lewy bodies. *Neurology* **63**, 1093–1095.

Kertelge, L., Bruggemann, N., Schmidt, A., et al. 2010. Impaired sense of smell and color discrimination in monogenic and idiopathic Parkinson's disease. *Movement Disorders* **25**, 2665–2669.

Khan, N.L., Katzenschlager, R., Watt, H., et al. 2004. Olfaction differentiates parkin disease from early-onset parkinsonism and Parkinson disease. *Neurology* **62**, 1224–1226.

Killgore, W.D.S., McBride, S.H., 2006. Odour identification accuracy declines following 24 h of sleep deprivation. *J Sleep Res* **15**, 111–116.

Kim, H.J., Jeon, B.S., Lee, J.Y., et al. 2011. Taste function in patients with Parkinson disease. *Journal of Neurology* **258**, 1076–1079.

Kishikawa, M., Iseki, M., Sakae, M., Kawaguchi, S., Fujii, H., 1994. Early diagnosis of Alzheimer's? *Nature* **369**(6479), 365–366.

Klein, C., Schneider, S.A., Lang, A.E., 2009. Hereditary parkinsonism: Parkinson disease look-alikes–an algorithm for clinicians to "PARK" genes and beyond. *Movement Disorders* **24**(14), 2042–2058.

Klimek, L., 1998. Sense of smell in allergic rhinitis. *Pneumologie* **52**, 196–202.

Knupfer, L., Spiegel, R., 1986. Differences in olfactory test performance between normal aged, Alzheimer and vascular type dementia individuals. *International Journal of Geriatric Psychiatry* **1**(1), 3–14.

Kobal, G., Plattig, K.H., 1978. [Objective olfactometry: Methodological annotations for recording olfactory EEG-responses from the awake human]. *EEG EMG Z eitschrift Fur Elektroenzephalographie, Elektromyographie Und Verwandte Gebiete* **9**, 135–145.

Koss, E., Weiffenbach, J.M., Haxby, J.V., Friedland, R.P., 1988. Olfactory detection and identification performance are dissociated in early Alzheimer's disease. *Neurology* **38**(8), 1228–1228.

Kovacs, T., Papp, M.I., Cairns, N.J., Khan, M.N., Lantos, P.L. 2003. Olfactory bulb in multiple system atrophy. *Movement Disorders* **18**, 938–942.

Kovacs, G.G., Trabattoni, G., Hainfellner, J.A., et al. 2002. Mutations of the prion protein gene phenotypic spectrum. *Journal of Neurology* **249**, 1567–1582.

Kovács, T., 2013. The olfactory system in Alzheimer's disease: Pathology, pathophysiology and pathway for therapy. *Translational Neuroscience* **4**(1), 34–45.

Kovacs, T., Cairns, N.J., Lantos, P.L., 2001. Olfactory centres in Alzheimer's disease: Olfactory bulb is involved in early Braak's stages. *Neuroreport* **12**, 285–288.

Krismer, F., Wenning, G.K., Li, Y., Poewe, W., Stefanova, N. 2013. Intact olfaction in a mouse model of multiple system atrophy. *PLoS One*, **8**, e64625.

Krüger, R., Müller, T., Riess, O., 2000. Involvement of α-synuclein in Parkinson's disease and other neurodegenerative disorders. *Journal of Neural Transmission* **107**(1), 31–40.

Krüger, S., Haehner, A., Thiem, C., Hummel, T. 2008. Neuroleptic-induced parkinsonism is associated with olfactory dysfunction. *Journal of Neurology* **255**(10), 1574–1579.

Kumar, K.R., Weissbach, A., Heldmann, M., et al. 2012. Frequency of the D620 N mutation in VPS35 in Parkinson disease. *Archives of Neurology* **69**, 1360–1364.

Kurtenbach, S., Wewering, S., Hatt, H., Neuhaus, E.M., Lubbert, H. 2013., Olfaction in three genetic and two MPTP-induced Parkinson's disease mouse models. *PLoS One* **8**, e77509.

Landis, B.N., Burkhard, P.R., 2008. Phantosmias and Parkinson disease. *Archives of Neurology* **65**, 1237–1239.

Lang, C.J., Leuschner, T., Ulrich, K. et al. 2006. Taste in dementing diseases and parkinsonism. *Journal of the Neurological Sciences* **248**, 177–184.

Lang, C., Schwandner, K., Hecht, M., 2011. Do patients with motor neuron disease suffer from disorders of taste or smell? *Amyotrophic Lateral Sclerosis* **12**, 368–371.

Larson, J., Kim, D., Patel, R.C., Floreani, C., 2008. Olfactory discrimination learning in mice lacking the fragile X mental retardation protein. *Neurobiology of Learning and Memory* **90**, 90–102.

Le Pichon, C.E., Valley, M.T., Polymenidou, M., et al. 2009. Olfactory behavior and physiology are disrupted in prion protein knockout mice. *Nature Neuroscience* **12**, 60–69.

Lee, D.H., Oh, J.S., Ham, J.H., et al. 2015. Is normosmic Parkinson disease a unique clinical phenotype? *Neurology* **85**(15), 1270–1275.

Lee, L.V., Munoz, E.L., Tan, K.T., Reyes, M.T., 2001. Sex linked recessive dystonia parkinsonism of Panay, Philippines (XDP). *Molecular Pathology* **54**, 362–368.

Lee, P.H., Yeo, S.H., Yong, S.W., Kim, Y.J., 2007. Odour identification test and its relation to cardiac 123I-metaiodobenzylguanidine in patients with drug induced parkinsonism. *Journal of Neurology, Neurosurgery, & Psychiatry* **78**, 1250–1252.

Lehman, C.D., Bartoshuk, L.M., Catalanotto, F.C., Kveton, J.F., Lowlicht, R.A., 1995. Effect of anesthesia of the chorda tympani nerve on taste perception in humans. *Physiology & Behavior* **57** (5), 943–51.

Lelan, F., Boyer, C., Thinard, R., et al. 2011. Effects of Human Alpha-Synuclein A53T-A30P Mutations on SVZ and Local Olfactory Bulb Cell Proliferation in a Transgenic Rat Model of Parkinson Disease. *Journal of Parkinson's Disease* 987084.

Lesage, S., Anheim, M., Condroyer, C., et al 1995. French Parkinson's Disease Genetics Study Group. Large-scale screening of the Gaucher's disease-related glucocerebrosidase gene in Europeans with Parkinson's disease. *Human Molecular Genetics* 2011; **20**(1), 202–10.

Lesage, S., Durr, A., Brice, A., 2007. LRRK2: A link between familial and sporadic Parkinson's disease? *Pathologie Biologie (Paris)*, **55**, 107–110.

Li, A.A., Mink, P.J., McIntosh, L.J., Teta, M.J., Finley, B., 2005. Evaluation of epidemiologic and animal data associating pesticides with Parkinson's disease. *Occupational and Environmental Medicine* **47**(10), 1059–1087.

Liberini, P., Parola, S., Spano, P.F., Antonini, L., 2000. Olfaction in Parkinson's disease: Methods of assessment and clinical relevance. *Journal of Neurology* **247**, 88–96

Liou, H.H., Tsai, M.C., Chen, C.J., et al. 1997. Environmental risk factors and Parkinson's disease: a case-control study in Taiwan. *Neurology* **48**(6), 1583–1588.

Lohmann, E., Leclere, L., De Anna, F., et al. 2009. French Parkinson's Disease Genetics Study Group. A clinical, neuropsychological and olfactory evaluation of a large family with LRRK2 mutations. *Parkinsonism & Related Disorders* **15**(4), 273–276.

Louis, E.D., Bromley, S.M., Jurewicz, E.C., Watner, D., 2002. Olfactory dysfunction in essential tremor: A deficit unrelated to disease duration or severity. *Neurology*, **59**(10), 1631–1633.

Louis, E.D., Jurewicz, E.C., 2003. Olfaction in essential tremor patients with and without isolated rest tremor. *Movement Disorders* **18**(11), 1387–1389.

Louis, E.D., Rios, E., Pellegrino, K.M., et al. 2008. Higher blood harmane (1-methyl-9H-pyrido [3,4-b]indole) concentrations correlate with lower olfactory scores in essential tremor. *Neurotoxicology* **29**, 460–465.

Louis, E.D., Vonsattel, J.P., Honig, L.S., et al. 2006. Neuropathologic findings in essential tremor. *Neurology* **66**(11), 1756–1759.

Louis, E.D., Faust, P.L., Ma, K.J., et al. 2011. Torpedoes in the Cerebellar Vermis in Essential Tremor Cases vs. *Controls. Cerebellum* **10**, 812–819.

Lovell, M.A., Jafek, B.W., Moran, D.T., Rowley, J.C., 1982. Biopsy of human olfactory mucosa: An instrument and a technique. *Archives of Otolaryngology* 247–249.

Lucassen, E.B., Sterling, N.W., Lee, E.Y., et al. 2014. History of smoking and olfaction in Parkinson's disease. *Movement Disorders* **29**(8), 1069–1074.

Luzzi, S., Snowden, J.S., Neary, D., Coccia, M., Provinciali, L., Lambon Ralph, M.A., 2007. Distinct patterns of olfactory impairment in Alzheimer's disease, semantic dementia, frontotemporal dementia, and corticobasal degeneration. *Neuropsychologia* **45**(8), 1823–1831.

Macknin, J.B., Higuchi, M., Lee, V.M.Y., Trojanowski, J.Q., Doty, R.L., 2004. Olfactory dysfunction occurs in transgenic mice overexpressing human τ protein. *Brain Research* **1000**(1), 174–178.

Magerova, H., Vyhnalek, M., Laczo, J., et al. 2014. Odor Identification in Frontotemporal Lobar Degeneration Subtypes. *American Journal of Alzheimer's Disease and Other Dementias.*

Mann, D.M., 1988. Alzheimer's disease and Down's syndrome. *Histopathology* **13**, 125–137.

Mann, D.M., 1989. The pathogenesis and progression of the pathological changes of Alzheimer's disease. *Annals of Medicine* **21**(2), 133–136.

Markesbery, W.R., Jicha, G.A., Liu, H., Schmitt, FA. 2009. Lewy body pathology in normal elderly subjects. *Journal of Neuropathology and Experimental Neurology* **68**, 816–822.

Markopoulou, K., Larsen, K.W., Wszolek, E.K., et al. 1997. Olfactory dysfunction in familial parkinsonism. *Neurology* **49**, 1262–1267.

Marras, C., Goldman, S., Smith, A., et al. 2005. Smell identification ability in twin pairs discordant for Parkinson's disease. *Movement Disorders* **20**(6), 687–693.

Martel, G., Simon, A., Nocera, S., et al. 2015. Aging, but not tau pathology, impacts olfactory performances and somatostatin systems in THY-Tau22 mice. *Neurobiology of Aging* **36**(2), 1013–1028.

Masucci, MG. 2004.Epstein-Barr virus oncogenesis and the ubiquitin-proteasome system. *Oncogene* **23**, 2107–2115.

McAuley, J.H., Gregory, S., 2012. Prevalence and clinical course of olfactory hallucinations in idiopathic Parkinson's disease. *Journal of Parkinson's Disease* **2**, 199–205.

McKeith, I.G., 2006. Consensus guidelines for the clinical and pathologic diagnosis of dementia with Lewy bodies (DLB): Report of the Consortium on DLB International Workshop. *Journal of Alzheimer's Disease* **9** (3 Suppl), 417–423.

McKeown, D.A., Doty, R.L., Perl, D.P., Frye, R.E., Simms, I., Mester, A., 1996. Olfactory function in young adolescents with Down's syndrome. *Journal of Neurology, Neurosurgery, & Psychiatry* **61**, 412–414.

McLaughlin, N.C., Westervelt, H.J., 2008. Odor identification deficits in frontotemporal dementia: a preliminary study. *Archives of Clinical Neuropsychology* **23**(1), 119–123.

McNeill, A., Duran, R., Proukakis, C., et al. 2012. Hyposmia and cognitive impairment in Gaucher disease patients and carriers. *Movement Disorders* **27**, 526–532.

McShane, R.H., Nagy, Z., Esiri, M.M., et al. 2001. Anosmia in dementia is associated with Lewy bodies rather than Alzheimer's pathology. *Journal of Neurology, Neurosurgery, & Psychiatry* **70**, 739–743.

Mesholam, R.I., Moberg, P.J., Mahr, R.N., Doty, R.L., 1998. Olfaction in neurodegenerative disease: a meta-analysis of olfactory functioning in Alzheimer's and Parkinson's diseases. *Archives of Neurology* **55**, 84–90.

Meusel, T., Westermann, B., Fuhr, P., Hummel, T., Welge-Lussen, A., 2010. The course of olfactory deficits in patients with Parkinson's disease–a study based on psychophysical and electrophysiological measures. *Neuroscience Letters* **486**, 166–170.

Mirelman, A., Alcalay, R.N., Saunders-Pullman, R., et al. 2015. Nonmotor symptoms in healthy Ashkenazi Jewish carriers of the G2019S mutation in the LRRK2 gene. *Movement Disorders* **30**, 981–986.

Mitchell, I.J., Heims, H., Neville, E.A., Rickards, H., 2005. Huntington's disease patients show impaired perception of disgust in the gustatory and olfactory modalities. *The Journal of Neuropsychiatry and Clinical Neurosciences* **17**, 119–121.

Miwa, T., Watanabe, A., Mitsumoto, Y., et al. 2004. Olfactory impairment and Parkinson's disease-like symptoms observed in the common marmoset following administration of 1-methyl-4-phenyl-1 2 3 6-tetrahydropyridine. *Acta Otolaryngologica Suppl.* (553): 80–84.

Moberg, P.J., Doty, R.L., 1997. Olfactory function in Huntington's disease patients and at-risk offspring. *International Journal of Neuroscience*; **89**, 133–139.

Moberg, P.J., McGue, C., Kanes, S.J., et al. 2007. Phenylthiocarbamide (PTC) perception in patients with schizophrenia and first-degree family members: Relationship to clinical symptomatology and psychophysical olfactory performance. *Schizophrenia Research* **90**(1–3), 221–228.

Moberg, P.J., Pearlson, G.D., Speedie, L.J., et al. 1987. Olfactory recognition: differential impairments in early and late Huntington's and Alzheimer's disease. *Journal of Clinical Experimental Neuropsychology* **9**, 650–664.

Moccia, M., Picillo, M., Erro, R., et al. 2014. How does smoking affect olfaction in Parkinson's disease? *Journal of the Neurological Sciences* **340**(1), 215–217.

Montgomery, E.B., Jr., Baker, K.B., Lyons, K., Koller, W.C., (1999) Abnormal performance on the PD test battery by asymptomatic first-degree relatives. *Neurology* **52**, 757–762.

Montgomery, E.B., Jr., Koller, W.C., LaMantia, T.J., et al. (2000) Early detection of probable idiopathic Parkinson's disease: I. Development of a diagnostic test battery. *Movement Disorders*, **15**, 467–473.

Morgan, C.D., Murphy, C., 2002. Olfactory event-related potentials in Alzheimer's disease. *Journal of the International Neuropsychological Society* **8**, 753–763.

Morley, J.F., Pawlowski, S.M., Kesari, A., et al. 2014. Motor and non-motor features of Parkinson's disease that predict persistent drug-induced Parkinsonism. *Parkinsonism & Related Disorders* **20**, 738–742.

Moscovich, M., Munhoz, R.P., Teive, H.A., et al. 2012. Olfactory impairment in familial ataxias. *Journal of Neurology, Neurosurgery, & Psychiatry* **83**, 970–974.

Mueller, A., Reuner, U., Landis, B. et al. 2006. Extrapyramidal symptoms in Wilson's disease are associated with olfactory dysfunction. *Movement Disorders* **21**, 1311–1316.

Muller, A., Mungersdorf, M., Reichmann, H., Strehle, G., Hummel, T., 2002. Olfactory function in Parkinsonian syndromes. *Journal of Clinical Neuroscience* **9**, 521–524.

Mundiñano, I.C., Hernandez, M., Dicaudo, C., et al. 2013, Reduced cholinergic olfactory centrifugal inputs in patients with neurodegenerative disorders and MPTP-treated monkeys. *Acta Neuropathologica* **126**, 411–425.

Mundinano, I.C., Caballero, M.C., Ordonez, C., et al. 2011. Increased dopaminergic cells and protein aggregates in the olfactory bulb of patients with neurodegenerative disorders. *Acta Neuropathologica* **122**, 61–74.

Murphy, C., Gilmore, M.M., Seery, C.S., Salmon, D.P., Lasker, BR. (1990). Olfactory thresholds are associated with degree of dementia in Alzheimer's disease. *Neurobiology of Aging* **11**, 465–469.

Murphy, C., Jinich, S., 1996. Olfactory dysfunction in Down's Syndrome. *Neurobio Aging*, **17**, 631–637.

Murphy, C., Schubert, C.R., Cruickshanks, K.J., Klein, B.E., Klein, R., Nondahl, D.M., 2002. Prevalence of olfactory impairment in older adults. *Jama*, **288**(18), 2307–2312.

Najim al-Din, A.S., Wriekat, A., Mubaidin, A., Dasouki, M., Hiari, M., 1994. Pallido-pyramidal degeneration, supranuclear upgaze paresis and dementia: Kufor-Rakeb syndrome. *Acta Neurologica Scandinavica* **89**, 347–52.

Navarro-Otano, J., Gaig, C., Muxi, A., et al. 2014. 123I-MIBG cardiac uptake, smell identification and 123I-FP-CIT SPECT in the differential diagnosis between vascular parkinsonism and Parkinson's disease. *Parkinsonism & Related Disorders* **20**, 192–197.

Nee, L.E., Scott, J., Polinsky, R.J., 1993. Olfactory dysfunction in the Shy-Drager syndrome. *Clinical Autonomic Research* **3**, 281–282.

Nee, L.E., Lippa, C.F., 2001, Inherited Alzheimer's disease PS-1 olfactory function: A 10-year follow-up study. *American Journal of Alzheimer's Disease & Other Dementias*, **16**, 83–84.

Neudorfer, O., Giladi, N., Elstein, D., et al. 1996. Occurrence of Parkinson's syndrome in type I Gaucher disease. *QJM* **89**, 691–694.

Neumann, J., Bras, J., Deas, E., et al. 2009. Glucocerebrosidase mutations in clinical and pathologically proven Parkinson's disease. *Brain* **132**, 1783–1794.

Newman, R., Winans, S.S., 1980. An experimental study of the ventral striatum of the golden hamster. II Neuronal connections of the olfactory tubercle. *Journal of Comparative Neurology* **191**, 193–212.

Nijjar, R.K., Murphy, C., 2002. Olfactory impairment increases as a function of age in persons with Down syndrome. *Neurobiology of Aging* **23**(1), 65–73.

Nishioka, K., Ross, O.A., Ishii, K., et al. 2009. Expanding the clinical phenotype of SNCA duplication carriers. *Movement Disorders* **24**, 1811–1819.

Nordin, S., Almkvist, O., Berglund, B., Wahlund, L.O., 1997. Olfactory dysfunction for pyridine and dementia progression in Alzheimer disease. *Archives of Neurology* **54**, 993–998.

Nordin, S., Paulsen, J.S., Murphy, C., 1995b. Sensory- and memory-mediated olfactory dysfunction in Huntington's disease. *Journal of the International Neuropsychological Society* 1, 281–290.

Nores, J.M., Biacabe, B., Bonfils, P., 2000. [Olfactory disorders due to medications: analysis and review of the literature]. *De Medecine Interne* 21, 972–977.

Nosrat, C.A., 1998. Neurotrophic factors in the tongue: expression patterns, biological activity, relation to innervation and studies of neurotrophin knockout mice. *Annals of the New York Academy of Sciences* 855, 28–49.

Noyce, A.J., Bestwick, J.P., Silveira-Moriyama, L., et al. 2014. PREDICT-PD: Identifying risk of Parkinson's disease in the community: Methods and baseline results. *Journal of Neurology, Neurosurgery, & Psychiatry* 85, 31–37.

Noyce, A.J., Mencacci, N.E., Schrag, A., et al. 2015. Web-based assessment of Parkinson's prodromal markers identifies GBA variants. *Movement Disorders* 30, 1002–1003.

Noyce, A.J., R'Bibo, L., Peress, L., Bestwick, J.P., Adams-Carr, K.L., Mencacci, N.E., Hawkes, C.H., Masters, J.M., Wood, N., Hardy, J., Giovannoni, G., 2017. PREDICT-PD: An online approach to prospectively identify risk indicators of Parkinson's disease. *Movement Disorders* 32(2), 219–226.

Oakley, B., Witt, M., 2004. Building sensory receptors on the tongue. *Journal of Neurocytology* 33, 631–646.

Okamoto, K., Hirai, S., Shoji, M., Takatama, M. 1990. Senile changes in the human olfactory bulbs. In Nagatsu, T (Ed), *Basic, Clinical, and Therapeutic Aspects of Alzheimer's and Parkinson's Diseases.* NY: Plenum Press, pp. 349–352.

Oleson, S., Murphy, C., 2015. Olfactory Dysfunction in ApoE ε4/4 Homozygotes with Alzheimer's Disease. *Journal of Alzheimer's Disease* 46(3), 791–803.

Olichney, J.M., Murphy, C., Hofstetter, C.R., et al. 2005. Anosmia is very common in the Lewy body variant of Alzheimer's disease. *JM* 76, 1342–1347.

Oliver, C., Holland, A.J., 1986. Down's syndrome and Alzheimer's disease: a review. *Psychological Medicine* 16, 307–322.

Omar, R., Mahoney, C.J., Buskley, A.H., Warren, J.D. 2013. Flavour identification in frontotemporal lobar degeneration. *Journal of Neurology, Neurosurgery, & Psychiatry* 84(1), 88–93.

Ondo, W.G., Lai, D., 2005. Olfaction testing in patients with tremor-dominant PD: Is this a distinct condition? *Movement Disorders* 20: 471–475.

Oyanagi, K., The nature of the parkinsonism-dementia complex and amyotrophic lateral sclerosis of Guam and magnesium deficiency. *Parkinsonism & Related Disorders* 11 Suppl 1: S17–23.

Paisan-Ruiz, C., Li, A., Schneider, S.A., Holton, J.L., Johnson, R., Kidd, D., Chataway, J., Bhatia, K.P., Lees, A.J., Hardy, J, Revesz, T., 2010. Widespread Lewy body and tau accumulation in childhood and adult onset dystonia-parkinsonism cases with PLA2G6 mutations. *Neurobiology of Aging* 33(4), 814–823.

Papaioannou, N., Tooten, P.C., van Ederen, A.M., et al. 2001. Immunohistochemical investigation of the brain of aged dogs. I. Detection of neurofibrillary tangles and of 4-hydroxynonenal protein, an oxidative damage product, in senile plaques. *Amyloid* 8(1), 11–21.

Pardini, M., Huey, E.D., Cavanagh, A.I., Grafman, J., 2009. Olfactory function in corticobasal syndrome and frontotemporal dementia. *Archives of Neurology* 66, 92–96.

Park, J.S., Blair, N.F., Sue, C.M., 2015. The role of ATP13A2 in Parkinson's disease: Clinical phenotypes and molecular mechanisms. *Movement Disorders* 30, 770–779.

Parkkinen, L., Kauppinen, T., Pirttilä, T., Autere, J.M., Alafuzoff, I. 2005. Alpha-synuclein pathology does not predict extrapyramidal symptoms or dementia. *Annals of Neurology* 57, 82–91.

Paschen, L., Schmidt, N., Wolff, S., et al. 2015. The olfactory bulb volume in patients with idiopathic Parkinson's disease. *European Journal of Neurology* 22, 1068–1073.

Paulsen, J.S., Langbehn, D.R., Stout, J.C., et al. 2008. Detection of Huntington's disease decades before diagnosis: the Predict-HD study. *Journal of Neurology, Neurosurgery, & Psychiatry* 79, 874–880.

Pearce, R.K., Hawkes, C.H., Daniel, S.E., 1995. The anterior olfactory nucleus in Parkinson's disease. *Movement Disorders* **10**, 283–287.

Petzold, G.C., Einhaupl, K.M., Valdueza, J.M., 2003. Persistent bitter taste as an initial symptom of amyotrophic lateral sclerosis. *Journal of Neurology, Neurosurgery, & Psychiatry* **74**, 687–688.

Pirogovsky, E., Gilbert, P.E., Jacobson, M., et al. 2007. Impairments in source memory for olfactory and visual stimuli in preclinical and clinical stages of Huntington's disease. *Journal of Clinical Experimental Neuropsychology* **29**, 395–404.

Pittock, S.J., Joyce, C., O'Keane, V., et al. 2000. Rapid-onset dystonia-parkinsonism: A clinical and genetic analysis of a new kindred. *Neurology* **55**, 991–995.

Piwnica-Worms, K.E., Omar, R., Hailstone, J.C., Warren, J.D., 2010. Flavour processing in semantic dementia. *Cortex* **46**, 761–768.

Poddighe, S., Bhat, K.M., Setzu, M.D., et al. 2013. Impaired sense of smell in a Drosophila Parkinson's model. *PLoS One* **8**, e73156.

Politis, M., Wu, K., Molloy, S., et al. 2010. Parkinson's disease symptoms: The patient's perspective. *Movement Disorders* **25**, 1646–1651.

Ponsen, M.M., Stoffers, D., Booij, J., et al. 2004. Idiopathic hyposmia as a preclinical sign of Parkinson's disease. *Annals of Neurology* **56**, 173–181.

Postuma, R.B., Gagnon, J.F., Montplaisir, J., 2010. Clinical prediction of Parkinson's disease: planning for the age of neuroprotection. *Journal of Neurology, Neurosurgery, & Psychiatry* **81**, 1008–1013.

Postuma, R.B., Gagnon, J.F., Vendette, M., Desjardins, C., Montplaisir, J.Y., 2011. Olfaction and color vision identify impending neurodegeneration in rapid eye movement sleep behavior disorder. *Annals of Neurology* **69**, 811–818.

Postuma, R.B., Montplaisir, J., 2010. Transcranial ultrasound and olfaction in REM sleep behavior disorder: testing predictors of Parkinson's disease. *Sleep Med* **11**, 339–340.

Quagliato, L.B., Viana, M.A., Quagliato, E.M., Simis, S., 2009. Olfaction and essential tremor. *Arquivos de Neuro-Psiquiatria* **67**(1), 21–24.

Quinn, N.P., Rossor, M.N., Marsden, C.D., 1987. Olfactory threshold in Parkinson's disease. *Journal of Neurology, Neurosurgery, & Psychiatry* **50**, 88–89.

Quinn, N.P., Rossor, M.N., Marsden, C.D., 1987. Olfactory threshold in Parkinson's disease. *Journal of Neurology, Neurosurgery, & Psychiatry* **50**, 88–89.

Rajput, A.H., Gibb, W.R., Zhong, X.H., et al. 1994. Dopa-responsive dystonia: Pathological and biochemical observations in a case. *Annals of Neurology* **35**, 396–402.

Rebeck, G.W., Hyman, B.T., 1993. Neuroanatomical connections and specific regional vulnerability in Alzheimer's disease. *Neurobiology of Aging* **14**(1), 45–47.

Reuber, M., Al-Din, A.S., Baborie, A., Chakrabarty, A., 2001. New variant Creutzfeldt-Jakob disease presenting with loss of taste and smell. *Journal of Neurology, Neurosurgery, & Psychiatry* **71**, 412–413.

Rial, D., Castro, A.A., Machado, N., et al. 2014. Behavioral phenotyping of Parkin-deficient mice: looking for early preclinical features of Parkinson's disease. *PLoS One* **9**, e114216.

Ritz, B., Lee, P-C., Lassen, C.F., Arah, O.A., 2014. Parkinson disease and smoking revisited Ease of quitting is an early sign of the disease. *Neurology*, **83**(16), 1396–1402.

Roberts, R.O., Christianson, T.J., Kremers, W.K., et al. 2016, Association between olfactory dysfunction and amnestic mild cognitive impairment and Alzheimer disease dementia. *JAMA Neurology* **73**, 93–101.

Roberts, E., 1986. Alzheimer's disease may begin in the nose and may be caused by aluminosilicates. *Neurobiology of Aging* **7**, 561–567.

Rosenberg, A., Gurevich, T., Mirelman, A., et al. 2011. Multivariate features associated with presence of "severe" mutations in the GBA gene in a cohort of asymptomatic first degree relatives of patient with Parkinson's disease. *Neurology* IN4–1.003.

Ross, G.W., Abbott, R.D., Petrovitch, H., Tanner, C.M., White, L.R., 2012. Pre-motor features of Parkinson's disease: The Honolulu-Asia Aging Study experience. *Parkinsonism and Related Disorders* **18**, 199–202.

Ross, G.W., Petrovitch, H., Abbott, R.D., et al. 2004. Parkinsonian signs and substantia nigra neuron density in descendants elders without PD. *Annals of Neurology* **56**, 532–539.

Ross, G.W., Abbott, R.D., Petrovitch, H., et al. 2006. Association of olfactory dysfunction with incidental Lewy bodies. *Movement Disorders* **21**, 2062–2067.

Ross, G.W., Petrovitch, H., Abbott, R.D., et al. 2008. Association of olfactory dysfunction with risk for future Parkinson's disease. *Annals of Neurology* **63**, 167–173.

Royall, D.R., Chiodo, L.K., Polk, M.S., Jaramillo, C.J., 2002. Severe dysosmia is specifically associated with Alzheimer-like memory deficits in nondemented elderly retirees. *Neuroepidemiology* **21**(2), 68–73.

Rutty, C.J., 1996. The middle-class plaque: Epidmic polio and the Canadian State, 1936–1937. *CBMH/BCHM* **13**, 277–314.

Sabin, A.B., Olitsky, P.K., Cox, H.R., 1936. Protective action of certain chemicals against infection of monkeys with nasally instilled poliomyelitis virus. *Journal of Experimental Medicine* **63**, 877–892.

Sabin, A.B., Ward, R., 1941. The natural history of human poliomyelitis. I. Distribution of virus in nervous and non-nervous tissues. *Journal of Experimental Medicine.*, **73**, 771–793.

Sagawa, M., Takao, M., Nogawa, S., et al. 2003. [Wilson's disease associated with olfactory paranoid syndrome and idiopathic thrombocytopenic purpura]. *No To Shinkei* **55**, 899–902.

Sajjadian, A., Doty, R.L., Gutnick, D., Chirurgi, R.J., Sivak, M., Perl, D., 1994. Olfactory dysfunction in amyotrophic lateral sclerosis. *Neurodegeneration* **3**, 153–157.

Salerno-Kennedy, R., Cusack, S., Cashman, K.D., 2005. Olfactory function in people with genetic risk of dementia. *Irish Journal of Medical Science Journal* **174**, 46–50.

Salihoglu, M., Kendirli, M.T., Altundag, A., et al. 2014. The effect of obstructive sleep apnea on olfactory functions. *Laryngoscope* **124**, 2190–2194.

Samaranch, L., Lorenzo-Betancor, O., Arbelo, J.M., et al. 2010. PINK1-linked parkinsonism is associated with Lewy body pathology. *Brain* **133**, 1128–1142.

Sandyk, R., 1981. Olfactory hallucinations in Parkinson's disease. *South African Medical Journal* **60**, 950.

Satya-Murti, S., Crisostomo, E. (1988). Olfactory threshold in Friedreich's ataxia. *Muscle & nerve*, **11**(4), 406–407.

Saunders-Pullman, R., Hagenah, J., Dhawan, V., et al. 2010. Gaucher disease ascertained through a Parkinson's center: imaging and clinical characterization. *Movement Disorders* **25**, 1364–1372.

Saunders-Pullman, R., Mirelman, A., Wang, C., et al. 2014. Olfactory identification in LRRK2 G2019S mutation carriers: a relevant marker? *Annals of Clinical and Translational Neurology* **1**, 670–678.

Saunders-Pullman, R., Stanley, K., Wang, C., et al. 2011. Olfactory dysfunction in LRRK2 G2019S mutation carriers. *Neurology* **77**, 319–324.

Schertler, C., Schocke, M.F., Seppi, K., et al. 2006. Voxel-wise analysis of diffusion weighted imaging reveals disruption of the olfactory tract in Parkinson's disease. *Brain* **129**, 538–542.

Schiffman, S.S., Clark, C.M., Warwick, Z.S., 1990. Gustatory and olfactory dysfunction in dementia: Not specific to Alzheimer's disease. *Neurobiology of Aging* **11**, 597–600.

Schiffman, S.S., Graham, B.G., Sattely-Miller, E.A., Zervakis, J., Welsh-Bohmer, K., 2002. Taste, smell and neuropsychological performance of individuals at familial risk for Alzheimer's disease. *Neurobiology of Aging* **23**, 397–404.

Schilit, N.A., Stackpole, E.E., T.L., et al. 2015. Fragile X mental retardation protein regulates olfactory sensitivity but not odorant discrimination. *Chemical Senses* **40**, 345–350.

Schlitt, M., Chronister, R.B., Whitley, R.J., 1991. Pathogenesis and pathophysiology of viral infections of the central nervous system. In Scheld, W.M., Whitley, R.J., Durack, D.T. (Eds.), *Infections of the Central Nervous System*. Raven Press, pp. 7–18.

Schubert, C.R., Carmichael, L.L., Murphy, C., Klein, B.E., Klein, R., Cruickshanks, K.J., 2008. Olfaction and the 5-year incidence of cognitive impairment in an epidemiological study of older adults. *Journal of the American Geriatrics Society* **56**(8), 1517–1521.

Schultz, E.W., Gebhardt, L.R., 1936. Prevention of intranasally inoculated poliomyelitis in monkeys by previous intranasal irrigation with chemical agents. *Proceedings of the Society for Experimental Biology and Medicine* **34**, 133–135.

Schultz, E.W., Gebhardt, L.R., 1937. Zinc sulfate prophylaxis in poliomyelitis. *Journal of the American Podiatric Medical Association* **108**, 2182–2184.

Schwartz, B.S., Doty, R.L., Monroe, C., Frye, R., Barker, S., 1989. Olfactory function in chemical workers exposed to acrylate and methacrylate vapors. *American Journal of Public Health* **79**(5), 613–618.

Schwartz, B.S., Ford, D.P., Bolla, K.I., et al. 1990. Solvent-associated decrements in olfactory function in paint manufacturing workers. *American Journal of Industrial Medicine* **18**(6), 697–706.

Semchuk, K.M., Love, E.J., Lee, R.G., Parkinson's disease and exposure to agricultural work and pesticide chemicals. *Neurology* **42**(7), 1328–1335.

Serby, M., Mohan, C., Aryan, M., et al. 1996. Olfactory identification deficits in relatives of Alzheimer's disease patients. *Biological Psychiatry* **39**, 375–377.

Shackelford, J., Pagano, J.S., Targeting of host-cell ubiquitin pathways by viruses. *Essays in Biochemistry* **41**, 139–154

Shah, M., Deeb, J., Fernando, M., et al. 2009. Abnormality of taste and smell in Parkinson's disease. *Parkinsonism & Related Disorders* **15**(3), 232–237.

Shah, M., Findley, L.J., Muhammed, N., Hawkes, C.H., 2005.Olfaction is normal in essential tremor and can be used to distinguish it from Parkinson's disease. *Movement Disorders* **20**, S10.Abs: 563.

Shah, M., Muhammed, N., Findley, L.J., Hawkes, C.H., 2007. Olfactory tests in the diagnosis of essential tremor. *Journal of Neurology Neurosurgery and Psychiatry*. In press.

Sharer, J.D., Leon-Sarmiento, F.E., Morley, J.F., Weintraub, D., Doty, R.L., 2015. Olfactory dysfunction in Parkinson's disease: Positive effect of cigarette smoking. *Movement Disorders* **30**, 859–862.

Sherer, T.B., Betarbet, R., Testa, C.M., et al. 2003. Mechanism of toxicity in rotenone models of Parkinson's disease. *Journal of Neuroscience* **23**, 10756–10764.

Shi, F., Liu, B., Zhou, Y., Yu, C., Jiang, T., 2009. Hippocampal volume and asymmetry in mild cognitive impairment and Alzheimer's disease: Meta-analyses of MRI studies. *Hippocampus* **19**, 1055–1064.

Shimoji, A., Miyakawa, T., Watanabe, K., et al. 1987. Wilson's disease with extensive degeneration of cerebral white matter and cortex. *The Japanese Journal of Psychiatry and Neurology* **41**, 709–717.

Shipley, M.T., 1985. Transport of molecules from nose to brain: Transneuronal anterograde and retrograde labelling in the rat olfactory system by wheatgerm agglutin-horseradish peroxidase applied to the nasal epithelium. *Brain Research Bulletin* **15**, 129–142.

Siderowf, A., Jennings, D., Eberly, S., et al. 2012. Impaired olfaction and other prodromal features in the Parkinson At-Risk Syndrome Study. *Movement Disorders* **27**, 406–412.

Siderowf, A., Newberg, A., Chou, K.L., et al. 2005. [99mTc]TRODAT-1 SPECT imaging correlates with odor identification in early Parkinson disease. *Neurology* **64**, 1716–1720.

Sienkiewicz-Jarosz, H., Scinska, A., Kuran, W., Ryglewicz, D., Rogowski, A., Wrobel, E., Korkosz, A., Kukwa, A., Kostowski, W., Bienkowski, P., 2005. Taste responses in patients with Parkinson's disease. *Journal of Neurology, Neurosurgery & Psychiatry* **76**(1), 40–46.

Sienkiewicz-Jarosz, H., Scinska, A., Swiecicki, L., et al. 2013. Sweet liking in patients with Parkinson's disease. *Journal of the Neurological Sciences* **329**(1–2), 17–22.

Sierra, M., Sanchez-Juan, P., Martinez-Rodriguez, MI., et al. 2013. Olfaction and imaging biomarkers in premotor LRRK2 G2019S-associated Parkinson disease. *Neurology* **80**, 621–626.

Silveira-Moriyama, L., Guedes, L.C., Kingsbury, A., et al. 2008. Hyposmia in G2019S LRRK2-related parkinsonism: clinical and pathologic data. *Neurology* **71**(13), 1021–1026.

Silveira-Moriyama, L., Holton, J.L., Kingsbury, A., et al. 2009. Regional differences in the severity of Lewy body pathology across the olfactory cortex. *Neuroscience Letters* **453**, 77–80.

Silveira-Moriyama, L., Hughes, G., Church, A., et al. 2010. Hyposmia in progressive supranuclear palsy. *Movement Disorders* **25**, 570–577.

Silveira-Moriyama, L., Mathias, C., Mason, L., et al. 2009, Hyposmia in pure autonomic failure. *Neurology*, **72**, 1677–1681.

Silveira-Moriyama, L., Munhoz, R.P., de, J.C., et al. 2010. Olfactory heterogeneity in LRRK2 related Parkinsonism. *Movement Disorders* **25**, 2879–2883.

Silveira-Moriyama, L., Munhoz, R.P., Carvalho, M.J., et al. 2010 Olfactory Loss in LRRK2 Related Parkinsonism. *Neurology* Suppl. Abstract P03.189

Silveira-Moriyama, L., Schwingenschuh, P., O'Donnell, A., et al. 2009. Olfaction in patients with suspected parkinsonism and scans without evidence of dopaminergic deficit (SWEDDs). *Journal of Neurology, Neurosurgery, & Psychiatry* **80**(7), 744–748.

Silveira-Moriyama, L., Williams, D., Katzenschlager, R., Lees, A.J., 2005. Pizza, mint, and licorice: Smell testing in Parkinson's disease in a UK population. *Movement Disorders* **20**, S139.

Singleton, A., Gwinn-Hardy, K., Sharabi, Y., et al. 2004. Association between cardiac denervation and parkinsonism caused by alpha-synuclein gene triplication. *Brain* **127**(Pt 4), 768–772.

Sliger, M., Lander, T., Murphy, C., 2004. Effects of the ApoE epsilon4 allele on olfactory function in Down syndrome. *Journal of Alzheimer's Disease* **6**(4), 397–402.

Smith, C.A.D, Gough, A.C., Leigh, P.N., Summers, et al. 1992. Debrisoquine hydroxylase gene polymorphism and susceptibility to Parkinson' disease. *Lancet* **339**, 1375–1377.

Smith, D.H., Uryu, K., Saatman, K.E., Trojanowski, J.Q., McIntosh, T.K., 2003. Protein accumulation in traumatic brain injury. *NeuroMolecular Medicine* **4**, 59–72.

Smutzer, G.S., Doty, R.L., Arnold, S.E., Trojanowski, J.Q., 2003. Olfactory system neuropathology in Alzheimer's Disease. In Doty R.L., (Ed.), *Parkinson's Disease and Schizophrenia. Chapter 24 in: Handbook of olfaction and gustation.* Second edition. New York: Marcel Dekker.

Sobel, N., Thomason, M.E., Stappen, I., et al. 2001. An impairment in sniffing contributes to the olfactory impairment in Parkinson's disease. *Proceedings of the National Academy of Sciences of the United States of America* **98**, 4154–4159.

Sommer, U., Hummel, T., Cormann, K., et al., 2004. Detection of presymptomatic Parkinson's disease: combining smell tests, transcranial sonography and SPECT. *Movement Disorders* **19**, 1196–1202.

Spiegel, J., Hellwig, D., Mollers, M.O., et al. Transcranial sonography and [123I]FP-CIT SPECT disclose complementary aspects of Parkinson's disease. *Brain* **129**(Pt 5), 1188–1193.

Stadlan, E., Duvoisin, R., Yahr, M., 1965. The pathology of Parkinsonism. *Fifth International Congress of Neuropathologists*, Zurich, Excerpta Medica., pp 569–571.

Stamps, J.J., Bartoshuk, L.M., Heilman, K.M., 2013. A brief olfactory test for Alzheimer's disease. *Journal of the Neurological Sciences* **333**(1), 19–24.

Stamps, J.J., Doty, L., Wade, C.I., Heilman, K.M., 2016. The Left versus Right Nostril Odor Detection Test for Early Alzheimer's Disease: Increased Sample Size, Changes with Progression of Alzheimer's, and Performance with other Neurodegenerative Diseases. *Abstract.* Bonita Springs, FL: Association for Chemosensory Research.

Steinbach, S., Hundt, W., Vaitl, A., et al. 2010. Taste in mild cognitive impairment and Alzheimer's disease. *Journal of Neurology* **257**, 238–246.

Stern, M.B., Doty, R.L., Dotti, M., et al. 1994. Olfactory function in Parkinson's disease subtypes. *Neurology* **44**, 266–268.

Stiasny-Kolster, K., Doerr, Y., Moller, J.C., et al. 2005. Combination of "idiopathic" REM sleep behaviour disorder and olfactory dysfunction as possible indicator for alpha-synucleinopathy demonstrated by dopamine transporter FP-CIT-SPECT. *Brain* **128**, 126–137.

Strang, R.R., 1965. The association of gastro-duodenal ulceration and Parkinson's disease. *Medical Journal of Australia* **52**, 842–843.

Svensson, E., Horvath-Puho, E., Thomsen, R.W., et al. 2015. Vagotomy and Subsequent Risk of Parkinson's Disease. *Annals of Neurology* **78**, 1012–1013.

Swan, G.E., Carmelli, D., 2002, Impaired olfaction predicts cognitive decline in nondemented older adults. *Neuroepidemiology* 21, 58–67.

Tabaton, M., Monaco, S., Cordone, M.P., et al. 2004. Prion deposition in olfactory biopsy of sporadic Creutzfeldt–Jakob disease. *Annals of Neurology* 55(2), 294–296.

Tabert, M.H., Liu, X., Doty, R.L., et al. 2005, A 10-item smell identification scale related to risk for Alzheimer's disease. *Annals of Neurology* 58, 155–160.

Takeda, T., Iijima, M., Uchihara, T., et al. 2015. TDP-43 Pathology Progression Along the Olfactory Pathway as a Possible Substrate for Olfactory Impairment in Amyotrophic Lateral Sclerosis. *Journal of Neuropathology and Experimental Neurology* 74, 547–556.

Talamo, B.R., Rudel, R., Kosik, K.S., et al. 1989. Pathological changes in olfactory neurons in patients with Alzheimer's disease. *Nature 23*, 337(6209), 736–739.

Tanner, C.M., Goldman, S.M., Aston, D.A., et al. 2002. Smoking and Parkinson's disease in twins. *Neurology* 58(4), 581–588.

Thomann, P.A., Dos, S.V., Seidl, U., et al. 2009. MRI-derived atrophy of the olfactory bulb and tract in mild cognitive impairment and Alzheimer's disease. *Journal of Alzheimer's Disease* 17, 213–221.

Thomann, P.A., Dos, S.V., Toro, P., et al. 2009. Reduced olfactory bulb and tract volume in early Alzheimer's disease–a MRI study. *Neurobiology of Aging* 30, 838–841.

Tijero, B., Gomez-Esteban, J.C., Llorens, V., et al. 2010. Cardiac sympathetic denervation precedes nigrostriatal loss in the E46 K mutation of the alpha-synuclein gene (SNCA). *Clinical Autonomic Research* 20, 267–269.

Tissingh, G., Berendse, H.W., Bergmans, P., et al. 2001. Loss of olfaction in de novo and treated Parkinson's disease: Possible implications for early diagnosis. *Movement Disorders* 16(1), 41–46.

Tjalve, H., Henriksson, J., 1999. Uptake of metals in the brain via olfactory pathways. *Neurotoxicology* 20, 181–195.

Tjalve, H., Henriksson, J., Tallkvist, J., Larsson, B.S., Lindquist, N.G., 1996. Uptake

of manganese and cadmium from the nasal mucosa into the central nervous system via olfactory pathways in rats. *Pharmacology & Toxicology* 79, 347–356.

Tomlinson, A.H., Esiri, M.M., 1983. Herpes Simplex encephalitis: Immuno-histological demonstration of spread of virus via olfactory pathways in mice. *Journal of Neurological Science* 60, 473–484.

Toomey, J.A., 1935. Intranasal or gastrointestinal portal of entry in poliomyelitis. *Science* 82(2122), 200–201.

Toomey, J.A., 1936. The gastrointestinal portal of entry in poliomyelitis. *Jorunal of Pediatrics* 8, 664–675.

Travers, J.B., Akey, L.R., Chen, S.C., Rosen, S., Paulson, G., Travers, S.P., 1993. Taste preferences in Parkinson's disease patients. *Chemical Senses* 18, 47–55

Trojanowski, J.Q., Newman, P.D., Hill, W.D., Lee, V.M., 1991. Human olfactory epithelium in normal aging, Alzheimer's disease, and other neurodegenerative disorders. *Journal of Comparative Neurology*., 310, 365–376.

Tsuboi, Y., Wszolek, Z.K., Graff-Radford, N.R., Cookson, N., Dickson, D.W., 2003. Tau pathology in the olfactory bulb correlates with Braak stage, Lewy body pathology and apolipoprotein epsilon4. *Neuropathology & Applied Neurobiology*, 29, 503–510.

Tyas, S.L., Manfreda, J., Strain, L.A., Montgomery, P.R., 2001. Risk factors for Alzheimer's disease: A population-based, longitudinal study in Manitoba, Canada. *International Journal of Epidemiology*, 30(3), 590–597.

Tysnes, O.B., Kenborg, L., Herlofson, K., et al. 2015. *Does vagotomy reduce the risk of Parkinson's disease? Annals Neurology* 78, 1011–1012.

Tzen, K.Y., Lu, C.S., Yen, T.C., Wey, S.P., Ting, G., 2001. Differential diagnosis of Parkinson's disease and vascular parkinsonism by (99 m)Tc-TRODAT-1. *Journal of Nuclear Medicine* 42(3), 408–413.

Ubeda-Bañon, I., Saiz-Sanchez, D., de la Rosa-Prieto, C., et al. 2010a. Alpha-Synucleinopathy in the human olfactory system in Parkinson's disease: Involvement of calcium-binding protein- and substance P-positive cells. *Acta Neuropathologica* **119**, 723–735.

Ubeda-Banon, I., Saiz-Sanchez, D., de la Rosa-Prieto, C., et al. 2010b. Staging of alpha-synuclein in the olfactory bulb in a model of Parkinson's disease: cell types involved. *Movement Disorders* **25**, 1701–1707.

Ubeda-Banon, I., Saiz-Sanchez, D., de la Rosa-Prieto, C., Martinez-Marcos, A., 2012. alpha-Synuclein in the olfactory system of a mouse model of Parkinson's disease: Correlation with olfactory projections. *Brain Structure and Function* **217**, 447–458.

Uchida, K., Kihara, N., Hashimoto, K., et al. 2003. Age-related histological changes in the canine substantia nigra. *Journal of Veterinary Medical Science* **65**(2), 179–185.

Uchiyama, T., Fukutake, T., Arai, K., Nakagawa, K., Hattori, T., 2001. Machado-Joseph disease associated with an absence of fungiform papillae on the tongue. *Neurology* **56**, 558–560.

van der Goes van Naters, W., Carlson, J.R., 2006. Insects as chemosensors of humans and crops. *Nature* **444**(7117), 302–307.

Veeriah, S., Taylor, B.S., Meng, S., et al. 2010. Somatic mutations of the Parkinson's disease-associated gene PARK2 in glioblastoma and other human malignancies. *Nature Genetics* **42**, 77–82.

Velayudhan, L., Lovestone, S., 2009. Smell identification test as a treatment response marker in patients with Alzheimer disease receiving donepezil. *Journal of Clinical Psychopharmacology* **29**, 387–390.

Velázquez-Pérez, L., Fernandez-Ruiz, J., Díaz, R., et al. 2006. Spinocerebellar ataxia type 2 olfactory impairment shows a pattern similar to other major neurodegenerative diseases *Journal of Neurology* **253**(9), 1165–1169.

Vemula, S.R., Puschmann, A., Xiao, J., et al. 2013. Role of Galpha(olf) in familial and sporadic adult-onset primary dystonia. *Human Molecular Genetics* **22**, 2510–2519.

Verbaan, D., Boesveldt, S., van Rooden, S.M., et al. 2008. Is olfactory impairment in Parkinson's disease related to phenotypic or genotypic characteristics? *Neurology* **71**, 1877–1882.

Vogt, B.A., Van Hoesen, G.W., Vogt, L.J., 1990. Laminar distribution of neuron degeneration in posterior cingulate cortex in Alzheimer's disease. *Acta Neuropathologica* **80**(6), 581–589

Vucic, S., Tian, D., Chong, P.S., et al. 2006. Facial onset sensory and motor neuronopathy (FOSMN syndrome): a novel syndrome in neurology. *Brain* **129**(Pt 12), 3384–3390.

Wakabayashi, K., Takahashi, H., Ohama, E., Ikuta, F., 1990. Parkinson's disease: An immunohistochemical study of Lewy body-containing neurons in the enteric nervous system. *Acta Neuropathologica* **79**, 581–583.

Wakabayashi, K., Takahashi, H., 1997. Neuropathology of autonomic nervous system in Parkinson's disease. *European Neurology* **38**, Suppl 2, 2–7.

Waldton, S., 1974. Clinical observations of impaired cranial nerve function in senile dementia. *Acta Psychiatrica Scandinavica* **50**, 539–547.

Warner, M.D., Peabody, C.A., Berger, P.A., 1988. Olfactory deficits in Down's syndrome. *Biological Psychiatry*, **23**, 836–839.

Waters, C.H., Faust, P.L., Powers, J., et al. 1993. Neuropathology of lubag (x-linked dystonia parkinsonism). *Movement Disorders* **8**, 387–390.

Wenning, G.K., Shephard, B., Hawkes, C.H., et al. 1995. Olfactory function in typical parkinsonian syndromes. *Acta-Neurologica Scandinavica* **91**, 247–250.

Wesson, D.W., Levy, E., Nixon, R.A., Wilson, D.A., 2010. Olfactory dysfunction correlates with amyloid-beta burden in an Alzheimer's disease mouse model. *Journal of Neuroscience* **30**, 505–514.

Westervelt, H.J., Carvalho, J., Duff, K., 2007. Presentation of Alzheimer's disease in patients with and without olfactory deficits. *Archives of Clinical Neuropsychology* **22**, 117–122.

Wetter, S., Murphy, C., 2001. Apolipoprotein E epsilon4 positive individuals demonstrate delayed olfactory event-related potentials. *Neurobiology of Aging* **22**, 439–447.

Wetter, S., Peavy, G., Jacobson, M., et al. 2005. Olfactory and auditory event-related potentials in Huntington's disease. *Neuropsychology* **19**(4), 428–436.

Wetter, S., Murphy, C., 1999. Individuals with Down's syndrome demonstrate abnormal olfactory event-related potentials. *Clinical Neurophysiology*, **110**, 1563–1569.

Wider, C., Skipper, L., Solida, A., et al. 2008. Autosomal dominant dopa-responsive parkinsonism in a multigenerational Swiss family. *Parkinsonism & Related Disorders* 14, 465–470.

Williams, S.S., Williams, J., Combrinck, M., et al. 2009. Olfactory impairment is more marked in patients with mild dementia with Lewy bodies than those with mild Alzheimer's disease. *Journal of Neurology, Neurosurgery, & Psychiatry* 80(6), 667–670.

Williams, D.R., de Silva, R., Paviour, D.C., et al. 2005. Characteristics of two distinct clinical phenotypes in pathologically proven progressive supranuclear palsy: Richardson's syndrome and PSP-parkinsonism. *Brain* 128, 1247–1258.

Wilson, R.S., Arnold, S.E.,Schneider, J.A.,Tang, Y., Bennett, D.A., 2007a. The relationship between cerebral Alzheimer's disease pathology and odour identification in old age. *Journal of Neurology, Neurosurgery, and Psychiatry* 78, 30–35.

Wilson, R.S., Schneider, J.A., Arnold, S.E., et al. 2007b. Olfactory identification and incidence of mild cognitive impairment in older age. *Archives of General Psychiatry* 64, 802–808.

Wilson, R.S., Arnold, S.E., Schneider, J.A., et al. 2009. Olfactory impairment in presymptomatic Alzheimer's disease. *Annals of the New York Academy of Sciences* 1170, 730–735.

Wilson, R.S., Yu, L., Schneider, J.A., et al. 2011. Lewy bodies and olfactory dysfunction in old age. *Chemical Senses* 36, 367–373.

Wisniewski, K.E., Wisniewski, H.M., Wen, G.Y., 1985. Occurrence of neuropathological changes and dementia of Alzheimer's disease in Down's syndrome. *Annals of Neurology* 17, 278–282.

Witoonpanich, P., Cash, D.M., Shakespeare, T.J., et al. 2013. Olfactory impairment in posterior cortical atrophy. *Journal of Neurology, Neurosurgery, & Psychiatry* 84, 588–590.

Witt, M., Bormann, K., Gudziol, V., et al. 2009. Biopsies of olfactory epithelium in patients with Parkinson's disease. *Movement Disorders* 24, 906–914.

Wood, N.I., Goodman, A.O., van der Burg, J.M., et al. 2008. Increased thirst and drinking in Huntington's disease and the R6/2 mouse. *Brain Research Bulletin* 76, 70–79.

Wu, N., Rao, X., Gao, Y., Wang, J., Xu, F., 2013. Amyloid-beta deposition and olfactory dysfunction in an Alzheimer's disease model. *Journal of Alzheimer's Disease* 37, 699–712.

Yahr, M.D., Orosz, D., Purohit, D.P., 2003. Co-occurrence of essential tremor and Parkinson's disease: Clinical study of a large kindred with autopsy findings. *Parkinsonism & Related Disorders* 9(4), 225–231.

Yamada, M., Onodera, M., Mizuno, Y., Mochizuki, H., 2004. Neurogenesis in olfactory bulb identified by retroviral labeling in normal and 1-methyl-4-phenyl-1,2,3,6-tetrahydropyridine-treated adult mice. *Neuroscience* 124(1), 173–181.

Yamagishi, M., Ishizuka Y., Seki, K., 1994. Pathology of olfactory mucosa in patients with Alzheimer's disease. *Annals of Otology, Rhinology, and Laryngology* 103, 421–427.

Yousem, D.M., Oguz, K.K., Li, C., 2001. Imaging of the olfactory system. *Seminars in Ultrasound, CT and MRI* 22, 456–472.

Zanusso, G., Ferrari, S., Benedetti, D., et al. 2009. Different prion conformers target the olfactory pathway in sporadic Creutzfeldt-Jakob disease. *Annals of the New York Academy of Sciences* 1170, 637–643.

Zanusso, G., Ferrari, S., Cardone, F., et al. 2003. Detection of pathologic prion protein in the olfactory epithelium in sporadic Creutzfeldt-Jakob disease. *The New England Journal of Medicine* 348, 711–719.

Ziegler-Graham, K., Brookmeyer, R., Johnson, E., Arrighi, H.M., 2008. Worldwide variation in the doubling time of Alzheimer's disease incidence rates. *Alzheimer's & Dementia* 4(5), 316–323.

Zijlmans, J.C., Thijssen, H.O., Vogels, O.J., et al. 1995. MRI in patients with suspected vascular parkinsonism. *Neurology* 45(12), 2183–2188.

Ziso, B., Williams, T.L., Walters, R.J., et al. 2015. Facial onset sensory and motor neuronopathy: Further evidence for aTDP-43 proteinopathy. *Case Reports in Neurology* 7, 95–100.

Zucco, G.M., Negrin, N.S., 1994. Olfactory deficits in Down subjects: A link with Alzheimer's disease. *Perceptual and Motor Skills* 78(2), 627–631.

8 Assessment, Treatment, and Medicolegal Aspects of Chemosensory Disorders

General Assessment

A thorough history is essential to establish the probable cause of smell or taste impairment and to select the most appropriate investigations. The majority of people who complain of taste loss will, in fact, have olfactory impairment. Before administering either taste or smell tests, it is useful to ask the patient the following questions: Do you experience the sweetness of sugar on breakfast cereal or when added to coffee or tea? Can you detect the saltiness of potato chips or when salt is added to your food from a salt-shaker? Do you appreciate the sour taste of grapefruit or lemon juice? Can you perceive the bitterness in tonic water (quinine)? If a patient reports "yes" to most or all of these questions, then their primary problem is likely to be olfactory and smell testing should be initiated. Such enquiries have high negative predictive value, i.e., they are sensitive to detection of those who have no taste problem. Conversely, the same questions are not very sensitive in detecting persons who have a true taste problem, i.e., they have low positive predictive value (Soter et al., 2008). Therefore, when true gustatory deficits are suspected, they must be verified by quantitative taste tests.

Olfaction

History and Investigation. A detailed history may identify the underlying cause of smell dysfunction. Many causes relate to local nasal disease such as polyps, allergic rhinitis, a severely deviated septum, and granulomas (Wegener's granulomatosis, sarcoidosis, syphilis). Head injury or radiotherapy to the head for brain tumor or nasal cancer may be relevant. It is rare to find medication that is responsible for impaired olfaction, but the main culprits appear to be calcium channel blockers, antibiotics, and anti-thyroid agents. Hyposmia is recognized in immune-related conditions such as multiple sclerosis, Sjögren's disease, myasthenia gravis, and vasculitic disorder, as well as endocrinopathies that include diabetes, myxedema, and Kallman's syndrome. On rare occasion hyposmia is the presenting feature of a neurodegenerative disorder such as multiple sclerosis, Parkinson's disease or Alzheimer's disease.

Validated olfactory tests are now widely available to assess olfaction, as detailed in Chapter 3. For screening purposes, there has to be a compromise between the time required for the test, its reliability, and its validity. In general, the reliability of a test is proportional to the number of items or trials it contains (Doty et al., 1995); lengthy procedures, such as some threshold tests, can be impractical for office screening. Since many olfactory procedures correlate relatively well with one another (e.g., tests of odor identification, detection, and discrimination; Doty et al., 1994), simple measures of odor identification with forced-choice responses are commonly employed. Although brief (e.g., 3-item) odor identification tests can be sensitive to total anosmia (Jackman & Doty, 2005), their sensitivity and specificity in detecting the severity of olfactory loss is compromised. Longer screening procedures, such as the 12-item Sniffin' Sticks and the 12-item Brief Smell Identification Test (B-SIT), are more sensitive and specific, although these measures still have limited ability to differentiate between categories of dysfunction and may not detect malingering. Whenever possible, longer tests should be employed. Procedures amenable to self-administration should still be administered by an examiner to those with disability from poor eyesight or movement disorder, to ensure the validity of the testing.

Once it is clear that an olfactory deficit is present, the next step is to decide whether the abnormality is conductive, due to local nasal disease or problems with the olfactory nerve or its connections, or both. Exclusion of sinonasal disease is achieved best by nasal endoscopy. This will overlook only about 10 percent of nasal pathologies. The presence of local nasal disease may be detected also by acoustic rhinometry, rhinomanometry, ciliary motility, and skin tests, although micro-inflammation within the olfactory epithelium cannot be determined by simple endoscopy. If there is still doubt, a high resolution CT scan of the nose and paranasal sinuses should be performed. In general, for investigation of smell deficits, CT scanning is often the preferred procedure for suspected local nasal problems because it displays bony structures well. MRI yields good images of the nose and sinuses, as well as the brain itself and provides acceptable definition of bone structure, but sometimes it overemphasizes the magnitude of sinus disease.

For evaluation of suspected central causes of anosmia, there is a choice of CT, MRI, and SPECT. MRI has particular value for determining the integrity of the olfactory bulbs and tracts, and special imaging with multiple cuts through the cribriform plate region can usually establish whether these structures are grossly abnormal. Functional MRI (fMRI) and positron emission tomography (PET), as detailed in Chapter 3, still belong to the domain of research. If the patient describes an olfactory aura with or without associated seizure, then epilepsy needs to be considered. Here electroencephalography (EEG) and MRI brain scan are the preliminary investigations of choice. Usually high resolution coronal slices through the medial temporal lobes are required to detect the presence of sclerosis or congenital lesions residing in the medial temporal zone.

A blood screen should be performed, testing in particular: the blood cell count (for anemia, drug effects); sedimentation rate and C-reactive protein (for infection, vasculitic disease, malignancy); B12 and folate level (nutritional state); glucose (diabetes, pituitary disease, Addison's and Cushing's disease); calcium and phosphate (parathyroid function, Paget's disease); thyroid function (myxedema); urea and electrolytes (renal disease, Addison's or Cushing's disease); liver function (cirrhosis); autoimmune tests (cANCA for Wegener's granulomatosis; Ro and La antibodies for Sjögren's disease); and IgE (allergic rhinitis). Further investigation depends on complexity and whether there is a question of malingering, as may be the case in compensation claims.

Treatment of Olfactory Disorders. Therapy directed to the underlying cause is the obvious treatment for local nasal inflammatory disease and tumor, whether growing in the nose, sinuses, or intracranially. Any process that obstructs airflow to the olfactory mucosa should be corrected, either with surgery, steroids, or anti-inflammatory sprays. Surgery for polyps is usually reserved for large medically refractory polyps or where there is diagnostic uncertainty, although therapy with the Interleukin-5 blocker (mepolizumab) is currently showing promise in this context. Predictably, steroids are used for granulomata affecting the nose, such as Wegener's granulomatosis or sarcoidosis. Wegener's granulomatosis usually needs more vigorous immunosuppression than steroids alone can provide, e.g., cylcophosphamide, azathioprine, or methotrexate, although some report that sulphonamides such as cotrimoxazole may be just as effective (Stegeman, 1996). The efficacy of steroid sprays or drops can be enhanced by administering them with the head in the inverted position, where the bridge of the nose is perpendicular to the floor (e.g., Moffett's position), thereby allowing the drops to enter the olfactory meatus.

Unconfirmed reports suggest that vitamin A might aid recovery in chronic nasal sinus disease (Steck-Scott et al., 2004). Use of this vitamin has been suggested frequently for treatment of olfactory problems (e.g., Duncan & Briggs, 1962), but in the absence of vitamin A deficiency such therapy is unlikely to be effective. The original idea that vitamin A would be helpful stemmed from the now outdated concept that pigmentation within the olfactory neuroepithelium is an important element of olfactory transduction (Briggs & Duncan, 1961). Nevertheless, bioactive vitamin A derivatives (retinoids) play an important role in the survival of mature olfactory neurons (Hagglund et al., 2006). Other agents, such as zinc and α-lipoic acid, an over-the-counter antioxidant, have been reported to mitigate smell loss (Schechter et al., 1972; Hummel et al., 2002). Unfortunately, these investigations lacked appropriate controls. Double-blind studies of zinc have shown no benefit (Henkin et al., 1976; Lill et al., 2006). More research is needed to determine whether α-lipoic acid is effective in some cases.

It is well recognized that calcium ions play an important role in regulating the sensitivity of the olfactory receptor cell (ORC). This is mediated through cyclic adenosine monophosphate (cAMP). Sodium citrate delivered as an intra-nasal solution binds to free calcium ions in the nasal mucus and would be expected to lower intracellular calcium levels. In theory this could lower ORC threshold and improve olfactory sensitivity. In the only published trial so far, Panagiotopoulos et al. (2005) administered sodium citrate to 31 subjects with olfactory impairment, of whom all but one displayed significant improvement in olfactory identification on the Sniffin' Sticks test. The beneficial effect was observed within one hour of treatment but little or no change was recorded with intranasal saline or adrenaline. These interesting findings were extended in a randomized double blind trial of sodium citrate nasal spray in 55 subjects with non-conductive olfactory loss (Philpott et al., 2017). At two hours, a significant improvement in thresholds was observed for phenylethyl alcohol, 1-butanol and eucalyptol. The benefit lasted for about one hour only but this is clearly an interesting new avenue for further research. Another compound undergoing open-label trial is n-acetyl cysteine, a substance that acts as a scavenger of free radicals and may promote nerve recovery. It is applied as a nasal spray.

For the patient who has become hyposmic from head injury, steroids are tried often, but there are no large randomized trials to validate their use. Many clinicians give prednisolone in high dose for the first few weeks followed by a taper for the following three weeks. The rationale is that scarring around the cribriform plate area may impede the growth of regenerating centripetal olfactory neurones and if the scarred tissue can be softened then connection with the bulb might be re-established (Jafek et al., 1989). More research on this point is clearly needed, although the steroid-related benefit may well reflect reduction of local nasal edema rather than an effect on olfactory receptor cell regeneration

There are a number of studies, all lacking double-blind procedures and most lacking appropriate control groups, that suggest that "olfactory training" may improve olfactory function in hyposmic patients (for review, see Patel, 2017). While perithreshold sensitivity is improved after repeated trials in normosmic persons (Engen, 1989; Doty et al., 1989; Wysocki et al., 1989; Dalton & Wysocki, 1995), it is not known how long this effect remains and whether it is simply a function of practice. The clinical initiative for "olfactory training" was a study based on repeated testing of 40 persons in a "training" group and 16 persons who received no such training (Hummel et al., 2009). Those exposed to the 12-week-long structured program of smelling rose oil (phenylethyl alcohol or PEA), clove oil (eugenol), eucalyptus (eucalyptol), and lemon (citronellal) in the evening and early morning significantly improved scores on olfactory thresholds to three of these agents (the eugenol thresholds did not differ significantly from baseline). Tests of odor identification and discrimination were not influenced by the training. Subsequent studies have been more equivocal but remain suggestive. For example, Geissler et al. (2014), in a study of 39 patients, found no influence of 12 weeks of training with the aforementioned four odors on the PEA threshold (other thresholds were not determined) or on tests of odor discrimination or identification. However, after 32 weeks of training, improvement on a discrimination test was noted (p = 0.021), but not on the threshold or odor identification tests. No control group was employed. Atundag et al. (2015) expanded the number of odorants from 4 to 12 and for 36 weeks of exposure/training. The additional odors had relatively little effect. Again, odor thresholds were not affected, but odor discrimination and identification improved over the course of the study. In the most recent study on this topic (Poletti et al., 2017), 26 post-traumatic hyposmic subjects and 70 post-viral hyposmic subjects were given olfactory training over the course of 5 months. Half were trained on "heavy weight molecules" [cis-3-hexenol (grass), ethyl maltol (carmelized sugar), alpha pinene (pine), and ocimene (citrus)] and half on "light weight molecules" [fructone (green apple), ethyl vanilline (vanilla), gardocyclene (herbaceous, woody), and alpha irone (floral)]. Within the post-viral group, post-training thresholds were lower in those who received heavy weight molecule training but not those who received light weight molecule training. No other effects were apparent. Again, blinding was absent and no control group receiving no training or blank stimuli was tested

While the evidence for olfactory training in improving smell function is suggestive, the magnitude of such effects, if present, is not large and the duration of the effect is unknown. More research is needed on this interesting concept before one can conclude that such "training" is of general clinical value.

Hyperosmia. Treatment of hyperosmia is not easy. Anecdotally the only compounds that appear beneficial are the anti-epileptic preparations, which are given on the assumption that there is increased firing activity possibly with ephaptic (short-circuiting) transmission somewhere along the olfactory pathway. The selection of medication is a matter of personal choice, but many use Carbamazepine (Tegretol®); Sodium Valproate (Epilim®, Depakene®), Gabapentin (Neurontin®), or Pregabalin (Lyrica®). With all these medications it is important to start at low dose then build up to the maximum tolerable. On basic principles, an antidepressant might help whether used alone or in conjunction with an anticonvulsant. That being said, there are no published empirical studies demonstrating an effect of any drug on apparent hyperosmia, distorted or phantom smells.

Case Report 8.1: A 23-Year-Old Housewife with Hyperosmia following Minor Head Injury. This lady was involved in a rear end collision while stationary in her car at traffic lights. She was in the driver's seat, the seat belt was applied correctly, and there were head restraints, but the airbag did not inflate. The impact caused her to bang the head on the sun visor, resulting in a laceration of the forehead. There was no alteration of consciousness.

Over the next few days she became headachy and noticed hypersensitivity to smells, particularly perfume and deodorants. She had experienced a similar degree of hyperosmia during the early months of pregnancy and consulted her GP on two occasions, each time thinking she might be pregnant again but the appropriate urine tests were negative. When examined five months after the accident she was still complaining of hyperosmia but no abnormality of the nose or sinuses was detected. A basic taste identification test was normal and on the UPSIT she scored 37/40 (normal). After the test she remarked "I hope I never have to do this test again as I feel very sick now." An MRI brain scan showed no sino-nasal disease and gradient-echo sequences did not disclose any areas of petechial hemorrhage (signs of severe head injury).

Comment. The initial injury was clearly minor, but it is likely there was slight damage to the olfactory tracts from shearing forces at the time of accident. The proximity of hyper-osmia to the time of accident gives credulity to her story, and so does her initial belief that she might have been pregnant. Another possibility would be triggering of migraine by the head trauma and the associated hyperosmia that is occasionally reported by migraineurs. She gave no history of migraine or prior hyperosmia apart from that experienced during early pregnancy. No treatment was requested by the patient. As mentioned in Chapter 3 there is some doubt about the existence of true hyperosmia and many apparent cases are really hyper-reactivity rather than increased power of detection. Her UPSIT score was unremarkable and no threshold test data were available to confirm her complaint of hypersensitivity. There is little available guidance on the prognosis for hyperosmia, but most complaints of hyperosmia tend to resolve gradually over the course of several years.

Gustation

History and Investigation. As mentioned in earlier chapters, medication is far more likely to influence the ability to taste than to smell, thus a detailed history of recent medication is essential. Major offenders include: antibiotics for helicobacter; chemotherapy for breast and gynecological cancers, particularly the taxane group; chlorhexidine mouthwash; hypnotics, terbinafine (Lamisil), ACE inhibitors, beta-blockers, anti-lipid drugs; and Chinese pine nuts. Enquiry should be made into peripheral causes of dysgeusia including facial palsy, third-molar tooth extraction, head injury, middle ear surgery, radiotherapy, and chemotherapy.

Examination of the oral cavity will help identify local causes of dysgeusia such as poor oral hygiene, dental disorder, dry mouth, smoking, etc. Central causes of taste dysfunction are rare and include brain stem vascular and neoplastic disorders, as well as lesions in the thalamus and cerebral hemispheres. The presence of metabolic and immune disease may be relevant, in particular, liver and kidney disease, diabetes, and Sjögren's syndrome.

As emphasized in Chapter 3, no matter how "perfect" a given test procedure may be, if it takes hours to evaluate just one subject it is unlikely to be used in any context, clinical or even research. For the busy but enthusiastic clinician, the number of commercially available tests is severely limited – in contrast to the much wider choice for olfactory evaluation. Electrogustometry is very practical because it does not require mixing or storage of chemicals. If just a basic threshold measure is all that is needed, both sides of the anterior tongue may be assessed in about 10 minutes, but more accurate testing requires a staircase approach and 20–30 minutes of someone's time. Care must be made in placement of the electrode, as slight variation in positioning can result in significant differences in sensitivity, given the uneven distribution of taste bud-containing papillae. The commercial choice rests between electrogustometry, taste sprays or taste filter strips. One might consider single solution assessments such as that developed for NHANES or dissolvable taste strips made from the polymer, hydroxypropyl methyl cellulose. Whole-mouth procedures reflect a patient's general perception and are less time consuming than regional taste tests, although they can overlook unilateral or regional damage to localized taste bud fields of CN VII and CN IX.

A blood screen analogous to that mentioned above in the olfactory deficit section should be performed, in particular autoimmune tests (protein electrophoresis; anti-Ro and anti-La antibodies for Sjögren's disease) and IgE (allergic rhinitis). Further investigation will depend on the suspected underlying cause. Measurement of salivary flow is valuable in cases of dry mouth. If CN VII is affected, a thorough examination of the external and middle ear is required, supplemented by CT or MRI scan of the petrous temporal bone. If there is a suspected neurological disorder affecting the brain stem or cortex (e.g., vascular, neoplastic, or traumatic), then MRI of the brain should be performed. Disorder of Cranial Nerves IX, X, or XI requires MRI of the posterior fossa, possibly supplemented by special views of the jugular foramen. Functional imaging by fMRI and PET belong to the domain of research.

Treatment. The drugs that have been used for ageusia are mostly zinc salts, but these should be given only where there is good evidence of deficiency, e.g., secondary to renal or liver disease (Weisman et al., 1979; Mahajan et al., 1980). Despite this, zinc salts are regularly prescribed out of therapeutic desperation if nothing else.

For all other cases, treatment is directed toward the underlying problem. If the patient is troubled by dysgeusia or phantogeusia, there is more likelihood of a local problem in the mouth. Candida infection is easily eradicated with an antifungal mouthwash such as Nystatin. A history of facial palsy or surgery to the ear or neck would lead one to suspect damage of the chorda tympani, although repair of this nerve is rarely attempted. Artificial saliva such as Xerolube may help those with xerostomia. Pilocarpine, the cholinergic drug, promotes salivary flow and is worth trying in these patients. The initial dose of 5 mg four times daily has been found to alleviate the dry mouth associated with radiation to the head and neck region. Subjects with dysgeusia as part of the burning mouth syndrome may be helped by application of topical anesthetic, e.g., Dyclonine 1.0% as a mouthwash. Antidepressants or antiepileptic drugs may be tried for this syndrome; of these we find gabapentin (Neurontin) and Pregabalin (Lyrica) in standard doses to be most effective. Individuals who are refractory to this approach may have a psychogenic disorder and need psychiatric help. In theory, it should be possible to assist those with familial dysautonomia by treatment with the suspected missing growth factor – BDNF. If there is damage to a peripheral nerve concerned with taste, conceptually BDNF might assist recovery, given the gustatory deficits in BDNF mutant mice (Nosrat et al., 1997).

A drug history is very relevant and reference should be made to Table 6.2. Even if the drug is not listed, a trial of withdrawal would be appropriate in many instances.

Medicolegal Aspects of Chemosensory Disorders

Head injury is a common cause of anosmia as described in Chapter 5. It should be recalled that severe trauma can lead to damage of the frontal and temporal poles, each of which is concerned with olfaction. Thus, damage to the temporal pole may injure the amygdala or piriform nucleus, which are primary olfactory regions. Frontal pole injury may involve the orbitofrontal cortex, which is an association area for smell (and taste). Anosmia can develop from mild trauma in the absence of skull fracture and possibly after whiplash injury (Kramer,

1983). Medical experts working for insurance companies who deal with head injured patients often forget to ask about smell impairment and, if any tests are done at all, they are usually inadequate. If injury involves the face directly, there may be conductive anosmia from fracture of nasal bones, displacement of the septum, or nasal congestion from blood and debris, etc. This type may resolve after surgical correction and resolution of edema, so further testing is desirable, say, 6–12 months after the trauma. Such patients may demonstrate unilateral anosmia over the initial months, but it can be persistent and will be overlooked if the nostrils are not tested independently. It is not sufficient just to ask a head-injured (or indeed any) patient about their smell perception. By analogy with cognitively normal Parkinson's disease patients, only 15 to 40 percent will be aware of a defect (Doty et al., 1988; Hawkes et al., 1997) and if there is cognitive impairment, which is often the case in brain injury, the figure will be higher still. Although practical brief olfactory tests are available for preliminary vetting in outpatient practice (see Chapter 3 and the beginning of this chapter), more comprehensive assessment is necessary to detect malingerers reliably. Assuming a deficit is not simulated or exaggerated, then further evaluation or repeated measurement would be appropriate at say, yearly intervals, although the prognosis for recovery is poor overall and depends upon the patient's age and severity of initial loss (London et al., 2008).

During the recovery phase a number of patients complain of distorted smell perception such that everyday odors induce a bland or unpleasant sensation (parosmia/dysosmia). Most parosmias or dysosmias resolve spontaneously, although this can take years and, when due to damage of the olfactory epithelium, may indicate further injury to the remaining olfactory receptor cells that signal the aberrant information (e.g., from viral infections). Treatment is problematic but, in a few cases antiepileptic or antidepressant medication may be of value, as described above for the management of hyperosmia.

On the industrial front, there are numerous olfactory toxins that may cause damage, as described in Chapter 5 (Section 14). Unquestionably, there is an association between many of those listed, but several reports are anecdotal or based on small numbers from financially motivated claimants. Some odor symptoms related to pollutants are primarily the result of sensory properties of the pollutants themselves which should resolve spontaneously, once the individual is removed from the workplace. Those exposed to pollutants may be receiving or have taken medication that by itself can affect smell sense or they may suffer coexisting disease known to alter olfaction. Note should be made of the compound alleged to have caused the olfactory defect and whether multiple substances were involved simultaneously. For most compounds there is a published Threshold Limit Value (TLV) established by the American Conference of Governmental Hygienists (ACGIH) that gives an idea of max-imum safe exposure levels and from this the magnitude of exposure can be estimated. This is of most relevance in cases of acute exposure, but for chronic exposure there may be individual susceptibility. The duration of exposure, latency of onset to first symptoms, their progression, and presence of dysosmia need to be recorded as well as the quality of ventilation, efficiency of filtration, and whether one or more workers had comparable symptoms at the same time. Importantly, TLVs are generally determined for non-olfactory end-points and rarely is olfaction considered when such guidelines are established.

According to guidance given by Sumner (1976), the law courts will wish to satisfy themselves on several counts in relation to anosmia:
1. that trauma or industrial exposure can produce anosmia itself –now an incontrovertible fact.
2. that there was no evidence of anosmia before the episode

3. that local causes of anosmia have been excluded
4. that there is no sign of amplification of symptoms or frank malingering
5. that the prognosis for recovery is based on reasoned assessment.

The same criteria could be applied to the loss of taste function, although as noted elsewhere in this book reports of taste loss usually reflect damage to the olfactory system. When true taste loss is present, i.e., an ability to detect sweet, sour, bitter, salty, or savory (umami) sensations, it is rarely salient and almost never identified by the patient.

It is sometimes difficult to know when to finalize a claim for anosmia, as there may be some prospect for recovery after a prolonged period. In broad terms, an interval of not exceeding three years from the date of injury would be reasonable. If the sense of smell has not recovered by then, the deficit is likely to be permanent. An exception appears to be parosmia, the prevalence of which in one series decreased from 41.1% to 15.4% over eight years post-trauma (Doty et al., 1997). Few people are happy to wait that long and the specialist may have to compromise by serial assessment at yearly intervals to determine the point at which no further improvement has taken place.

Case Report 8.2: **A Heavy Goods Vehicle Driver and Amateur Chef with Post-Traumatic Anosmia.** A 56-year-old man was hit just above the left eyebrow by a piece of protruding scaffolding. There was no laceration or impairment of consciousness. Later that day, he noted lack of smell when using deodorant, and during the evening when eating a curry dish, there was no smell from the food although it tasted spicy. On the following day, he experienced a peculiar burning odor, described as an "acid sharp burning" sensation which persisted for one week. It sometimes woke him from sleep. A further week later, the smell sense disappeared completely. He specifically mentioned lack of odor from onions, ammonia, or bleach; all food tasted bland. When interviewed two years after the accident he reported no improvement in the sense of smell and no recurrence of the parosmic burning sensation. One of his hobbies was to cook meals for friends each weekend. Following the accident, it became difficult to mix sauces by their smell or taste and he resorted to cooking simpler dishes. He took the precaution of installing smoke and gas detectors throughout his house and a special malodor detector in his refrigerator. General neurological examination was unremarkable; likewise, a brief identification test to five tastants was normal. His score on the UPSIT was within the anosmic (but not malingering) range at 16/40.

Comment. The most reasonable explanation is post-traumatic anosmia, as a result of a relatively minor blow to the head. It is now accepted that even minor blows to the head may damage the sense of smell. The history is convincing because of the relatively immediate appearance of smell loss and its association with transient parosmia. The UPSIT scores are within the anosmic range and show no sign of malingering (range usually 0–4). His test scores and medical history are convincing and would strongly support his claim for anosmia and disruption of his main hobby as an amateur chef. Assuming the smell loss to be complete, the likelihood of recovery of useful smell function is poor.

Case Report 8.3: **A Manual Laborer and Amateur Archer with Microsmia and Probable Parkinson's Disease following Head Trauma.** This 59-year-old manual laborer, who was a keen amateur archer, was involved in an accident at work. He slipped on a wet floor surface, striking the left side of his head on a metal girder. He was concussed but did not lose consciousness. There was blood oozing from the left ear and subsequent examination revealed a perforation injury of the ear drum. Two weeks later he noted shaking of the left hand. During archery practice, he found it difficult to operate the bow and maintain the arrow steady because of tremulous movement. He was referred for a neurological opinion one year after the accident. Examination revealed an intermittent rest tremor without any increase of tone. MRI brain scan was normal but the DATScan showed bilateral reduction of transporter uptake in the putamen on both sides. The UPSIT score was 26/40 which is within the microsmic range for a male of 59 years. The Mini-Mental Status Examination Score was normal at 28/30 and so were tests of taste threshold.

Comment. This man had good evidence on neurological examination, smell testing, and DATScan of tremulous Parkinson's disease. The UPSIT score was within a range suggestive of significant, but not total, loss of function, without evidence of malingering or amplification of symptoms. The medicolegal question posed was whether the accident could have caused a tremor which emerged after just two weeks. There is a large and confusing literature on post-traumatic PD without any clear consensus, apart from those rare instances of parkinsonism resulting from repeated blows to the head, as in boxing. The latent period of two weeks from accident to tremor is far too short for the development of classical PD. Furthermore, an injury to the left skull, if it caused tremor at all, would be more likely to do so on the right side of the body unless there was a contre-coup effect, which would be unusual for subcortical structures. One possibility is that the subject was in the early stages of PD at the time of accident and that the injury unmasked latent PD. The abnormal smell tests are compatible with a diagnosis of PD. A normal UPSIT score would have been more in keeping with a parkinsonian syndrome (e.g., progressive supranuclear palsy, corticobasal degeneration, vascular parkinsonism) or essential tremor. If the smell defect is secondary to PD, it will be permanent.

Malingering

The 4th edition of the American Psychiatric Association's Diagnostic and Statistical Manual (DSM-IV) defines malingering as "the intentional production of false or grossly exaggerated physical or psychological symptoms motivated by external incentives" (2000). Many patients claim to have smell or taste disturbances when, in fact, they have normal or relatively normal function. Forced-choice tests, such as the UPSIT, are capable of detecting most patients who feign illness, because malingerers often deliberately deselect the correct answers more frequently than expected by chance. Those with non-organic disorders variously termed "functional," "hysterical," or psychogenic may also score badly on tests, but in our experience such patients are extremely rare. At one extreme is the patient with true hysteria, where there may be no deliberate deception but the patient has assumed the features of disease – so-called conversion hysteria. Between true hysteria and malingering are people who, because of various stressors (anxiety, depression, etc.), score badly. This may be unintentional but nonetheless extremely difficult to detect.

In a unique study, the responses to general medical history and demographic items on a 350-item questionnaire were obtained from 22 chemosensory malingerers who provided improbable responses on the UPSIT and other forced-choice tests and 66 with genuine symptoms matched to the malingerers on the basis of etiology (Doty & Crastnopol, 2010). Variables that best predicted false or exaggerated illness were identified using logistic regression. Relative to genuine subjects, malingerers reported significantly fewer dental problems, allergies, surgical operations, cigarettes smoked, and nasal sinus problems. Malingerers also described use of fewer medications and reported experiencing more weight loss, decreased appetite, taste loss, interference with daily activities, and putative symptom-related psychological duress. They were more likely to be involved in litigation than their non-malingering counterparts. Interestingly, age, sex, education, and length of symptom description in the questionnaire did not differentiate malingerers from genuine responders.

An example of a woman who was found to malinger is presented in the following case report.

Case Report 8.4: **A Female Chef with Impaired Chemosensation after Nasal Surgery.** A 23-year-old woman, reportedly working as a chef, presented with complaints of decreased smell and taste function secondary to a nasal operation undertaken three years earlier. She mentioned subsequent operations in an effort to mitigate pain, poor cosmetic result, and nasal stuffiness. On the first visit for chemosensory assessment, the UPSIT score was suggestive of severe microsmia (22/40). Phenylethyl alcohol (PEA) detection thresholds were mildly elevated, and the score on the 12-item Odor Memory Test was at chance level (3/12). Her score on the Beck Depression inventory was high (36), suggesting significant psychological depression. While electrogustometric thresholds on the left and right sides of the anterior tongue were within normal limits, whole-mouth identification testing of sweet, sour, bitter, and salty stimuli were at chance level and suprathreshold ratings of taste intensity and hedonics were atypically flattened across ascending concentrations. In contrast, her regional tongue tests were within normal limits. This pattern of taste test response was difficult to explain on the basis of a nasal operation and raised the specter of malingering. A year later she was re-tested because her court case was due and the attorney wanted to know whether the deficit was long-lasting. On this occasion she scored 3/40 on the UPSIT, in keeping with malingering. When repeated, the score was zero. By chance alone she should have scored around 10 on the UPSIT on both occasions. Based on these two test scores, the probability of her having true anosmia and not avoiding the correct answer was roughly 4.7 in one billion. Similar improbable responses were observed on the re-administration of the PEA detection threshold test which, like the UPSIT, is a forced-choice procedure. In this case, the binomial probability of missing so many trials was less than 1.2 in 100,000 for someone with no smell function. Her taste scores were also suspect, just as they were on the first occasion. The best interpretation of these findings is that on the first assessment there was probably some smell loss that subsequently improved over the course of a year. On the second test occasion, she must have deliberately avoided answers she knew to be correct on both the olfactory and gustatory tests, thus confirming evidence of malingering.

Detection of Malingering and Patients with Non-organic Psychiatric Disorders

Traditionally, it has been assumed that malingering can be detected reliably by asking a patient to inhale a strong trigeminal stimulant, such as ammonia, and enquiring whether a smell is perceived. If this is denied, the assumption was made that malingering is present. Unfortunately, this procedure is unreliable, since ammonia usually evokes reflex coughing, secretion from nasal membranes, or other rejection reactions which the patient obviously cannot deny. Furthermore, trigeminal thresholds vary considerably; some may experience little reaction to the ammonia and truthfully report perceiving no sensations. Indeed, anosmia has been associated with heightened trigeminal thresholds (Gudziol et al., 2001). The clever malingerer may be smart enough to report the irritant effect, so the accuracy of the procedure is questionable and, in the authors' view, this test should not be employed.

Table 8.1. Probabilities (not p values) of a particular UPSIT score by chance based on a single test. This table is relevant to detection of malingering. A person with complete anosmia by chance would, on average, have a mean score of 10/40, given that there of 4 alternative odors to be selected. Thus a value of 10/40 would be found by chance in 144/1000 true anosmics, whereas 0/40 would happen just once in every 100,000 people and should provide strong evidence of malingering. Subjects scoring within the gray-shaded area are probably malingering. Table courtesy of DR Altmann, Institute of Hygiene and Tropical Medicine, London.

Score/40	Probability of this score by chance alone	Number of people/1000 who might score this value by chance alone
0	0.00001	0.01
1	0.00013	0.13
2	0.00087	0.87
3	0.00368	3.68
4	0.01135	11.35
5	0.02723	27.23
6	0.05295	52.95
7	0.08573	85.73
8	0.11788	117.88
9	0.13971	139.71
10	0.14436	144.36

The results of longer forced-choice tests, including identification and detection threshold measures, can be examined for improbable responses that usually signify malingering. On the UPSIT, for example, malingerers typically score between zero and 4 out of 40 (see Table 8.1). The probability of achieving 4/40 by chance is 0.011, i.e., an occurrence of 11 people in 1000, whereas a value of zero corresponds to a probability of 0.0001, i.e., an occurrence of 1 person in 10,000. To achieve such a low score, the patient must first identify the odor and then avoid the correct answer. In general, if a patient scores within the probable malingering region on the UPSIT, the test should be repeated, to confirm the apparent avoidance of correct responses. Multiplication of the two probabilities is then used to establish the statistical likelihood of malingering. Some true anosmics scratch the UPSIT pad so hard that they abrade the strip down to its cardboard backing (Doty et al., 1998) – a feature not seen in malingering. Some malingerers (and genuine anosmics) repetitively choose the same response to every test item, i.e., they always indicate for example, the first option in each set of four response alternatives on the UPSIT and this will result in a score around 10/40, which is in the true anosmic range. Prior to testing it is therefore important to advise subjects against selecting the same response option for each question and to inspect the pattern of choices for each question, but at present there is no formula to distinguish whether the pattern of selection is that of deliberate deselection by a malingerer or response-variable preference by a genuine anosmic.

For the Sniffin' Sticks screening test or B-SIT, in both of which there are 12 odors with a forced choice of one from 4 possible answers, the chances of a genuine low score are higher (Table 8.2). The likelihood of scoring 0/12 is 0.03 or three people in 100. The total probability

Table 8.2. The 12 odor Sniffin' Stick and B-SIT probabilities of a low score in a genuine anosmic subject. Courtesy DR Altmann, Institute of Hygiene and Tropical Medicine, London.

Score out of 12	Probability of score in genuine anosmic
0	0.032
1	0.127
2	0.232

of getting less than three is the sum of these at 0.39. Hence, nearly 40% of genuinely anosmic people will score less than three. Although the odds are higher than the UPSIT, a score of 0/12 should nevertheless raise suspicion of malingering and call for further evaluation.

Some patients with genuine smell impairment but preserved taste may deliberately avoid correct answers on forced-choice taste tests. This pattern reflects a naïve attempt to embellish the "taste loss" which in reality stems from lack of retronasal stimulation of the olfactory receptors. Such behavior usually confirms a normal ability to taste.

Non-psychological Procedures. The Olfactory Event-Related Potential (OERP) is of potential value in detecting a malingerer as long as (1) the technical difficulties can be overcome, (2) the patient cooperates with the examiner (e.g., does not exhibit significant body movements), and (3) the subject is not unduly stressed by the obvious importance and complexity of the procedure. In theory, olfactory agnosia in such cases cannot be ruled out so that a patient with a temporal lobe defect could have difficulty naming odors in the presence of a normal OERP. Brain imaging by MRI, CT, or SPECT may show post-traumatic change in a relevant area, e.g., temporal, insular, or orbitofrontal cortices. The gradient echo MRI sequence is particularly useful in revealing petechial areas of hemorrhage which can persist for several years after head trauma and may be invisible on conventional MRI. There may be atrophy of the olfactory bulb (Yousem et al., 1999), a point of relevance where there is a suspicion of amplification or malingering. Even with this procedure there are added difficulties as there are no healthy control measurements that take into account the effect of age and sex, and it is unknown whether the olfactory bulbs regress in size in a uniform manner over time among different individuals. Nonetheless, there is growing evidence of strong associations between MRI-determined olfactory bulb volumes and olfactory function in both normal individuals and in persons with olfactory deficits (see Doty, 2015, for review). For example, a -0.86 correlation was noted by Turetsky et al. (2000) between MRI-determined olfactory volumes and detection thresholds for phenylethyl alcohol in a group of 22 healthy subjects. Theoretically, malingering might be detected by fMRI or PET studies using olfactory stimuli. Such measures may not be reliable because activity could be present in primary olfactory areas and not in tertiary regions, making it possible that the subject is genuinely unaware of odors, All this assumes, as noted above, that a malingerer will co-operate with a complex test – which is unlikely.

Several cognitive tests are used by neuropsychologists on which amnesic patients perform well, yet malingerers fail to do so. One example is the Rey's Memory Test, also known as Rey's 3×5 test, and the Rey 15-item memory test (Rey, 1964). The rationale behind this is that malingerers will fail at a memory task that all but the most retarded or severely brain-damaged persons perform easily. This is a highly specialized area of evaluation for which the reader is referred elsewhere (e.g., Hall & Pritchard, 1996).

Case Report 8.5: **An Office Worker with Probable Malingering.** An 18-year-old lady reported loss of taste and smell after an accident in which she fell from the back of a pickup truck, striking her head on the ground. There was concussion and amnesia for the entire event. The CT brain scan revealed a transverse fracture of the left temporal bone predominantly through the mastoid bone. There was transient decrease in hearing on the left, as well as mild positional vertigo. She was referred for assessment by her lawyer three years after the accident. According to the patient records, she had previously reported to an otolaryngologist (who was following up her case) that her sense of smell was improving. Upon testing, the UPSIT score was 1, which was well within the probable malingering range. The UPSIT was repeated, giving a score of 3, a value that similarly fell within the probable malingering range. On a two-alternative forced-choice odor detection threshold test, in which a blank and an odor were presented in random fashion, the patient performed correctly on only 24 of the 96 trials (25%; chance level). On a forced-choice regional taste test, in which six trials each of sweet-, sour-, bitter-, and salty-tasting substances are presented to four regions of the tongue (6 trials × 4 tastants × 4 tongue regions = 96 trials), this patient missed 79 of the 96 trials; i.e., she only provided correct responses on 17 of the 96 trials (18%). On this test, a forced-choice response is also required to four response alternatives (sweet, sour, bitter, and salty).

Comment. This lady most likely suffered transient loss of smell from head trauma, but had subsequently improved and was malingering for litigation purposes. A true anosmic would correctly answer, on average, one-quarter of the UPSIT items, or have a predicted average score of 10. There is a sampling distribution around this value, but the binomial probability of achieving a score of 1 out of 40 on this 4-alternative forced choice test by an anosmic is 0.0001. On the second administration, she scored 3/40, which has a binomial probability of occurrence of 0.0037. The combined probability of her being a true anosmic based on these test responses alone is $0.0001 \times 0.0037 = 3.70^{-6}$. On the olfactory threshold test, the binomial probability of missing 72 of 96 trials by chance is <0.000001. Her taste tests also suggested she was deliberately avoiding correct responses. For example, on a test in which 25 percent of 96 trials would be expected on the basis of random responding (i.e., 24), she detected correctly only 17. The probability of performing this badly and not avoiding the correct responses would be less than 1 in a 1000. Olfactory event-related potentials were not done but presumably they would be normal in this case.

Case Report 8.6: A 57-Year-Old Housewife with Smell and Taste Impairment Related to Fungal Sinus Infection. This was a graduate in psychology who suffered recurrent urinary tract infection for several years and was placed on a long-term antibiotic, Nitrofurantoin (Furadantin®, Macrodantin®, Macrobid®). The treatment worked well, but after three years use she developed chronic active hepatitis, a recognized complication of long-term use of this drug. This was treated by long-term steroids, but after two months she developed progressive blurring of vision and a lower altitudinal field defect in the left eye. Investigation showed a fungal infection (aspergillus) in the sphenoid and ethmoid sinuses. Treatment with an antifungal drug, amphotericin B (Fungilin®; Fungisome®) and spheno-ethmoidotomy resulted in improved vision. Two weeks after surgery, she returned home and noticed for the first time that her smell sense was impaired. Sweet food and chocolates tasted normal, but there was no sensation from flowers or shrubs and she lost all interest in cooking. There was some odorous sensation if garlic was held close to the nose. Formerly, she was able to tell if her urine was infected by its abnormal odor, but this was impossible. On one occasion, her husband came home to find the house full of gas. A writ had been served on her primary care physicians for (1) failing to monitor liver function while taking long-term Nitrofurantoin, (2) subsequent development of chronic active hepatitis, and (3) complications of steroid use.

Detailed evaluation was performed about three years after surgery at the request of her solicitor. The taste threshold over the tongue tip using a Rion electrogustometer was elevated significantly at 64µA (normal below 25 µA). The UPSIT score was 12/40 which is well within the anosmic range. She was distressed throughout this test, commenting that everything smelled the same. Evaluation of thresholds to phenylethyl alcohol with the Sensonics' Smell Threshold Test using the single staircase method was also abnormal at over minus 2.00 log vol/vol (normal, minus 6.0 to minus 5.5). Olfactory event-related potential recordings (OERP) showed a *normal* latency to H_2S of 412mS, recorded from Pz.

Comment. Several interesting points are raised by this case. Most likely, long-term steroid exposure caused the fungal infection in the sinuses. Such infection could easily have impaired the sense of smell, but so could the surgical decompression and the use of the antifungal agent, amphotericin B. On questioning she affirmed that smell impairment was first noticed only on arriving home after she would have completed 16 days of amphotericin therapy. She did not think it occurred after surgery. The first question is whether the smell loss was genuine. The history alone is convincing in many respects; her inability to detect the smell of infected urine and of the house filled with gas unknown to her. Her score on UPSIT was at chance level, and the smell threshold value was elevated markedly, in keeping with a diagnosis of anosmia. Although no problem with taste was declared, the electro-gustometer suggested partial impairment. Despite the fact that this patient had a degree in psychology and therefore might have sufficient knowledge to fabricate some of her symptoms, there was no evidence that this occurred. It is of interest, however, that the OERP, which should have been a deciding "objective" test, was within normal limits. The final opinion offered was that the anosmia was in fact genuine and the delay in reporting a problem related to general malaise in hospital where she was recovering from major surgery. It was considered that when she had fully recuperated from inpatient treatment, she would have been better placed to detect other, less severe problems. It was advised that the normal OERP may have been a technical issue caused by inadvertent stimulation of healthy nasal trigeminal afferent fibers. The cause of anosmia was thought to be a mixture of fungal infection, possibly sinus surgery and exposure to a drug (Amphotericin B) known to produce anosmia. Amphotericin B may have caused the mild impairment of taste as well. Useful recovery of smell sense in someone with such severe loss is unlikely to occur three years after the initiating event. This case was eventually settled in the claimant's favor, out of court.

General Advice and Vocational Issues

Olfaction. The medicolegal and indeed everyday clinical importance of anosmia or hyposmia relates to occupation. A wine taster or chef may well be unemployable if there is even the smallest reduction in olfactory identification or threshold and the potential for legitimate financial compensation is high. This contrasts with the unskilled laborer, who would be entitled to less. Where a workman may be exposed to natural gas, e.g., a plumber, continued employment would be difficult unless a gas detector was carried on site. In general, a plaintiff's former employment should be allowed to continue unless a good sense of smell is essential or the person had to work alone in a potentially dangerous environment. A retired person would command less financial reward, but the dangers in everyday life must not be underestimated, nor the lack of enjoyment from food or drink and the overall reduction in the quality of life.

Disability awards and compensations are provided in the USA under the 1963 amendment to the Workman's Compensation Law. Where a diminution of future earning power is apparent, the Veterans Administration awards a 10 percent disability for total anosmia. In general, there is considerable inter-state variability in workman compensation payment and the results of private individual settlements are hardly ever made public. Up to a 5 percent compensation for anosmia is suggested by the 6th edition of the American Medical Association's Guides to the Evaluation of Permanent Impairment: "Only rarely does complete loss of the closely related senses of olfaction and taste seriously affect an individual's performance of the usual activities of daily living. For this reason, a 1% to 5% impairment of the whole person is suggested for use in cases involving partial or complete bilateral loss of either sense due to peripheral lesions" (Anderson & Cocchiarella, 1995). This is surprising, given that anosmia or dysosmia disqualifies applicants for service in the US Armed Forces, including the Coast Guard, and can be a basis for discharge or retirement (Air Force Directive 48–123 Vol 2, 2006). Private accident insurance policies in the United Kingdom recompense their clients by less than 10 percent of that awarded for parallel cases in the United States. In the United Kingdom, an average level of compensation for non-vocational smell disorder is £12,000 for partial loss of smell and £18,000 for complete loss.

In the case of negligence by health professionals, published median settlements and awards to claimants for olfactory loss in the United States were found to range from $300,000 to $412,000 (Svider et al., 2014). Otolaryngologists were the most frequently named defendants (68.0%), with most iatrogenic cases (55.0%) related to rhinologic procedures. Complications that accompanied anosmia included dysgeusia, cerebrospinal fluid leaks, and meningitis.

Anosmic patients and even those experiencing natural decline of smell function through aging should be given guidance on simple precautions. A disproportionate number of elderly people die from accidental gas poisonings (Chalke & Dewhurst, 1956) and, presumably, had they been advised properly, this tragedy would not have occurred. Inadvertent consumption of stale or infected food probably causes minor ailments in the elderly and on occasion, food poisoning. Nutritional problems and weight loss in the aged may relate to anosmia, as food loses its appeal. Indeed, it is suspected that the frequent finding of weight loss in patients with advanced Parkinson's disease relates to hyposmia, which, as mentioned in Chapter 4, affects at least 80 percent of these individuals (Hawkes et al., 1997). A smoke detector is essential for the kitchen and in every room where there is the potential for fire. It is preferable to have a detector in all bedrooms, particularly in those belonging to smokers. An electric cooker (range) is preferable to one operated by gas. If the household has a gas supply, patients should purchase a gas detector for this as well. Propane, butane, and petroleum spirit (gasoline) are heavier than air and because of this, detectors for them should be placed near the ground. Natural gas and smoke are lighter than air so the detectors for this need to be situated near the ceiling or top of the stairwell. An anosmic person may have difficulty appreciating spoiled food, which can be hazardous to eat even if kept in the refrigerator. Such people should be encouraged to discard leftover food and milk products and ideally ask someone with normal smell sense to check before consumption. Finally, advice ideally from a dietician should be given on how to enhance the appeal of food with artificial flavorings, without inducing weight gain. A book written by a chef and a neurologist that is supported by the American Academy of Neurology provides several recipes designed to make more food appealing to persons with smell deficits (DeVere and Calvert, 2011).

A frequently underappreciated fact is that simply quantifying the degree of olfactory loss and ruling out serious causes is extremely beneficial for the psychological well-being of a patient, whether or not treatment is possible. Helping the patient place into perspective the magnitude of his or her loss is very therapeutic, and in some cases mitigates depression and other symptoms produced by fear or by uncaring medical providers. Many patients feel alienated and are unaware that others suffer the same predicament. Meeting other individuals with similar problems in a waiting room, for example, has proven in our experience to be most helpful, since the patient becomes directly aware they are not "suffering alone." It can be pointed out to an older person who has significant smell loss (in an absolute sense) that their olfactory test scores are actually above the 50th percentile relative to individuals of their same age and sex. This patient may leave with the understanding that while loss has occurred, he or she is still "hanging in there" and is outperforming the majority of his or her peers.

Importantly, patients who fear safety issues, such as inability to detect leaking natural gas and fire, can be counseled about smoke and gas detectors, as well as changing from gas to electrical appliances where economically possible. Psychological strategies to help patients cope with their disability are beyond the scope of this book, but are described in elsewhere (Tennen et al., 1991).

Gustation. Some taste complaints relating to pollutants are simply a result of the sensory properties of the pollutants themselves rather than direct pathological change in the taste receptor or neural pathway. Recovery is to be expected once the person is removed from the workplace. Persons exposed to pollutants may be taking or have received medication that can affect taste sense or they may suffer from coexisting disease known to alter gustation. It is important to quantify the degree of loss and for this, referral to a specialist center or clinic is essential, especially where the claimant is suspected to be fabricating their taste problem. The overall approach is similar to that concerning anosmia claims. Head injury rarely causes ageusia, but if there has been a blow to the head, even trivial in nature, an MRI brain scan would be essential. Particular attention must be paid to the insula area, orbitofrontal cortex, and temporal lobes. If functional imaging can be performed, that would be ideal in problematic cases. There are few examples of industrial gas or chemical exposure in association with ageusia but organophosphates, paint solvents, selenium, and other sulfur-containing chemicals have been incriminated. As mentioned above, the threshold limit value (TLV) or equivalent may provide a useful guide to the magnitude of exposure.

Detection of malingering in ageusic individuals is a major problem and once more should be addressed in specialist centers. Threshold and identification tests are the most important initial procedures. Suspicion would be aroused if the subject claimed to detect no taste for all substances irrespective of concentration, although a number of older persons have considerable difficulty detecting tastants presented to small regions of the tongue. Note that there is crude taste appreciation from lingual nerve somatosensory fibers, thus an ageusic may report something even if it is just burning or irritation mediated by the trigeminal nerve. As in the case of smell loss, rating scales can be used to compare the relationship between concentration and perceived intensity. In general, monotonically increasing intensity functions should occur as stimulus intensity increases. Persons with no taste generally exhibit relatively flat functions. Variations from monotonicity, assuming an adequate number of test trials, would arouse suspicion. Recording of gustatory evoked cortical responses would be an ideal and objective approach, but this procedure is still under development.

The impact of even a small degree of taste impairment on a wine taster or chef, for example, will command a major award as a career change will be essential. Even for those whose occupation does not depend on it, taste disturbance will have an important effect on the quality of life. It is likely that minor gastro-intestinal ailments will result from hypogeusia, although there are no specific studies of this. There is a conspicuous lack of literature and guidance for ageusia claims, particularly its prognosis for recovery but it is usually stated that taste impairments recover better than smell impairment, deficits possibly because of the multiple neural innervation of taste buds in different regions of the oral cavity.

Summary. Smell and taste complaints both require a thorough initial assessment by history and general investigations. For taste disorders in particular, a thorough medication history is essential. A general blood screen is advisable for all and so is imaging by CT or MRI. Specific chemosensory investigations should be initiated to decide whether the defect is conductive, due to disease in the nose or mouth, or sensorineural thereby relating to problems with the olfactory/taste nerves and their central connections. Treatment of chemosensory disorders is directed to the underlying disease and to assist the patient to cope with their problem from the psychological perspective. Steroids, zinc supplements, and various antioxidants are commonly tried, but their value is dubious. Steroids are beneficial only for local nasal conditions, particularly where there is conductive anosmia from polyps or hay fever. Some benefit may accrue from nasal operations that facilitate sinus drainage and reduce infection, although topical steroids are usually required to minimize local inflammation and such operations can have unexpected consequences. Measures to alleviate oral infection or dry mouth are often required to help dysgeusia. Where compensation is pursued the patient is best directed to a unit specializing in chemosensory problems, particularly where there is a question of malingering. It is important to help sufferers cope psychologically with their problem and to put their deficit in perspective, as well as to provide them with general advice about their occupation, safety in the home, and how to make food more palatable.

References

Air Force Instructions 48–123, Accession, Retention and Administration. *Medication Examination and Standards* Volume **2**, 5 June 2006.

Altundag, A.A., Cayonu, M., Kayabasoglu, G., Salihoglu, M., Tekeli, H., Saglam, O., et al., 2015. Modified olfactory training in patients with postinfectious olfactory loss. *Laryngoscope* **125**, 1763–1766.

Anderson, G.B.J., Cocchiarella, L., 1995. *Guides to the Evaluation of Permanent Impairment*, 6th Edition. Chicago: American Marketing Association Press.

Briggs, M.H., Duncan, R.B., 1961. Odor receptors. *Nature* **91**, 1310–1311.

Chalke, H.D., Dewhurst, J.R., Loss of smell in old people. *Publ. Health (London)* **72**, 223.

DeVere, R., Calvert, M., *Navigating Smell and Taste Disorders*. Saint Paul, MN, AAN Enterprises, Inc.

Dalton, P., Wysocki, C.J., 1995. The effects of long-term exposure to odorants on olfactory thresholds and perceived odor intensity. *Chemical Senses* **20**, 49.

Doty, R.L., 2015. Clinical disorders of olfaction. In: Doty, R.L. (Ed.), *Handbook of Olfaction and*

Gustation. Hoboken, NJ: John Wiley and Sons, pp. 375–401.

Doty, R.L., Crastnopol, B., 2010. Correlates of chemosensory malingering. *Laryngoscope* **120**(4), 707–711.

Doty, R.L., Snyder, P.J., Huggins, G.R., Lowry, L.D., 1981. Endocrine, cardiovascular, and psychological correlates of olfactory sensitivity changes during the human menstrual cycle. *Journal of Comparative & Physiological Psychology* **95**, 45–60.

Doty, R.L., Deems, D., Stellar, S., 1988. Olfactory dysfunction in Parkinson's disease: A general deficit unrelated to neurologic signs, disease stage, or disease duration. *Neurology* **38**, 1237–1244.

Doty, R.L., Genow, A., Hummel, T., 1988. Scratch density differentiates microsmic from normosmic and anosmic subjects on the University of Pennsylvania Smell Identification Test. *Perceptual and Motor Skills* **86**(1), 211–216.

Doty, R.L., Smith, R., McKeown, D.A., Raj, J., 1994. Tests of human olfactory function: Principal components analysis suggests that most measure a common source of variance. *Perception and Psychophysics* **56**(6), 701–707.

Doty, R.L., McKeown, D.A., Lee, W.W., Shaman, P., 1995. A study of the test-retest reliability of ten olfactory tests. *Chemical Senses.* **20**(6), 645–656.

Doty, R.L., Yousem, D.M., Pham, L.T., Kreshak, A.A., Geckle, R., Lee, W.W., 1997. Olfactory dysfunction in patients with head trauma. *Archives of Neurology* **54**(9), 1131–1140.

Duncan, R.B., Briggs, M.H., 1962. Treatment of uncomplicated anosmia by vitamin A. *Archives of Otolaryngology* **75**, 116–124.

Engen, T., 1960. Effect of practice and instruction on olfactory thresholds. *Perceptual and Motor Skills* **10**, 195–198.

Geissler, K., Reimann, H., Gudziol, H., Bitter, T., Guntinas-Lichius, O., 2001. Olfactory training for patients with olfactory loss after upper respiratory tract infections. *European Archives of Oto-Rhino-Laryngology* **271**, 1557–1562.

Gudziol, H., Schubert, M., Hummel, T., 1996. Decreased trigeminal sensitivity in anosmia. *ORL Journal for Oto-Rhino-Laryngology and Its Related Specialties* **63**(2), 72–75.

Hall, H.V., Pritchard, D.A., 1996. *Detecting Malingering and Deception.* Delray Beach, FL: St. Lucie Press.

Hagglund, M., Berghard, A., Strotmann, J., Bohm, S., 2006. Retinoic acid receptor-dependent survival of olfactory sensory neurons in postnasal and adult mice. *Journal of Neuroscience* **26**, 3281–3291.

Hawkes, C.H., Shephard, B.C., Daniel, S.E., 1997. Olfactory dysfunction in Parkinson's disease. *Journal of Neurology Neurosurgery and Psychiatry* **62**, 436–446.

Henkin, R.I., Schechter, P.J., Friedewald, W.T., et al., 1976. A double-blind study of the effects of zinc sulfate on taste and smell dysfunction. *The American Journal of the Medical Sciences* **272**, 167–174.

Hummel, T., Heilmann, S., Huttenbriuk, K.B., 2002. Lipoic acid in the treatment of smell dysfunction following viral infection of the upper respiratory tract. *Laryngoscope* **112**, 2076–2080.

Hummel, T, Rissom, K., Reden, J., Hahner, A., Weidenbecher, M., Huttenbrink, K.B., 2009. Effects of olfactory training in patients with olfactory loss. *Laryngoscope* **119**, 496–499.

Jackman, A.H., Doty, R.L., 2005. Utility of a three-item smell identification test in detecting olfactory dysfunction. *Laryngoscope* **115**(12), 2209–2212.

Jafek, B.W., Eller, P.M., Esses, B.A., Moran, D.T., 1989. Post-traumatic anosmia. Ultrastructural correlates. *Archives of Neurology* **46**(3), 300–304.

Kramer, G., 1983. Diagnosis of neurologic disorders after whiplash injuries of the cervical spine. *Deutsche Medizinische Wochenschrift* **108**(15), 586–588.

Lill, K., Reden, J., Muller, A., Zahnert, T., Hummel, T., 2006. Olfactory function in patients with post-infectious and post-traumatic smell disorders before and after treatment with vitamin A: A double-blind, placebo-controlled, randomized clinical trial. *Chemical Senses* **31**(5), Abstract A33.

London, B., Nabet, B., Fisher, A.R., White, B., Sammel, M.D., Doty, R.L., 2008. Predictors of prognosis in patients with olfactory disturbance. *Annals of Neurology* **63**, 159–166.

Mahajan, S.K., Prasad, A.S., Briggs, W.A., et al. Improvement in uremic hypogeusia by zinc: a double-blind study. *American Journal of Clinical Nutrition* 1980; **33**, 1517–1521.

Nosrat, C.A., Blomlöf, J., El Shamy, W.M., Ernfors, P., Olson, L., 1997. Lingual deficits in BDNF and NT3 mutant mice leading to gustatory and somatosensory disturbances, respectively. *Development* **124**, 1333–1342.

Panagiotopoulos, G., Naxakis, S., Papavasiliou, A., Filipakis, K., Papatheodorou, G., Goumas, P., 2005. Decreasing nasal mucus Ca improves hyposmia. *Rhinology* **43**, 130–134.

Patel, Z.M., 2017. The evidence for olfactory training in treating patients with olfactory loss. *Current Opinion in Otolaryngology & Head and Neck Surgery* **25**, 43–46.

Philpott, C.M., Erskine, S.E., Clark, A., Leeper, A., Salam, M., Sharma, R., Murty, G.E., Hummel, T., 2017. A randomised controlled trial of sodium citrate spray for non-conductive olfactory disorders. *Clinical Otolaryngology*.

Poletti, S.C., Michel, E., Hummel, T., 2017. Olfactory training using heavy and light weight molecule odors. *Perception* **46**, 343–351.

Rey, A., 1964. *L'examen clinique en psychologie.* Paris: Presses Universitaires de France.

Schechter, P.J., Friedewald, W.T., Bronzert, D.A., et al. 1972. Idiopathic hypogeusia: a description of the syndrome and a single blind study with zinc sulfate. *International Review of Neurobiology* **1**, 125–140

Soter, A., Kim, J., Jackman, A., Tourbier, I., Kaul, A., Doty, R.L., 2008. Accuracy of self-report in detecting taste dysfunction. *Laryngoscope* **118**, 611–617.

Stegeman, C.A., Cohen Tervaert, J.W., de Jong, P.E., Kallenberg, C.G., 1996. Trimethoprim-sulfamethoxazole (co-trimoxazole) for the prevention of relapses of Wegener's granulomatosis. Dutch Co-Trimoxazole Wegener Study Group. *The New England Journal of Medicine* **335**, 16–20.

Steck-Scott, S., Forman, M.R., Sowell, A., Borkowf, C.B., Albert, P.S., Slattery, M., et al. 2004. Carotenoids, vitamin A and risk of adenomatous polyp recurrence in the polyp prevention trial. *International Journal of Cancer* **112**(2), 295–305.

Sumner, D., 1976. Disturbances of the senses of smell and taste after head injuries. In Vinken, P.J., Bruyn G.W. (Eds.).*Handbook of Clinical Neurology.* Elsevier Press Amsterdam. Eds Vol **24** Injuries of the Brain and Skull Part II Chapter 1, pp. 1–25.

Svider, P.F., Mauro, A.C., Eloy, J.A., Setzen, M., Carron, M.A., Folbe, A.J., 2014. Malodorous consequences: What comprises negligence in anosmia litigation?. *International Forum of Allergy & Rhinology* **4**(3), 216–222.

Tennen, H., Affleck, G., Mendola, R., Coping with smell and taste disorders. In Getchell T.V., Doty, R.L., Bartoshuk L.M., Snow, J.B., Jr, 1991. (Eds.). *Smell and Taste in Health and Disease.* NY: Raven Press, pp. 787–802.

Turetsky, B.I., Moberg, P.J., Yousem, D.M., Doty, R.L., Arnold, S.E., Gur, R.E., 2000. Reduced olfactory bulb volume in patients with schizophrenia. *American Journal of Psychiatry* **157**, 828–830.

Weisman, K., Christensen, E., Dreyer, V., 1979. Zinc supplementation in alcoholic cirrhosis: A double-blind clinical trial. *Acta Medica Scandinavica* **205**, 361–366.

Wysocki, C.J., Dorries, K.M., Beauchamp, G.K., 1989. Ability to perceive androstenone can be acquired by ostensibly anosmic people. *Proceedings of the National Academy of Sciences of the United States of America* **86**, 7976–7978.

Yousem, D.M., Geckle, R.J., Bilker, W.B., Kroger, H., Doty, R.L., 1999. Post-traumatic smell loss: Relationship of psychophysical tests and volumes of the olfactory bulbs and tracts and the temporal lobes. *Academic Radiology* **6**(5), 264–272.

Index

familial dysautonomia (FD), 366
familial PD, 321–33
FD. *See* familial dysautonomia
fetus, 67–68
filiform papillae, 48–49
flavor, 60. *See also specific flavors*
fMRI. *See* functional magnetic
    resonance imaging
foliate papillae, 48–49
FOSMN. *See* facial onset
    sensori-motor
    neuropathy
fragile X syndrome, 308
FRDA. *See* Friedreich's ataxia
free modulus method, 98
Friedreich's ataxia (FRDA),
    345–46
frontotemporal dementia
    (FTD), 305–6, 348
functional imaging, 116–22
    fMRI, 120–21
    MEG, 122
    overview, 116–18
    PET, 118–19
    SPECT, 121
functional magnetic resonance
    imaging (fMRI),
    120–21, 171
    assessment and, 388
fungal infections, gustation
    and, 252
fungal sinus infection case
    report, 399–400
fungiform papillae, 48–49
    in adults, 71

GABAergic periglomerular
    cells, OB and, 17
Gabapentin, 390
gamma oscillatory activity, in
    OB, 18
Gaucher-variant
    Parkinsonism, 328–29
gender, taste and, 71–72
general advise
    gustation, 402–3
    olfaction, 400–2
    prevention, 401–2
General Labeled Magnitude
    Scale (gLMS), 154–56
genetics
    environmental determinants
      versus, 356–57
    rare disorders of olfaction,
      228–29
    SZ and, 203–5

GEPs. *See* gustatory event-
    related potentials
giant cell arteritis, 220
gLMS. *See* General Labeled
    Magnitude Scale
glomerular layer, 13–14
glossopharyngeal nerve, 49–51
glutamate, OB and, 15–16
gonadotropin-releasing
    hormone (GnRH)
    nervus terminalis and, 4–5
    VNO and, 4–5
granule cell layer, 14
granulomatous disease, 190
greater (superficial) petrosal
    nerve, 49–51
Guam PD–dementia complex
    (PDC), 340–41
gustation. *See specific topics*
gustatory event-related
    potentials (GEPs),
    166–68

HADS. *See* Hospital Anxiety
    and Depression Scale
Hansen's disease. *See* leprosy
HCV. *See* hepatitis C virus
HD. *See* Huntington's disease
head trauma (HT)
    chef hit by van case report,
      196–97
    combat and, 192–93
    fall on ice case report, 196
    investigations, 194
    mild, effects of, 193–94
    as non-neurodegenerative
      disorder of olfaction,
      190–97
    prognosis, 194–96
    sports and, 192
    studies on, 191–92
    superficial siderosis of
      CNS, 197
hepatitis C virus (HCV), 251–52
hepatolenticular degeneration.
    See Wilson's disease
hereditary sensory and
    autonomic neuropathy
    type 3. *See* familial
    dysautonomia
Hg. *See* mercury
HIV. *See* human
    immunodeficiency virus
Hospital Anxiety and
    Depression Scale
    (HADS), 205–6

HT. *See* head trauma
human immunodeficiency
    virus (HIV)
    gustation and, 251
    olfaction and, 219
Huntington's disease (HD)
    olfaction and, 348–49
    taste and, 364
hydrocephalus
    classic, 200–1
    ICP and, 200–1
    IIH, 200–1
    NPH, 200
hypergeusia, 248–49
hyperosmia, 184
    case report on, 390–91
    treatment of, 390–91
hypertension, gustation
    and, 269
hypnotics, 279
hypogeusia, 248–49
hyposmia, 183
hypothyroidism
    gustation and, 267–68
    olfaction and, 208–9

ICP. *See* intracranial pressure
idiopathic hypogonadotropic
    hypogonadism (IHH),
    209–10
idiopathic intracranial
    hypertension (IIH),
    200–1
IHH. *See* idiopathic
    hypogonadotropic
    hypogonadism
IIH. *See* idiopathic intracranial
    hypertension
ILB. *See* incidental Lewy bodies
imaging
    CT, 113
    fMRI, 120–21, 171, 388
    functional, 116–22
    measurement of taste
      studies, 168–76
    MEG, 122, 171
    MRI, 114–16
    of olfactory structures,
      113–22
    PET, 118–19, 171
    SPECT, 121
    studies, 168–76
immune-related diseases
    of gustation
      MG and, 263
      MS, 262–63